Small Animal Soft Tissue Surgery

Small Animal Soft Tissue Surgery

Donald A. Yool

Royal (Dick) School of Veterinary Studies
The University of Edinburgh
Hospital for Small Animals
Easter Bush Veterinary Centre
Roslin, Scotland

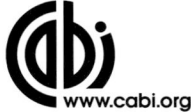
www.cabi.org

CABI is a trading name of CAB International

CABI
Nosworthy Way
Wallingford
Oxfordshire OX10 8DE
UK

Tel: +44 (0)1491 832111
Fax: +44 (0)1491 833508
E-mail: cabi@cabi.org
Website: www.cabi.org

CABI
875 Massachusetts Avenue
7th Floor
Cambridge, MA 02139
USA

Tel: +1 617 395 4056
Fax: +1 617 354 6875
E-mail: cabi-nac@cabi.org

A catalogue record for this book is available from the British Library, London, UK.

Library of Congress Cataloging-in-Publication Data

Yool, Donald A.
  Small animal soft tissue surgery / Donald A. Yool.
    p. ; cm.
  Includes bibliographical references and index.
  ISBN 978-1-84593-821-5 (alk. paper)
1. Veterinary surgery. 2. Pets--Surgery. I. Title.
  [DNLM: 1. Surgery, Veterinary--methods. 2. Pets--surgery. SF 911]

  SF911.Y66 2012
  636.089'7--dc23

                    2011026522

ISBN-13: 978 1 84593 821 5

Commissioning editor: Sarah Hulbert
Editorial assistant: Alexandra Lainsbury
Production editor: Holly Beaumont

Typeset by SPi, Pondicherry, India.
Printed and bound in the UK by Cambridge University Press, Cambridge.

Contents

Preface

This text is designed to support veterinary undergraduate students in the clinical years of their study, and new graduates, particularly those completing the Royal College of Veterinary Surgeons (RCVS) Professional Development Phase. I hope it is also of value to general practitioners with an interest in small animal soft tissue surgery. The intention of the text is to provide a comprehensive overview of the common procedures and conditions encountered in general practice, to enable inexperienced clinicians to begin to develop their clinical skills in these areas. It is not intended to provide a definitive commentary on small animal soft tissue surgery. The content has been matched to the RCVS year-one competency skills in this area (www.rcvs.org).

There is a strong emphasis on the application of basic principles that are defined in Part I. The rest of the text is divided into anatomic regions, and the surgical diseases and their treatment relevant to each part are discussed. A small number of key procedures suitable for a new graduate to perform are described in detail and illustrated with intra-operative photographs. Sufficient information is given about common, more complex conditions to enable the reader to instigate supportive therapy, discuss treatment options, and consider referral. Glossary terms are defined at the start of most chapters. Each chapter has a set of learning objectives aimed at supporting veterinary undergraduate students, and a bibliography providing the key reference sources and acting as a suggested further reading list. At the end of the text are Appendix 1 with a list of medical terminology, and Appendix 2 containing self-assessment sections covering each chapter.

Some notes on the use of drugs and intravenous fluids have been given in this text. These are intended as guidelines only. The prescribing veterinary surgeon must take into account the benefits and risks of treatment for the individual animal when making their selection. Some of the products listed in this text are not licensed for use in dogs or cats. These products are included because, to the author's knowledge, licensed products with an equivalent effect are not available in the UK. When this is the case, guidelines are based on evidence from the current veterinary literature as referenced in the bibliography of the appropriate sections. The prescribing veterinary surgeon must appreciate that unlicensed products may have unexpected, adverse effects. They must ensure that local prescribing regulations (e.g. the 'Prescribing Cascade' as defined by the Veterinary Medicines Directorate in the UK) are followed before deciding whether or not it is safe or appropriate to use these products. As with any treatment, drugs and other products should only be administered with the informed consent of the owner of the animal. New evidence is emerging continually on the treatment of veterinary patients. Drug licensing and datasheet information changes regularly. The reader should ensure that they have the relevant current information required when making these choices through the review of product datasheets and the current veterinary literature.

Donald Yool
November 2011

Acknowledgements

I would like to thank my colleagues at the Hospital for Small Animals, Royal (Dick) School of Veterinary Studies, University of Edinburgh, for help in the production of this text. In particular, I would like to thank Ana Marques, Smita Das, John Ryan, Lynne Wylie, Sam Woods, Henrique Silva, Nicki Reed, Martyn Camburn, Tobias Schwarz, Marcel Kovalik, and Gudrun Schoeffmann for assistance in collecting images for the book. Liz Welsh (Vets Now Referral Hospital, Glasgow) has also provided many of the images used in this text, having generously shared her image archive with me over the years, and I am very grateful to her for the help and support she has offered me. Similarly, W. Andrew Yool kindly proofread the text and Marion S. Yool provided much-needed encouragement. Finally, I must thank my employer, the University of Edinburgh, and in particular Ronnie Soutar, who together have generously permitted me to use the images in this text and supported me in this venture.

1   Applying Halsted's Principles

---

asepsis: absence of bacteria, viruses, and other microorganisms that may cause infection; methods used to prevent contamination of surgical sites with infectious agents

dead space: the potential space left between fascial planes after dissection

dehiscence: wound breakdown

haemostasis: the action of stopping haemorrhage during surgery

high-level disinfectant: a substance that destroys most infectious agents although resistant forms such as spores may remain

sterile: devoid of all infectious agents (microbes, viruses, and spores)

sterilization: a method of destroying all microbes, viruses, and spores

sterilizing disinfectants: a disinfectant that is sporicidal if contact time is long enough

---

The reader should be able to:

- list Halsted's principles and illustrate their application within the context of small animal surgery
- explain the common methods of sterilization of surgical instruments
- explain the methods employed to prepare the operating theatre, patient, and surgeon for aseptic surgery
- demonstrate hand scrubbing and patient preparation for aseptic surgery
- demonstrate gowning and closed gloving
- describe and compare the methods of haemostasis
- describe and compare the different surgical drains and the indications and complications of their use
- explain the importance of minimizing dead space, of sharp anatomic dissection, of tension-free wound closure and of careful tissue handling, and subsequently be able to demonstrate the application of the principles following review of chapter

---

Good surgical practice builds on a set of basic surgical principles that emphasize the importance of avoiding wound infection, minimizing tissue trauma, and creating a healthy wound environment to promote healing. The importance of key surgical principles was promoted by W.S. Halsted, an eminent human surgeon of the late 19th and early 20th century who pioneered modern surgical training. His philosophy of good surgical technique is often condensed into *Halsted's Principles*:

1. strict adherence to aseptic technique;
2. gentle tissue handling;
3. sharp anatomic dissection of tissues;
4. meticulous haemostasis;
5. obliteration of dead space;
6. avoidance of tension.

This chapter describes how these principles are broadly applied in veterinary surgery and is a critical starting point for understanding and using this text.

Aseptic Technique

Wound infection causes tissue damage and inflammation that impede healing and cause pain

---

and discomfort. Infection may also extend into surrounding tissues or spread systemically producing life-threatening complications. Surgical wounds can become contaminated with bacteria and other infectious agents from a variety of sources. These include surgical instruments, the skin and coat of the patient, the hands and clothing of the surgeon, and the environment where surgery is performed. Aseptic techniques are the methods used to prevent wound infection during surgery by removing infectious agents from the surgical field.

Cleaning and sterilization of instruments

Surgical instruments must be sterilized to remove infectious agents before use. This prevents contamination of the surgical site and cross-contamination between patients.

Cleaning instruments prior to sterilization

Organic debris impedes many sterilization processes and must be removed from the surface of instruments before they are sterilized. Dirty instruments are soaked in cold water to remove blood, saline, and tissue. The instruments are then cleaned manually (using a brush under running water) or automatically (using an ultrasonic instrument washer). Finally, they are dried and packaged for sterilization. If possible, instruments with moving parts should be disassembled for cleaning and ratchets should be left open for sterilization to ensure that all surfaces of the instrument come into contact with the sterilizing agent. Instruments with moving parts also require regular lubrication before they are sterilized. Water-based lubricant ('instrument milk') is used instead of oil-based lubricant as it does not leave a film on the instrument that could impede sterilization.

Sterilization

There are many sterilization methods but four are regularly encountered in veterinary practice.

IONIZING RADIATION Ionizing radiation is used to sterilize pre-packaged items such as needles, syringes, suture materials, and plastics. Radiation inactivates viruses, bacteria, spores, and yeasts by damaging nucleic acids. It is very effective but is only available industrially.

STEAM STERILIZATION Steam sterilization is used extensively in veterinary practice to sterilize instruments, drapes, gowns, and some plastic-ware. It is the preferred method of sterilization. To steam sterilize an object, it must be exposed to superheated steam for a minimum period of time. This is achieved using a pressurized steam chamber called an *autoclave* (Figs. 1.1 and 1.2). By pressurizing the chamber, the boiling point of water is increased enabling superheated steam to be generated. Typical sterilization protocols range from heating to 121°C for 30 min to heating to 132°C for 4 min although these times are dependent on the type of autoclave and the materials being sterilized.

Instruments may be sterilized on open trays and stored in the autoclave until required. Alternatively, instruments can be packed in steam-permeable bags or drapes for sterilization and then removed from the autoclave for longer-term storage. These instruments are double-bagged or double-wrapped before sterilization to limit the risk of contamination of the instrument if the outer packaging

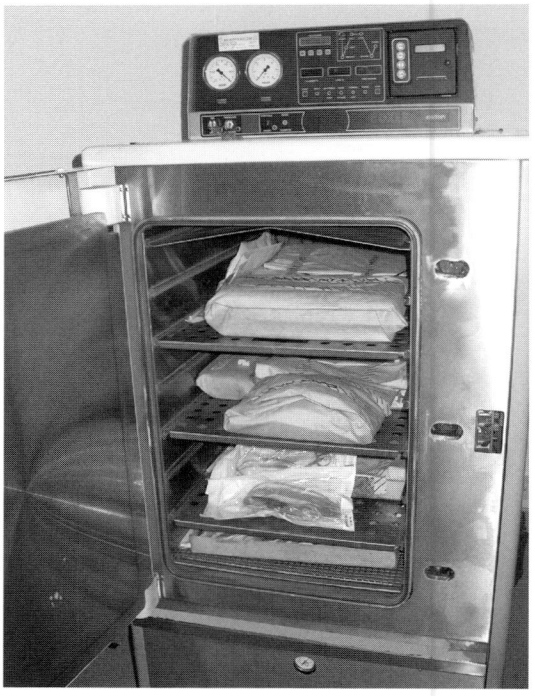

Fig. 1.1. Large hospital autoclave loaded with several instrument trays in preparation for sterilization. Once sterilized, the packs can be removed and stored before use.

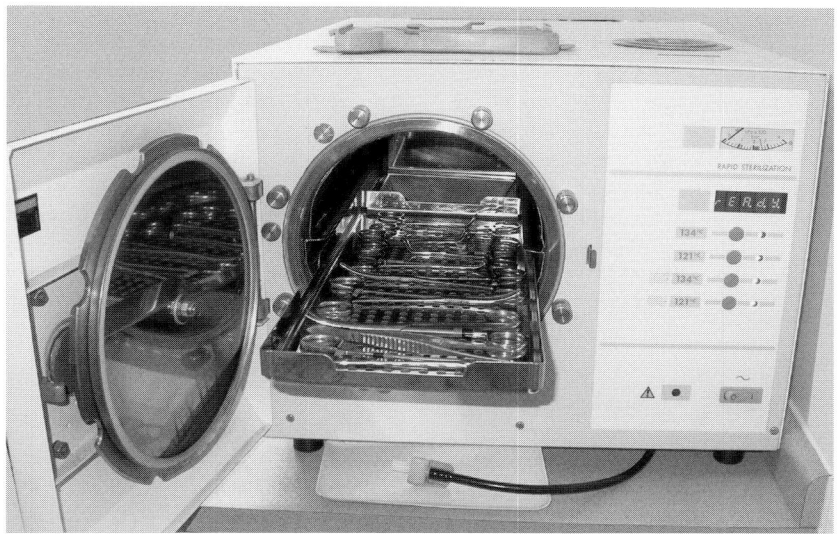

Fig. 1.2. Small bench-top autoclave loaded with unbagged instruments on a tray. These instruments must be stored in the autoclave with the door shut until required.

becomes damaged. To open double-bagged items, a non-sterile assistant opens the outer layer, taking care not to contaminate the inner packaging, then either delivers the inner packaging directly onto the sterile field or allows the surgeon to retrieve it (Fig. 1.3). Appropriately packaged and sterilized items should remain sterile indefinitely providing that the packaging is not compromised.

COLD CHEMICAL STERILIZATION Cold sterilization is used for instruments and materials that will be damaged at high temperatures (e.g. endoscopes). The instruments are soaked in a disinfectant for a minimum period of time. Most disinfectants are not sporicidal so this method is less effective than other forms of sterilization and may only achieve high-level disinfection. Modern 'sterilizing disinfectants' can be sporicidal if left in contact with objects for long enough and these provide more effective sterilization.

ETHYLENE OXIDE GAS STERILIZATION Ethylene oxide is a gas that is used to sterilize items such as plastic-ware that are heat or moisture sensitive and cannot be steam sterilized. It is used commercially to sterilize many pre-packaged items and is available in some larger veterinary hospitals. Items are placed in gas-permeable bags and exposed to ethylene oxide gas for several hours. Ethylene

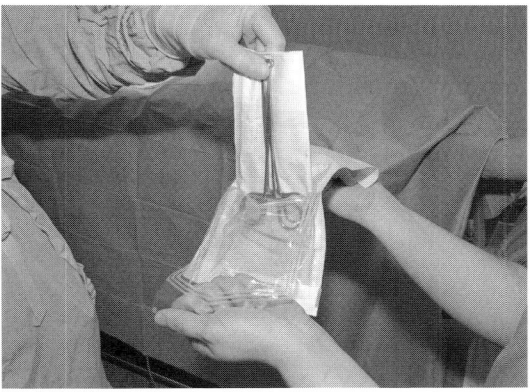

Fig. 1.3. Opening a double-bagged instrument: the inner bag and instrument can either be delivered directly onto the instrument trolley or retrieved by the surgeon from the outer packaging, as shown.

oxide sterilizes surfaces as it causes DNA damage and microbial death but the gas is irritant, carcinogenic, and flammable. Gas sterilization units must be carefully vented to prevent workplace contamination and instruments must be aerated to allow desorption of ethylene oxide from their surfaces prior to use. If aeration is not performed, ethylene oxide retained on the instruments will cause injury to tissues, delaying wound healing. Depending on the unit, aeration can take from less than 24 h to several days.

QUALITY CONTROL OF STERILIZATION METHODS
Commercially sterilized items are guaranteed to be sterile unless the packaging is damaged. In-house sterilization cycles should be quality controlled to limit the risk of non-sterile instruments being used. Autoclaves and ethylene oxide sterilizers incorporate internal monitors of temperature, pressure, and cycle length to ensure that each sterilization cycle has been completed appropriately. However, these are not fool-proof and additional measures should be taken.

For autoclaved items, *autoclave tape* is used to seal packs. Pigments in the tape change colour when they are heated to high temperature indicating that the pack has been through an autoclave heat cycle (Fig. 1.4). Although this is an inexpensive

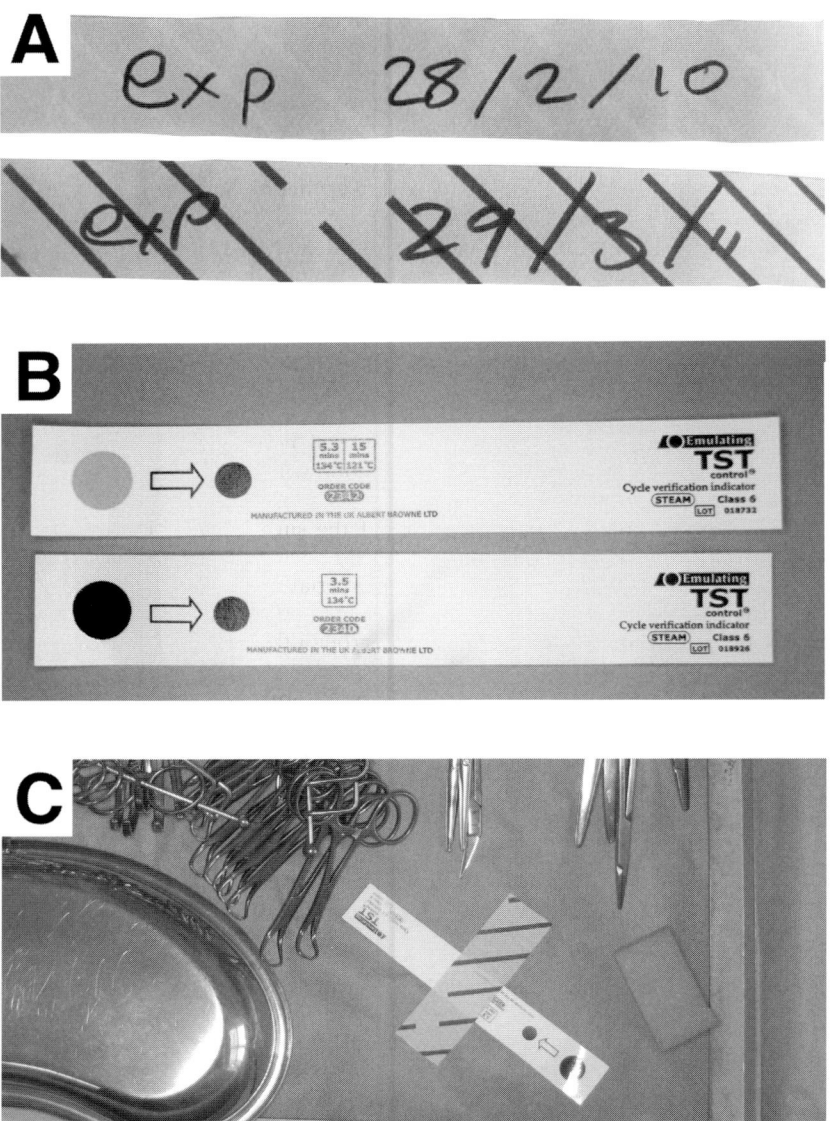

Fig. 1.4. Sterilization markers: (A) autoclave tape before and after sterilization; (B) chemical indicator strip before and after sterilization; (C) example of use of these within a pack to indicate that the pack has been through one autoclave cycle.

and effective way of recording that a pack has been through one autoclave cycle, it does not actually indicate that the pack has been effectively sterilized because infectious agents may survive if the autoclave is faulty and the optimal conditions are not met. More sophisticated chemical indicator strips are time and temperature dependent and are more reliable indicators of sterilization (Fig. 1.4). *Biological indicators* contain bacterial spores that are killed during effective sterilization cycles. Biological indicators must be incubated following sterilization to see if spores remain active so there is a delay between use and interpretation of the results. Biological indicators are better indicators of effective sterilization as they directly test sporicidal action after sterilization.

A standard operating procedure for a veterinary practice might include the use of chemical indicator tapes and strips on the outside and inside of all instrument packs to indicate that the pack has been autoclaved, and weekly use of a biological indicator to confirm that the autoclave is working appropriately. Chemical indicator strips and tapes are also available for ethylene oxide-sterilized items.

Preparing theatre

Custom-designed theatres incorporate many features to limit the risk of environmental contamination, such as controlled ventilation limiting turbulent airflow and preventing dust from being blown into the theatre. These sophisticated theatre features are rarely incorporated into veterinary theatres although basic design features still reduce the potential sources of contamination. For example, all surfaces should be covered with impermeable, easily cleaned coverings. Surfaces that accumulate dust should be avoided (e.g. items should be stored in sealed cupboards rather than on open shelves). The patient preparation area, scrub sink area, and operating room should be in separate rooms adjacent to each other.

Regardless of the design of the theatre, strict attention to theatre cleaning is important and an established cleaning schedule should be developed and implemented, tailored to the individual practice. This is likely to include wiping down all surfaces that will collect dust with a surface disinfectant at the start of each day, disinfecting items that come into close proximity or direct contact with the patient (e.g. theatre table) between patients, thoroughly scrubbing the floors (moving mobile items such as tables and anaesthetic trolleys) and soiled areas at the end of each day, and thorough weekly cleaning of the facility.

Antiseptic solutions for surgeon and patient preparation

Preparation of the patient's skin and the surgeon's hands is a major element of aseptic technique. The aim of skin preparation is to reduce the bacterial load as much as possible prior to surgery, but it is impossible to destroy all bacteria and the surface of the skin rapidly recolonizes. The aqueous-based products chlorhexidine gluconate and povidone-iodine are commonly used in veterinary practice. Alcohol-based products are gaining in popularity and offer some advantages over aqueous-based products.

Chlorhexidine gluconate

Chlorhexidine gluconate is an antimicrobial soap applied diluted in water. It is bactericidal and has a rapid onset of action. It has a sustained antimicrobial effect preventing recolonization of skin for several hours after use. It also has a cumulative action with repeated applications, as it binds to the superficial layers of skin. This means that the skin of the surgeon's hand will not rapidly recolonize with bacteria during a surgical procedure, and the bacterial load on hands will reduce with subsequent applications of chlorhexidine gluconate through the course of the day, increasing the effectiveness of hand preparation with subsequent applications. As with all aqueous-based antimicrobial soaps, activity is dependent on the concentration and the contact time. During hand washing using sufficient water to generate lather is desirable, but excess water will dilute the active agent and may reduce its effectiveness. Contact times of 5 min are recommended for maximum effect.

Povidone-iodine

Povidone-iodine is also an antiseptic applied diluted in water. It has a rapid onset of action and a similar activity to chlorhexidine gluconate when first applied. However, it has less residual effect and no cumulative effect so skin recolonizes more quickly with bacteria. Contact times of 5 min are recommended and, like chlorhexidine gluconate, over-dilution during hand washing may reduce its efficacy.

Alcohol-based products

Alcohol-based gels and liquids quickly kill more bacteria than aqueous products and are highly effective. However, they have no residual effect so bacteria will recolonize the surface of the skin more quickly. For hand washing, alcohol-based gels are applied without water using a hand-rubbing technique to ensure that all surfaces of the hand and forearm come into contact with the alcohol. They may also be used for surgical site preparation. Contact times of 3 min are generally recommended for maximum effect, and the alcohol-based products cause the fewest contact dermatitis problems.

Alcohol scrubs with additional active ingredients

These are alcohol-based gels that typically have chlorhexidine gluconate added. They still have a rapid onset of action and are as effective as the pure alcohol products. However, they have the additional feature of a sustained antimicrobial effect due to the inclusion of chlorhexidine gluconate. This makes them attractive alternatives to more traditional antiseptic solutions for hand and surgical site preparation, combining the best features of both products.

Preparing the surgeon

Shedding of bacteria from the skin, hair, respiratory secretions, and clothing of theatre staff may contribute to wound contamination. To counter this, in the surgical suite dedicated theatre attire is worn that includes a clean scrub suit, dedicated theatre footwear, hats, and masks. Theatre masks may also protect the surgeon from contamination from the patient. Surgical hats are demonstrably effective at reducing shedding from the scalp but the efficacy of theatre masks is questionable. Before every surgery, the surgeon must also perform a surgical hand scrub and don a sterile gown and gloves.

Hand washing for aseptic surgery

Before hand washing starts, rings and nail varnish should be removed and nails should be trimmed short as these may harbour bacteria. Antimicrobial washes are not very effective at removing gross contaminants. If hands are grossly soiled, they should be washed with non-medicated soap before performing a surgical hand scrub, and dirt should be removed from beneath fingernails.

Traditionally, scrub brushes were used to clean hands and forearms but there is evidence that brushes should not be used. Using scrub brushes is no more effective at reducing the level of bacteria on skin compared to other techniques and may be detrimental through abrasion of the skin surface encouraging rapid bacterial recolonization. Instead, a hand-washing sponge can be used to generate lather without causing skin abrasion. A common hand-'scrubbing' technique using a sponge (Fig. 1.5) and a recommended hand-washing technique (Fig. 1.6) are illustrated.

Hand washing reduces the population of bacteria on the skin but resident microbes will persist and lead to recolonization of the surface of the skin over time. After a surgical hand preparation has been performed, a sterile gown and sterile gloves should be put on to further reduce the risks of

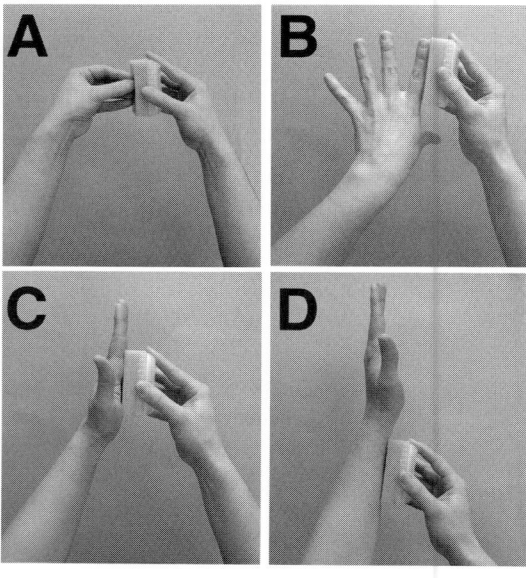

Fig. 1.5. Hand scrubbing (using sponge): (A) scrub the nails with 30 strokes; (B) divide the fingers and the thumb into dorsal, palmar, medial, and lateral surfaces and scrub each in turn – 20 strokes; (C) with fingers closed, divide the surface of the hand into four surfaces and scrub each in turn – 20 strokes; (D) divide the forearm from above the elbow into four surfaces and scrub each in turn – 20 strokes. Repeat for other arm, discard scrub sponge and rinse in running water from fingertips to elbows, ensuring that water runs away from fingers towards elbow.

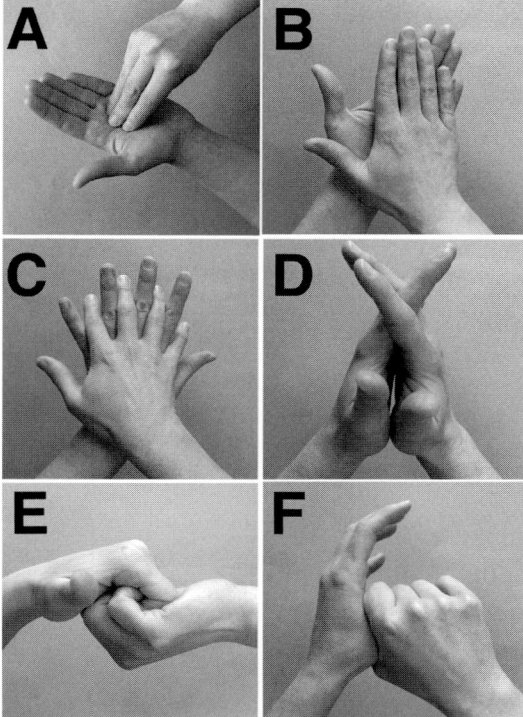

Fig. 1.6. Hand washing without brushing suitable for clean technique. Repeat each step five times before moving to the next manoeuvre and ensure that lather is generated: (A) rotate fingertips of right hand into pool of scrub solution in left hand – repeat for left hand; (B) rub palm to palm, fingers closed; (C) rub right hand over left hand; repeat left hand over right hand; (D) rub palm to palm, fingers interlaced; (E) rub back of fingers with sideways back-and-forth movement; (F) rub thumb of left hand with palm of right hand (rotatory movement); repeat for right thumb. To perform a hand rub for aseptic technique using alcohol gels, this technique is modified to include forearm preparation and minimum contact times following the manufacturer's guidelines.

wound contamination during surgery. The surgical gown should have long sleeves extending to the wrist to enable *closed gloving* to be performed. The gown should wrap around the surgeon's body, overlapping at the back and extending below the level of the knees. The cuffs of the gown do not provide an adequate barrier to prevent contamination and must be covered by sterile gloves.

Gowning (Fig. 1.7) and closed gloving (Fig. 1.8) are demonstrated. During closed gloving, the hands remain covered by the sleeves of the gown until the gloves are in place. Closed gloving is preferred over open gloving (where hands are exposed prior to gloving) as closed gloving limits the risk of inadvertent contamination of the outer surfaces of the gown or gloves as they are put on. *Open gloving* (Fig. 1.9) should be reserved for donning sterile gloves when a gown is not being worn. No system is perfect; gloves become punctured during around one-fifth of all surgeries, exposing the wound to bacteria on the surgeon's hands. Sterile gloving in isolation cannot be used as a substitute for thorough hand washing prior to gloving.

Preparing the patient

Veterinary patients are heavily contaminated with bacteria and dirt that collect on their coats and skin. Some areas, such as the paw, are very difficult to clean thoroughly as they are heavily contaminated and physically harbour contaminants on nails and in pad beds. Patient preparation is crucial to limit wound contamination.

Preparation prior to scrubbing

The patient should be encouraged to defecate and urinate shortly before being anaesthetized to prevent contamination with body effluent during surgery. If the patient is likely to defecate during surgery (e.g. if it has diarrhoea) or if perineal surgery is being performed, a purse-string suture can be placed in the anus (see p. 50). If the bladder is full, this may be expressed or catheterized once the patient is anaesthetized.

If the coat is heavily soiled, it should be washed the day before surgery to limit the amount of dirt that is carried into theatre. Clipping away fur exposes the surgical field and removes much of the detritus and potential contaminants from the area. Patients should be clipped rather than shaved as shaving causes more trauma, contributing to skin inflammation and increasing the risk that a contaminated wound will become infected. Clipping patients before anaesthesia leads to a threefold increase in the rate of surgical site infection through colonization of the injured skin, so clipping should generally be performed after the patient has been anaesthetized for surgery. The clip should extend well beyond the proposed surgical field to enable draping of the patient with adequate exposure of the site and to prevent hair at the periphery of the wound contaminating the surgical field.

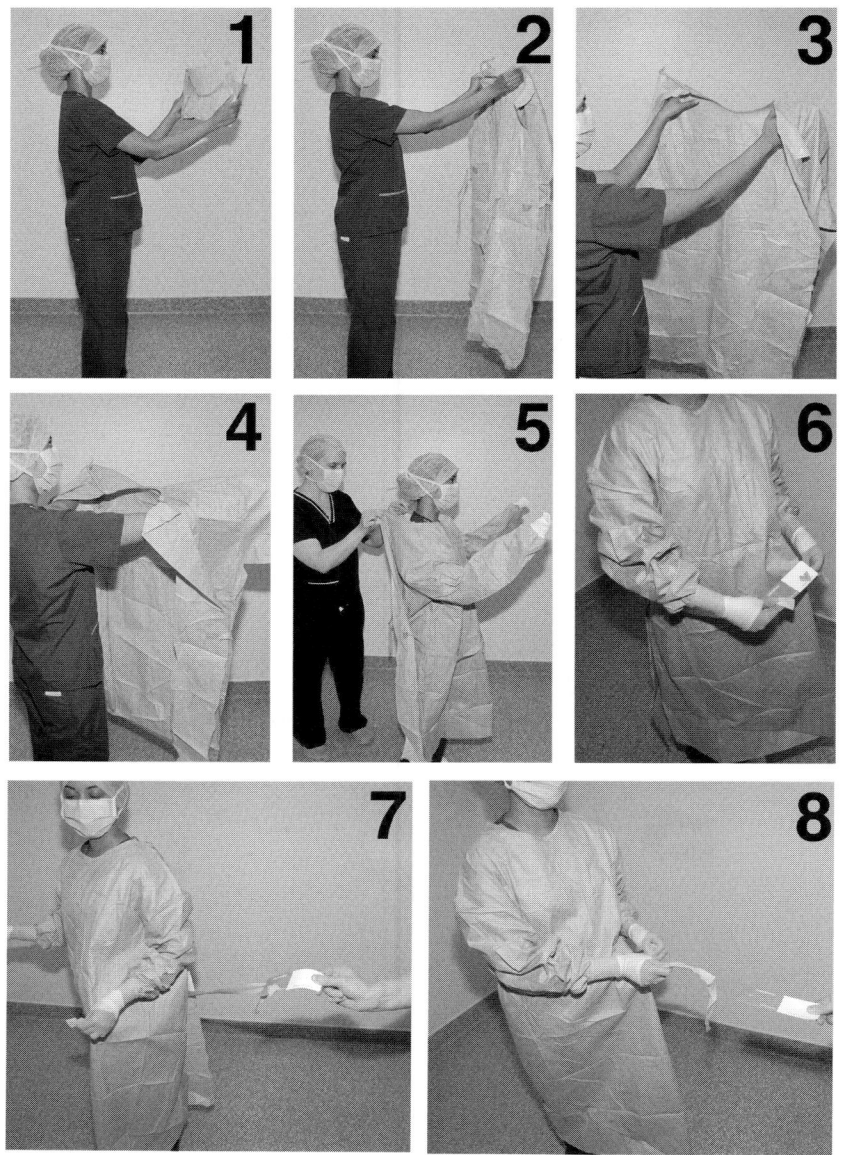

Fig. 1.7. Closed gowning: (1 and 2) hold gown by top with the inside surface facing you and let the rest unravel, ensuring that it does not touch the ground; (3 and 4) push hands and arms into sleeves in a fluid movement but do not allow hands to protrude through the cuffs; (5) wait for an assistant to secure back ties – NOW PERFORM CLOSED GLOVING; (2 and 6) after gloving, pull card with waist tie off front of gown and hand it to the assistant without contaminating the gown; (7 and 8) turn clockwise to wrap your body around the waist tie, retrieve the waist tie from the card and tie it at your side. The gown is folded so only the inside of the gown is exposed to you – avoid handling the outer surface of the gown at all times. The cuffs do not provide adequate protection so do not push hands through the cuffs until they are covered by sterile gloves. Gowning technique may be modified a little depending on the precise design of the gown.

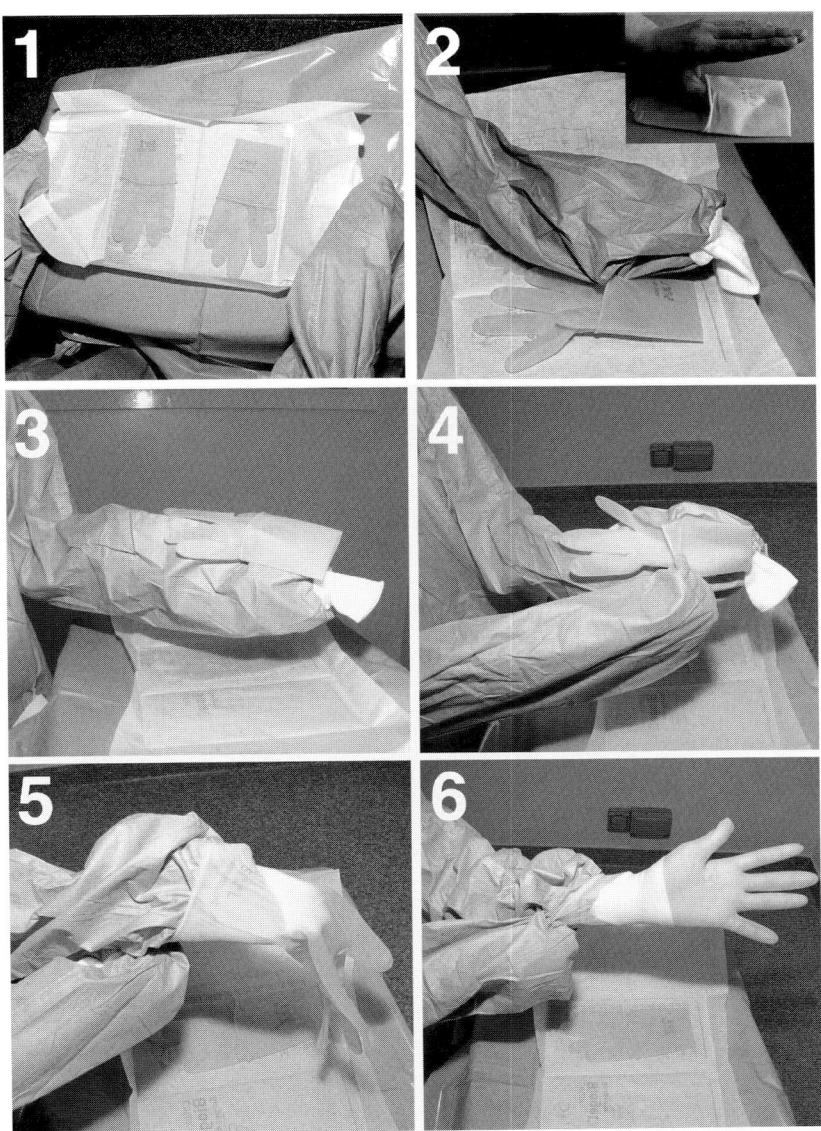

Fig. 1.8. Closed gloving. Keep hands inside the sleeves of the gown until the gloves are engaged over the gown cuffs: (1) orientate gloves with fingers facing you; (2) pick up the left glove by the cuff using your left thumb and index finger (as shown in insert); (3) turn hand over so glove lies along wrist; (4) grasp the glove cuff with your right hand; (5) pull it over the end of your left hand; (6) grasp the gown sleeve through the cuff with your right hand and pull both together over your left hand (engage your fingers as the glove slides over your hand). The cuff of the gown should remain covered by the sterile glove. Repeat for the right hand.

Preparing the surgical site

The surgical site is prepared using antiseptic-soaked swabs to scrub the skin without causing abrasion. For aqueous products such as chlor-hexidine gluconate and povidone-iodine, scrubbing starts at the centre of the clipped area and works out in concentric circles to the clip margin. The dirty swab is discarded and the process is

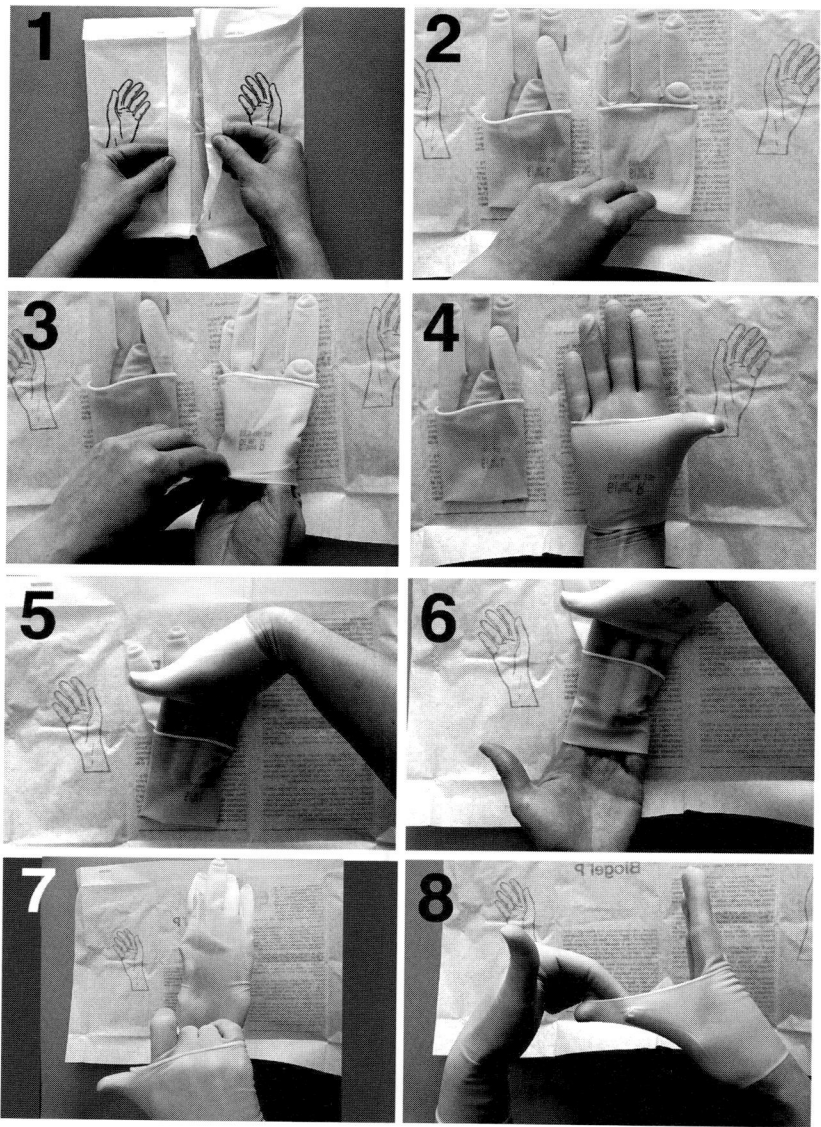

Fig. 1.9. Open gloving. The gloves are packaged with the cuff folded over, exposing the inner surface of the glove. During open gloving, flesh should only touch the inside surface of the glove, and gloved fingers should only touch the external surface of the glove. To achieve this: (1) orientate pack with cuffs facing you and open to create a sterile work field; (2) pick up the cuff of the right glove with your left hand; (3) slide the fingers of the right hand into the glove; (4) catch the cuff with your thumb as you pull the glove over your palm; (5) with your gloved right hand, slide your fingers into the folded cuff of the left glove; (6) slide the fingers of your left hand into the left glove; (7) use your right hand to pull the cuff over the left hand without touching the inside surface of the glove; (8) slide left hand into cuff of right glove and pull it over hand.

repeated until the minimal contact time for the disinfectant has elapsed (generally 5 min) and the swabs are no longer lifting dirt off the skin. Excess disinfectant is removed with saline or an alcohol-based wash before the patient is transferred to theatre. Once positioned for surgery, additional scrubbing may be performed if contamination of the surgical site has occurred during transport, and the site is finally sprayed with an alcohol solution.

Draping the surgical site

Drapes isolate the prepared surgical site from the surrounding haired skin and extend the sterile working area for the surgeon. They may be cloth, plastic or non-woven 'disposable' fabrics (often referred to as 'paper drapes' although their chemical composition varies) (Fig. 1.10). Drapes may also be coated with disinfectant and may be adhesive. They must be resistant to moisture penetration during normal surgical conditions as strike-through of fluid enables infectious agents on the other side of the drape to penetrate through into the surgical field. The composition of disposable and plastic drapes ensures that they have these properties but reusable cloth drapes probably provide less protection when exposed to moisture.

When draping, it is important to ensure that contaminants are not dragged from beneath the drapes forward into the surgical field, and all draping actions should work from the centre of the surgical site outwards to avoid this. In other words, it is acceptable to place the edge of the drape in the centre of the scrub site and drag it backwards towards the clipped margin to reposition it, but it is never acceptable to move a drape from the periphery of a surgical site in towards the centre as this may drag contaminants into the surgical field.

When placing drapes, the surgeon avoids contaminating their gloves by cuffing them into the drape (Fig. 1.11). Drapes should not be passed over the patient as this risks contaminating the surgical field. Instead, the surgeon moves around the table in order to drape all sides of the field (Fig. 1.12). Drapes are secured to the patient using towel clips (Fig. 1.13). As the towel clip penetrates the skin under the drape, the tips are considered to be contaminated so the clip should not be removed and reused. Similarly, towel clips should not be tucked underneath the drapes as the surgeon cannot guarantee the sterility

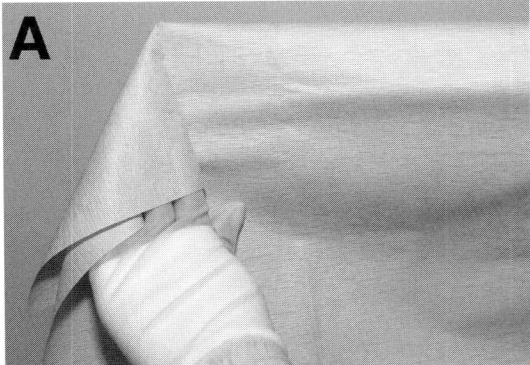

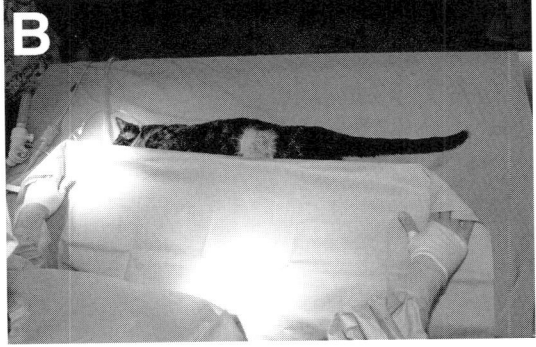

Fig. 1.11. To place drapes, turn the top quarter of the drape over on itself to generate a double layer and cuff the hands into the drape (A) before placing, to prevent glove contamination (B).

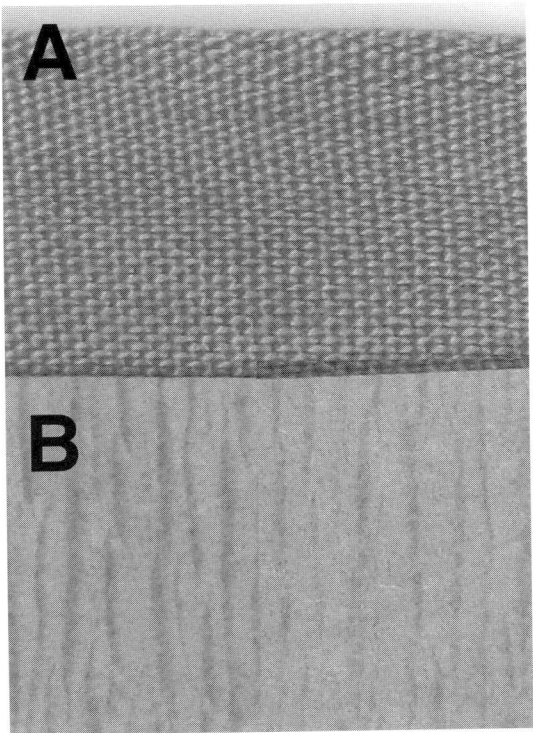

Fig. 1.10. (A) cloth drape; (B) non-woven, disposable drape.

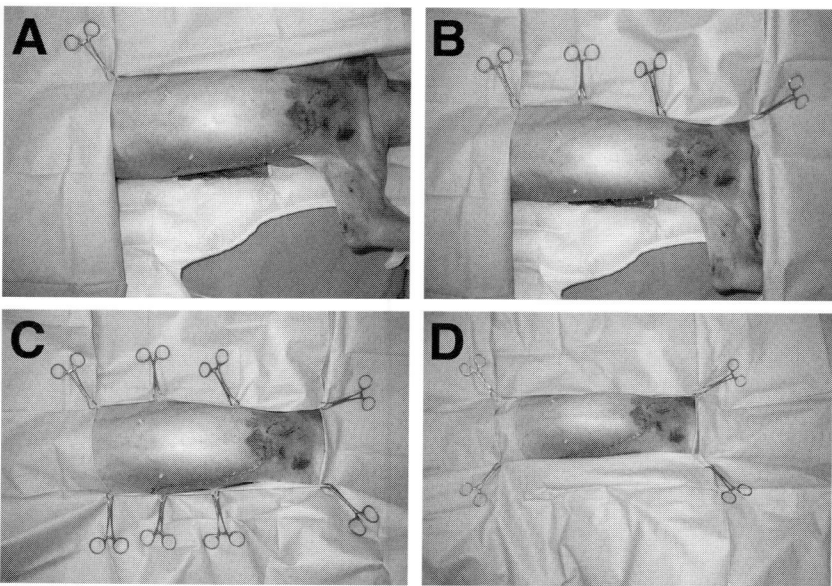

Fig. 1.12. Four-quadrant draping: (A–C) work round the table, placing drapes along the four sides of the surgical field in turn and securing them with towel clips; (D) over-drape with a second layer of large drapes to provide additional protection and extend the sterile field.

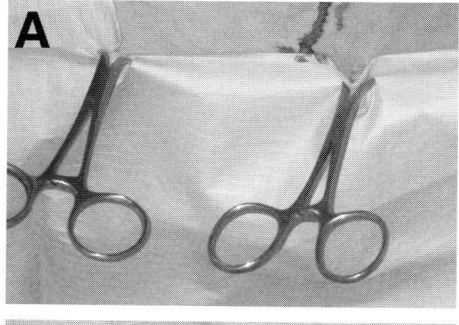

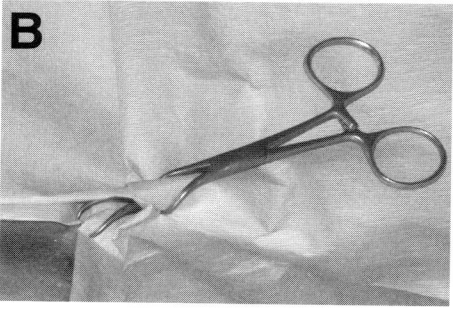

Fig. 1.13. (A) The first layer of drapes is secured to the skin using towel clips; (B) The second layer of drapes is secured using towel clips anchored to the lower layer of towel clips.

of the area covered by the drape and may contaminate their hands by doing this. A single layer of drapes is used to isolate the surgical field. Over-draping with a second layer of drapes is recommended and can be used to extend the sterile field by covering more of the patient and table (Fig. 1.12D).

It is often necessary to include an entire limb within the surgical field (so-called '*draping in*' of the limb). The entire limb including the foot can be clipped and scrubbed for inclusion within the sterile field. However, this is laborious and the foot-pads, interdigital spaces, and nails of the foot make thorough cleaning and aseptic preparation difficult. Alternatively, for surgery that does not require direct access to the foot, the foot is left unclipped but is covered with a non-sterile bandage while the rest of the limb is being prepared. When the surgical field is being draped, the distal foot is draped separately within a sterile, plastic foot bandage that is held in place with towel clips and an outer, sterile, cohesive bandage (Fig. 1.14).

Maintaining the sterile field

The *sterile field* is the safe operating field defined by the area covered by sterile drapes where all

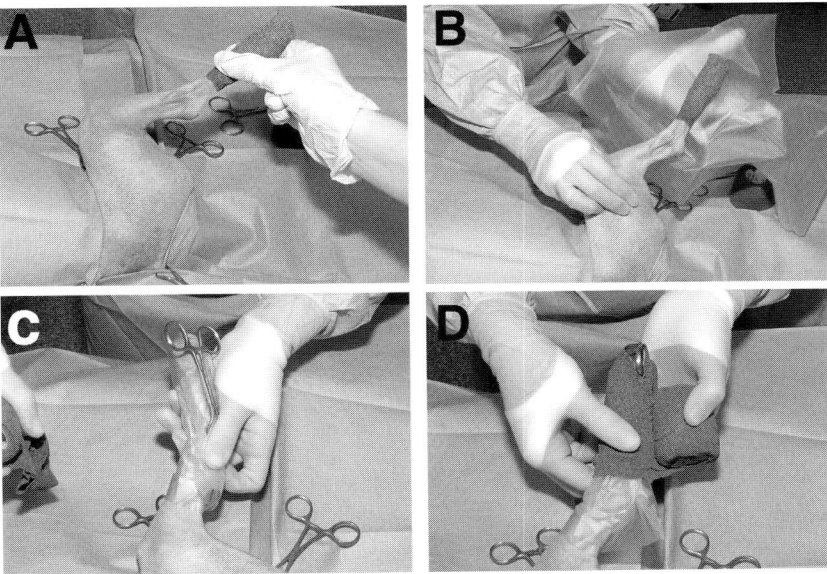

Fig. 1.14. Foot drape: (A) the distal foot, which has not been clipped, has been covered in a non-sterile bandage to prevent shedding during draping. Get a non-sterile assistant to hold the foot while you place the first layer of drapes around the surgical field; (B) then wrap the foot in an impervious plastic drape to prevent strike-through from the unprepared skin of the foot; (C) hold the plastic drape in place with towel clips; (D) finally, secure the plastic drape under a sterile, cohesive bandage (autoclaved).

surfaces should be aseptic. If a second layer of drapes has been used to cover the entire patient and table, the sterile field extends from the exposed surgical field across the entire table drape. The instrument trolley drape can be secured to the table drape to extend the sterile field further (Fig. 1.15). When the table is fully draped and the surgeon is gloved and gowned, the sterile field extends from the point of contact between the surgeon's body and the table (generally the waist) up to below the surgeon's neck, and from the surgeon's gloved hands to 2 cm distal to the elbows. The sterile field does not extend below the level of the tabletop or out of the field of view of the surgeon. It does not include the surgeon's axillae or the cuffs of the gown (these must be covered by sterile gloves).

Post-operative surgical wound management

The surgical site may also become contaminated or infected following surgery, and preventing wound infection extends into the post-operative period. Intact skin is a good barrier to bacterial infection but a surgical wound is at risk of infection until it re-epithelializes. Despite meticulous attention to hygiene, the hospital environment harbours a higher than normal flora of pathogens that may cause wound infection, due to the high throughput of patients. To prevent surface contamination of the wound during hospitalization, the wound can be covered with a padded film dressing (see Chapter 7).

Clean technique

A range of procedures may be performed using 'clean', rather than aseptic, technique. Examples include placing intravenous catheters, changing wound dressings and examining surgical sites post-operatively. Clean technique involves taking reasonable precautions to prevent cross-contamination between the operator or environment and the patient. Clean technique includes wearing suitable, clean protective clothing (e.g. white coat), washing hands and donning clean examination gloves, changing gloves as they become contaminated, working on clean surfaces, and cleaning surfaces before and after use. It is part of best practice and should be promoted. Like aseptic technique, donning clean examination gloves should be performed in combination with, rather than instead of, hand washing.

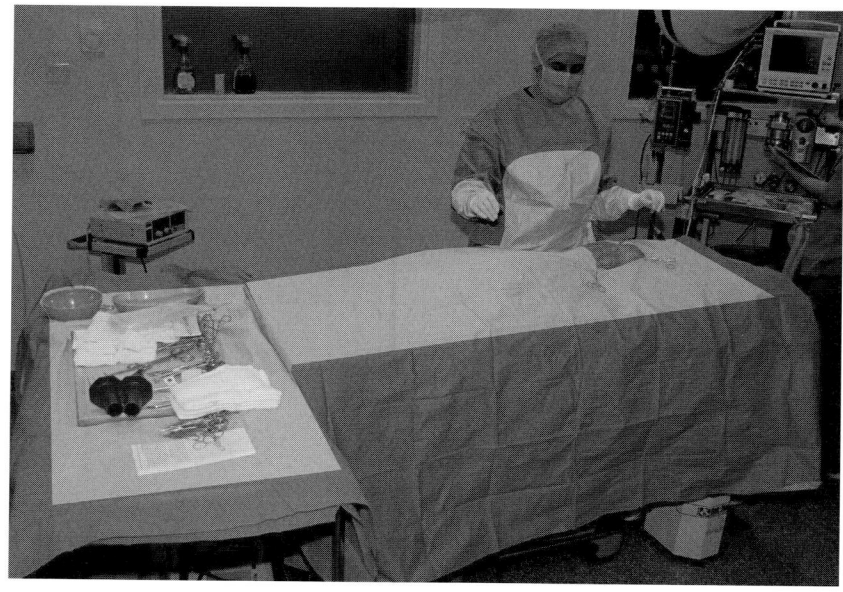

Fig. 1.15. Sterile field: the non-shaded area demonstrates the sterile field that has been extended by over-draping the surgical field with a large table drape and clipping this to the instrument trolley drape. The front of the surgeon's gown from the point of contact with the table upwards is also included in the sterile field. Note that the sterile field does not extend below the level of the table top, into areas that the surgeon cannot see, or above the surgeon's elbows.

Anatomic Dissection and Reconstruction

Sharp anatomic dissection along natural tissue planes and anatomic reconstruction of wounds promote healthy wound healing. They do this by minimizing unnecessary trauma and damage to tissues, by closing dead space, and by limiting the inflammatory phases of wound healing.

Sharp dissection

Sharp dissection minimizes injury to tissues adjacent to the plane of dissection and should be used in preference to blunt dissection whenever possible (see Chapter 5, Fig. 5.8). In contrast to blunt dissection, sharp dissection also reduces dead space and maintains continuity between adjacent tissue planes facilitating anatomic reconstruction. *Dead space* is the cavity generated in tissues by dissection between tissue planes or left after removal of masses. It is a potential space that may fill with fluid post-operatively, impeding wound healing (see below).

Sharp dissection is achieved using cutting instruments such as scalpel blades and fine dissecting scissors. Of the commonly available surgical cutting devices, the scalpel produces least collateral tissue injury and should be used to make skin incisions and to carry out much of the subsequent dissection. Scalpel blades blunt quickly, particularly when making long skin incisions or incising through collagen-rich fascial planes (e.g. linea alba). Disposable scalpel blades must be replaced intra-operatively if they begin to blunt.

Anatomic dissection along tissue planes

There are natural cleavage planes through tissues that should be used for separating tissues where possible. For example, the plane between the subcutaneous fat and underlying muscle separates easily with minimal effort and offers a good dissection plane during skin tumour excision. This is preferable to incising through the centre of the fat layer, which does not separate naturally and becomes bruised and oedematous. Similarly, natural cleavage planes are found between, rather than through, muscle bellies. When muscle bellies must be split, dissecting parallel to, rather than across, the muscle fibres reduces tissue trauma and haemorrhage.

Anatomic reconstruction

Precise, layered reconstruction of incised tissues provides anatomic reconstruction of the disrupted tissue planes. This reduces dead space and facilitates early healing and a return to normal function of the incised tissues.

Careful Tissue Handling

Handling tissue during surgery causes trauma. This leads to inflammation, delays wound healing, and may increase the risk of wound infection. To minimize tissue trauma, avoid unnecessary handling of tissue and select instruments carefully (see Chapter 5). Exposed tissues become desiccated during surgery and this also causes injury. The tissues should be kept moist using isotonic sterile saline (0.9% NaCl), by flushing the surface of the wound, or by covering it with saline-soaked swabs (Fig. 1.16). The action of swabbing wound surfaces to remove blood causes tissue abrasion. Use moistened swabs and dab, rather than rub, the surface of the wound to limit this.

Haemostasis

Good haemostasis (control of bleeding) should be promoted during surgery for many reasons. Blood pooling obscures the base of the wound, and blood on the surface of tissues obscures the natural dissection planes. Maintaining a bloodless surgical field improves visualization of the surgical site, facilitating precise dissection and reconstruction. Post-operatively, haematomas from uncontrolled bleeding also contribute to tension along suture lines and will delay wound healing. Finally, excessive blood loss can lead to haemorrhagic shock.

For haemostasis to be most effective, pre-emptive steps should be taken whenever possible to prevent bleeding before a blood vessel is cut. For example, the advantages of ligating the ovarian pedicle during ovariohysterectomy before it is cut are obvious. While it is important to control haemorrhage to prevent blood loss and improve exposure, it is also important to ensure that the blood supply to the tissues being preserved is not compromised. To achieve this, *pinpoint haemostasis* should be performed whenever possible. Pinpoint haemostasis describes methods that stop bleeding from ruptured vessels but which avoid causing collateral injury to tissues. Several techniques are used for achieving haemostasis.

Direct pressure

Direct pressure is the simplest of all haemostatic techniques and is extremely effective when applied

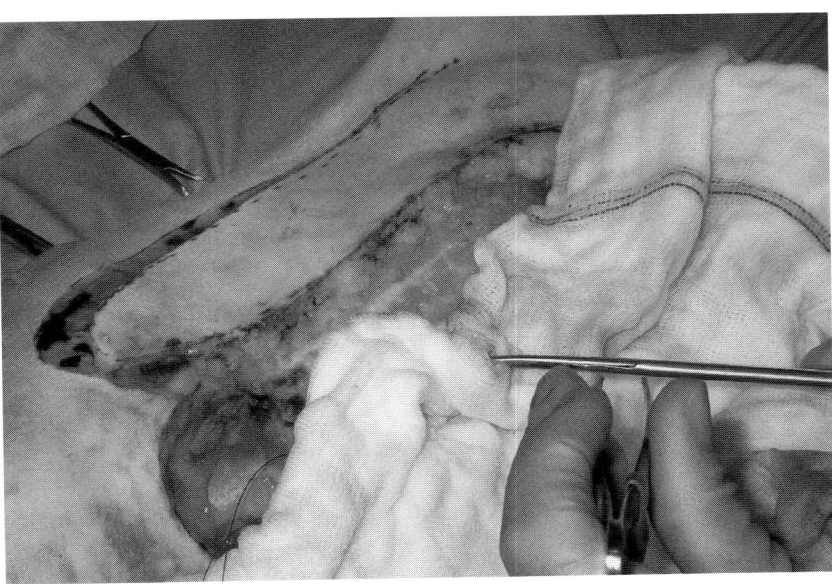

Fig. 1.16. Large, saline-soaked swab being used to partly cover an extensive wound to prevent desiccation during reconstructive surgery.

to bleeding capillaries and small vessels. Pressure is applied to the bleeding surface or cut vessel using either *direct digital pressure* or by *packing the wound* with swabs and applying pressure to these for up to 5 min. This allows the primary clot to form through slowing blood flow in small vessels enabling platelet aggregation. Once formed, the primary clot may be dislodged by excessive force of lavage or by swabbing over tissues and further haemorrhage from the same vessel may occur. Direct digital pressure gives focused pressure to a small area and is suitable when the point of haemorrhage is directly visualized. Packing the wound and applying pressure distributes pressure more widely and evenly across the wound surface. This may be less effective than direct digital pressure but it is extremely useful when used in a wound in which the point of bleeding cannot be directly visualized or space is limited.

Crushing haemostasis

Crushing haemostasis is produced when a haemostatic forceps (see Chapter 5) is clamped onto a vessel and left for several minutes. This causes injury to the vessel and activates coagulation. This method is very effective when applied to small vessels and capillaries (e.g. in the cut subcutaneous fat) (Fig. 1.17). However, it is unreliable when applied to larger vessels.

Ligation

Ligation ('tying off' a cut vessel with suture material) is a very effective form of haemostasis when the bleeding vessel or vascular pedicle can be isolated from the surrounding tissue (e.g. splenic artery during splenectomy; ovarian pedicle during ovariohysterectomy). The advantages of ligation are that it is very effective for large vessels and vascular pedicles, and that it is not reliant on normal coagulation to be effective (it is effective in patients with coagulopathies). The main disadvantage of ligation is that foreign material is placed in the wound and may act as a nidus for infection or inflammation.

There are two basic suture patterns used to achieve haemostasis and these are often used in combination (Fig. 1.18). The *circumferential ligature* encircles the vessel completely and is tied tightly, constricting the vessel and preventing blood flow. This constricts the vessel to the minimum diameter possible, achieving maximum haemostasis. However, this ligature may slide off the vessel, particularly if the vessel has a strong arterial pulse that pushes the ligature distally. The *transfixing ligature* is similar to the circumferential ligature but is anchored into the wall of the vessel before encircling it. This prevents the ligature from slipping but the ligature does not occlude the vessel as efficiently

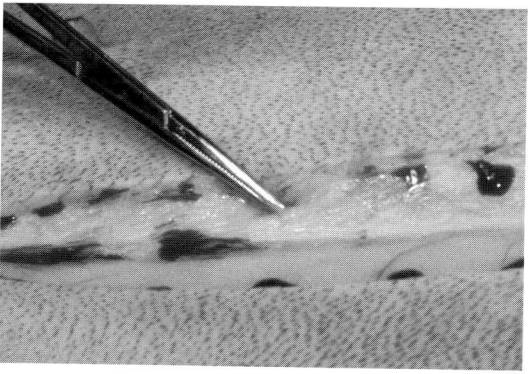

Fig. 1.17. Haemostat applied to subcutaneous capillary – an example of pinpoint haemostasis.

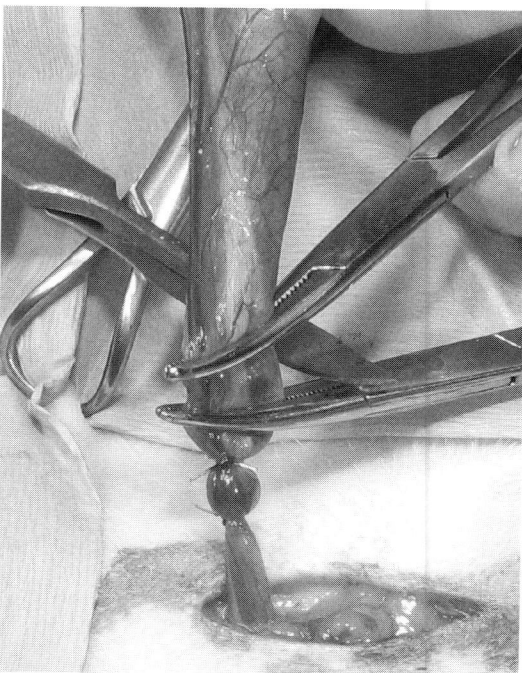

Fig. 1.18. Applying ligatures: a combination of a circumferential and a transfixing ligature has been used to achieve haemostasis during castration.

as a circumferential ligature. A combination of the two ligatures is often used when large vessels or vascular pedicles are transected. These ligatures are described in detail in Chapter 4.

Vessel clips

Stainless steel or titanium vessel clips can be used in place of ligatures. They are applied across the vessel with an applicator and crush the vessel wall to achieve haemostasis (Fig. 1.19). This is a fast and convenient method of haemostasis but the surgeon must be familiar with the limitations of the products stocked as, if applied incorrectly, the vessel clip may slip and lead to bleeding.

Vasoconstriction

It is possible to achieve haemostasis by causing vasoconstriction of a cut vessel. As blood flow

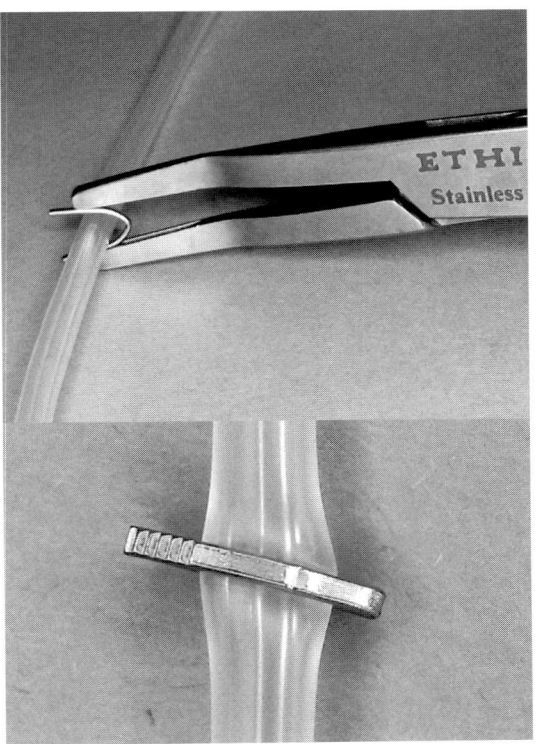

Fig. 1.19. A popular and inexpensive haemostatic clip used extensively in veterinary medicine (Ligaclip®; Ethicon Endo-Surgery Inc., Cincinnati, Ohio, USA). Clips are retrieved from a multi-clip cassette and applied using a special applicator.

slows, platelets aggregate in the damaged vessel and initiate coagulation. Ice-cold saline can be used to flood the surgical field. Chilled saline is produced by storing 1 l of sterile saline at −20°C in a freezer for 1 h or at 4°C in a fridge overnight. The advantages of this technique are that it controls bleeding from medium to small vessels and is effective throughout the area flooded with saline. However, it causes detrimental heat loss from the patient and is reliant on normal coagulation to have a sustained effect. Alternatively, adrenaline can be applied topically (1:10,000 dribbled over the bleeding surface or applied by soaking a swab in the solution and applying this to the bleeding surface). This technique does not cause patient cooling but absorption of adrenaline into the bloodstream through the cut vessels may have systemic effects. Both techniques are effective but are generally used during advanced nasomaxillary surgery and have little application in general practice.

Diathermy

Diathermy (also referred to as electrocautery) achieves haemostasis by passing an electric current through tissue. Some of the electrical energy converts to heat, causing protein coagulation within vessels and stopping haemorrhage. The current is modulated to limit nerve excitation and muscle activity. Diathermy is widely used and is a convenient and effective method of achieving haemostasis of small vessels. There is some damage to the surrounding tissue through charring but, if applied correctly, pinpoint haemostasis can be achieved with diathermy. However, diathermy is only effective when applied to veins less than 2 mm in diameter and arteries less than 1 mm in diameter. If it is applied to larger vessels, it may damage the vessel leading to rupture and more bleeding. Char can also build up on the electrodes and this reduces conduction and makes the unit ineffective. The char must be removed periodically, for example by using a sterile scourer. The use of diathermy carries some risk of electrical injury to the patient or the surgeon (e.g. electrical burns). When units are used correctly, this risk is minimized and most machines have safeguards to limit the risk.

Monopolar diathermy

Monopolar units pass electric current from the diathermy handpiece into the target tissue where it causes haemostasis. The current then passes through the patient's body to an earth plate (or indifferent electrode) that is in contact with the animal (Fig. 1.20). The earth plate connects to the unit completing the circuit. The earth plate offers the path of least resistance for the current to discharge through, and dissipates the current over a large area of the body to prevent electrical burns. If contact between the patient and earth plate is poor, the lead connecting the plate to the unit is broken, or the earth plate is not used, the current will dissipate through any point of contact between the patient and the table (usually bony prominences such as the greater trochanter). This is likely to lead to electrical burns as the current dissipates through a small area of skin. Monopolar diathermy is ineffective when applied in a pool of blood as the current is conducted over too wide an area. Despite these concerns, monopolar units are popular. The tip of the handpiece can be applied directly to the point of haemorrhage and the current turned on using a switch on the handpiece, making the unit easy to use (Fig. 1.20).

Bipolar diathermy

Bipolar units pass the current between the two jaws of a forceps-shaped handpiece (Fig. 1.21). The bleeding vessel is grasped lightly between the jaws of the handpiece, leaving a small gap between the jaws to allow current to flow through the tissue. The circuit is completed within the handpiece meaning that an earth plate is not required and the risk of electrical burn is greatly reduced. The handpiece design facilitates pinpoint haemostasis and limits collateral damage. However, the unit is generally activated by a foot pedal and this is a little more awkward to use than a monopolar unit.

Topical haemostatic agents

Topical haemostatic agents act by stimulating primary and secondary clot formation. Agents include gelatin sponge, oxidized-cellulose mesh, collagen mesh, and microporous polysaccharide powder (Fig. 1.22).

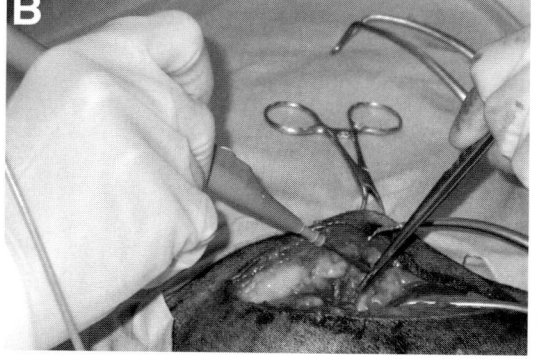

Fig. 1.20. Monopolar diathermy: (A) handpiece and earth plate; (B) in use.

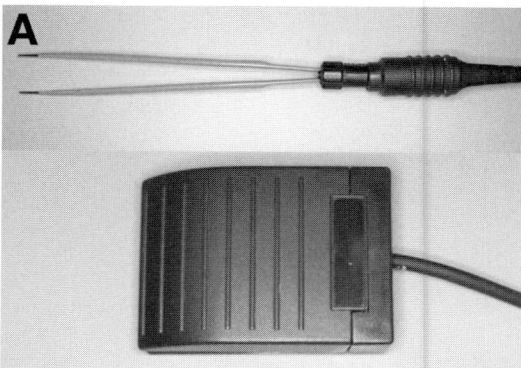

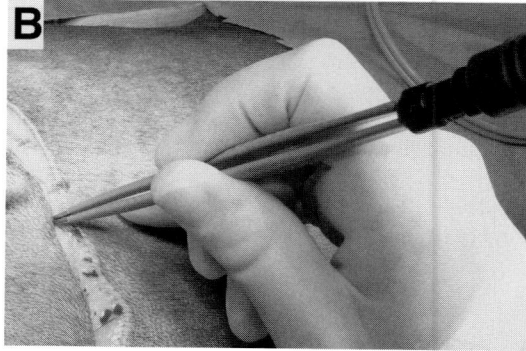

Fig. 1.21. Bipolar diathermy: (A) handpiece and foot pedal; (B) in use.

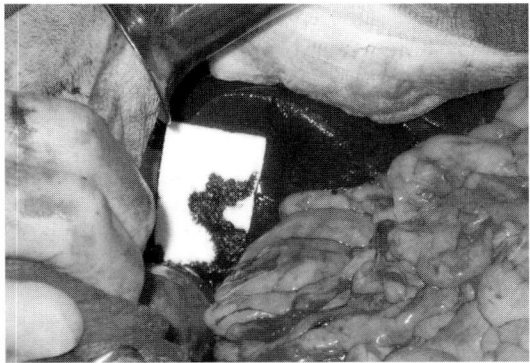

Fig. 1.22. Collagen swab being used to stop bleeding from a liver laceration: the collagen activates the coagulation cascade.

Patients with bleeding disorders

Achieving haemostasis in patients with bleeding disorders is not as challenging as it may sound, but techniques that rely largely on promoting normal blood clotting in the cut vessel (i.e. direct pressure; vessel crush; collagen swab) are less reliable. Techniques that rely on other methods to stop blood flow are effective and should be used in preference (i.e. ligation; diathermy). More attention needs to be paid to pinpoint haemostasis of small capillaries in the subcutaneous tissues, as these may continue to bleed post-operatively, leading to haematoma formation or significant blood loss.

Minimizing Dead Space

Dead space is the potential space left between fascial planes after dissection. Interstitial fluid and blood may pool in dead space leading to seroma or haematoma formation, respectively. Both inhibit wound healing because tissues are not anatomically apposed and the swelling generates tension across the suture line. The fluid also acts as a nidus for infection. There are several approaches to minimizing dead space and all should be employed during surgery.

Avoid unnecessary dissection

Undermining tissues (separating them from the underlying fascia) may be necessary to expose tissues or to facilitate wound reconstruction, but generates a large amount of dead space. Undermining should be avoided when it is not necessary (e.g. fat should not be undermined from the linea alba during abdominal entry).

Anatomic apposition of tissues

All surgical wounds have some dead space. Anatomic reconstruction of wounds closes down the dead space. The incised edges of each disrupted fascial plane should be sutured together individually. Sutures can also be placed between the undermined tissues and the deeper fascial plane to close the dead space further (Fig. 1.23).

Surgical drains

Surgical drains prevent fluid accumulation in dead space and help to maintain contact between the cut edges of fascial planes. Drains are used in wounds where dead space is difficult to close, or where a large dead space has been created (e.g. following removal of a large subcutaneous mass that leaves a void in the tissues). Drains may also be used to remove exudate from infected or inflamed wounds and to remove fluid or air from the pleural or peritoneal cavities.

Types of drains

There are two simple methods of classifying drains: they may be *open or closed*, and *passive or active*.

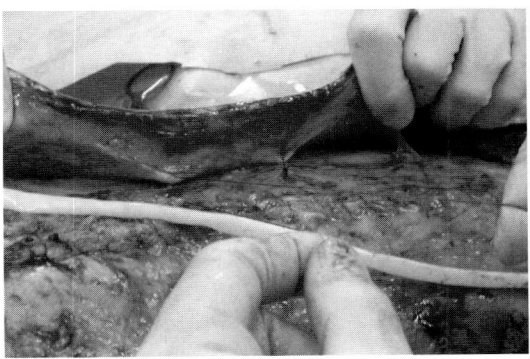

Fig. 1.23. Large mammary tumour excision demonstrating sutures placed between the subcutaneous fat and external rectus fascia to close the dead space generated by blunt dissection.

Open drains drain to the environment. *Closed drains* drain to a sealed collection system. Open drains are associated with a higher rate of secondary infection following drain placement due to ascending infection (Fig. 1.24).

Passive drains allow passive drainage of fluid from the wound through gravity flow and capillarity between the drain and surrounding tissues. Most passive drains are open drains. *Penrose drains* are popular passive drains that are made from soft, thin, collapsible rubber or silicone tubes. Penrose drains are inexpensive, comfortable, and effective. As they are open drains, they must be covered with a sterile dressing to prevent ascending infection. The drain should exit the wound and skin at a dependent point to encourage gravity-assisted drainage (Fig. 1.24).

Active drains apply a vacuum to the drain to encourage active drainage of fluid into a reservoir. These are closed drains as the reservoir and drain form a sealed unit so the risk of ascending infection is reduced. The vacuum is generated with a self-expanding reservoir (Fig. 1.25). The reservoir is collapsed when it is applied to the drain and generates negative pressure as it re-expands. The reservoir is emptied intermittently, and negative pressure is re-established. The drain itself may be a fenestrated tube or a channel drain. Channel drains are soft drains with channels along their length that connect to a collection tube (Fig. 1.25). These are more comfortable and more compliant than fenestrated tube drains and the channels are designed to stay open even when compressed by surrounding tissues.

The advantages of closed, active drains over passive drains are: (i) that they do not need to be covered by a dressing (making them easier to use in sites which are awkward to dress); (ii) that they are not gravity dependent and can exit any part of the wound; and (iii) that the vacuum actively holds tissues in apposition, obliterating dead space and maintaining apposition of tissues to promote healing. The disadvantages of closed active drains are that they are expensive and they may be more prone to failure due to the complexity of their design.

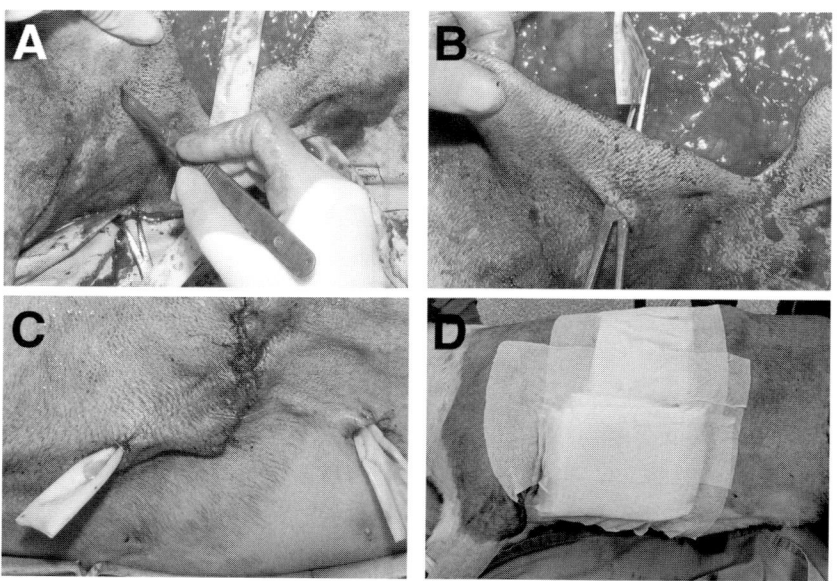

Fig. 1.24. Passive open drain placement – Penrose drain: (A) make a stab incision at a dependent point on the body close to the wound; (B) bluntly force a haemostat through the stab incision and grab the tip of the drain; (C) pull the drain out through the stab incision and secure it to the skin using sutures (ensure the stab incision is large enough); (D) cover the drain to prevent ascending infection.

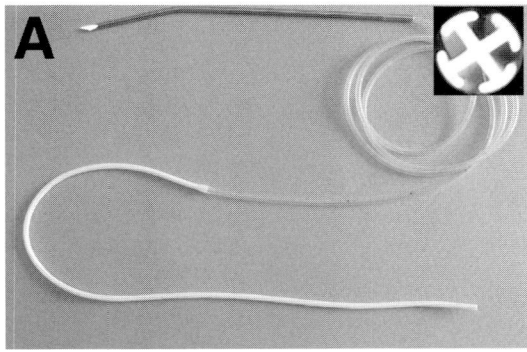

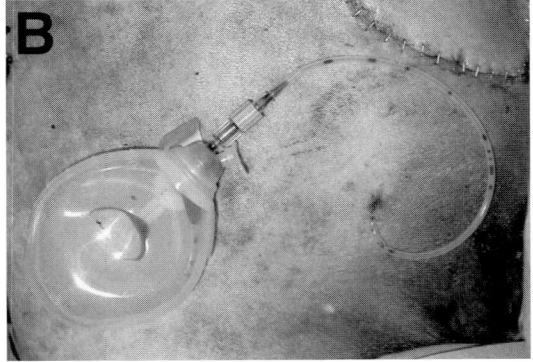

Fig. 1.25. Active, channel drain: (A) the drain is supplied attached to collection tube and placement needle – insert shows end of drain with channels that spiral along its length; (B) drain reservoir that generates suction.

Complications of drain use

Drains may allow ascending infection from the environment into the wound and are associated with an increased infection rate in clean wounds. Drains act as foreign bodies, stimulating some tissue reaction and fluid production. Drains exiting the body through the primary incision will impede wound healing and may lead to dehiscence. They may also cause discomfort. Rarely, drains can rub against and traumatize vessels, leading to haemorrhage. Although drains may be beneficial, they should be removed as soon as possible.

Placing drains

To maximize the effectiveness and limit complications of wound drainage, these basic principles of drain placement should be followed:

1. **Use soft, compliant drains** to reduce tissue reaction.
2. **Exit the drain through a separate stab incision from the primary incision:** drains exiting through the primary incision may delay healing and promote bacterial colonization of the primary incision.
3. **Exit passive drains in dependent positions** to encourage gravity-assisted drainage.
4. **Cover open drains** with sterile dressings to prevent ascending infection.
5. **Remove drains as soon as possible** to limit the risk of drain-associated complications (see below).
6. **Do not place drains directly over large vessels.**
7. **Do not fenestrate Penrose drains:** this reduces their surface area and their efficacy.

Step-by-step guides to drain placement are shown in Fig. 1.24. Drains should be secured to skin using a Roman sandal suture (tubular drains) or skin sutures (flat drains) (see p. 51).

Removing drains

Drains are removed when the volume of fluid produced drops and the fluid itself becomes serous or serosanguinous. The drain will induce some fluid production so it is unlikely that a wound will stop producing fluid completely until the drain is removed. Most drains can be removed easily by removing retaining sutures and applying gentle traction. The drain exit site should be covered until it has formed a dry scab (usually within 24 h) and should be left to heal by second intention.

Closure Without Tension

Tension along suture lines is one of the commonest reasons for wound breakdown. Tension distracts tissues increasing dead space and disrupting granulation tissue. Tension at suture lines leads to compression and ischaemia of the ensnared tissue, which impedes wound healing. During surgery, great care must be taken to avoid closing areas of the wound under tension by careful preoperative planning and wound reconstruction. These areas are discussed in detail in Chapter 8.

Bibliography

AEAPS Committee (2008a) AST recommended standards of practice for surgical drapes. www.ast.org/pdf/Standards_of_Practice/RSOP_Surgical_Drapes.pdf, accessed 17 April 2010.

AEAPS Committee (2008b) Recommended standards of practice for gowning and gloving. www.ast.org/pdf/Standards_of_Practice/RSOP_Gowning_Gloving.pdf, accessed 17 April 2010.

Alexander, J.W. (1984) Bacteriologic comparison of closed suction and Penrose drainage. *American Journal of Surgery* 148, 699.

Anon (2006) Recommended practices for maintaining a sterile field. *AORN Journal* 83, 402–404, 407–410, 413–416.

Baines, S. (1996) Surgical asepsis: principles and protocols. *In Practice* 18, 23–33.

Berg, J. (1998) Principles of oncologic orofacial surgery. *Clinical Techniques in Small Animal Practice* 13, 38–41.

Brown, D.C., Conzemius, M.G., Shofer, F. and Swann, H. (1997) Epidemiologic evaluation of postoperative wound infections in dogs and cats. *Journal of the American Veterinary Medical Association* 210, 1302–1306.

Dougherty, S.H. and Simmons, R.L. (1992) The biology and practice of surgical drains. Part 1. *Current Problems in Surgery* 29, 559–623.

Dudley, H. and Pories, W. (1982) Operative techniques. In: Dudley, H. and Pories, W. (eds) *Rob & Smith's Operative Surgery. General Principles, Breast and Extracranial Endocrines*, 4th edn. Butterworth, London, pp. 98–138.

Durai, R., Mownah, A. and Ng, P.C. (2009) Use of drains in surgery: a review. *Journal of Perioperative Practice* 19, 180–186.

Erne, J.B. and Mann, F.A. (2003) Surgical hemostasis. *Compendium of Continuing Education for the Practicing Veterinarian* 25, 732–740.

Hansen, J.M. and Shaffer, H.L. (2001) Sterilization and preservation by radiation sterilization. In: Block, S.S. (ed.) *Disinfection, Sterilization, and Preservation*. Lippincott, Williams and Wilkins, Philadelphia, Pennsylvania, pp. 729–746.

Howard, J.L. and Hanssen, A.D. (2007) Principles of a clean operating room environment. *Journal of Arthroplasty* 22, 6–11.

Jankauskas, S., Cohen, I.K. and Grabb, W.C. (1991) Basic techniques in plastic surgery. In: Smith, J.W. and Anton, S.J. (eds) *Grabb and Smith's Plastic Surgery*, 4th edn. Lippincott, Williams and Wilkins, London, pp. 3–90.

Mangram, A.J., Horan, T.C., Pearson, M.L., Silver, L.C. and Jarvis, W.R. (1999) Guideline for prevention of surgical site infection, 1999. Centers for Disease Control and Prevention (CDC) Hospital Infection Control Practices Advisory Committee. *American Journal of Infection Control* 27, 97–132; quiz 133–134; discussion 196.

McHugh, D. (2007) Theatre practice. In: Lane, D., Cooper, B. and Turner, L. (eds) *BSAVA Textbook of Veterinary Nursing*. British Small Animal Veterinary Association, Gloucester, UK, pp. 561–589.

Moyle, J. (2002) Surgical diathermy. *Surgery* 20, 112–114.

Niles, J. (1999) Surgical haemostasis. *In Practice* 21, 196–204.

Raves, J.J., Slifkin, M. and Diamond, D.L. (1984) A bacteriologic study comparing closed suction and simple conduit drainage. *American Journal of Surgery* 148, 618–620.

Rutala, W.A. and Weber, D.J. (2001) A review of single-use and reusable gowns and drapes in health care. *Infection Control and Hospital Epidemiology* 22, 248–257.

Rutala, W.A., Weber, D.J. and HCPAC (2008) Guideline for disinfection and sterilization in healthcare facilities, 2008. Department of Health and Human Services – USA. www.cdc.gov/ncidod/dhqp/pdf/guidelines/Disinfection_Nov_2008.pdf, accessed 17 May 2011.

Rutkow, I.M. (2001) History of surgery. In: Townsend, C.M., Beauchamp, D.R., Evers, M.B. and Sabiston, D.C. (eds) *Sabiston Textbook of Surgery: The Biological Basis of Modern Surgical Practice*, 16th edn. W.B. Saunders Co., London, pp. 1–12.

Tanner, J., Swarbrook, S. and Stuart, J. (2008) Surgical hand antisepsis to reduce surgical site infection. *Cochrane Database of Systematic Reviews* 23 1, DOI: 10.1002/14651858.CD004288.pub2.

Tanner, J., Khan, D., Walsh, S., Chernova, J., Lamont, S. and Laurent, T. (2009) Brushes and picks used on nails during the surgical scrub to reduce bacteria: a randomised trial. *Journal of Hospital Infection* 71, 234–238.

Targett, M. (1992) The right diathermy unit for you. *In Practice* 14, 232–236.

Toombs, J.P. and Clarke, K.M. (2003) Basic operative techniques. In: Slatter, D.H. (ed.) *Textbook in Small Animal Surgery*, 3rd edn. Saunders, Philadelphia, Pennsylvania, pp. 199–222.

Vince, K.J., Lascelles, B.D., Mathews, K.G., Altier, C. and Roe, S.C. (2008) Evaluation of wraps covering the distal aspect of pelvic limbs for prevention of bacterial strike-through in an *ex vivo* canine model. *Veterinary Surgery* 37, 406–411.

Whyte, W. (1988) The role of clothing and drapes in the operating room. *Journal of Hospital Infection* 11, 2–17.

Widmer, A.F., Rotter, M., Voss, A., Nthumba, P., Allegranzi, B., Boyce, J. and Pittet, D. (2010) Surgical hand preparation: state-of-the-art. *Journal of Hospital Infection* 74, 112–122.

Williams, J., McHugh, D. and White, R. (1992) Use of drains in small animal surgery. *In Practice* 14, 73–81.

2 Prophylactic, Perioperative Antimicrobials

elective procedure: a planned procedure
prophylactic treatment: treatment to prevent disease
therapeutic treatment: treatment to treat current disease

The reader should be able to:

- define the difference between prophylactic, perioperative antimicrobial administration, and therapeutic antimicrobial treatment
- explain the National Research Council (NRC) wound classification system (clean, clean-contaminated, contaminated, and dirty) and how it is applied to common veterinary surgical procedures
- summarize how the NRC wound classification system is used to select veterinary patients that may benefit from perioperative antimicrobial treatment
- list intrinsic and extrinsic factors that increase the risk of surgical site infection
- explain the ideal properties of an antibiotic used for prophylactic, perioperative antimicrobial therapy
- select appropriate antimicrobials and formulate treatment schedules for patients undergoing a range of procedures including elective gastrointestinal surgery, abscess drainage, traumatic wound reconstruction, and elective neutering
- criticize the administration of antimicrobials in the perioperative period to animals undergoing clean procedures
- criticize the selection of non-standard dosing regimes for perioperative, prophylactic antimicrobials in clean-contaminated procedures

Prophylactic, perioperative antimicrobials (given shortly before and up to 24 h after surgery) may reduce the incidence of surgical site infection but are controversial. Their use risks adverse drug reactions and selection for resistant strains of organisms that may lead to post-operative complications. In many elective procedures, they may not reduce the risk of surgical site infection and they add to treatment costs. Factors including the expected level of contamination of a wound during surgery, intrinsic patient factors, and extrinsic factors that affect the patient should be taken into account when deciding whether or not to administer antimicrobials. For most elective surgeries in veterinary practice, perioperative antimicrobials are probably unnecessary and may be of little or no benefit to the patient. This chapter reviews the key concepts and makes broad recommendations based on current veterinary practice and the available evidence. Ultimately, the decision as to whether or not to use perioperative antimicrobials, which drugs to use, and how to administer them should be decided on an individual patient basis taking into account local prescribing policies.

Surgical Wound Classification

In human surgery, a classification system was developed to grade surgical procedures on the expected level of intra-operative bacterial contamination and the likelihood of post-operative wound infection. This system has been modified and used to develop guidelines for the administration of prophylactic, perioperative antimicrobials in animals. Procedures are classified as clean, clean-contaminated, contaminated, or dirty.

Clean

Clean procedures have a low level of bacterial contamination and the risk of infection is low. Prophylactic antimicrobials do not reduce the risk of post-operative infection and are not indicated.

Clean procedures are characterized by having all of these characteristics:

- non-traumatic, elective procedures;
- no inflammation;
- no break in aseptic technique;
- no entry into the respiratory, gastrointestinal, and oropharyngeal tracts; and
- no entry into the genitourinary tract (apart from elective neutering procedures).

Elective neutering procedures are classified as clean procedures even though the genital tract is transected. The healthy uterine lumen has very low numbers of bacteria and transecting it is unlikely to increase the level of bacterial contamination of the surgical site. Prophylactic antimicrobials are not indicated in uncomplicated ovariohysterectomy or castration in the dog or cat.

Examples of clean procedures: (i) excision of a lipoma from the flank; (ii) elective ovariohysterectomy; (iii) elective castration; and (iv) splenectomy.

Clean-contaminated

Clean-contaminated procedures have low levels of bacterial contamination but have increased risks of surgical site infection. Prophylactic antimicrobials may reduce the incidence of surgical site infection and are generally indicated in veterinary patients.

Clean-contaminated surgeries are classified as surgeries that otherwise would meet the criteria to be called 'clean' except for:

- entry into the digestive or respiratory tracts under controlled conditions without gross spillage of contents;
- entry into the genitourinary tract in the absence of infection (excluding elective neutering);

- oropharyngeal surgery; and
- minor break in aseptic technique.

Examples of clean-contaminated surgery: (i) enterotomy to remove a jejunal foreign body; (ii) tonsillectomy; (iii) cystotomy to remove a bladder stone in the absence of urinary tract infection; and (iv) Caesarean section.

Contaminated

Contaminated surgeries have moderate levels of bacterial contamination and prophylactic antimicrobials are indicated to reduce the incidence of surgical site infection.

Contaminated wounds are characterized by one of the following features:

- inflamed tissues are incised in the absence of purulent discharge;
- entry into and spillage from the gastrointestinal or respiratory tracts;
- entry into the genitourinary or biliary tracts in the presence of infected bile or urine;
- fresh traumatic wounds; and
- a major break in aseptic technique.

Examples of contaminated surgery: (i) enterotomy to remove a jejunal foreign body with spillage of intestinal contents intra-operatively; (ii) closure of a dog bite wound; and (iii) anal sacculectomy for anal sacculitis.

Dirty

Dirty surgical sites are infected at the time of surgery or are heavily contaminated and likely to become infected. Therapeutic antimicrobial therapy is indicated.

Dirty wounds are characterized by one of the following features:

- presence of a perforated viscus encountered at surgery;
- acute bacterial inflammation with or without pus; and
- traumatic wounds that are not fresh.

Examples of dirty surgery: (i) enterectomy to remove a ruptured portion of intestine following pressure necrosis over a jejunal foreign body; and (ii) lancing a cat bite abscess.

Summary

Prophylactic antimicrobials are not recommended in dogs and cats undergoing clean, elective procedures unless there are additional intrinsic or extrinsic factors that may contribute to surgical site infection. There is reasonable evidence to support the use of prophylactic antimicrobials in dogs and cats undergoing clean-contaminated and contaminated procedures. Animals undergoing dirty procedures are likely to require therapeutic antimicrobial therapy and are at highest risk of surgical site infection.

Although this classification system has proved useful for studying surgical site infection in veterinary patients, the groupings are too broad to allow the easy prediction of risk of surgical site infection in an individual patient. In the medical profession, additional classification systems have been introduced and studies evaluating the role of prophylactic antimicrobials for specific procedures have been used to modify these broad recommendations. To date, there are few procedure-specific recommendations in veterinary surgery.

Intrinsic Factors Contributing to Surgical Site Infection

Intrinsic factors may increase the likelihood of surgical site infection, and may prompt the use of prophylactic antimicrobials for procedures for which they would not routinely be given. Intrinsic factors include local wound factors and concurrent diseases.

Placement of a drain

Placement of wound drains increases the risk of surgical site infection in dogs and cats although the risk of infection may reduce if closed suction drains are used.

Placement of a surgical implant

A surgical implant (e.g. a bone plate) acts as a nidus for infection. Organisms grow in a biofilm of extracellular matrix that coats the implant. The organisms enter a slow growth state due to environmental factors within the biofilm and this renders them relatively resistant to antimicrobial therapy. Organisms trapped in the biofilm can lead to infections emerging in the early post-operative period or several months later. Perioperative prophylactic antimicrobials reduce the rate of implant-associated infection in people and are generally given when orthopaedic implants are placed. This practice has been widely adopted in veterinary orthopaedic surgery.

Endocrine disorders

Endocrine disorders in general have been associated with an increased risk of surgical site infection in dogs and cats through alteration of host defences. In man, diabetes mellitus specifically increases the risk of post-operative infection, but the effects of specific endocrinopathies have not been established in animals.

Concurrent diseases

In humans, a range of additional patient factors increases the risk of surgical site infection. *Distant sites of infection* (e.g. tooth root abscess) have been associated with increased infection rates and may also be important in veterinary patients. *Concurrent systemic illness*, *poor nutritional status*, or *immunosuppressive therapy* may increase the risk of surgical site infection, and the presence of *multiple risk factors* further increases the risk. Direct evidence is lacking to show that these factors also increase surgical site infections in animals, but a reasonable argument can be made for administering perioperative antimicrobials to patients with similar additional disease processes.

Extrinsic Factors Contributing to Surgical Site Infection

Extrinsic factors may also increase the incidence of surgical site infection and, if present, may prompt the use of prophylactic antimicrobials.

Prolonged surgery

Prolonged surgical time is associated with an increased risk of surgical site infection in veterinary patients. For every additional 70–90 min of surgery time, the risk of surgical site infection doubles. Administration of prophylactic antimicrobials can be justified for clean procedures that are expected to exceed 90 min of operating time.

Prolonged anaesthesia

Patients that are anaesthetized for protracted periods of time (e.g. for investigative procedures prior to surgery), even if they subsequently undergo a short surgical procedure, are at increased risk of surgical site infection.

Other external factors

Breaks in aseptic technique and poor patient, surgeon, and theatre preparation may all contribute to surgical site infection. Examples include the use of non-sterile instruments or inadvertent contamination of the surgeon, surgical field, or instruments. In these scenarios, an otherwise clean wound will be reclassified as clean-contaminated and prophylactic antimicrobials would be justified. In addition, clipping of fur in advance of anaesthesia for surgery leads to a threefold increase in the incidence of surgical site infection and should be avoided.

Selection and Administration of Drugs

Several factors should be taken into consideration when selecting prophylactic antimicrobials for perioperative use:

1. **Select an antimicrobial effective against the organisms expected to contribute to surgical site infection.** Surgical site infections are most often caused by *Staphylococcus* spp. in animals. Gram-negative organisms, including *Escherichia coli*, are also frequently implicated and commonly cause surgical site infections in people. Gram-negative organisms may be more likely to contribute to surgical site infection following enteric surgery due to their high numbers in the gastrointestinal tract. Antimicrobials with action against *Staphylococcus* spp. and enteric bacteria are suitable choices for prophylaxis in general surgery. *First generation cephalosporins* and *penicillin derivatives* are most commonly used. These have a time-dependent bactericidal effect. Bacteria must be exposed to at least the minimum effective concentration of antibiotic for a minimum period of time for the drug to be effective.

2. **Administer antimicrobials using a route and dose that will maintain high tissue levels from the start of surgery.** The goal is to achieve bactericidal levels of drug in tissues by the time bacteria contaminate the wound, to reduce the numbers of bacteria below the level necessary to allow colonization and infection. Antimicrobials should be given *intravenously 20–30 min before the onset of surgery* to ensure high tissue levels at the times of surgery.

3. **Repeat dosing may be required during protracted surgeries.** Repeated dosing of antimicrobials may be necessary to ensure a sustained bactericidal effect throughout protracted surgeries. For example, cefazolin dosed at 20 mg/kg every 120 min maintains high tissue levels adequate to have a sustained bactericidal effect against *E. coli*. However, it is worth noting that this dose schedule is excessive when considering more sensitive organism such as the Gram-positive *Staphylococcus* spp. and some protocols recommend repeat dosing after 4 h. In general practice, most procedures are unlikely to exceed these times and repeat dosing is generally unnecessary.

4. **Prophylactic antimicrobial therapy should not extend into the post-operative period.** Post-operative antimicrobial therapy is only indicated in wounds that are infected at the time of surgery or heavily contaminated and likely to become infected (e.g. ruptured abdominal viscus), where antimicrobials are being used for therapeutic rather than prophylactic effect.

Cephalosporins

The first generation cephalosporin, *cefazolin*, has been extensively evaluated as a prophylactic antimicrobial for use in veterinary patients. It has a suitable range of activity against Gram-positive and Gram-negative organisms, can be administered intravenously, and distributes rapidly from serum to achieve high concentrations in tissues. When given at *20 mg/kg intravenously 20 min before the start of surgery*, cefazolin concentrations will reach bactericidal levels in tissues for *E. coli* by the time of surgery and these levels will be maintained for up to 120 min. Repeat dosing *every 90–120 min* may be considered in animals undergoing prolonged surgeries.

Although cefazolin is a good choice for prophylactic antibiosis, local licensing and availability issues may make it an impractical choice in some countries. For example, in the UK, cefazolin is not licensed for use in any veterinary species and can be difficult to source.

Amoxicillin/Clavulanic Acid

Amoxicillin, like first generation cephalosporins, has a suitable range of antimicrobial activity for prophylactic use and is frequently augmented with clavulanic acid to extend its spectrum to include beta-lactamase-producing organisms. Amoxicillin/clavulanic acid administered *intravenously at 20 mg/kg* also reaches peak serum concentrations exceeding the levels required to produce a bactericidal effect within 20 min.

Amoxicillin/clavulanic acid has not been evaluated for its ability to reduce surgical site infection in dogs and cats. However, it is widely used for surgical prophylaxis in human surgery and its pharmacokinetics in dogs and cats indicate that it is likely to be effective. Amoxicillin/clavulanic acid is not licensed for use intravenously in dogs and cats in the UK but it is licensed for use by other routes, and is available as an intravenous preparation licensed for use in man. Following the RCVS prescribing cascade, the use of intravenous amoxicillin/clavulanic acid preparations for surgical prophylaxis appears to be justifiable.

Use of Other Drugs and Other Routes of Administration

The use of first generation cephalosporins and amoxicillin/clavulanic acid by other routes, such as by intramuscular injection, has not been described for preventing surgical site infections in animals. Although these drugs are widely available in licensed formulations for administration by these routes, peak serum concentrations are likely to be lower than those achieved by intravenous administration and may be too low to produce a sustained bactericidal effect for resistant organisms such as the Gram-negative enterobacteria. If considering the use of these drugs for surgical prophylaxis, veterinary surgeons should be aware of the lack of evidence demonstrating their efficacy, and must appreciate that serum concentrations are likely to peak as late as 2 h following injection when timing the administration of drugs prior to surgery.

A range of other drugs has been described for provision of surgical prophylaxis by intravenous injection in veterinary patients that includes penicillin G, ampicillin, and cefalexin.

Summary of Recommendations

1. Do not administer perioperative antimicrobials to patients undergoing clean, elective surgeries unless specific intrinsic or extrinsic factors exist that justify their use.
2. Give perioperative antimicrobials to patients that will have a drain or surgical implant placed during surgery.
3. Intrinsic factors that justify the use of perioperative antimicrobials in patients undergoing clean procedures include concurrent endocrine disorders, debilitating disease, or distant sites of infection.
4. Extrinsic factors that justify the use of perioperative antimicrobials in patients undergoing clean procedures include procedures that are likely to exceed 90 min and protracted periods of general anaesthesia for investigative procedures prior to surgery.
5. Administer perioperative antimicrobials to patients undergoing clean-contaminated, contaminated, or dirty procedures.
6. Use cefazolin at 20 mg/kg given intravenously 20 min before the start of surgery. If cefazolin cannot be given, consider amoxicillin/clavulanic acid at 20 mg/kg given intravenously 20 min before the start of surgery.
7. Consider repeat dosing if surgery exceeds 90 min.
8. Delay elective surgery if possible until intrinsic factors increasing the risk of surgical site infection have been treated. For example, delay surgery until distant sites of infection have been treated or diabetes mellitus has been stabilized.

Bibliography

Alexander, J.W. (1984) Bacteriologic comparison of closed suction and Penrose drainage. *American Journal of Surgery* 148, 699.

Beal, M.W., Brown, D.C. and Shofer, F.S. (2000) The effects of perioperative hypothermia and the duration of anesthesia on postoperative wound infection rate in clean wounds: a retrospective study. *Veterinary Surgery* 29, 123–127.

Berard, F. and Gandon, J. (1964a) Postoperative wound infections: the influence of ultraviolet irradiation of the operating room and of various other factors. Chapter III: organization, methods and physical factors of the study. *Annals of Surgery* 160, 1–31.

Berard, F. and Gandon, J. (1964b) Postoperative wound infections: the influence of ultraviolet irradiation of the operating room and of various other factors. Chapter IV: factors influencing the incidence of wound infection. *Annals of Surgery* 160, 32–81.

Berard, F. and Gandon, J. (1964c) Postoperative wound infections: the influence of ultraviolet irradiation of the operating room and of various other factors. Chapter V: bacteriological studies. *Annals of Surgery* 160, 82–113.

Brown, D.C., Conzemius, M.G., Shofer, F. and Swann, H. (1997) Epidemiologic evaluation of postoperative wound infections in dogs and cats. *Journal of the American Veterinary Medical Association* 210, 1302–1306.

Bubenik, L.J. and Smith, M.M. (2003) Orthopaedic infections. In: Slatter, D.H. (ed.) *Textbook of Small Animal Surgery*, 3rd edn. Saunders, Philadelphia, Pennsylvania, pp. 1862–1875.

Budsberg, C.S. and Kirsch, J.A. (2001) Antibiotic prophylaxis in veterinary orthopedic surgery. *Veterinary and Comparative Orthopedics and Traumatology* 14, 184–189.

Clemetson, L.L. and Ward, A.C. (1990) Bacterial flora of the vagina and uterus of healthy cats. *Journal of the American Veterinary Medical Association* 196, 902–906.

Culver, D.H., Horan, T.C., Gaynes, R.P., Martone, W.J., Jarvis, W.R., Emori, T.G., Banerjee, S.N., *et al.* (1991) Surgical wound infection rates by wound class, operative procedure, and patient risk index. National Nosocomial Infections Surveillance System. *American Journal of Medicine* 91, 152S–157S.

Dunning, D. (2003) Surgical wound infection and the use of antimicrobials. In: Slatter, D.H. (ed.) *Textbook of Small Animal Surgery*, 3rd edn. Saunders, Philadelphia, Pennsylvania, pp. 113–122.

Eugster, S., Schawalder, P., Gaschen, F. and Boerlin, P. (2004) A prospective study of postoperative surgical site infections in dogs and cats. *Veterinary Surgery* 33, 542–550.

Gould, I. (2008) *Antibiotic Prophylaxis in Surgery – a National Clinical Guideline 104*. Scottish Intercollegiate Guidelines Network, Edinburgh, pp. 1–71.

Howe, L.M. and Boothe, J.H.W. (2006) Antimicrobial use in the surgical patient. *Veterinary Clinics of North America Small Animal Practice* 36, 1049–1060.

Humphreys, H. (2009) Preventing surgical site infection. Where now? *Journal of Hospital Infection* 73, 316–322.

Jaegar, M., Maier, D., Kern, W.V. and Südkamp, N.P. (2006) Antibiotics in trauma and orthopedic surgery – a primer of evidence-based recommendations. *Injury* 37, S74–S80.

Mangram, A.J., Horan, T.C., Pearson, M.L., Silver, L.C. and Jarvis, W.R. (1999) Guideline for prevention of surgical site infection, 1999. Centers for Disease Control and Prevention (CDC) Hospital Infection Control Practices Advisory Committee. *American Journal of Infection Control* 27, 97–132; quiz 133–134; discussion 196.

Nicholson, M., Beal, M., Shofer, F. and Brown, D.C. (2002) Epidemiologic evaluation of postoperative wound infection in clean-contaminated wounds: a retrospective study of 239 dogs and cats. *Veterinary Surgery* 31, 577–581.

Papich, M.G. (2000) Antimicrobial drugs. In: Ettinger, S.J. and Feldmen, E.C. (eds) *Textbook of Veterinary Internal Medicine*, 5th edn. W.B. Saunders, Philadelphia, Pennsylvania, pp. 301–307.

Rosin, E., Ebert, S., Uphoff, T.S., Evans, M.H. and Schultz-Darken, N.J. (1989) Penetration of antibiotics into the surgical wound in a canine model. *Antimicrobial Agents and Chemotherapy* 33, 700–704.

Trampuz, A. and Zimmerli, W. (2006) Diagnosis and treatment of infections associated with fracture-fixation devices. *Injury* 37, S59–66.

Vasseur, P.B., Paul, H.A., Enos, L.R. and Hirsh, D.C. (1985) Infection rates in clean surgical procedures: a comparison of ampicillin prophylaxis vs. a placebo. *Journal of the American Veterinary Medical Association* 187, 825–827.

Vasseur, P.B., Levy, J., Dowd, E. and Eliot, J. (1988) Surgical wound infection rates in dogs and cats. Data from a teaching hospital. *Veterinary Surgery* 17, 60–64.

Watts, J.R., Wright, P.J. and Whithear, K.C. (1996) Uterine, cervical and vaginal microflora of the normal bitch throughout the reproductive cycle. *Journal of Small Animal Practice* 37, 54–60.

Wendelburg, K. (1993) Surgical wound infection. In: Bojrab, M.J. (ed.) *Disease Mechanisms in Small Animal Surgery*, 2nd edn. Lea and Febiger, Philadelphia, Pennsylvania, pp. 54–65.

3 Suture Materials, Staples, and Tissue Adhesive

The reader should be able to:

- describe the different characteristics of suture materials using the terms natural, synthetic, monofilament, multifilament, absorbable, non-absorbable, memory, knot security, tensile strength, capillarity, dyed, and coated, and explain how these characteristics affect suture selection
- describe the properties of the ideal suture material
- list the generic names and characteristics of common short-lasting, long-lasting, and non-absorbable suture material
- select suture materials suitable for closure of bladder, linea alba, subcutaneous fat, and skin
- explain the USP and EP suture size classification systems
- define the different types of suture needle and their application using the terms straight, curved, eyed, swaged-on, cutting, reverse cutting, taperpoint, and tapercut

Suture Material Properties

Suture materials are used to reconstruct wounds and form ligatures. A wide range is available and each suture has different properties that dictate how it will perform. Suture materials can be classified by their chemical and physical properties and by their handling and knotting characteristics. These basic features are used to select the best suture for each application.

Natural versus synthetic

Natural suture materials are composed of organic material such as collagen or silk. These sutures were among the first materials used to reconstruct wounds and continue to be widely used today. They remain popular because of familiarity with them and because of their handling characteristics. However, natural suture materials are more antigenic than synthetic materials, cause more inflammation, and degrade in a less predictable fashion.

Synthetic suture materials are chemically manufactured and behave consistently in tissues. They induce little tissue reaction as they are non-antigenic and are not subject to enzymatic degradation. For these reasons, synthetic suture materials are preferred over natural suture materials.

Absorbable versus non-absorbable

Absorbable suture materials degrade over time losing tensile strength first and then being completely absorbed. Synthetic, absorbable suture material is absorbed through *hydrolysis*. Water penetrates the suture material disrupting the covalent bonds within the polymer and leading to its dissolution. Hydrolysis occurs in a consistent fashion and is not influenced greatly by the local wound environment. Synthetic materials lose tensile strength in a predictable fashion and perform reliably in tissues. Natural absorbable suture materials are degraded by both *hydrolysis* and *enzymatic degradation*. During degradation, natural materials invoke more tissue reaction because their breakdown products are more antigenic. The enzymatic absorption of natural suture materials may be influenced by the local wound environment and this makes the loss of tensile strength less predictable. For these reasons, synthetic absorbable suture materials should be chosen in preference to natural absorbable materials.

Non-absorbable suture materials undergo minimal degradation over time and retain most of their tensile strength throughout the lifetime of the patient. As they are not absorbed, they persist as foreign material within the body. Non-absorbable sutures should be reserved for wound reconstruction where long-term suture support is required or where suture material will be routinely removed (e.g. skin sutures).

Multifilament versus monofilament

Multifilament suture material is composed of thousands of very fine strands that are braided or twisted to produce a thick band of suture material (Fig. 3.1). Multifilament materials generally have good knot security and low memory (see below) but the multifilament construction creates a multifaceted surface that can harbour bacteria and shield them from host defences. These materials also have increased capillarity (see below). Both these characteristics mean a multifilament suture may act as a nidus for infection. In addition, the irregular surface leads to increased friction as the suture passes through tissues, producing high tissue drag (see below).

In comparison, monofilament suture material is manufactured as a single strand of suture material (Fig. 3.1). It has no surface features that harbour bacteria and has low capillarity. Monofilament materials do, however, have higher memory and poorer knot security than multifilament materials (see below). Many of the newer, synthetic, monofilament suture materials have improved handling and knotting characteristics, and monofilament suture materials are generally used in preference to multifilament materials.

Memory

Memory refers to the tendency of suture to retain the shape to which it has been conformed. For example, following bending or packaging, suture material with high memory will retain the bends along its length (Fig. 3.2). Memory is disadvantageous as it makes suture handling and knotting more difficult. High memory is a feature of monofilament suture materials in comparison to multifilament suture materials.

Knot security

Knot security is a feature of friction between adjacent strands of suture in a knot. Multifilament suture materials generally have better knot security than monofilament suture materials as they have less memory and higher coefficients of friction between adjacent strands of material within the knot.

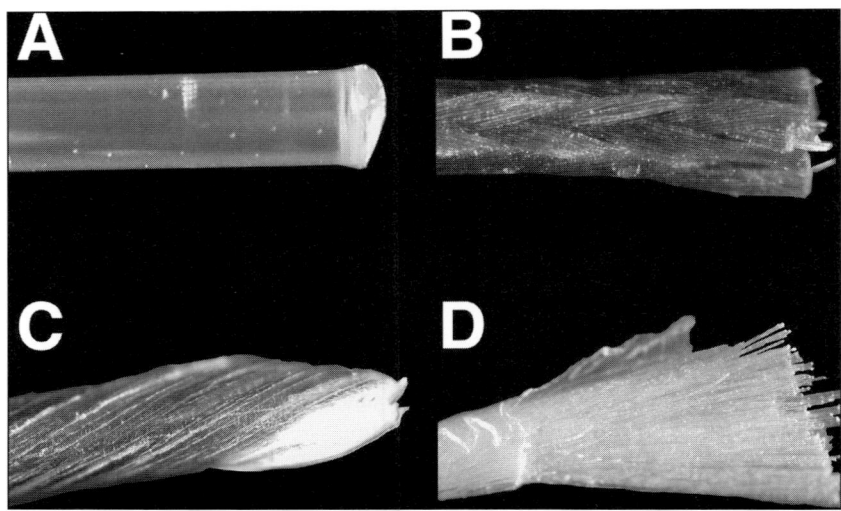

Fig. 3.1. Monofilament and multifilament suture materials: (A) monofilament, synthetic (poliglecaprone 25); (B) multifilament, braided, synthetic (polyglactin 910); (C) multifilament, twisted, natural (chromic catgut); (D) multifilament, sheathed, synthetic (nylon).

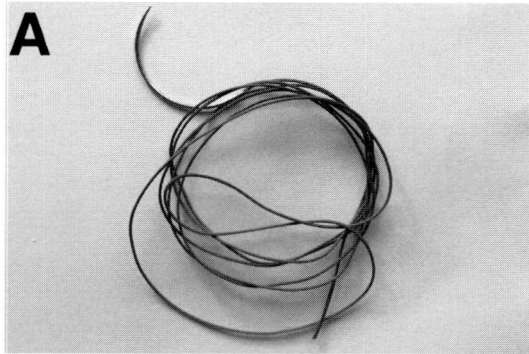

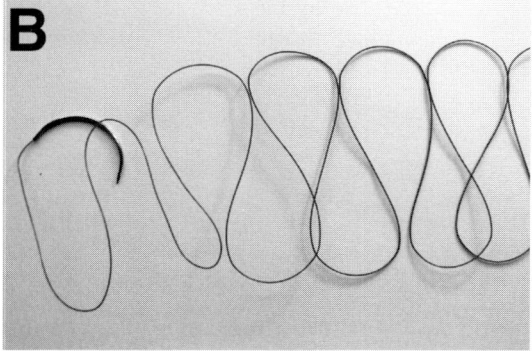

Fig. 3.2. Memory: (A) suture with low memory – multifilament, braided material (polyglactin 910); (B) suture with high memory that retains kinks from packaging – monofilament material (polydioxanone).

Tissue drag

Tissue drag is created by friction between the surface of the suture and the tissue through which it is moving. High tissue drag is a feature of multifilament suture materials and causes tissue trauma. Some multifilament sutures are coated to reduce tissue drag.

Capillarity

Capillarity allows wicking of fluid and bacteria across suture lines, potentially leading to wound contamination and infection. Multifilament suture materials have high capillarity because the spaces between the filaments provide conduits for capillary action. Monofilament suture materials have low capillarity.

Tensile strength

Suture materials are manufactured to have predictable tensile strengths when first placed in wounds.

Non-absorbable suture materials retain most of their tensile strength indefinitely. Absorbable suture materials lose tensile strength over time and ultimately will be completely absorbed. The chemical composition, size, and coating of suture material dictate its initial tensile strength and the rate of loss of tensile strength in a wound. A suture material should be at least as strong as the tissues that it is reconstructing and should retain tensile strength for sufficient time to support the tissues until they have regained their strength.

Coated suture material

Some suture materials are coated to confer additional properties to the material. Braided suture materials may be coated to reduce tissue drag. Some sutures are coated with antiseptics such as triclosan to reduce the potential for the material to act as a nidus for infection.

Dyed suture material

Suture materials may be dyed to help distinguish between different types during surgery and to aid visualization of smaller suture materials. However, the dye will remain at the site of implantation and in some situations (e.g. corneal surgery) undyed suture material may be preferred.

The 'Ideal' Suture Material

The ideal suture material is one which: (i) has adequate tensile strength during wound healing; (ii) is rapidly absorbed once it is no longer required; (iii) has low memory, good tissue handling, good knot security and low tissue drag; and (iv) induces minimal tissue reaction. It also has low capillarity and will not act as a nidus for infection. Unfortunately, no suture material has all of these features, as good knot security and low memory are achieved at the expense of reduced capillarity and low tissue drag. However, many of the modern, synthetic, monofilament suture materials have reasonable handling and knot security while maintaining low tissue drag and low capillarity and do not act as niduses for infection. *Monofilament, synthetic, absorbable* suture materials should be selected whenever possible.

Different Types of Suture Material

There are a wide variety of suture materials. Most manufacturers produce a range that covers common applications and there is little to separate the performance of equivalent suture materials produced by different manufacturers. For practical purposes, suture materials can be separated into three broad groups that help to define when they might be selected. These are: (i) short-acting absorbable; (ii) long-acting absorbable; and (iii) non-absorbable suture materials.

The following sections describe commonly available suture materials used in general practice. The monofilament, synthetic materials are described before other materials in each group as these generally have the most favourable characteristics.

Short-acting absorbable suture materials

Short-acting suture materials retain most of their tensile strength for 5–14 days. After this time, remaining tensile strength is lost rapidly although the suture will take several weeks to be completely absorbed. Short-acting absorbable suture is suitable for ligatures and for apposing well-vascularized tissue that will regain its strength rapidly. Examples of use include: (i) subcutaneous fat apposition; (ii) intradermal skin closure; (iii) muscle apposition; (iv) bladder closure; (v) ligation of ovarian pedicle during ovariohysterectomy; and (vi) ligation of splenic vessels during splenectomy.

Synthetic monofilament

Poliglecaprone 25 (e.g. Monocryl™, Ethicon Inc., West Somerville, New Jersey, USA) is a short-acting, monofilament suture material that has high initial tensile strength, low tissue drag, and reasonable knotting and handling properties. It performs better than braided short-acting suture material in intradermal closures, producing less inflammatory reaction, and is a versatile product.

Glycomer™ 631 (e.g. Biosyn™, Covidien plc, Dublin, Ireland) (a polymer of glycolide, dioxanone, and trimethylene carbonate) shares many of the features of poliglecaprone 25 but retains tensile strength for longer.

Both are good choices for short-term wound support and have favourable handling properties and physical features.

Synthetic multifilament

Polyglactin 910 (e.g. Vicryl™, Ethicon Inc., West Somerville, New Jersey, USA) is a popular braided suture material that has moderate tensile strength and retains most of this for 10–14 days. It has low memory and good knot security. It may be coated to reduce tissue drag. Partly hydrolysed polyglactin 910 (Vicryl Rapide™, Ethicon Inc., West Somerville, New Jersey, USA) is one of the shortest-acting suture materials as the partial hydrolysis speeds loss of tensile strength and absorption. It loses 50% of tensile strength after 5 days and all of its strength by 14 days. When placed in skin, Vicryl Rapide will fall out after 7–10 days, making suture removal unnecessary. It is suitable for short-term wound support and the manufacturers recommend it for use in oral mucosa and for skin closure.

Polyglycolic acid has also been used to produce multifilament, short-acting synthetic suture material with similar properties.

Natural

Collagen ('catgut' or **surgical gut**) is a multifilament, twisted suture material that is collagen-rich and manufactured from the intestinal submucosa of ruminants. Chromium salts may be incorporated to slow absorption and increase strength producing **chromic catgut**. It is popular, particularly for ligation, as it is inexpensive and forms knots easily. However, it invokes an inflammatory tissue reaction and is absorbed by proteolysis giving it an unpredictable pattern of absorption. In addition, absorption is accelerated if it is placed in enzymatic environments such as the gastrointestinal tract, or if it used in infected sites. It induces moderate inflammatory reaction when used in subcutaneous tissues. It has comparatively low tensile strength and loses tensile strength rapidly, making it unsuitable for closure of fascia.

Although gut is popular, modern synthetic monofilament suture materials are as effective and more versatile and should be used in preference. Gut should not be used for linea alba closure, for gastrointestinal surgery or for other hollow organ closure. Gut should not be used in contaminated or infected sites.

Long-acting absorbable suture materials

Long-acting absorbable suture materials retain most of their tensile strength beyond the first 4 weeks of placement. They then gradually lose tensile strength and are usually completely absorbed within 1 year. They are suitable for reconstructing fascia that regains strength slowly (e.g. linea alba; tensor fascia lata). They are also used extensively for gastrointestinal surgery.

Synthetic monofilament

Polydioxanone (e.g. PDS™ II, Ethicon Inc., West Somerville, New Jersey, USA) is a monofilament, long-acting, absorbable suture material. It has moderate memory but little tissue drag and reasonable knot security. It retains most of its tensile strength for 4 weeks and is completely absorbed by 8 months following placement.

Polyglyconate (e.g. Maxon™, Covidien plc) is a monofilament suture material that has similar properties to PDS II.

Non-absorbable suture materials

The non-absorbable suture materials remain in the body permanently. They retain most of their tensile strength throughout the lifetime of the patient. The synthetic non-absorbable materials generally induce very little tissue reaction as they are not antigenic and interact minimally with tissue. They have good tensile strength but tend to have high memory making handling more difficult. Steel wire and metal surgical staples are also classified in this group.

The non-absorbable, synthetic, monofilament suture materials are used extensively for skin sutures as they induce least tissue reaction, have low tissue drag, and are easy to remove. Non-absorbable suture materials may also be used in tissues within the body that require long-term support (e.g. perineal hernia repair) or when minimum tissue reaction is essential (e.g. vascular surgery to prevent thrombosis). In general practice, it is rarely necessary to leave non-absorbable suture materials buried within the body, and the long-acting, synthetic, absorbable materials are usually selected instead.

Synthetic monofilament

Monofilament nylon (polyamide) (e.g. Ethilon™, Ethicon Inc., West Somerville, New Jersey, USA) is a popular and inexpensive suture used predominantly for skin closure. It is moderately elastic enabling it to conform to changing wound shape (e.g. wound swelling post-operatively). It does not adhere to tissues so it is easy to remove once the skin wound has healed adequately. Like most monofilament materials, it has moderate memory that affects handling and knot security, but it remains a good choice for skin closure and for securing drains and tubes to skin.

Polypropylene (e.g. Prolene™, Ethicon Inc., West Somerville, New Jersey, USA), like nylon, is a monofilament suture material that retains elasticity making it suitable for skin closure. However, it has high memory that impedes handling and knot tying. It remains popular, not least because it is considered to be one of least reactive of all suture materials. The low tissue reactivity associated with polypropylene makes it a good choice when non-absorbable suture material is left buried in tissues, and for vascular surgery.

Synthetic multifilament

Multifilament nylon is a twisted multifilament material encased in a thin outer sheath to reduce tissue drag (Fig. 3.1). It is inexpensive, has low memory, and good knot security. However, it is usually supplied on spools requiring that it is used with eyed needles (see below).

Another example of a non-absorbable, synthetic, multifilament material is polyethylene teraphthalate, which has poor knot security.

Natural

Silk is classed as a non-absorbable suture material. Unlike the other non-absorbable materials, it loses much of its tensile strength within the first year. It is a multifilament suture material that has low memory, good handling, and good knot security. However, it has high tissue drag, may act as a nidus for infection and, as it is a natural material, it induces more tissue reaction than synthetic materials. Silk remains popular for permanent ligation of vessels although other suture materials may be better choices.

Suture Size

Recommended standards for minimal tensile strength and for suture size have been developed by the United States Pharmacopeia (USP) and the European Pharmacopoeia (EP). These bodies have developed two suture size scales, the USP scale and the metric scale. The metric scale is easiest to use as each unit represents suture diameter of one tenth of a millimetre. The USP scale incorporates the metric scale but also denotes minimum tensile strength of the material under standard test conditions. Table 3.1 summarizes the USP and metric scales and the legend provides additional information about conversion between these scales.

Table 3.1. Suture size chart: comparison of USP and metric scales. The USP scale runs from the smallest (12-0) to largest (10) sizes. For sizes less than size 0, each stepwise decrease in size is denoted by adding an additional '0' to the label. However, this is abbreviated and the number preceding the zero indicates the number of zeros in an annotation (e.g. 4-0 is an abbreviation of '0000'). The USP scale defines standard suture size and minimal tensile strength for a given class of suture and three separate standards are used for different classes of suture (collagen, synthetic absorbable, and non-absorbable). The metric system is a direct measure of suture diameter and each unit represents 0.1 mm. Most commercially supplied sutures come close to matching the USP and EP standard classifications.

USP	11-0	10-0	9-0	8-0	7-0	6-0	5-0	4-0	3-0	2-0	0	1	2	3	4	5	6
Metric: absorbable synthetic; non-absorbable	0.1	0.2	0.3	0.4	0.5	0.7	1.0	1.5	2.0	3.0	3.5	4.0	5.0	6.0	6.0	7.0	8.0
Metric: collagen	–	0.2	0.3	0.5	0.7	1.0	1.5	2.0	3.0	3.5	4.0	5.0	6.0	7.0	8.0	–	–

Needle Type and Selection

There are many different types of suture needle designed for a variety of uses. However, only a few are regularly used in veterinary surgery. Needles are classified by their shape, cutting point, and method of attachment to the suture.

Eyed needles versus swaged-on needles

Eyed needles are supplied separately from suture material. They have an eye to thread suture through and may be reused. *Swaged-on needles* are permanently fixed to lengths of suture during manufacture. They are supplied in individual suture packages containing a short length of suture material with needle designed for single use (Fig. 3.3).

Eyed needles are inexpensive and can be reused but they are associated with more tissue trauma than swaged-on needles. When the needle passes through tissue, it drags the bulky loop of suture material passing through the eye. This generates a large channel in the tissue that is considerably wider than the suture material itself. This leads to more potential for wicking across the suture line. Eyed needles also become blunted with repeated use.

Swaged-on needles have suture secured within a hollow channel at the end of the needle that reduces the bulk of the needle/suture junction. As the needle and suture pass through tissue, a small channel is created that is largely filled by suture material reducing tissue trauma and the potential for wicking. Trauma associated with needle blunting is less of an issue as swaged-on needles cannot be reused.

Although using pre-packaged lengths of suture with swaged-on needles is more expensive than using suture with eyed needles, it offers significant advantages and should be used in preference. Swaged-on needles and suture material should be used without exception in gastrointestinal and other hollow-organ surgery to reduce the risk of leakage and wicking across the suture line.

Needle shapes and tips

Curved needles are designed to be held with needle holders and to be pushed through tissues in an arc that matches the movement created by wrist action. Straight needles are designed to be held in the hand and to be pushed through tissues in a straight line that suits the natural trajectory created by hand suturing. The leading tip of the needle is also important to the way it functions. Three versatile needle tips are demonstrated in Fig. 3.4.

Taperpoint needles have a round body that narrows to a fine, sharp point. These penetrate easily through less dense tissues (e.g. subcutaneous fat) and are easy to control. They blunt quickly, particularly if forced through more collagen-dense tissue. They are used mostly for suturing subcutaneous fat.

Tapercut needles are similar to taperpoint needles but have a short, cutting tip engineered into the very tip of the needle. These penetrate collagen-dense tissues easily but, because only the tip is cutting, they are easy to control, preventing unwanted deeper tissue penetration and limiting unintended tissue laceration. They are used predominantly in collagen-rich fascia (e.g. linea alba), in oral mucosa, and for closing hollow organs where the balance between fine control and easy penetration of tougher tissues is good.

Cutting needles have a longer cutting edge and are designed to penetrate tough tissue such as skin. The cutting edge may be on the inside aspect of the needle arc (standard '*cutting*') or the outside aspect ('*reverse cutting*'). Standard cutting needles create a

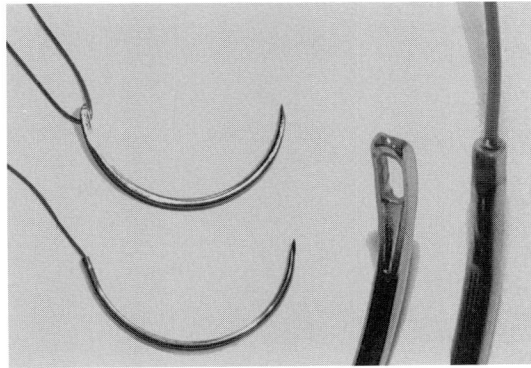

Fig. 3.3. Eyed and swaged-on needles.

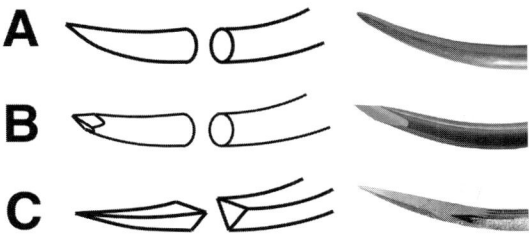

Fig. 3.4. Needle tips: (A) taperpoint; (B) tapercut; (C) reverse cutting.

'V'-shaped channel on the inside of the suture arc that may encourage suture pull-through if tension is applied to the tissues. Reverse cutting needles overcome this problem by reversing the direction of the channel so that suture pull-through is less likely to occur. The reverse cutting needles are most popular and are ideal for skin and intradermal suturing.

Suture Packaging

Suture material is packaged either as long spools of suture in multi-use dispensers (cassettes) or as short lengths of suture in individual packages for single use (Fig. 3.5). Suture material may be sterilized by gamma-irradiation, ethylene oxide, or alcohol and

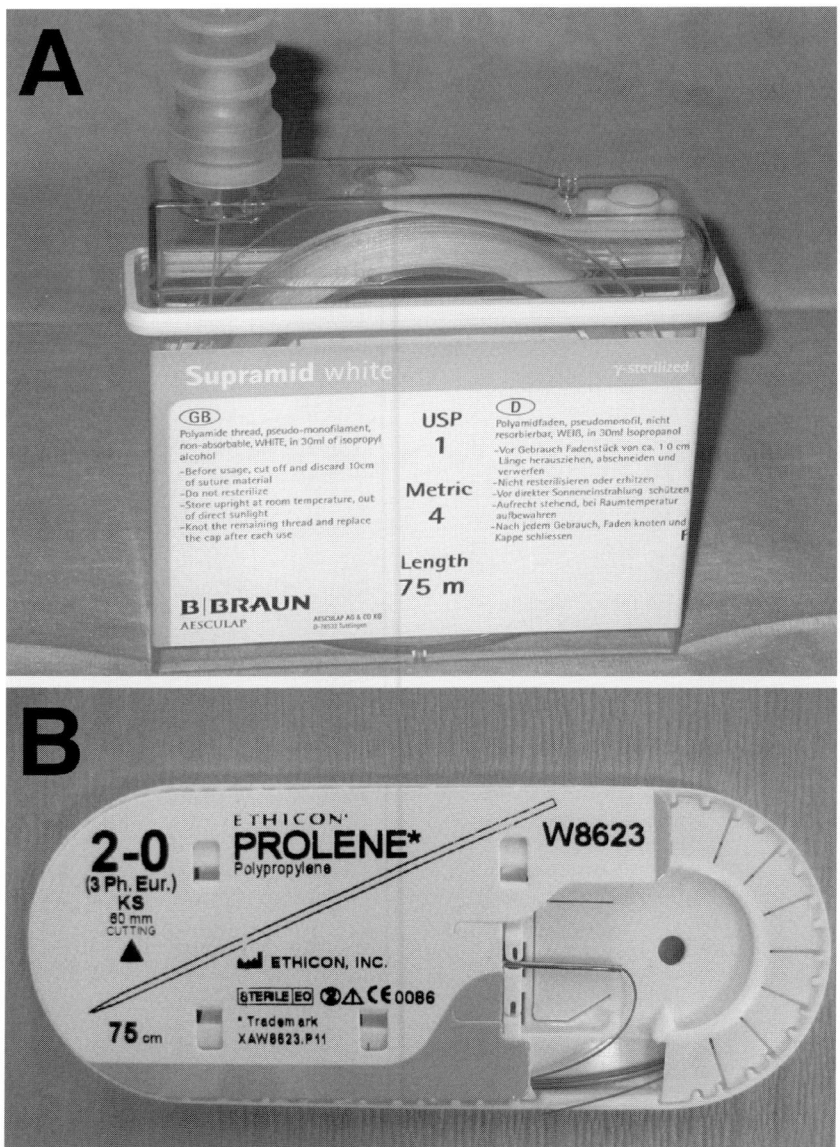

Fig. 3.5. Suture packaging: (A) multi-use suture cassette containing alcohol; (B) suture pack with a short length of suture and a swaged-on needle.

should not be resterilized as this may affect its physical properties.

Suture cassettes are popular because they are inexpensive. However, only a few suture materials are available on cassettes and they are not compatible with swaged-on needles. Suture cassettes increase the risk of the suture becoming contaminated, as suture cannot be delivered from a sterile pack directly into the surgical field. Instead, the suture must be withdrawn from the cassette away from the sterile field and transferred to the surgical site. Also, the free end of the suture is left outside the protective environment of the cassette between uses and becomes contaminated. It must be disposed of before a new strand of material is used. These features increase the potential for contamination of the suture during use.

Pre-packaged suture materials with swaged-on needles are preferred over the use of suture cassettes and eyed needles. There is minimal risk of contamination of the suture prior to use and the pack can be opened directly onto the sterile field. Individual packs of suture also enable the use of swaged-on needles and encourage frequent changes of needle, limiting trauma induced by needle blunting. The main disadvantage is that the packs are expensive.

Surgical Staples

Stainless steel surgical staples invoke minimal tissue reaction and have a variety of uses. They are used extensively in general practice for skin closure and for vessel ligation. Special staple devices can also be used for more complex procedures (e.g. enterectomy; lung lobectomy). The use of skin staples for skin closure will be discussed in more detail (see p. 100).

Tissue Adhesive

Cyanoacrylate-based compounds polymerize on contact with moisture to form an adhesive that can be used for skin closure. The incised skin edges are held in apposition, adhesive is applied across the incision line (ensuring that it does not seep into the wound), and the adhesive is allowed to dry for a few moments. Cyanoacrylate adhesives are painless to apply and achieve good skin apposition. However, skin wounds closed with adhesives are not as strong as sutured wounds and, if the adhesive seeps into the incision below the epidermis, it may impede wound healing. Cyanoacrylate adhesives are sometimes used to augment other methods of closure (e.g. to appose a gaping portion of intradermal skin closure).

Bibliography

Anon (1998) Opinion and report on the equivalency of alternative products to intestines of animal origin for use as surgical sutures adopted by the Scientific Committee on Medicinal Products and Medical Devices on 16 September 1998. http://ec.europa.eu/health/ph_risk/committees/scmp/docshtml/scmp_out05_en.print.htm, accessed 16 March 2010.

Anon (2007a) *USP Monographs: Absorbable Surgical Suture*. www.pharmacopeia.cn/v29240/usp29nf24s0_m80190.html, accessed 20 March 2010.

Anon (2007b) *USP Monographs: Non-absorbable Surgical Suture*. www.pharmacopeia.cn/v29240/usp29nf24s0_m80200.html, accessed 20 March 2010.

Bichon, D., Borloz, W. and Cassano-Zoppi, A.L. (1984) *In vivo* evaluation of a new polyurethane-coated catgut suture. *Biomaterials* 5, 255–263.

Boothe, H.W. Jr (1998) Selecting suture materials for small animal surgery. *Compendium: Continuing Education for Veterinarians* 20, 155–163.

Dunn, D.L. (2007) *Ethicon Wound Closure Manual*. Ethicon Inc., West Somerville, New Jersey, USA.

Edlich, R.F. (2008) Absorbable suture. In: Edlich, R.F. *Surgical Knot Tying Manual*, 3rd edn. Covidien AG, Portland, Oregon, pp. 12–21.

Faria, M.C., De Almeida, F.M., Serrao, M.L., De Oliveira Almeida, N.K. and Labarthe, N. (2005) Use of cyanoacrylate in skin closure for ovariohysterectomy in a population control programme. *Journal of Feline Medicine and Surgery* 7, 71–75.

Hochberg, J., Meyer, K.M. and Marion, M.D. (2009) Suture choice and other methods of skin closure. *Surgical Clinics of North America* 89, 627–641.

Kirpensteijn, J., Maarschalkerweerd, R.J., Koeman, J.P., Kooistra, H.S. and Van Sluijs, F.J. (1997) Comparison of two suture materials for intradermal skin closure in dogs. *Veterinary Quarterly* 19, 20–22.

Marco, F., Vallez, R., Gonzalez, P., Ortega, L., De La Lama, J. and Lopez-Duran, L. (2007) Study of the efficacy of coated Vicryl plus antibacterial suture in an animal model of orthopedic surgery. *Surgical Infections* 8, 359–365.

Ming, X., Rothenburger, S. and Yang, D. (2007a) *In vitro* antibacterial efficacy of MONOCRYL plus antibacterial suture (Poliglecaprone 25 with triclosan). *Surgical Infections* 8, 201–208.

Ming, X., Nichols, M. and Rothenburger, S. (2007b) *In vivo* antibacterial efficacy of MONOCRYL plus antibacterial suture (Poliglecaprone 25 with triclosan). *Surgical Infections* 8, 209–214.

Ming, X., Rothenburger, S. and Nichols, M.M. (2008) *In vivo* and *in vitro* antibacterial efficacy of PDS plus (polidioxanone with triclosan) suture. *Surgical Infections* 9, 451–457.

Okada, T., Hayashi, T. and Ikada, Y. (1992) Degradation of collagen suture *in vitro* and *in vivo*. *Biomaterials* 13, 448–454.

Sanz, L.E., Patterson, J.A., Kamath, R., Willett, G., Ahmed, S.W. and Butterfield, A.B. (1988) Comparison of Maxon suture with Vicryl, chromic catgut, and PDS sutures in fascial closure in rats. *Obstetrics and Gynecology* 71, 418–422.

Singer, A.J., Quinn, J.V. and Hollander, J.E. (2008) The cyanoacrylate topical skin adhesives. *American Journal of Emergency Medicine* 26, 490–496.

Tan, R.H., Bell, R.J., Dowling, B.A. and Dart, A.J. (2003) Suture materials: composition and applications in veterinary wound repair. *Australian Veterinary Journal* 81, 140–145.

Tian, F., Appert, H.E. and Howard, J.M. (1994) The disintegration of absorbable suture materials on exposure to human digestive juices: an update. *The American Surgeon* 60, 287–291.

Tobin, G.R. (1984) Closure of contaminated wounds. Biologic and technical considerations. *Surgical Clinics of North America* 64, 639–652.

Williams, D.F. (1980) The effect of bacteria on absorbable sutures. *Journal of Biomedical Material Research* 14, 329–338.

4 Suture Patterns and Knots

appositional suture pattern: a pattern that anatomically apposes wound edges
bite of tissue: portion of tissue ensnared by suture
everting suture pattern: a pattern that everts wound edges
inverting suture pattern: a pattern that inverts wound edges
surgeon's throw: a throw with two twists
suture ear: the cut end of suture material in a knot
tension relieving suture pattern: a pattern that distributes tension over a wider area than a simple interrupted suture
throw: the basic unit of a knot made by looping two strands of suture material around each other

The reader should be able to:

- list the components of a square knot
- contrast the properties of the square knot, surgeon's knot, and granny knot
- explain when a surgeon's throw might be used in preference to a single throw for ligation of a vascular pedicle, and explain how this might detract from the primary goal of haemostasis
- contrast the effect on wound healing of appositional, inverting, and everting suture patterns for the closure of a hollow organ
- contrast the effect on wound healing of using horizontal mattress sutures to close a skin wound that is under tension, compared with using simple interrupted appositional pattern to close a skin wound which is not under tension
- demonstrate a two-handed tie using string and a fixed hook
- demonstrate an instrument tie to generate a square knot to close a 1 cm incision in a skin suture pad model*
- demonstrate how to place simple continuous, horizontal mattress, vertical mattress, cruciate mattress, and Cushing suture patterns*
- demonstrate how to secure a tube to a fixed surface using a Roman sandal suture and an appropriate sham*

*materials list for suture exercises: skin suture pad model; Mayo-Hegar needle holders; Mayo scissors; Brown-Adson thumb forceps; 2-0 polyamide suture on a swaged-on reverse-cutting needle.

This chapter reviews common suture knots and patterns used in veterinary surgery; further advice on suture pattern selection is given in individual chapters relating to specific procedures. However, today most surgeons gravitate towards simple appositional suture patterns, as these encourage early wound healing, and square knots, as these are secure.

Surgical Knots

The knot is the weakest point of a suture line as the suture material weakens through handling as the knot is tied and because the knot can unravel. Each knot is composed of a series of throws made by looping one piece of suture around another. Knots have between four and seven throws stacked on top of each other. Each throw may be composed of a single or a double turn of the two suture ends around each other (Fig. 4.1). A throw with a double turn (the 'surgeon's throw') is more resistant to slippage as there is more contact between the two pieces of suture material. However, the surgeon's throw also creates a bulkier knot. The ears of the knot are the cut ends of suture material. These must be of sufficient length to prevent the knot from unravelling.

Square knot

The square knot is extremely secure and forms the basis of most knots used in veterinary surgery. The basic unit of the square knot is based on the 'reef knot' and is a symmetrical, flat knot that resists slippage (Fig. 4.2). If it is tied incorrectly, either an asymmetric knot (a 'granny knot') or a slipknot may form and neither is as secure. Surgical square knots are formed by three or four single throws.

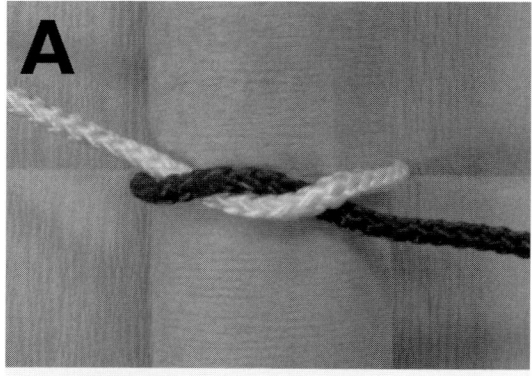

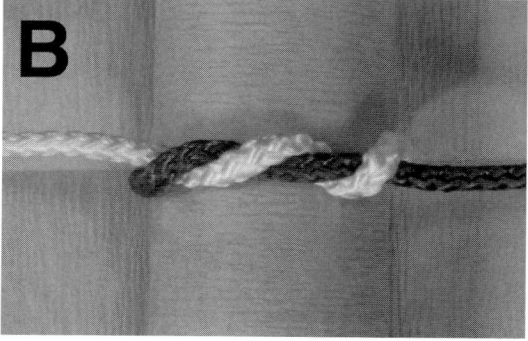

Fig. 4.1. Basic knot throws: (A) single turn; (B) double turn (surgeon's throw).

The first two throws dictate the tightness of the knot; the remaining throws add further security to the knot. To tie square knots follow the instructions for instrument-tied and hand-tied knots.

Surgeon's knot

The surgeon's knot is similar to the square knot but the first throw is a surgeon's throw (double turn). This is followed by three single throws tied in the same manner as a square knot (Fig. 4.3). The surgeon's throw is often used in preference to the single throw to start the knot, as it is less likely to loosen before the second throw is applied. It may be used to appose tissues that have slight tension pulling the wound edges apart. It may also be used to secure monofilament suture materials with high memory as the first throw is inclined to slip if a single turn is used. However, the surgeon's knot is bulkier and less secure than the classic square knot so it is advisable to reserve the surgeon's knot for situations where a square knot cannot be tied.

Knots for continuous suture lines

Knots for continuous suture lines require additional throws for security. Place five throws at the start and seven throws at the end of continuous suture lines.

Principles of tying square knots

Square knots can be tied by hand or by using instruments. The two-handed tie is demonstrated in Fig. 4.4. This method should be used whenever tying knots by hand during surgery, as it ensures that a square knot is always tied in a secure fashion. The surgeon also has greater control of suture tension than when performing an instrument tie.

Instruments are used to tie most surgical knots. A series of basic principles should be followed to ensure that a square knot is always formed:

1. Only the end of the suture material should be handled to avoid damaging the material that will form the knot.
2. Always place the instrument in the centre of the knot.
3. Always place the instrument into the knot from the surgeon's side.
4. Apply tension evenly to each end of the suture as the throws are laid.

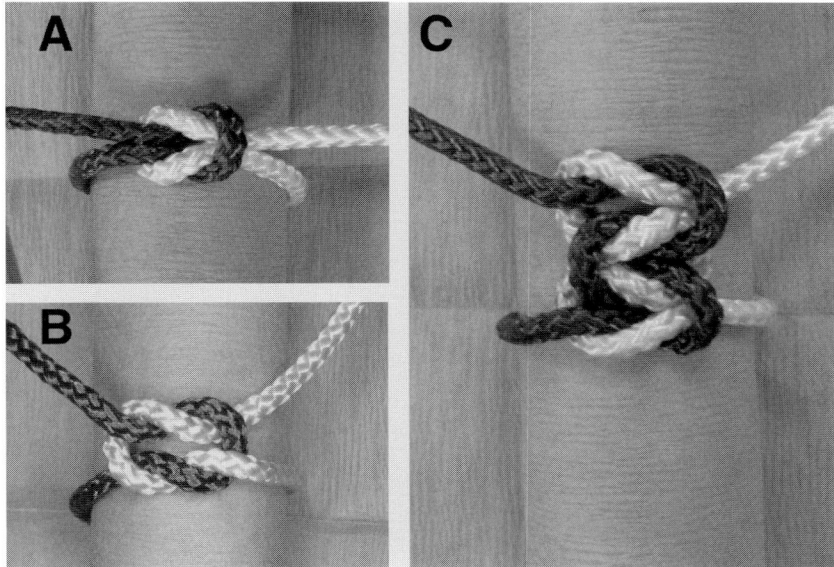

Fig. 4.2. (A) basic unit of the square knot; (B) granny knot – this is much less secure than the square knot and shou d not be used; (C) a four-throw square knot, the basis of most surgical knots.

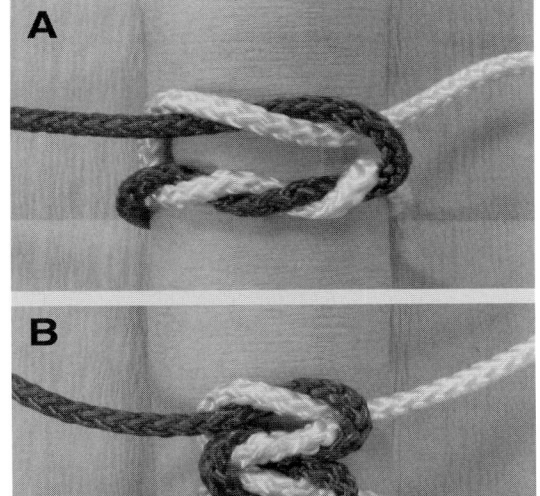

Fig. 4.3. Surgeon's knot: (A) basic unit of surgeon's throw with single throw (not tightened); (B) four-throw surgeon's knot (surgeon's throw with three single throws) – note that this knot is bulkier than the square knot because of the additional suture in the surgeon's throw (arrow).

5. Pull the ends of the suture material in opposite directions when laying a throw.
6. Apply tension perpendicular to the wound when tightening throws.
7. Suture ends always change sides as each throw of a square knot is tied.
8. When placing a series of sutures, right-handed surgeons should suture from right to left; left-handed surgeons should suture from left to right.
9. When placing continuous suture lines, place five throws at the start and seven throws at the end.

The steps required to tie a square knot using instruments are illustrated in Figs 4.5 and 4.6.

Ligatures

Ligatures are sutures tied around vessels and vascular pedicles to prevent bleeding. Circumferential and transfixing ligatures are used extensively in veterinary surgery.

Circumferential ligature

The circumferential ligature encircles and compresses a vessel to achieve haemostasis (Fig. 4.7). Suture material is passed around the structure to be ligated. A single throw is placed and tied as securely as possible.

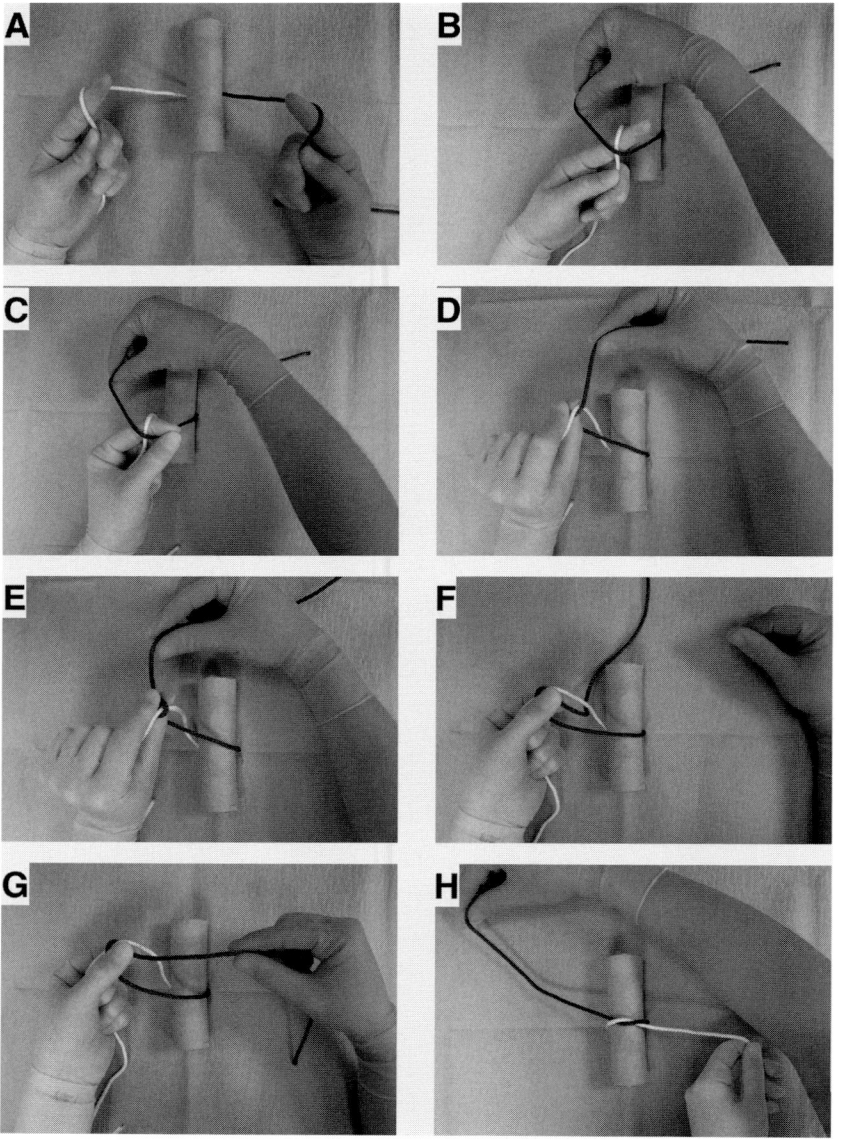

Fig. 4.4. Two-handed tie: right-handed version.

This crushes the vessel or vascular pedicle. Three additional single throws are placed to secure the ligature and the suture ends are cut short leaving a minimum of 3–5 mm (dependent on suture size and material) to prevent the knot unravelling. Occasionally, a surgeon's throw is required as the first throw to overcome resistance to compression by the tissues, but this produces a bulkier knot, leading to inferior haemostasis.

Transfixing ligature

A transfixing ligature is anchored into the wall of the vessel or pedicle to prevent it slipping (Fig. 4.8). Transfixing ligatures are commonly used on major vascular pedicles or larger arteries as they resist slippage along the vessel as might occur, for example, when the ligature is pushed by the action of the

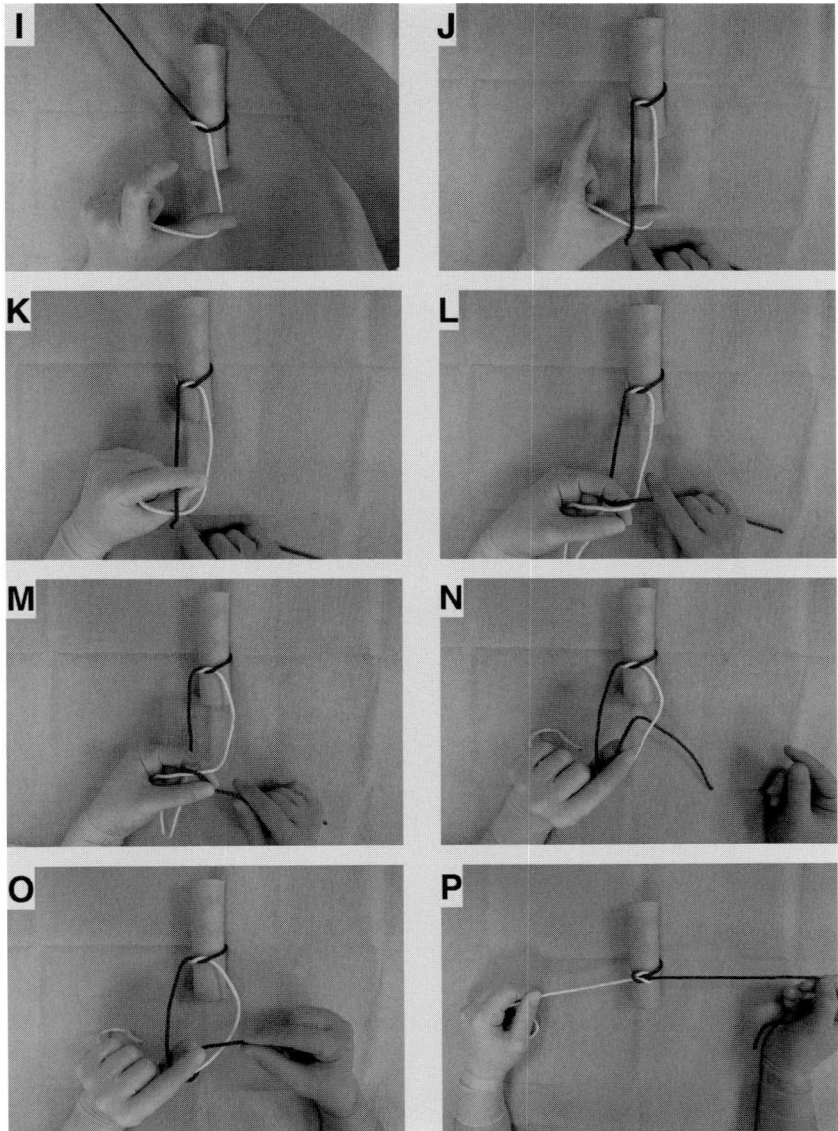

Fig. 4.4. Continued.

arterial pulse. Although transfixing ligatures are less likely to fall off than circumferential ligatures, they are bulkier, making them less effective at crushing and occluding the structure that they are tied round.

Ligature combinations

The circumferential ligature is less bulky and provides better haemostasis than a transfixing ligature. The transfixing ligature is more secure and less prone to slippage. A combination of both should be used to ligate large arteries and veins (e.g. femoral vessels for hind limb amputation) (Fig. 4.9):

1. Isolate the vessel from the surrounding tissues by blunt dissection.
2. Tie a circumferential ligature proximally to occlude blood flow.

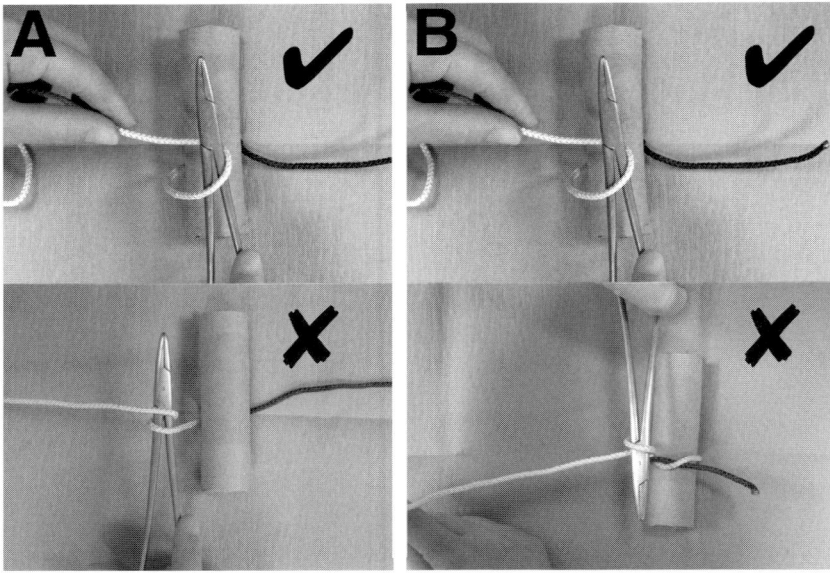

Fig. 4.5. Basic principles in knot tying: (A) place instruments in the centre of the knot or granny knots will be tied; (B) always work from the surgeon's side.

3. Tie a second circumferential ligature at least 15 mm distally to the first. This ligature remains on the distal end of the transected vessel to prevent back-bleeding (blood flowing back from the tissues being amputated).

4. Place a transfixing ligature between the two circumferential ligatures.

5. Transect the vessel between the transfixing (middle) and distal ligature. Leave at least a 5 mm stump of vessel distal to the transfixing ligature to provide further protection from ligature slippage.

Appositional Suture Patterns

Appositional patterns appose tissue edges precisely, reconstructing the wound anatomically and promoting early wound healing. They also hold tissues in close apposition without causing unnecessary crushing of tissue, which would compromise the blood supply to the wound edge. These patterns are used in preference to everting and inverting patterns and are often referred to as 'simple' patterns.

Simple interrupted patterns reconstruct the wound with a series of individually placed sutures (Fig. 4.10). *Simple continuous* patterns reconstruct the wound with a single, uninterrupted piece of suture that runs from one end of the wound to the other and only has knots at each end (Fig. 4.11). Interrupted patterns are most versatile and can accommodate closure of irregularly shaped wounds or tissues of unequal thickness. They also cause least compromise of the blood supply to the wound edge. Continuous patterns are quicker to place and use less suture material. They may also provide a better seal against leakage. However, continuous patterns may cause more compromise of the blood supply to the wound edge as they compress the capillary supply along the continuous length of the suture line. They are also entirely reliant on the two knots at either end for their integrity and the distal knot must be tied by creating a loop of suture material, which reduces its security (Fig. 4.12). Continuous suture patterns require additional throws on each knot in comparison to interrupted suture patterns. Place five throws at the start and seven throws at the end.

Both interrupted and continuous simple appositional patterns are highly versatile. Simple appositional interrupted patterns are used extensively for skin closure and for walking sutures. Continuous simple appositional patterns are used for most other applications including closure of the linea alba and subcutaneous tissues. Both simple interrupted and continuous suture patterns can be used

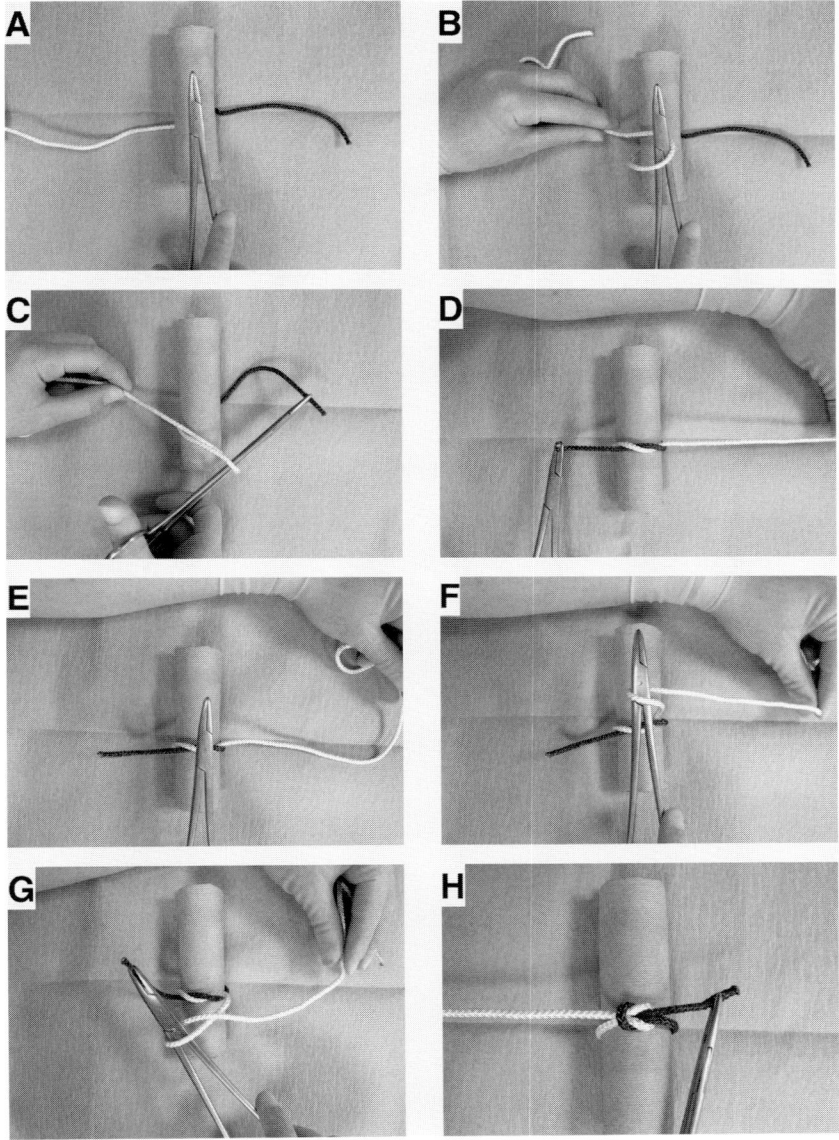

Fig. 4.6. Instrument tie: following the principles listed to generate a square knot.

to close hollow organs, but continuous closures may provide a better seal.

Intradermal pattern

The intradermal pattern is popular for skin closure as it produces a cosmetic result that does not rely on external skin sutures. This means that there are no exposed sutures for the patient to interfere with or which need to be removed. This pattern is also referred to as a *subcuticular* pattern.

The suture is placed in the tissues immediately between the dermis and subcutis. These tissues are collagenous, and a swaged-on, cutting needle is required. This is a continuous suture line. Use a short-acting, monofilament, absorbable suture

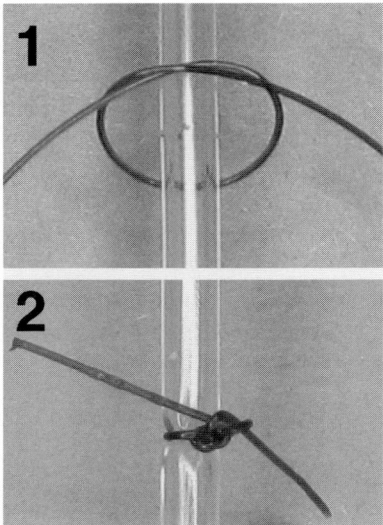

Fig. 4.7. Circumferential ligature: suture material is passed around the structure being ligated and tied with a square or a surgeon's knot.

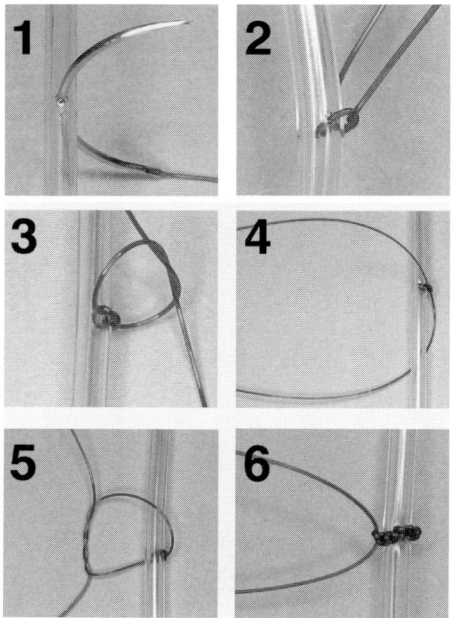

Fig. 4.8. Modified transfixing ligature: (1) take a bite of the vessel wall; (2 and 3) tie a surgeon's throw followed by a single throw to anchor the suture in the vessel wall; (4) pass the ends of the suture material around to the other side of the vessel (encircling it); (5 and 6) tie a four-throw surgeon's knot.

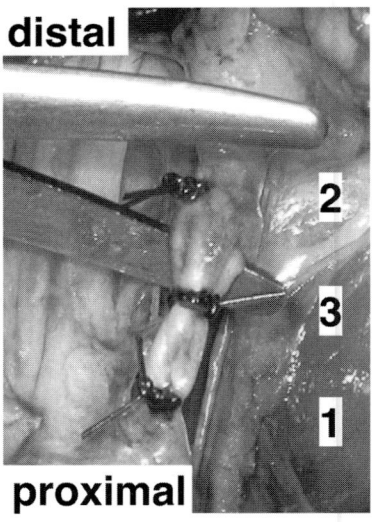

Fig. 4.9. Combination ligature pattern on femoral artery: ligature 1: circumferential ligature placed proximally to occlude the vessel; ligature 2: circumferential ligature placed distally to prevent back-bleeding; ligature 3: transfixing ligature placed between 1 and 2 for added security. Transect vessel between the middle (transfixing) and distal ligature leaving a 5 mm stump of vessel to further guard against ligature slippage. Repeat this process to ligate the femoral vein.

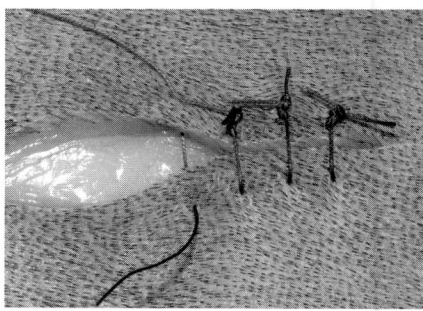

Fig. 4.10. Simple interrupted pattern. To place a simple interrupted suture, take a bite of tissue inserting the needle a few millimetres from the wound edge and exiting through the incision. Take a second bite of tissue from the opposite side of the wound, passing the needle into the incision and exiting it a few millimetres from the wound edge. The two bites of tissue should be perpendicular to the wound edge and directly opposite each other. The suture is secured by tying a four-throw square knot or a surgeon's knot. Cut the suture ends leaving 5 mm ears to prevent suture slippage. Repeat this process to create a line of sutures. Bites of tissue are 3–8 mm in width and are spaced 3–10 mm apart (depending on the thickness of the tissues being sutured).

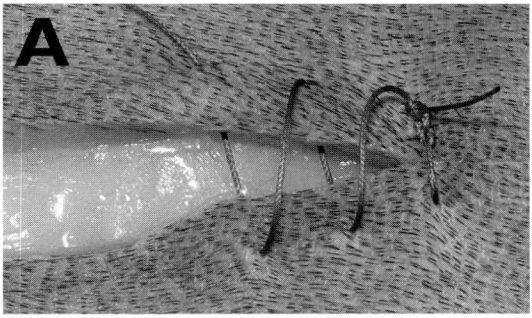

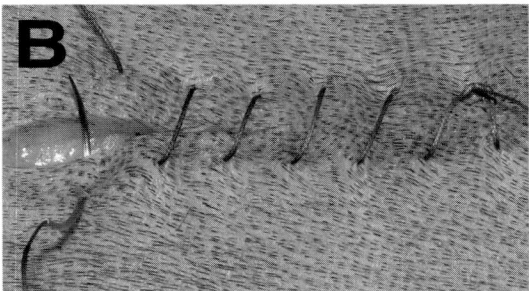

Fig. 4.11. Simple continuous pattern. This is an extension of the simple interrupted pattern: (A) anchor the start of the suture line with a five-throw square knot and place a series of simple sutures along the wound (this panel shows the sutures placed loosely for demonstration purposes – maintain tissue apposition as the suture is placed); (B) adjust tension as the sutures are placed to appose the tissue edges.

material on a reverse-cutting needle of size 4-0 or 3-0. Complete the incision line by suturing parallel to the skin surface just below the level of the dermis (the dense, pale layer that abuts the subcutaneous fat). Ensure that knots at the start and end are buried. Figures 4.13, 4.14, and 4.15 summarize placement of this suture pattern.

Tension-Relieving Suture Patterns

Mattress sutures are designed to relieve tension by distributing pressure over a wider area than simple interrupted sutures. However, most mattress sutures cause tissue eversion and this impedes wound healing. They also are inclined to cut into the skin under the suture material, causing pressure necrosis. These suture patterns are associated with a high complication rate due to their negative effects on wound healing. Avoid using mattress sutures to alleviate tension whenever possible.

Vertical and horizontal mattress sutures

Vertical and horizontal mattress sutures are tension-relieving sutures that cause wound eversion (Figs 4.16 and 4.17). These sutures compress the tissue, causing vascular compromise of the skin immediately below the suture. This can lead to the suture cutting into the tissue, and other wound

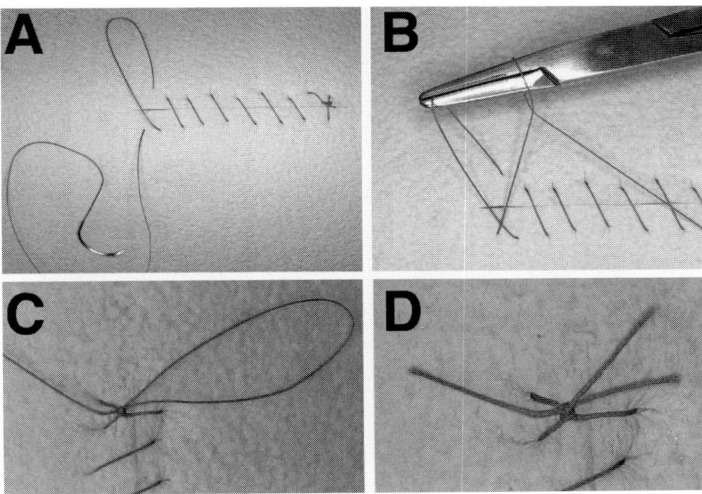

Fig. 4.12. Finishing a continuous suture line: (A) when the end of the suture line is reached, place the final suture but do not tighten it. This creates loop; (B and C) tie a seven-throw knot using the loop and the free end of the suture to secure the suture line; (D) trim the loop and the free end of suture.

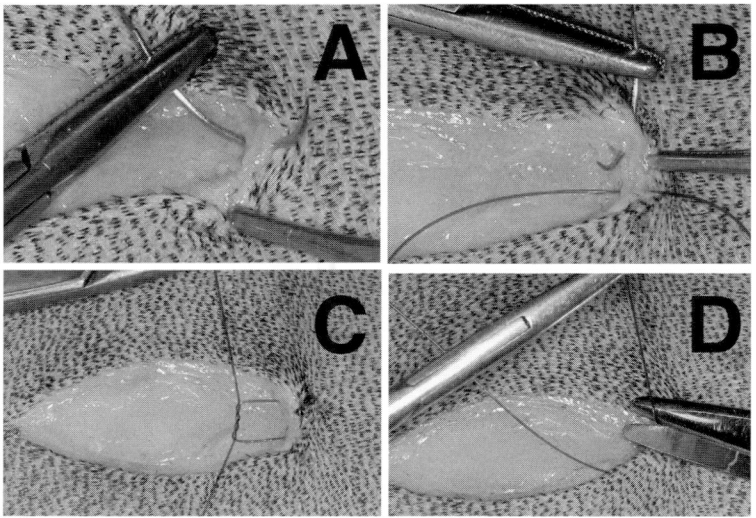

Fig. 4.13. Intradermal pattern – starting knot. All sutures are placed just below the dermis. Place the starting knot in the right-hand margin of the wound (reverse direction for left-handed surgeons). The knots of the intradermal suture line are buried below the surface of the skin: (A) place a suture perpendicular to the skin edge by taking a bite of tissue starting 3–4 mm deep to the dermis and running up to exit the tissues just below the dermis; (B) take a second bite of suture on the opposite skin margin, this time introducing the needle just below the dermis and exiting the needle 3–4 mm below this in the deeper intradermal tissues; (C) tie a square knot – the knot will be buried in the deeper layers below the dermis; (D) trim the free end of the suture short.

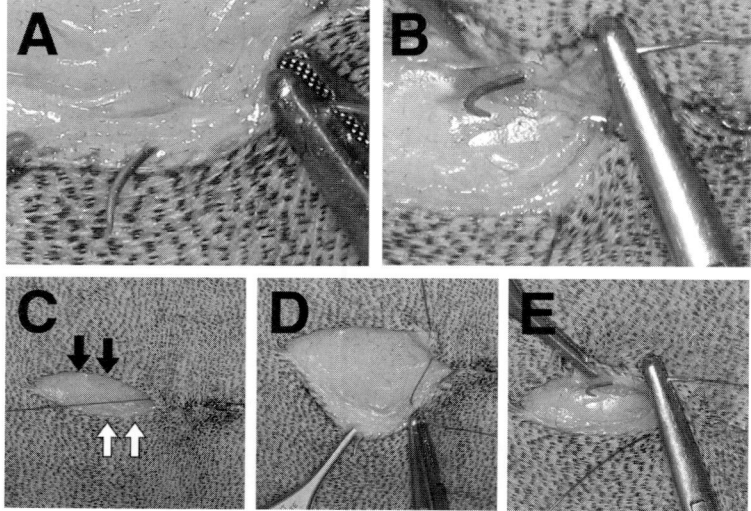

Fig. 4.14. Intradermal pattern – apposing the skin edges. To appose the skin edges, place a running suture (similar to a continuous, buried, horizontal mattress suture) just below the dermis advancing the needle with each tissue bite: (A) take a 4–6 mm bite of tissue running parallel to the skin surface just below the dermis; (B) take a second bite in the opposite tissue edge introducing the needle level with the exit point of the first bite (hence advancing the needle along the wound); (C) tighten the suture and repeat these steps until the entire wound is closed. White arrows demonstrate the entry and exit points of the third bite of tissue in this closure pattern; black arrows demonstrate the entry and exit points of the fourth bite of tissue in this closure pattern; (D) the third bite; (E) the fourth bite.

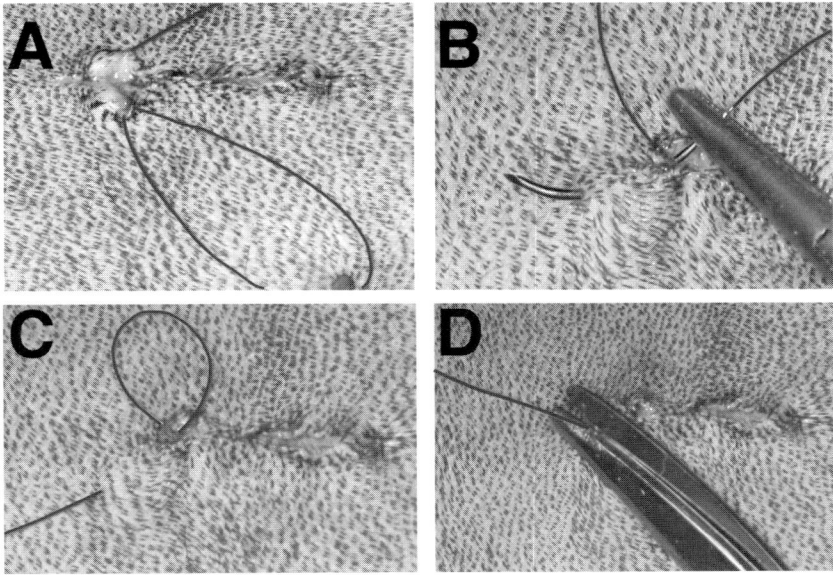

Fig. 4.15. Intradermal suture pattern – finishing the suture line: (A) at the end of the incision, repeat the processes performed to bury the starting knot (Fig. 4.13). This generates a loop and a free end of suture. Tie these together in a square knot, trim the loop short but leave the free end of suture with needle attached. To bury the knot: (B) introduce the needle into the apex of the wound and exit it a few millimetres away from the end of the incision; (C) draw the remaining suture tight; (D) tense the skin by applying traction to the end of the suture and trim the suture close to the skin edge. This effectively buries the free end of suture subcutaneously (the end retracts below the wound surface when it is cut).

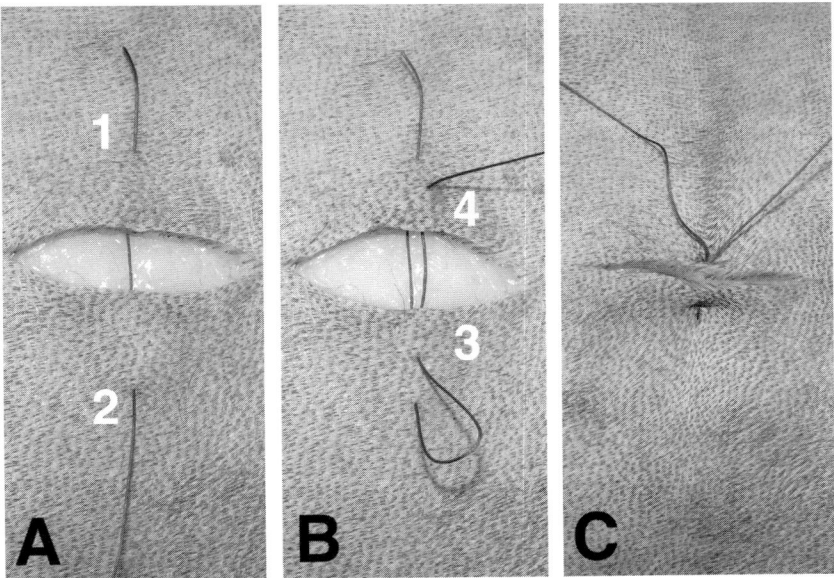

Fig. 4.16. Vertical mattress suture: (A) pass suture through the wound taking two large bites of tissue on either side; (B) pass the suture back through the wound taking bites midway between the first bites and the skin edges to lay the vertical mattress suture; (C) tie the suture everting the skin edges (numbers indicate order in which bites are taken).

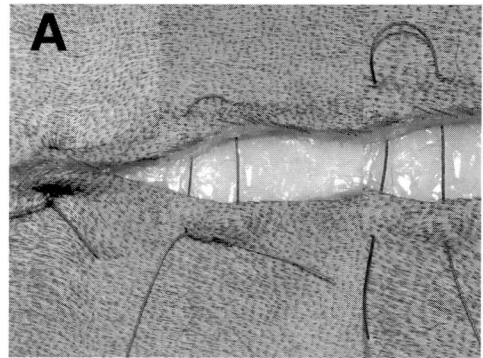

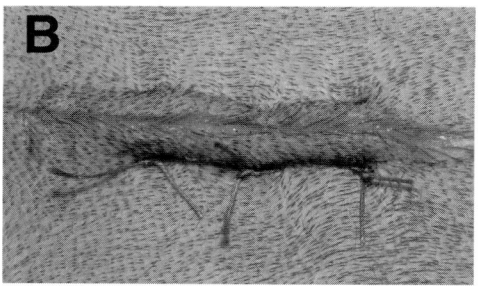

Fig. 4.17. Horizontal mattress suture: (A) pass the suture through the wound normally, move along the wound, pass suture back through the wound running parallel to the first pass of suture material and tie the knot; (B) the horizontal mattress suture causes marked wound eversion.

problems. To reduce the degree of skin damage, stents can be used to spread the pressure under the suture over a wider area (Fig. 4.18).

Cruciate mattress suture

The cruciate mattress suture resembles two simple interrupted sutures placed parallel to each other before the suture ends are tied. When the suture ends are tied, the visible suture forms a cross from which the suture gets its name (Fig. 4.19). Cruciate mattress sutures cause less wound eversion compared with other mattress sutures. Although these can be used as tension-relieving sutures, they have become popular for skin closure when they are not placed under tension (and hence do not cause skin injury or wound eversion). When used in this manner, they achieve reasonable tissue apposition and, as fewer knots are required, are quicker to place than an equivalent row of simple interrupted sutures. This suture is sometimes referred to as the *cross-stitch*.

Inverting (Cushing) Pattern

Inverting suture patterns are designed to invert the serosal surface of hollow organs. The serosa-to-serosa contact that this achieves leads to an

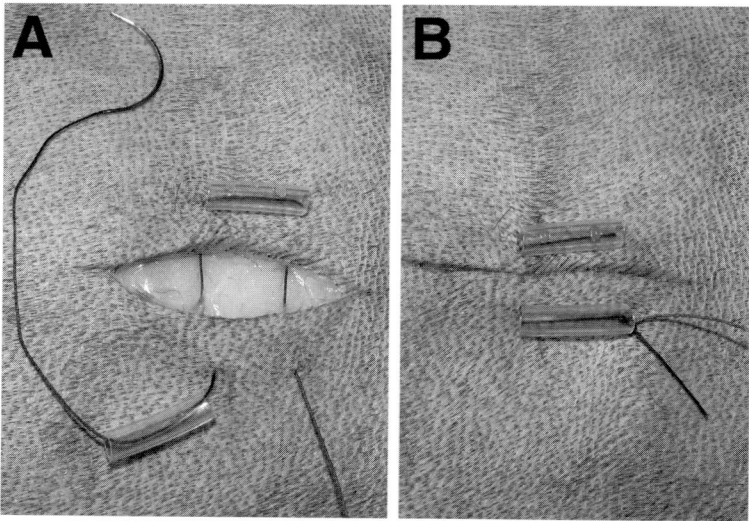

Fig. 4.18. Stented horizontal mattress suture: this horizontal mattress suture has been stented by feeding sections of drip tubing through the suture before tying. This distributes pressure under the suture over a much larger area, reducing the degree to which the suture cuts into the skin (which can cause pressure necrosis).

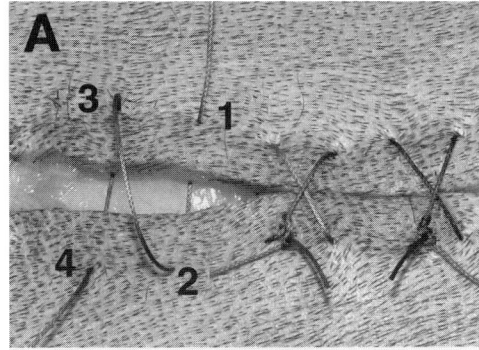

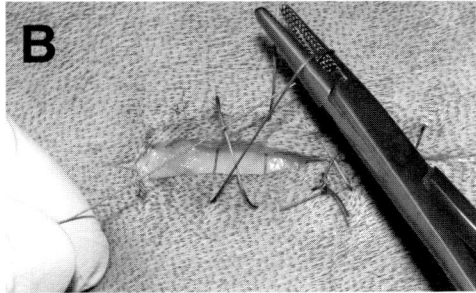

Fig. 4.19. Cruciate mattress suture: (A) numbers denote order of suture placement; when the suture is tied to appose the edges in wounds with minimal tension, these sutures achieve reasonable tissue apposition; (B) tying the suture.

early serosal seal that may resist leakage better than appositional suture patterns. The disadvantages of inverting patterns in comparison to appositional patterns are that they may lead to some delay in wound healing as the tissues are not anatomically reconstructed, and they cause more luminal narrowing. Inverting patterns can only be used to close incisions in large hollow organs (e.g. stomach; uterus; bladder) where luminal narrowing will not cause obstruction. In most situations, appositional suture patterns are as effective. The Cushing suture pattern is an inverting pattern that is suitable for hollow organ surgery (Fig. 4.20).

Purse-String Suture

The purse-string suture is a circular suture used to close an orifice or stoma (Fig. 4.21). It is used: (i) to prevent faecal spillage from the anus during perianal surgery; (ii) to prevent recurrence of rectal prolapse; and (iii) to create a snug-fitting stoma around tubes introduced into hollow organs (e.g. gastrostomy tube). Use 2-0 or 3-0 monofilament, synthetic suture material that is suitable for the location in which it is being placed (e.g. polydioxanone for gastrostomy tube; nylon for anus).

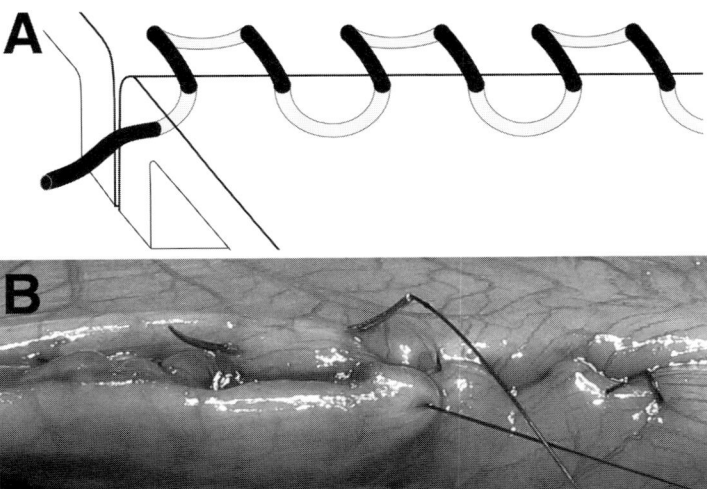

Fig. 4.20. Cushing suture pattern: start and finish the suture pattern in the same manner as a simple continuous suture. (A) Diagram demonstrating key features: 4–8 mm bites of tissue are taken running parallel to, and placed 4 mm lateral to, the incision edge. (B) Cushing suture pattern being placed in stomach: the needle penetrates the seromuscular layers but not the lumen of the organ. The completed section of suture line causes inversion of the serosal surface creating an early serosal seal.

Roman Sandal Suture

The Roman sandal suture is used to secure drains and other tubes to the body (Fig. 4.22). Use suture materials and sizes suitable for skin closure in the patient in which the tube is being placed. Adjust the size of suture material to the tube to avoid occluding the tube.

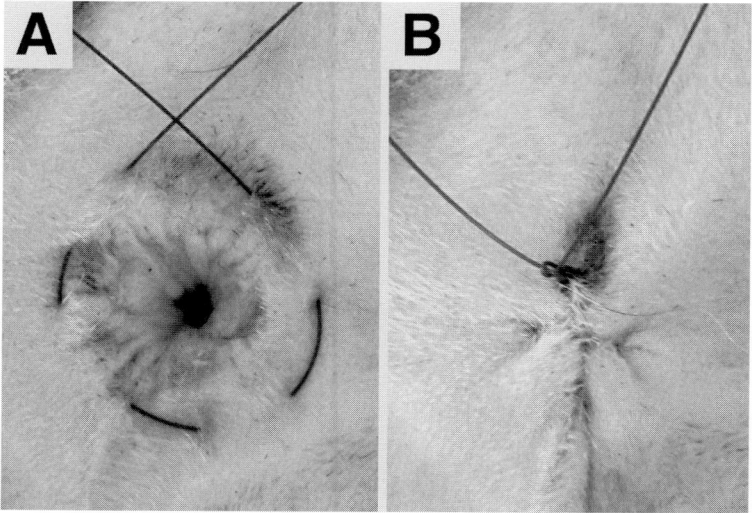

Fig. 4.21. Purse-string suture around the anus: (A) before tying; (B) after tying. Empty the anal sacs first and avoid the anal sac ducts when placing the suture.

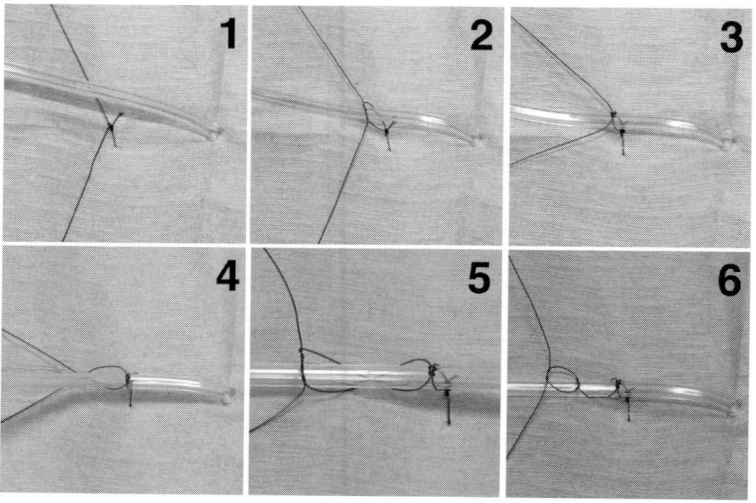

Fig. 4.22. Roman sandal suture: (1) anchor the middle of the length of suture to the skin close to the tube exit site using a square knot to generate two equal lengths of suture; (2) encircle the tube with the suture ends; (3) tie a surgeon's throw and tighten it snugly on to the tube; tie a single throw to anchor the first throw; (4) wrap the suture ends in opposite directions around the tube so that they cross underneath the tube; (5 and 6) bring the suture ends up and repeat steps 3 to 6 four or five times; (7 and 8) to finish the suture pattern, pass the suture ends to the underside of the tube and tie a secure square knot; (9+10) the completed suture. *Figure continued on page 53.*

Chapter 4

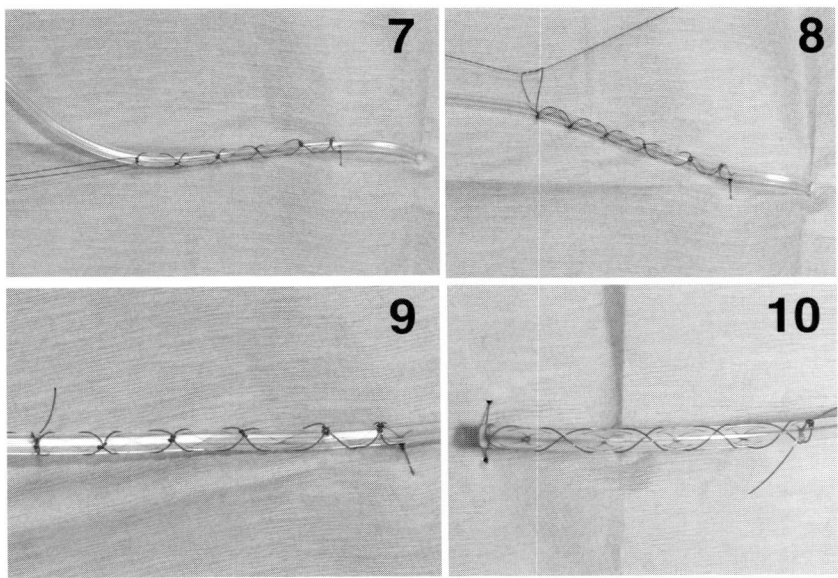

Fig. 4.22. Continued.

Bibliography

Adams, B., Anwar, J., Wrone, D.A. and Alam, M. (2003) Techniques for cutaneous sutured closures: variants and indications. *Seminars in Cutaneous Medicine and Surgery* 22, 306–316.

Annunziata, C.C., Drake, D.B., Woods, J.A., Gear, A.J., Rodeheaver, G.T. and Edlich, R.F. (1997) Technical considerations in knot construction. Part I. Continuous percutaneous and dermal suture closure. *Journal of Emergency Medicine* 15, 351–356.

Babar, A.Z. (1997) Interrupted skin suturing with 'cross stitch'. *Plastic and Reconstructive Surgery* 100, 1620–1621.

Dudley, H. and Pories, W. (1982) Operative techniques. In: Dudley, H. and Pories, W. (eds) *Rob & Smith's Operative Surgery. General Principles, Breast and Extracranial Endocrines*, 4 edn. Butterworth, London, pp. 98–138.

Dunn, D.L. (2007) *Ethicon Wound Closure Manual.* Ethicon Inc., West Sommerville, New Jersey.

Edlich, R.F. and Long (III), W.B. (2008) *Surgical Knot Tying Manual.* Covidien AG, Norwalk, Connecticut.

Johnston, D.E. (1990) Tension-relieving techniques. *Veterinary Clinics of North America Small Animal Practice* 20, 67–80.

Rosin, E. and Robinson, G.M. (1989) Knot security of suture materials. *Veterinary Surgery* 18, 269–273.

Smeak, D.D. (1990) The Chinese finger trap suture technique for fastening tubes and catheters. *Journal of the American Animal Hospital Association* 26, 215–218.

Smeak, D.D. (1992) Buried continuous intradermal suture closure. *Compendium of Continuing Education for the Practicing Veterinarian* 14, 907–919.

Toombs, J.P. and Clarke, K.M. (2003) Basic operative techniques. In: Slatter, D.H. (ed.) *Textbook in Small Animal Surgery*, 3rd edn. Saunders, Philadelphia, Pennsylvania, pp. 199–222.

5 Surgical Instruments

curette: an instrument used to debride the surface of tissue
forceps: an instrument for holding tissues (*plural form also forceps*)
haemostat: a forceps that causes haemostasis by crushing vessels
hand-held instrument: an instrument that has to be held in place
needle holder: an instrument for holding a needle
retractor: an instrument used to retract tissue
rongeur: an instrument used to detach small fragments of bone through a nibbling action
self-retaining instrument: an instrument that does not have to be held in place

The reader should be able to:

- list the components of a generic ratcheted instrument
- explain the advantages of instruments with tungsten carbide inserts over instruments without
- compare the properties of the various thumb forceps described in this chapter
- compare the properties of the various tissue forceps described in this chapter
- compare the properties of the various haemostatic forceps described in this chapter
- compare the properties of the various retractors described in this chapter
- list and contrast the different methods of cutting tissues described in this chapter
- derive a list of surgical instruments required to perform elective ovariohysterectomy in a bitch and justify their inclusion (assuming a detailed knowledge of that procedure obtained from Chapters 10 and 14)

The best results are achieved when the appropriate instrument is used for each specific task during surgery. This chapter overviews the common instruments used for general surgery. Towel clips and diathermy units are discussed in Chapter 1.

General Features of Instruments

Most surgical instruments are made of strong, high-quality, stainless steel. This has high levels of chromium that oxidizes to form *chromium oxide* in the surface layers. Chromium oxide is stain and corrosion resistant. It gives the steel its stainless properties and extends the life of the instrument. Some high-quality instruments also have *tungsten carbide*

inserts to provide the cutting or grasping surfaces (Fig. 5.1). Tungsten carbide is much harder than steel so the inserts do not blunt or wear down as quickly, and they extend the life of the instrument.

Instruments may be colour coded to give an indication of quality. The handles of instruments may be plain, gold, or black to indicate increasing quality. *Gold-handled* instruments often have tungsten carbide inserts but the colour coding is not synonymous with this and simply reflects the quality of the instrument. *Black-handled* ('*super cut*') instruments are of the highest quality. They have at least one precision-engineered, very sharp blade and are generally reserved for specialist applications such as vascular surgery. In general practice, a mixture

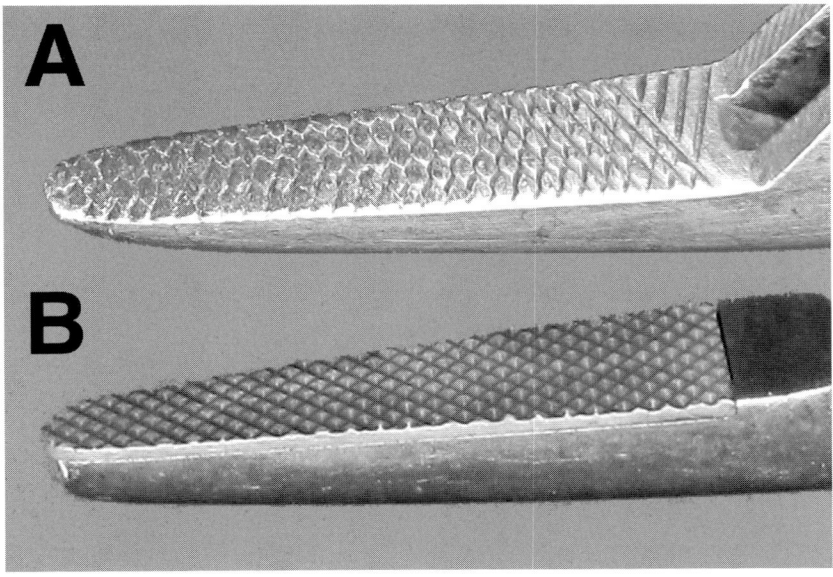

Fig. 5.1. Tungsten carbide inserts: (A) normal needle holder jaw with gripping surface engraved directly onto the stee jaw; (B) higher quality needle holder with gripping surface provided by hard-wearing tungsten carbide insert.

of plain and gold-handled instruments is more than adequate. Investing in some instruments with tungsten carbide cutting or grasping surfaces (e.g. needle holders; Metzenbaum dissecting scissors) is worth considering.

Scissors and ratcheted instruments are not designed for ambidextrous use. It is very difficult to open ratchets and to effectively cut using right-handed instruments in a left-handed grip, so it is worth investing in left-handed instruments if they are required.

Needle Holders

Ring-handled needle holders with locking ratchets are versatile and suitable for all general surgical applications (Fig. 5.2). Ring-handled instruments are held in the tripod grip that enables fine control (Fig. 5.3). The locking ratchet mechanism enables the needle to be gripped firmly to prevent it swivelling, so all of the surgeon's efforts can be concentrated on controlling the movement of the needle through tissues. The instruments are designed to hold curved needles that should be held between the midpoint and a third of the way from the suture end. To prevent blunting, avoid holding the tip of the needle.

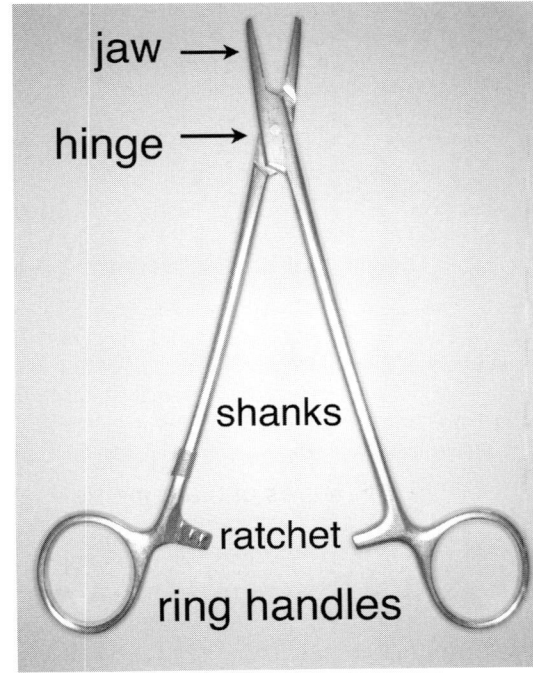

Fig. 5.2. Features of ring-handled ratcheted instruments.

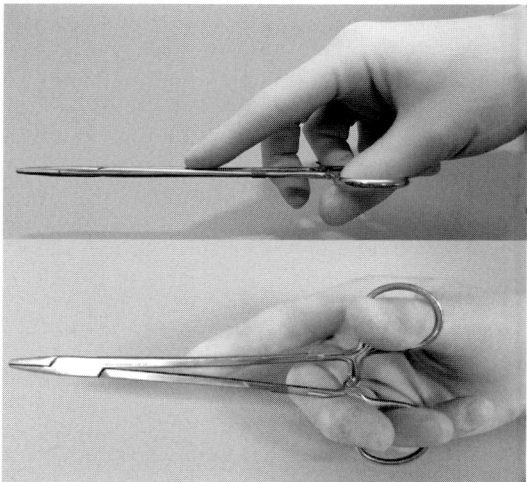

Fig. 5.3. Tripod grip: the thumb and third finger are inserted into the ring-handles, the index finger is extended along the shank to steady it, and the ratchet is closed to engage the first or second tooth. Note that the thumb and third finger are inserted to the most distal joint to improve control. This grip gives maximal control of the instrument enabling the jaws to be moved through a range of fine movements. The ratchet mechanism improves control as power is not required to hold the jaws closed.

Mayo-Hegar needle holder

The Mayo-Hegar needle holder is a versatile needle holder suitable for all general practice applications. It has crosshatched striations on the jaws to secure the needle, and a robust box hinge (Fig. 5.4).

Olsen-Hegar needle holder

The Olsen-Hegar needle holder is very similar to the Mayo-Hegar needle holder but has cutting blades incorporated behind the jaws, and a lap joint (Fig. 5.4). Some surgeons prefer this needle holder as sutures can be cut without changing instruments, but it is also easy to inadvertently cut the suture as the knot is being tied.

Gillie needle holder

Gillie needle holders have been used traditionally in veterinary surgery but are less versatile than the Mayo-Hegar needle holders. They are held in a modified tripod grip and, as there is no locking ratchet, they require constant effort to keep the

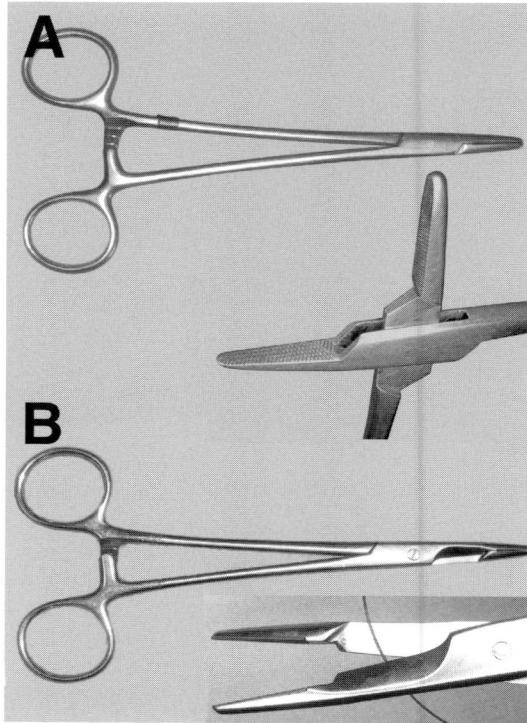

Fig. 5.4. Needle holders: (A) Mayo-Hegar; (B) Olsen-Hegar incorporating cutting blades behind the jaws for suture cutting. Fig. 5.1 illustrates the gripping surface of the jaws of these needle holders.

jaws clamped firmly on the needle. They are more difficult to control than the Mayo-Hegar needle holders but they do incorporate suture-cutting blades behind the jaw tips (Fig. 5.5). Mayo-Hegar or Olsen-Hegar needle holders should be used in preference.

Scalpels

Disposable scalpel blades are very sharp and inexpensive. They cause less tissue trauma than scissors and should be used to make all skin incisions and to incise into deeper tissues whenever possible. The blades should be replaced if they become blunt during surgery.

Scalpel blades are supplied either preloaded onto disposable handles or as individual blades for loading onto reusable metal handles. Preloaded disposable scalpels are safer as they avoid the risks of injury when scalpel blades are being loaded onto, or removed from, reusable handles. However, they are more expensive. When loading or removing blades from a scalpel handle, always work with the scalpel facing away from you and hold the blade with a needle holder to prevent injury to your hands (Fig. 5.6).

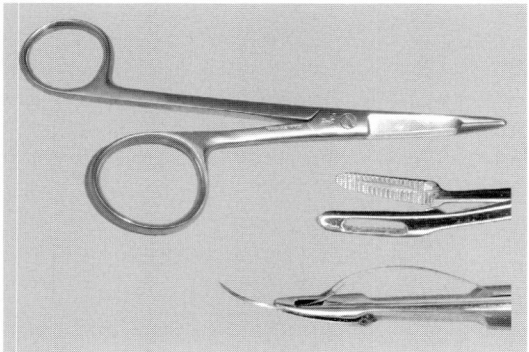

Fig. 5.5. Gillie needle holder. Insets show unusual jaw conformation that enables forward loading of needles. This feature is largely redundant and this needle holder has been superseded by the ratcheted needle holders.

There is a wide range of scalpel blades and scalpel handles. However, for general surgery in dogs and cats, blades no. 10, no. 11, and no. 15 (fitting onto a no. 3 scalpel handle) cover most surgical applications (Fig. 5.7). The no. 10 blade is a good choice for general use. It has a long, curved cutting edge along the bottom that is good for making long incisions using the palm grip (most incisions will be made using this grip). It also has a sharp cutting point at the front enabling it to be used to make short, fine incisions using the pencil grip (Fig. 5.6). The no. 15 blade has similar features to the no. 10 blade but has a scaled-down and modified cutting edge. It can be used in similar fashions to the no. 10 blade and is used when making smaller incisions through thin tissue (e.g. skin incision in puppies and small cats). The no. 11 blade ('dagger point' blade) is designed for making stab incisions held in the pencil grip and is used to make the initial incision into hollow organs (e.g. enterotomy).

Scissors

Surgical scissors are used predominantly for *sharp dissection* but the tips of smaller scissors may also

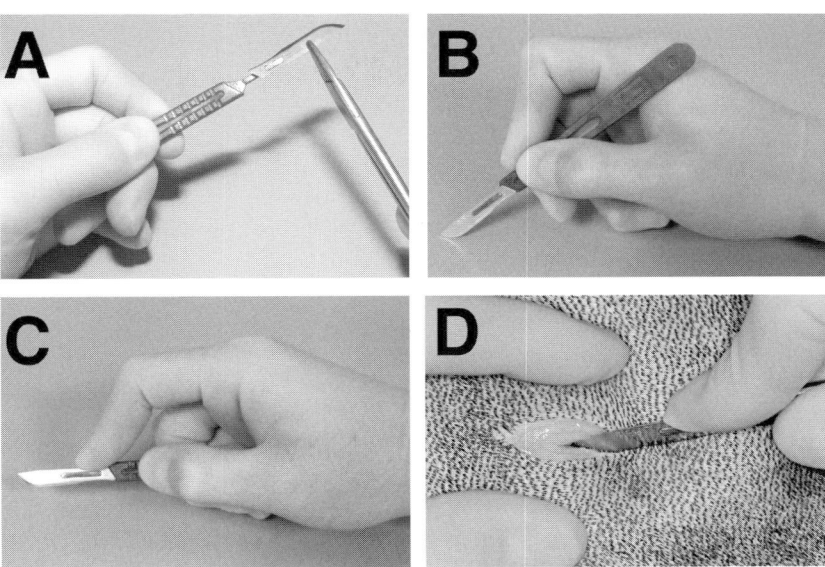

Fig. 5.6. Handling the scalpel and scalpel blade: (A) use a needle holder to attach and remove disposable scalpel blades; (B) the 'pencil grip' is suitable for making short incisions (<1 cm) with the tip of the blade; (C) the 'palm grip' is used most and is suitable for making long incisions with the curved portion of the blade. The scalpel handle is held in the palm of the hand and the index finger is used to apply pressure directly to the blade; (D) use your non-dominant hand to stretch the skin taut as you incise, to give a more controlled incision.

be used for *blunt dissection* (Fig. 5.8). When used for sharp dissection, scissors tend to cause more crush injury than a sharp scalpel blade, but they are easily controlled.

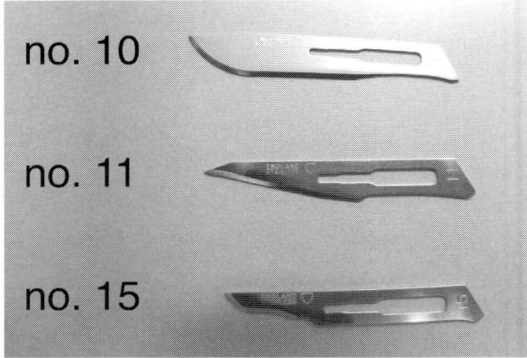

Fig. 5.7. Disposable scalpel blades used commonly in small animal practice.

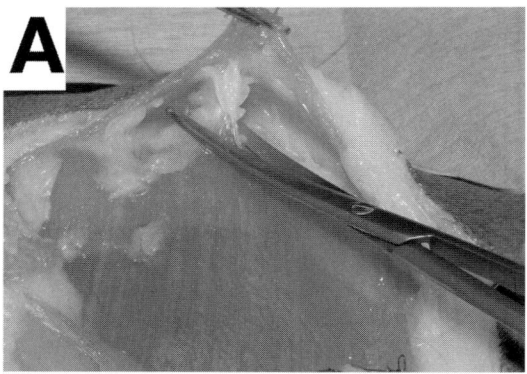

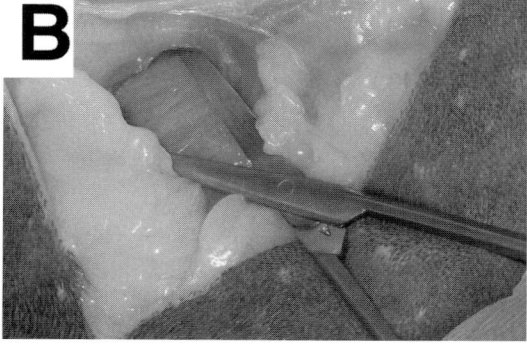

Fig. 5.8. Dissection using Metzenbaum scissors: (A) sharp dissection – cutting loose fascia; (B) blunt dissection – separating between fascial planes (also known as 'undermining').

Blunt dissection is used to separate fascial planes. Insert the scissor blades in the closed position into the natural dissection plane between adjacent tissues. Open the blades parallel to the plane of dissection, bluntly pushing the tissues apart and generating dead space (Fig. 5.8). Blunt dissection is useful for quickly dissecting between natural cleavage planes in tissues but is over-used. It generates more dead space than sharp dissection and causes more tissue trauma.

Scissors may have straight or curved blades. The curved blades are more versatile as they facilitate blunt dissection and perform well for sharp dissection. The blades require periodic sharpening, and fine dissection scissors should not be used to cut thick fascia or sutures (which causes them to blunt quickly).

Mayo dissecting scissors

Mayo scissors are heavy-duty scissors designed for cutting through thick fascia (e.g. linea alba; tensor fascia lata) (Fig. 5.9). They are not suitable for fine sharp or blunt dissection as they cause too much trauma. Mayo scissors are also used to cut sutures.

Metzenbaum scissors

Metzenbaum scissors are fine dissecting scissors designed primarily for fine, sharp dissection. They can also be used for fine blunt dissection (Fig. 5.9). They are sharper than Mayo scissors, have smaller blades, and cause less tissue trauma when used for sharp or blunt dissection. They are designed to cut light fascial planes (e.g. subcutaneous fat) and blunt quickly when used to cut heavy fascia (e.g. linea alba) or suture material.

Other scissors

Using a combination of Mayo and Metzenbaum scissors meets most requirements of general surgery. Other scissors may be used for specialist applications. For example, *iris scissors* are ophthalmic scissors designed for fine, sharp dissection. They are more robust than Metzenbaum scissors and can cut denser fascia and sutures. They are used for fine sharp dissection of dense tissue (e.g. thyroid capsule during thyroidectomy) (Fig. 5.9).

Dissecting ('Thumb') Forceps

Thumb forceps are sprung forceps with a tweezer action. They are the main instruments used for tissue

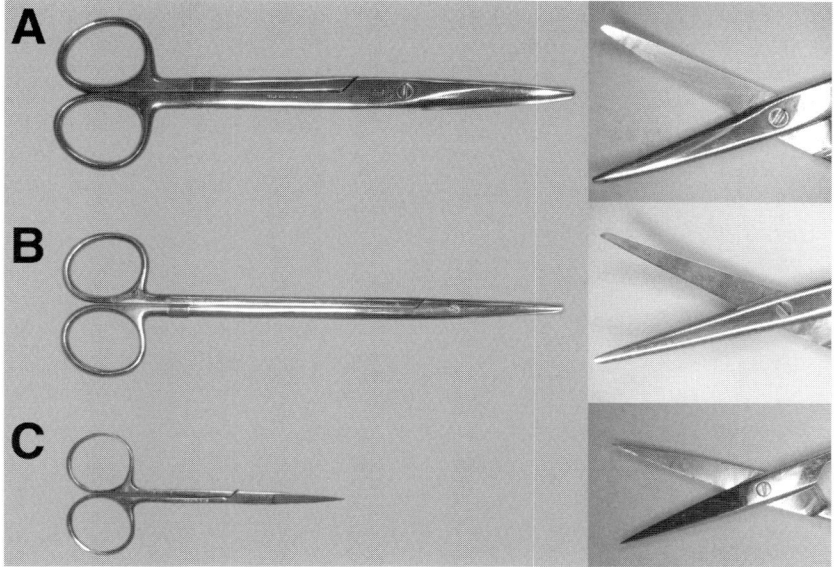

Fig. 5.9. Scissors: (A) Mayo; (B) Metzenbaum; (C) iris.

manipulation and should be selected carefully to avoid unnecessary tissue trauma. Thumb forceps should be held in the pencil grip. Some thumb forceps have sharp teeth that enable them to grip heavy or dense tissue without having to use excessive force, which prevents tissue crushing. However, these are classed as traumatic forceps as they puncture the tissues and they cannot be used to handle hollow organs or vessels. Atraumatic thumb forceps have tips with blunt ridges that are suitable for holding hollow organs without puncturing them.

Rat-toothed thumb forceps

Rat-toothed forceps have sharp teeth that interdigitate at the tips. They have two teeth on one jaw and one tooth on the other (Fig. 5.10). These are versatile forceps that are used extensively in small animal surgery. They are robust enough to hold heavy or fibrous tissues and their teeth enable tissues to be held firmly without causing excessive crushing. However, they should not be used to hold hollow organs or vessels.

DeBakey tissue forceps

DeBakey tissue forceps are suitable for holding delicate tissues (e.g. vessels), hollow organs (e.g. gastrointestinal tract; bladder), and subcutaneous fat.

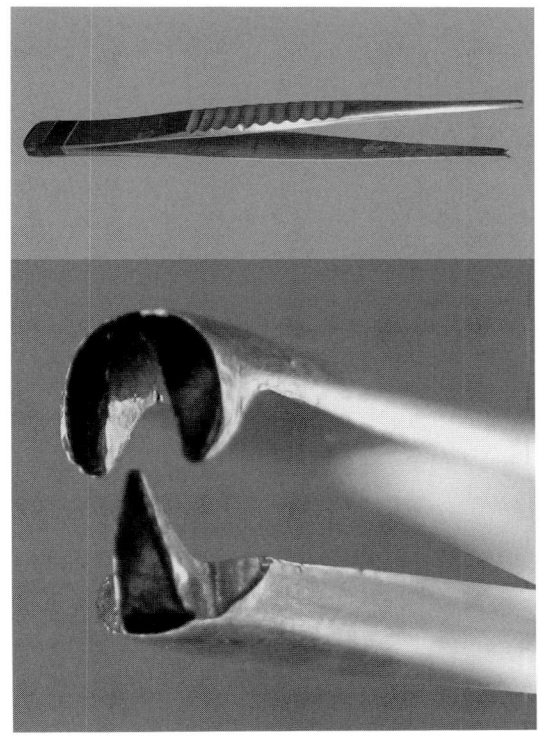

Fig. 5.10. Rat-toothed thumb forceps.

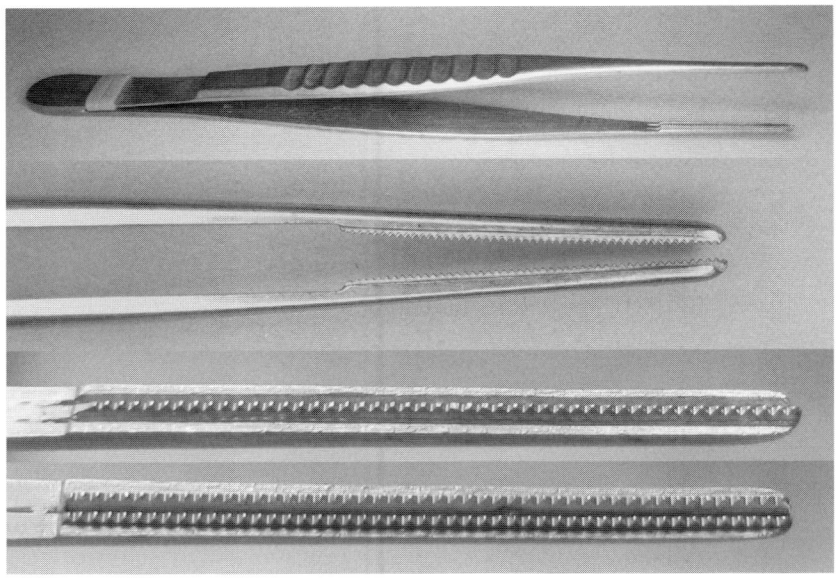

Fig. 5.11. DeBakey tissue forceps.

These are classed as atraumatic thumb forceps. The grasping surfaces of the jaws have longitudinal, raised ridges (one on one jaw; two on the other jaw) with shallow, transverse grooves cut into their surfaces (Fig. 5.11). The grooved ridges give more traction when holding tissue, enabling light tissues to be held securely without causing crushing. These forceps have a better grip than plain forceps and can also be used to hold hollow organs without puncturing them. However, they are too delicate to be used to handle skin or heavy fascia (e.g. linea alba).

Brown-Adson thumb forceps

Brown-Adson thumb forceps have two rows of fine interdigitate teeth on each jaw (Fig. 5.12). They are designed for holding fibrous tissue with a delicate grip that minimizes crush injury and are ideal for holding skin. These forceps are too delicate to hold heavy fibrous tissues (e.g. linea alba) and will puncture hollow organs.

Plain thumb forceps

Plain thumb forceps ('*dressing forceps*') (Fig. 5.13) are designed for holding dressing materials and do not have any teeth or grooved ridges that might shred dressing material. This gives them a poor grip on tissue. They are often used to hold hollow organs

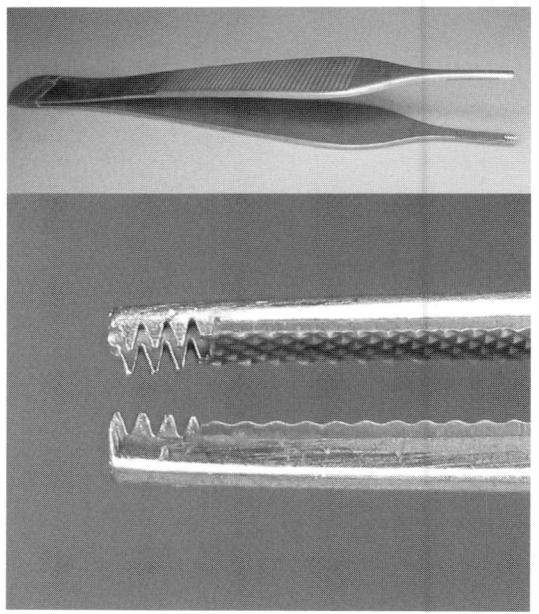

Fig. 5.12. Brown-Adson forceps.

when more appropriate forceps (e.g. DeBakey forceps) are not available, as they do not puncture the tissue. However, to hold tissues with plain forceps requires that excessive pressure be placed across the tips. This causes more crushing injury than is caused by other instruments such as the DeBakey forceps.

Haemostatic Forceps

Haemostatic forceps are used primarily for haemostasis, and fine haemostats may also be used for blunt dissection. The jaws are either curved or straight and have transverse ridges that crush and irreversibly

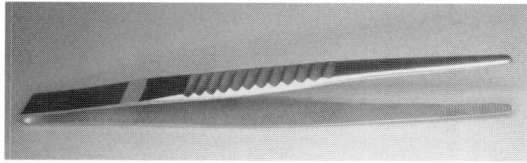

Fig. 5.13. Plain dressing forceps.

damage tissue. The forceps should only be applied to tissues that are not being preserved. Three sizes are used regularly in general surgery (Fig. 5.14).

Halsted mosquito forceps

The Halsted mosquito forceps is the smallest forceps used in general surgery (Fig. 5.14). It has fine jaws for pinpoint haemostasis of arterioles, venules, and capillaries. It is often used for fine, blunt dissection although the edge of the transverse ridges along its jaws may traumatize tissue.

Crile haemostatic forceps

The Crile haemostatic forceps is a medium-sized forceps for use on small arteries and veins and small vascular pedicles (e.g. feline ovarian pedicle; hilar

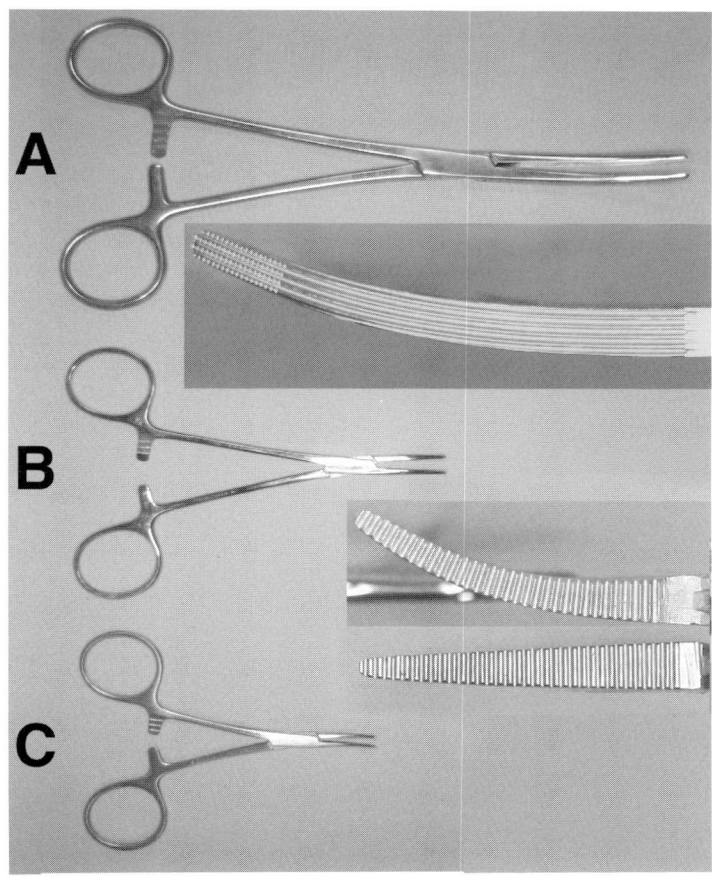

Fig. 5.14. Haemostatic forceps: (A) Rochester-Carmalt forceps – longitudinal ridges with checked pattern at tips; (B) Crile forceps – transverse ridges; (C) Halsted mosquito forceps.

splenic vessel; subcutaneous capillary). It has transverse ridges running the entire length of jaws (Fig. 5.14). The Kelly haemostatic forceps is similar but only has ridges extending halfway along the jaw. As the entire jaw of the Crile forceps can be used for haemostasis, it is preferred by many surgeons.

Large haemostatic forceps

Large haemostatic forceps are for crushing large vascular pedicles prior to ligature application (e.g. Rochester-Carmalt; Rochester-Péan; Kocher) (Fig. 5.14). The main application of these in small animal surgery is for crushing the canine ovarian pedicle during ovariohysterectomy, and these forceps are often referred to as 'bitch spay forceps'.

Other Tissue Forceps

Doyen intestinal forceps

Doyen intestinal forceps (Fig. 5.15) are used for occluding the intestine to prevent leakage during intestinal surgery. They have long, springy blades and a locking ratchet. They are used in pairs to isolate a section of intestine. The blades compress the intestine and occlude its lumen, preventing intestinal contents from leaking into the surgical site, without crushing the tissues.

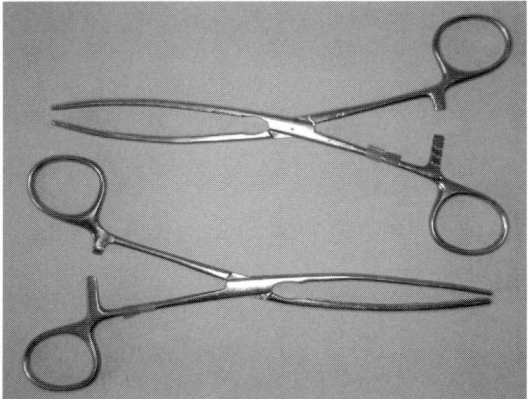

Fig. 5.15. Doyen intestinal forceps: used for atraumatic occlusion of the intestinal tract. These are often used with rubber sleeves placed over the jaws to provide further protection against iatrogenic injury, although many can be used without rubber sleeves.

Babcock forceps

Babcock forceps (or Babcock intestinal forceps) (Fig. 5.16) were designed to hold human bowel without causing trauma. The forceps have springy shafts and relatively atraumatic jaws with longitudinal ridges to improve tissue grip. In dogs and cats, they can be used to hold the stomach (e.g. during gastrotomy) but are used mostly to hold and retract soft tissue during general surgery as they cause minimal trauma.

Allis tissue forceps

Allis tissue forceps (Fig. 5.16) look similar to Babcock forceps but have sharp-toothed jaws and rigid shafts. Allis tissue forceps cause irreversible crushing and penetrating injuries to tissues and should not be used to hold tissue unless the tissue is being excised. They are often used to manipulate tissue as it is being removed from the body and may also be used to anchor cables and suction tubing to drapes.

Hand-Held Retractors

Hand-held retractors are used to expose tissues during surgery but a surgical assistant must be available to hold the retractor.

Langenbeck retractor

The Langenbeck retractor is a versatile instrument. It has a broad blade set perpendicular to the handle that is used to pull soft tissues away from the surgical field. Langenbeck retractors are generally used in pairs to hold wound edges apart, facilitating exposure (Fig. 5.17).

Hohmann retractor

The Hohmann retractor is designed for holding muscles away from bone during orthopaedic surgery. It has a wide blade that is used to push muscle away from tissue and a short beak at the tip of the blade that is hooked behind bone to act as a point of leverage (Fig. 5.17).

Self-Retaining Retractors

A self-retaining retractor has a ratchet mechanism that locks the retractor in position enabling it to be used without an assistant. There are numerous self-retaining retractors but examples of those used commonly in

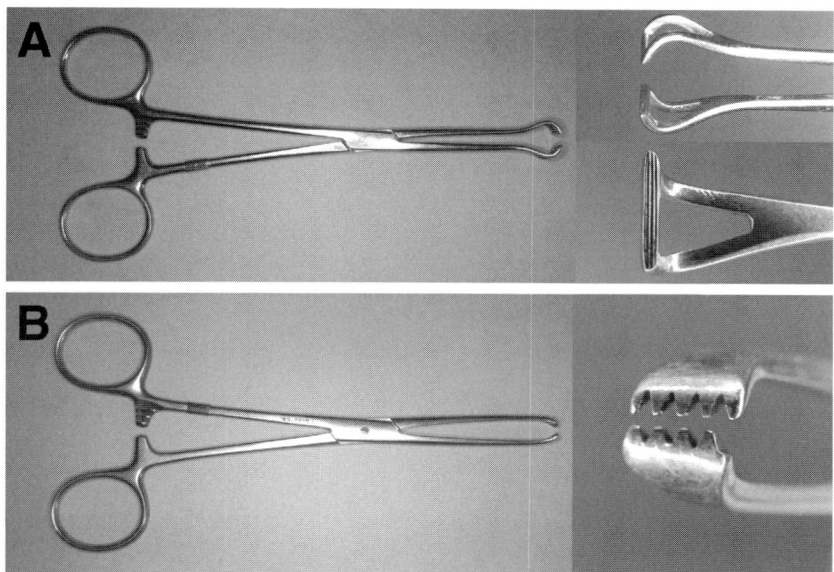

Fig. 5.16. (A) Babcock forceps; (B) Allis tissue forceps.

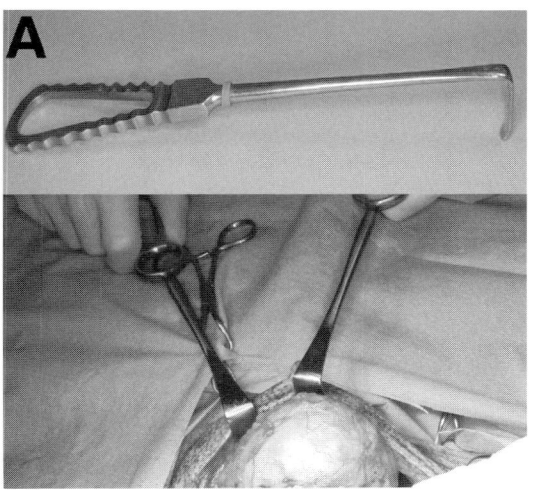

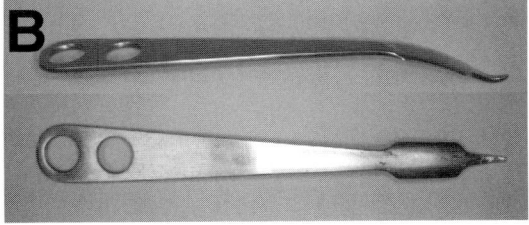

Fig. 5.17. Hand-held retractors: (A) Langenbeck;
(B) Hohmann.

veterinary surgery include the Gelpi retractor, the Gosset retractor, and the Balfour retractor.

Gelpi retractor

Gelpi retractors (Fig. 5.18), also known as Gelpi perineal retractors, are versatile retractors used to expose a variety of surgical fields. They are generally used in pairs placed perpendicular to each other to maximize exposure by holding the edges of incisions apart. The narrow, angled shafts enable these retractors to be placed in most wounds.

Abdominal retractors

Gosset and Balfour retractors are abdominal retractors that greatly facilitate abdominal surgery (Fig. 5.19). They are designed to retract the sides of the abdomen. The Gosset retractor has a pair of blades that push the sides of the abdominal incision laterally. It is available in a range of sizes for use in cats and small to medium size dogs. The Balfour retractor is similar to the Gosset retractor but also has a central spoon. The spoon is designed to fit under the xiphisternum and pull it forward, improving exposure to the cranial abdomen. The Balfour retractor also comes in a range

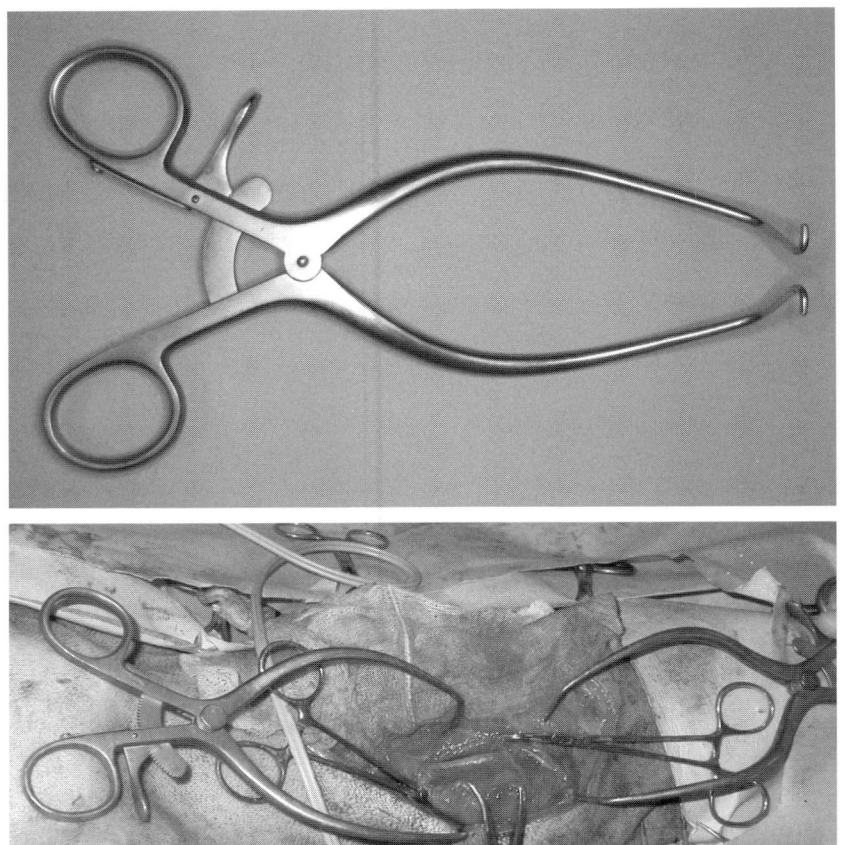

Fig. 5.18. Gelpi retractors.

of sizes suitable for use in medium and large breed dogs. These retractors are essential equipment to perform effective exploratory abdominal surgery, but a range of sizes is required to fit the variety of patients seen in general practice (see Chapter 11 for their use).

Rongeurs and Curettes

Rongeurs are designed for cutting away small pieces of bone in a nibbling action. They have sharp cutting jaws and long handles to give good leverage (Fig. 5.20). Rongeurs are used mainly for removing or reshaping small areas of bone in orthopaedic surgery.

Curettes are designed for debriding soft tissue and cancellous bone away from cortical bone (Fig. 5.20). They may also be used for debriding the lining of fibrous tracts (e.g. during surgery for cervical abscesses associated with penetrating pharyngeal stick injuries, see p. 332)

Suction Units

Suction units are very useful for removing blood and lavage fluid from wounds and the abdomen. Units may be electric or run off a piped gas supply. Different suction tips have different applications.

The *Poole* tip is designed for removing large volumes of fluid from the abdominal cavity. It has a central suction rod with an outer, removable fenestrated sleeve (Fig. 5.21). The fenestrated sleeve prevents abdominal organs such as the omentum from being sucked into the apparatus.

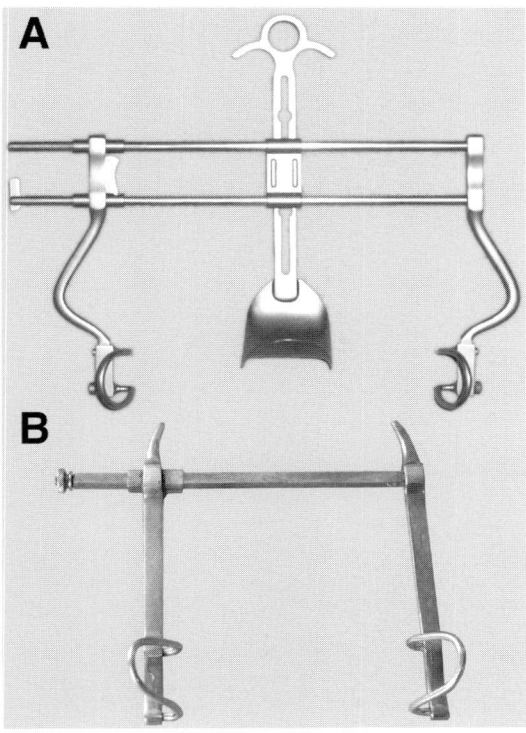

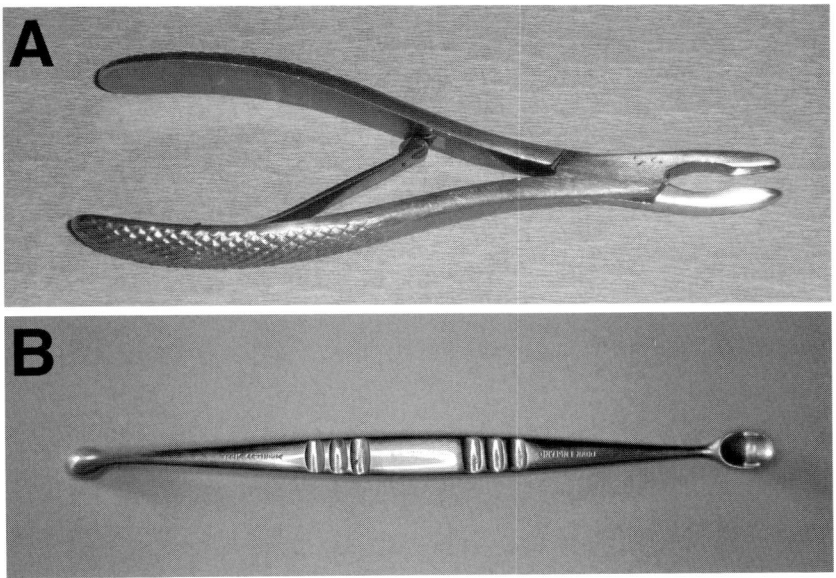

Fig. 5.19. Abdominal retractors: (A) Balfour; (B) Gosset.

The *Yankauer* and *Frazier* tips are general-purpose suction tips that do not have a protective outer sleeve (Fig. 5.21). The Yankauer tip is a large-bore tube that allows large volumes of fluid and viscous fluid to be removed rapidly. The Frazier tip is a fine suction tip for removing smaller volumes of blood or fluid from wound cavities.

Suction tips often incorporate a decompression hole into the handle. For maximum suction, the decompression hole is blocked with a thumb. To rapidly drop the suction pressure, the decompression hole is uncovered. This feature enables tissues that get sucked into the apparatus to be released rapidly and helps control the level of suction.

Swabs

Swabs are used to remove blood, fluid, and detritus from the surgical site. They are placed over the wound to prevent desiccation and contamination. They are used to isolate hollow organs before they are incised to prevent contamination of surrounding tissues. Most surgical swabs are made from absorbent cotton. Surgical swabs should not shed lint and should contain a radiographic marker to enable them to be identified post-operatively if they are left in tissues.

Fig. 5.20. (A) Lempert rongeur; (B) curette.

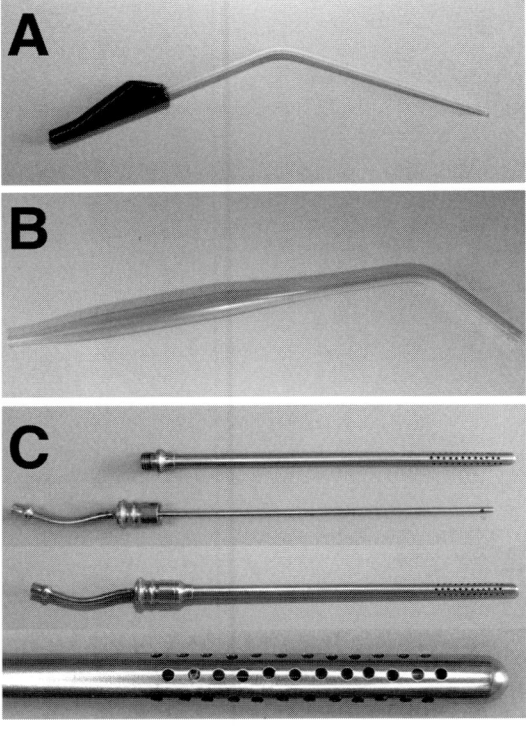

Fig. 5.21. (A) Frazier suction tip; (B) Yankauer suction tip; (C) Poole suction tip assembled and separated into central suction tube and outer fenestrated sheath (magnified view of fenestrated sheath).

Bibliography

Caw (College of Animal Welfare) (1997) *Veterinary Surgical Instruments: An Illustrated Guide*, 1st edn. Butterworth-Heinemann, Oxford, UK.

Fossum, T.W. (2007) Surgery instrumentation. In: Fossum, T.W. (ed.) *Small Animal Surgery*, 3rd edn. Mosby Elsevier, St. Louis, Missouri, pp. 47–56.

Hamilton, M.H. (2004) Dealing with fluids – swabs and suction. *UK Vet* 9, 27–35.

Kapczynski, H. (1997) *Surgical Instruments 101: An Introduction to KMedic Certified Instruments*. KMedic, Northvale, New Jersey.

Nieves, M.A. and Wagner, S.D. (2003) Surgical instruments. In: Slatter, D.H. (ed.) *Textbook in Small Animal Surgery*, 3rd edn. Saunders, Philadelphia, Pennsylvania, pp. 185–198.

Rutherford, C. (2005) *Differentiating Surgical Instruments*, 1st edn. F.A. Davis Co., Philadelphia, Pennsylvania.

6 Nutritional Support

aerophagia: swallowing of air leading to gastric dilatation

enteral nutrition: provision of nutrients into the digestive tract

Fr: abbreviation for 'French gauge' – a scale for measuring tube diameter that increases in increments of one-third of a millimetre (3 Fr = 1 mm; 6 Fr = 2 mm). This is sometimes referred to as the Charriere scale (1 Ch is equal to 1 Fr).

gastrostomy tube: tube inserted into the stomach through the abdominal wall

naso-oesophageal tube: tube inserted through the nose into the oesophagus

oesophagostomy tube: tube inserted into the oesophagus through the neck

parenteral nutrition: provision of nutrients intravenously

pexy: permanent fixation of an organ to the abdominal wall

The reader should be able to:

- compare the different types of nutritional support, their advantages and disadvantages, and the indications, contraindications, and complications of their use
- perform naso-oesophageal and oesophagostomy tube placement under the supervision of a qualified veterinary surgeon
- describe placement of a gastrostomy tube
- perform checks to ensure that a naso-oesophageal, oesophagostomy or gastrostomy tube is properly positioned and working
- formulate an appropriate plan for providing nutritional support to a patient taking into account its specific problems and requirements
- employ the calculations and information provided in the text to generate and implement a feeding plan for an individual patient

---

Veterinary patients are often unable or unwilling to eat. This may be because of alimentary tract disease (e.g. fractured jaw; oesophagitis) or systemic disease causing nausea and inappetence (e.g. renal failure). Other less obvious factors may also lead to inappetence, such as post-operative pain or stress during hospitalization. Inadequate nutrition has many negative effects. Animals with low calorie or protein intake enter a catabolic state that can lead to impaired wound healing and poor immune function. They also develop metabolic derangements such as hypokalaemia that can lead to lethargy and weakness. Within the digestive tract itself, the mucosal lining relies heavily on the direct nutrition supplied by the intestinal contents, and lack of feeding leads to villous atrophy and reduced intestinal immune responses. Part of the general healthcare of patients should include close attention to ensure that their nutritional needs are met to avoid these problems.

The importance of nutritional support for inappetent veterinary patients has become widely accepted but it can be difficult to decide which patients require it and when it should be started. Preferably, nutritional support should be started before the patient becomes debilitated. It should be considered for any patient that is inappetent for more than two or three days. Pre-emptive placement of a feeding tube should be considered for a patient that is likely to become inappetent during treatment (e.g. at the onset of treatment for a cat that is known to become inappetent during hospitalization).

Providing Nutritional Support

Methods of nutritional support range from encouraging normal intake of food (e.g. offering highly palatable food; warming food to body temperature; hand-feeding; using appetite stimulants) to provision of nutrients directly into the bloodstream (parenteral nutrition). The simpler methods that closely match normal eating are preferred over more complex techniques that bypass the normal digestive or absorptive mechanisms. This is because the simpler methods are easier to implement, have fewer complications, are most likely to meet the physiological needs of the patient, and are least expensive. In general practice, naso-oesophageal, oesophagostomy, and gastrostomy tubes provide versatility to manage most patients that require nutritional support.

It is important to identify what factors prevent the patient from eating normally and to select a method of feeding that overcomes these. For example, a patient with a fractured jaw will not maintain adequate food intake by mouth and placing a feeding tube that bypasses the oral cavity (such as an oesophagostomy tube) would be appropriate. In contrast, naso-oesophageal, oesophagostomy, and gastrostomy tubes are not suitable for an animal that has a large gastric tumour as none will bypass the problem.

Naso-oesophageal tube placement

The naso-oesophageal tube is a tube that is inserted through the nostril and passed into the distal oesophagus. Food is delivered into the distal oesophagus from where it quickly moves into the stomach.

Advantages

- The tube is easy to place.
- The tube can be inserted in conscious animals.

- The tube can be removed at any time without adverse consequences.
- The technique is inexpensive.

Disadvantages

- Only small-bore tubes can be used, limiting the rate and volume of food that can be fed. As a result, it is difficult to provide the full nutritional requirements of the patient.
- Tube blockage is common.
- The tube can be inhaled either during placement or if it becomes dislodged during vomiting.
- The patient may not start eating with the tube in place, making it difficult to judge when to remove the tube. This is because the tube passes through the pharynx causing irritation during swallowing.
- Premature removal by the patient is common as the tube causes nasal irritation.

Indications

- Short-term nutritional support until normal feeding is started or an alternative method of assisted feeding is provided.
- Nutritional support of patients that cannot tolerate general anaesthesia.

Contraindications

- Patients with nasal, oesophageal, or gastric lesions.
- Patients with facial trauma (e.g. fractured jaw) as these animals often have undiagnosed nasomaxillary injuries (e.g. fractured nasal turbinates).
- Patients that have uncontrolled vomiting.
- Naso-oesophageal tubes should not be placed in unconscious patients (the tube may pass into the trachea).

Technique

The naso-oesophageal tube is passed along the ventral nasal meatus, across the pharynx, and into the oesophagus. Naso-oesophageal tubes range in size from 3.5 Fr (small cats) to 12 Fr (large dogs). The tubes have blunt tips with side ports to limit trauma during insertion and capped ends to prevent aerophagia.

Position: sit the patient down and hold the head in a neutral position. The patient must be conscious and not sedated during placement.

1. **Pre-measure and mark the tube from the nares to the eighth rib** (Fig. 6.1). This ensures that the tip of the tube sits in the distal oesophagus and does not enter the stomach. If the tube passes into the stomach, the oesophageal cardia will remain open and gastric contents may reflux into the oesophagus leading to oesophagitis.

2. **Instill local anaesthetic into the nasal cavity and lubricate the tube** (Fig. 6.1). Anaesthetize the nostril using local anaesthetic spray or drops. Lubricate the tube with a water-soluble lubricant (e.g. K-Y jelly) or a local anaesthetic gel.

3. **Insert the tube into the nasal cavity to the pre-measured point.** In cats, insert the tube ventromedially through the nostril and direct it ventromedially and caudally. Push it steadily into the nasal cavity until the pre-measured point is reached. There should be no resistance to tube passage. The anatomy of the canine nostril differs to the cat and the nasal turbinates are easily traumatized. To prevent this, insert the tube into the ventromedial area of the nostril but, as soon as the tube reaches the median septum, push the rhinarium dorsally with the thumb before continuing to push the tube into the nasal cavity. This opens the ventral nasal meatus preventing nasal trauma (Fig. 6.2).

The patient may swallow and gag a little as the tip of the tube passes through the pharynx before running into the oesophagus. If the patient coughs during placement, this indicates that the tube has passed into the trachea and the tube should be removed completely before the process is repeated.

4. **Secure the tube to the patient.** Run the tube laterally under the wing of the nostril then pass it up along the dorsal aspect of the nose and between the eyes. Secure the tube using sutures or tissue adhesive to the skin of the nose. Tape the tube to an Elizabethan collar or cover it with a light neck bandage to secure it (Fig. 6.3).

5. **Check the position of the tube prior to use.** Before the tube is used for the first time, flush a small volume of radio-opaque contrast agent into it

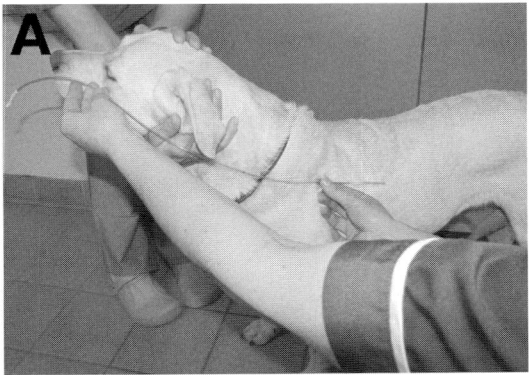

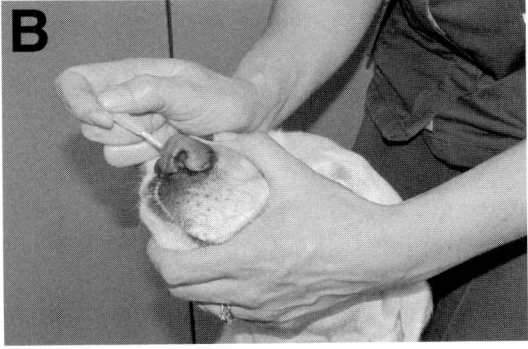

Fig. 6.1. Naso-oesophageal tube 1: (A) pre-measure tube; (B) instill local anaesthetic into nostril.

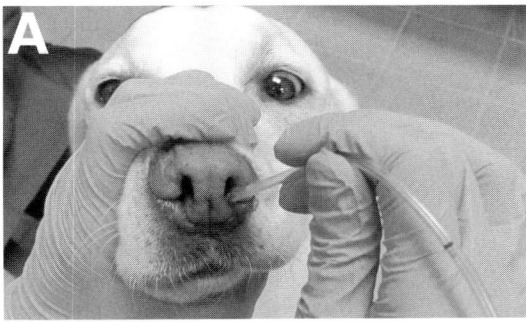

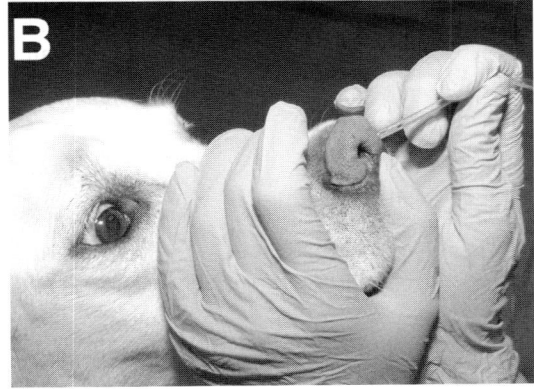

Fig. 6.2. Naso-oesophageal tube 2: (A) insert tip ventromedially into nostril; (B) push rhinarium dorsally (dogs only) and advance catheter.

and radiograph the neck and thorax. Ensure that the tube is not in the trachea and that contrast is moving rapidly from the oesophagus into the stomach (Fig. 6.3). Before each subsequent use, instill a small volume of water into the tube. If this induces coughing, assume the tube has been inhaled and do not use it.

Complications

The main problems associated with the naso-oesophageal tube are the limited volume of food that can be administered and the tendency of the tube to block. The tubes may cause discomfort and epistaxis. They may be dislodged by vomiting or may be misplaced leading to inhalation into the trachea. If this occurs and the tube is used, life-threatening aspiration pneumonia will develop. The patient may interfere with the tube and remove it prematurely.

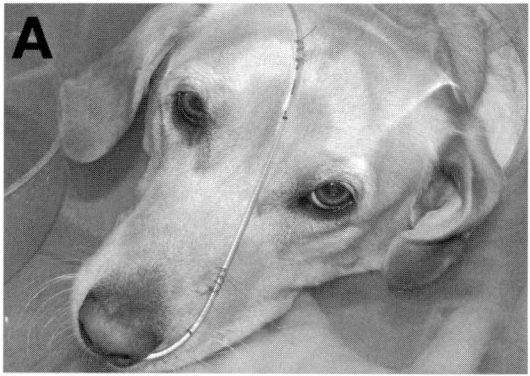

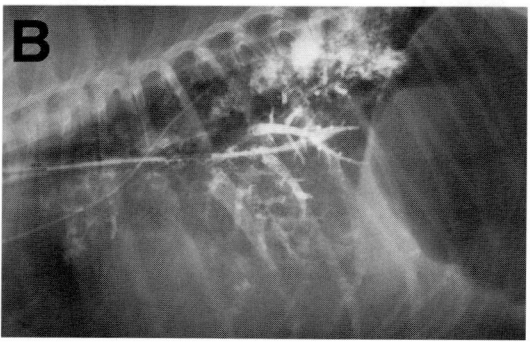

Fig. 6.3. Naso-oesophageal tube 3: (A) securing the tube; (B) example of inhaled nasogastric tube during radiographic check – contrast can be seen outlining the bronchi and alveoli.

Oesophagostomy tube placement

The oesophagostomy tube is placed into the oesophagus through a skin incision in the neck and is passed down into the terminal oesophagus. This is an extremely versatile form of feeding tube and is considered to be the first choice for most dogs and cats. The tube has the advantages over the gastrostomy tube (see below) that it is easier to place, is less invasive, and can be removed immediately without risking life-threatening complications.

Advantages

- The tube is easy to place.
- Large-bore tubes are used, enabling the full nutritional requirements to be met with bolus feeding.
- Liquidized normal diets can be fed via the tube.
- The tube is less likely to block than the naso-oesophageal tube.
- The tube can be removed at any time without adverse consequences.
- There is little risk of inhalation of the tube.
- As the tube bypasses the pharynx, it does not impede normal eating.

Disadvantages

- The patient must be anaesthetized to place the tube.
- Minor neck surgery is required to place the tube.

Indications

- Short- to long-term nutritional support of patients.

Contraindications

- Patients with oesophageal or gastric lesions.
- Patients that have uncontrolled vomiting.
- Patients that cannot tolerate general anaesthesia.
- Patients with concurrent neck injuries.

Technique

Oesophagostomy feeding tubes range in size from 12 Fr (kittens) to 24 Fr (large dogs). The tubes are long, soft, and pliable and have blunt-tipped distal ends with side ports which limit trauma during placement. The tubes have wide syringe connectors to accommodate catheter-tip syringes.

Position: Anaesthetize the patient, place it in right lateral recumbency and put a pad under its neck to elevate the mid-cervical region. Clip the left side of the neck from the midline to the cervical spine and from the angle of the jaw to the shoulder (Fig. 6.4). Prepare the site for surgery. Place a mouth gag in the right hand side. Drape the surgical site ensuring that access to the mouth is still possible. This is a contaminated procedure as the oral cavity and oesophagus are entered and breaks in aseptic technique are unavoidable.

1. **Pre-measure and mark the tube from the mid-neck to the eighth rib.** This ensures that food is delivered into the distal oesophagus and not the stomach, preventing reflux oesophagitis (Fig. 6.4).
2. **Insert a closed, long, curved haemostat through the mouth and direct it above the larynx and into the oesophagus.** The haemostat should pass easily into the oesophagus without resistance. Pass the haemostat down the oesophagus to the midpoint of the cervical oesophagus. For larger dogs, a longer forceps (e.g. Mixter forceps – long-handled, right-angled forceps) may be required.

3. **Use the tips of the haemostat to push the oesophageal wall up and tent the overlying skin in the mid-cervical region.** Raise the jugular vein to locate it and ensure that tips of the haemostat are positioned above the jugular furrow to avoid damaging the vein.
4. **Make a stab incision through the skin into the oesophageal lumen.** With the oesophagus and skin tented, use a no. 11 scalpel blade to make a stab incision through the skin onto the closed haemostat jaws. Push the haemostat tips firmly through the oesophageal wall and out of the skin incision. This ensures that a small hole in the oesophagus is made to accommodate the feeding tube and limits the risk of leakage around the tube (Fig. 6.5).
5. **Pull the distal end of the oesophageal feeding tube into the oesophagus and out through the**

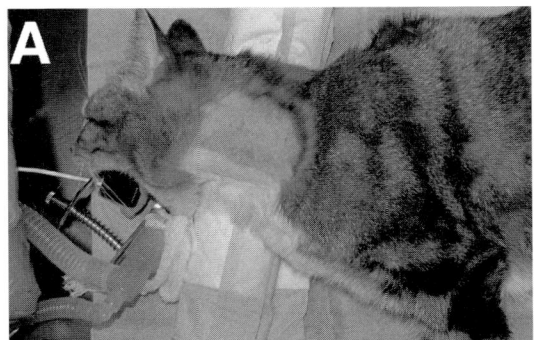

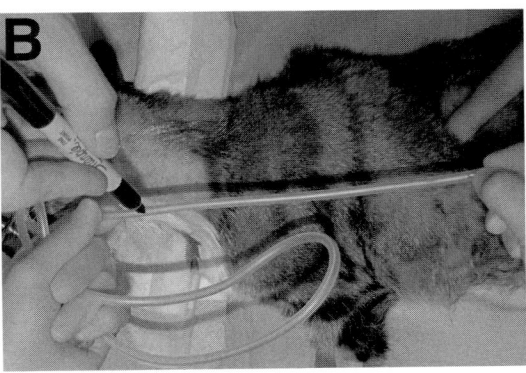

Fig. 6.4. Oesophagostomy tube 1: (A) patient positioning; (B) pre-measure the tube.

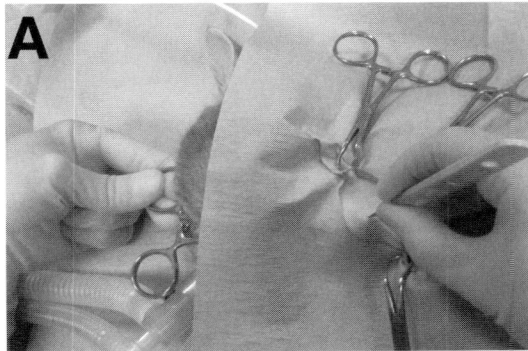

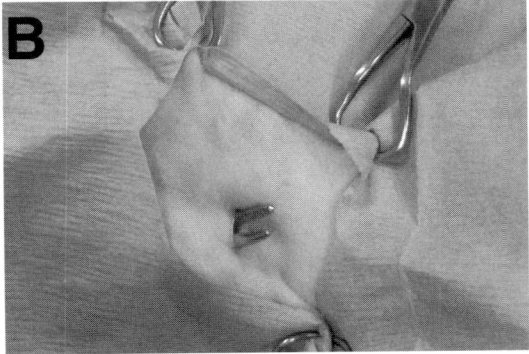

Fig. 6.5. Oesophagostomy tube 2: (A) use the haemostat to tent the oesophageal wall and overlying skin and make a stab incision; (B) push the haemostat through the wall of the oesophagus and out of the skin incision.

mouth using the haemostat. Open the jaws of the haemostat and feed the distal tip of the feeding tube into them. Firmly grasp the tube with the haemostat and pull the haemostat out of the oral cavity, dragging the distal tip of the feeding tube into the oesophagus and out of the oral cavity. Continue to pull the feeding tube into the oesophagus and out of the mouth in this manner until the pre-measured point on the tube reaches the skin (Fig. 6.6).

6. **Feed the oesophagostomy tube back into the oesophagus and down to the distal portion of the thoracic oesophagus.** Remove the haemostat from the end of the tube. Pass the tube back into the oesophagus by looping it back on itself and directing the tip dorsally above the larynx (Fig. 6.7). Continue to push the tube down the oesophagus beyond the point where it has entered until the loop in the tube untwists and all of the tube runs distally towards the stomach. Reposition the tube so that the pre-measured point on the tube sits at the skin incision site.

7. **Secure the tube to the skin using a Roman sandal suture and neck bandage** (see p. 51) (Fig. 6.7). Cover the tube exit site with a sterile dressing and secure the tube under a light bandage (Fig. 6.8). Put an Elizabethan collar on the patient.

8. **Check the position of the tube prior to use.** Radiograph the neck and thorax to check the position of the tube (Fig. 6.8). If the patient is conscious, flush a small volume of radio-opaque contrast agent into the tube to confirm that contrast rapidly enters the stomach and that the tube is not misplaced into the trachea.

Complications

The main problems associated with oesophagostomy tubes are premature removal of the tube by the patient and tube blockage. The tube may be dislodged during vomiting but is unlikely to be inhaled. Infection of the stoma may occur but subcutaneous leakage of food is very uncommon.

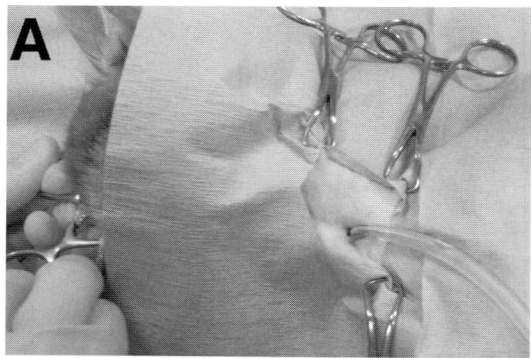

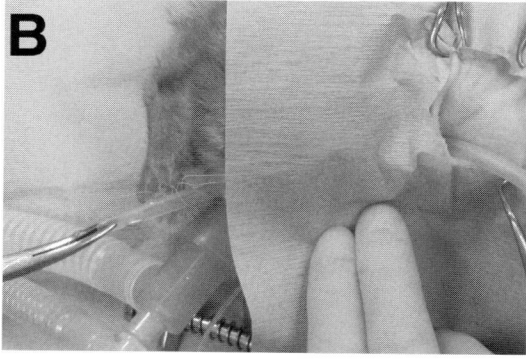

Fig. 6.6. Oesophagostomy tube 3: (A) grasp the tip of the tube in the haemostat; (B) pull the tube into the oesophagus and out of the mouth.

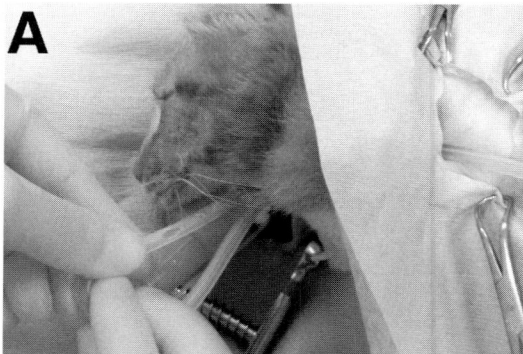

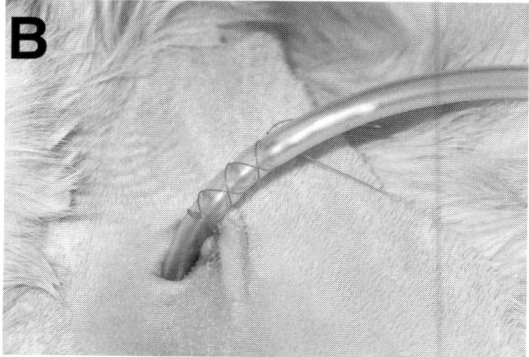

Fig. 6.7. Oesophagostomy tube 4: (A) reverse the tip of the tube and feed it back into the oesophagus to the pre-measured point; (B) secure the tube to the skin.

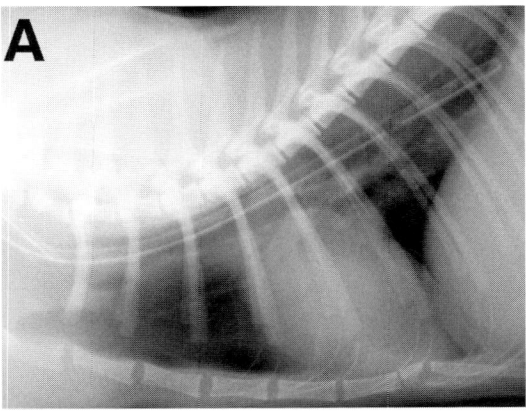

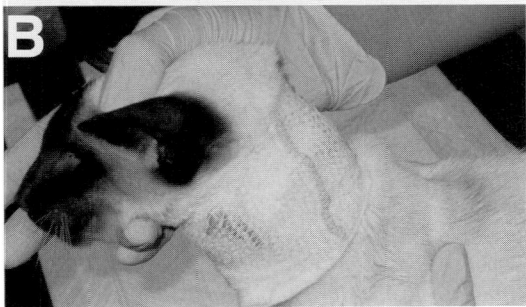

Fig. 6.8. Oesophagostomy tube 5: (A) check positioning – this tube is ideally positioned in the distal oesophagus; (B) secure tube under a neck bandage.

There is a small risk of damage to jugular vein, carotid artery, or vagosympathetic trunk.

Gastrostomy tube placement

Gastrostomy tubes are placed directly into the stomach through the abdominal wall. The tubes can be used to provide the patient's full nutritional requirements and are preferred to oesophagostomy tubes for patients with oesophageal disease. Unlike the other feeding tubes, gastrostomy tubes should not be removed in the first ten days following placement, or leakage from the stomach may cause peritonitis.

Advantages

- Large-bore tubes can be used, enabling the full nutritional requirements to be met with bolus feeding.
- Normal dog and cat food can be liquidized and fed via the tube.

- The tube is less likely to block than the naso-oesophageal tube.
- There is no risk of aspiration or respiratory obstruction.
- The tube will not interfere with normal eating.

Disadvantages

- General anaesthesia is required for placement.
- Abdominal surgery is required for placement.
- Early tube removal may lead to leakage and peritonitis.

Indications

- Medium- to long-term nutritional support of patients.
- Patients that are not candidates for oesophagostomy tube placement (e.g. patients with oesophagitis).

Contraindications

- Patients with gastric or intestinal disease.
- Patients with vomiting that cannot be suppressed.
- Patients that cannot tolerate general anaesthesia.

Technique

Special catheters, like the mushroom-tipped De Pezzer catheter, must be used. Use sizes from 14 Fr (kittens) to 24 Fr (large dogs). Balloon catheters designed for use in the urinary tract (e.g. Foley catheter) should not be used as the bulb is not designed to survive in the acidic environment of the stomach and may rupture, leading to early tube failure and peritonitis. Gastrostomy tubes are usually inserted into the left side of the stomach (fundus) as this mimics food entering the stomach from the oesophagus. Occasionally tubes are placed into the right side of the stomach (into the pylorus) for the management of gastric dilatation and volvulus (see Chapter 12) but this is not performed routinely as feeding directly into the pylorus can stimulate vomiting. The patient is anaesthetized, clipped, and prepared for abdominal surgery (see Chapter 11).

1. Make a midline coeliotomy incision from the xiphisternum to the umbilicus.
2. Select areas on the left side of the stomach and on the left body wall to insert the tube through. Select an area of the parietal surface of the stomach

midway between the greater and lesser curvatures that can easily be lifted to the left body wall behind the costal arch. Push this portion of stomach up against the peritoneal surface of the left body wall caudal to the last rib and at least 2 cm lateral to the midline. The points of contact between the stomach and the body wall are the landmarks for tube placement.

3. **Introduce the gastrostomy tube into the abdomen through the body wall.** Make a small stab incision (~0.5 cm) with a no. 11 scalpel blade through the peritoneum and abdominal muscles at the proposed tube insertion site. It is important to make a small incision to prevent herniation. Push the closed tips of a straight haemostat through the incision until the tips of the haemostat tent the skin on the other side of the abdominal wall. Make a short (<1 cm) skin incision over the tips of the haemostat and push the haemostat so that it protrudes through the skin incision. Open the haemostat and grasp the tip of the gastrostomy tube in the jaws (place the clamp across the mushroom tip of the catheter to collapse it). Use the haemostat to pull the gastrostomy tube through the abdominal wall.

4. **Place a purse-string suture at the proposed insertion site in the stomach and make a stab incision into the lumen.** Using 2-0 to 4-0 long-lasting, absorbable suture material (e.g. polydioxanone), place a purse-string suture (see p. 50) into the stomach wall at the selected insertion site but do not tighten it. Isolate the stomach from the surrounding abdominal viscera with moistened swabs to limit contamination (Fig. 6.9). Use a no. 11 scalpel blade to make a stab incision in the centre of the purse-string suture into the gastric lumen.

5. **Pass the tip of the feeding tube into the stomach through the stab incision and tighten the purse-string suture.** Once the purse string suture is tightened around the tube, the mushroom tip will prevent the catheter from dislodging from the stomach (Fig. 6.9).

6. **Place pexy sutures between the stomach and body wall to encircle the tube as it passes between them.** The stomach and body wall bordering the tube are sutured together with four simple interrupted sutures that encircle the tube penetration sites. These anchor the stomach to the body wall around the stoma, creating an early serosal seal and limiting the risk of leakage. Include a bite of the transverse abdominis muscle and a bite of the seromuscular layer of the stomach in each suture (Fig. 6.10).

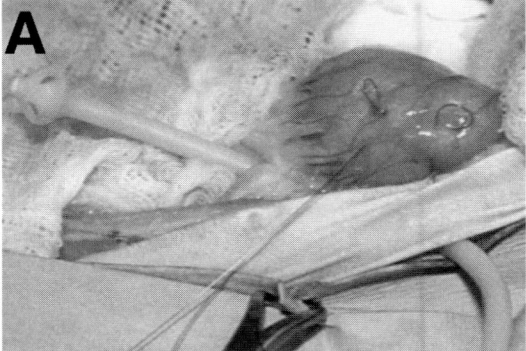

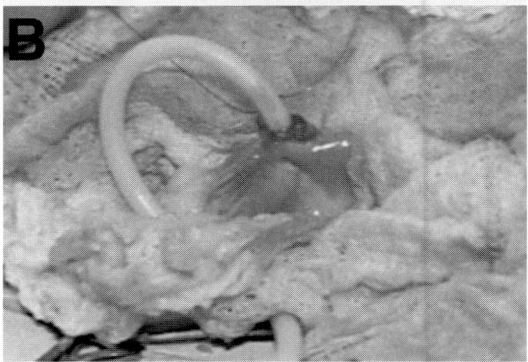

Fig. 6.9. Gastrostomy 1: (A) the tube has been introduced through the left body wall and a purse-string suture has been placed in the gastric fundus; (B) make a stab incision into the gastric lumen through the centre of the purse-string suture, insert the tube, and tighten the suture.

Preplace all four sutures first before tying them: take bites of the stomach and body wall and pass suture through them; leave the suture ends long and clamp them with a haemostat. Once all the sutures are preplaced, tie them in turn (Fig. 6.10). Preplacing the sutures in this restricted area facilitates placement as the tissues can still be manipulated while the remaining sutures are placed. Once the final pexy suture is tied, loosely wrap the omentum around the body wall and stomach stoma site and tack it in position with a suture.

7. **Secure the tube to the skin** using a Roman sandal suture and close the abdominal incision (see p. 51).

8. **Bandage the tube to the body wall** and put an Elizabethan collar on the patient. It is critical to prevent the patient from removing the tube prematurely.

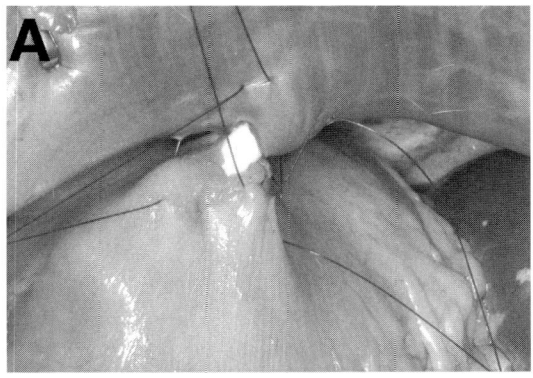

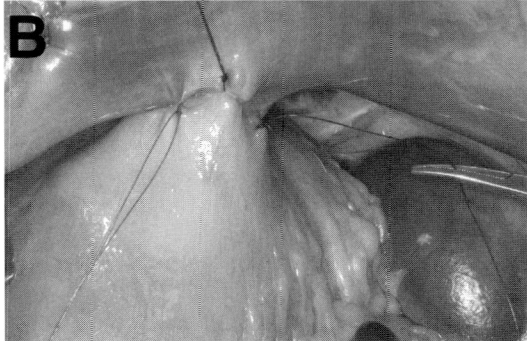

Fig. 6.10. Gastrostomy 2: (A) preplace four pexy sutures; (B) tie the pexy sutures to seal the gap between the stomach and the body wall.

9. **Check the position of the tube prior to use.** Before using the tube for the first time, instill a small volume of radio-opaque contrast agent through the tube and radiograph the abdomen to ensure that contrast is contained within the stomach.

Complications

Early tube removal may lead to leakage from the gastrostomy site and peritonitis. By ten days, scar tissue forms between the stomach and body wall creating a sealed tract from the stomach to the skin and preventing leakage. Other complications include tube blockage and discharge from the stoma.

Removing feeding tubes

To remove a feeding tube, cut the securing sutures and pull the tube out of the patient. This generally does not require sedation. Mushroom-tipped gastrostomy tubes are designed so that the mushroom tip will collapse when moderate traction is applied. The stomas from gastrostomy and oesophagostomy tubes are left to heal by second intention (suturing the stomas increases the risk of wound complications such as abscesses). Discharge from the stoma will stop after 24 or 48 h and a dry scab will form.

Feeding Using a Tube

Types of diet

There are several veterinary diets for nutritional support of critically ill patients that are suitable for tube feeding. Liquid diets must be used with small-bore tubes (e.g. naso-oesophageal; feline oesophagostomy). Liquidized tinned food may be given through large-bore tubes (e.g. canine oesophagostomy; gastrostomy). Debilitated or critically ill patients require a diet with a high protein content and a minimum calorie density of 1 kcal/g. Diets designed for supporting critically ill patients incorporate these features. Animals receiving long-term tube feeding can be fed standard diets that have been liquidized. Most tinned pet foods that do not contain chunks of meat can be liquidized in a food processor by adding a small amount of water. This generates a sloppy slurry that can be administered through large, catheter-tip syringes.

Calculating daily nutritional requirements

Current guidelines recommend initially providing the *resting energy requirement* (RER) for critically ill patients. This is the calorific requirement to support normal physiological processes during minimal activity. Previously, to calculate the daily calorie intake the RER was multiplied by a 'disease factor' that estimated the increased metabolic requirements of a sick patient. However, this practice is thought to overestimate the optimal nutritional intake of ill patients and may lead to detrimental metabolic derangements.

RER can be calculated using two formulae in dogs and cats (Eqns 6.1 and 6.2):

RER (kcals)
= 70 × *(current body weight in kg)*$^{0.75}$ (6.1)

or, for patients weighing between 2 and 30 kg:

RER (kcals)
= 70 × *(30 x current body weight in kg)*   (6.2)

Veterinary diets formulated for nutritional support of critically ill patients state the kilocalorie content per millilitre of food, enabling the quantity of food required to be calculated.

The nutritional requirements of a patient should be monitored continually and the calorie intake and type of diet should be adjusted as necessary. It is good practice for the body weight and food intake of patients receiving nutritional support to be monitored daily. For patients receiving long-term nutritional support, maintaining optimal body weight and body condition are appropriate goals.

Initiating tube feeding

Patients take a few days to adjust to tube feeding and will not tolerate being fed large meals initially. To overcome this, feeding is introduced gradually. One-third of the calculated daily ration is fed on the first day. This is divided into six small meals spaced regularly through the day. If this is tolerated, two-thirds of the calculated ration is fed on the second day and the full ration is fed on the third day. Subsequently, the number of meals can be reduced and the volume of each meal increased until the daily ration is given in three or four meals through the day.

Each meal is fed slowly. If the patient shows signs of nausea (salivating, licking excessively, retching) or vomits during feeding, the volume of each feed and the speed of feeding should be reduced for a period to give further time for adaptation. Food should be allowed to warm to room temperature before being fed (cold food may induce vomiting).

To prevent the feeding tube from blocking, it must be flushed with water before and after each feed. To prevent aerophagia, the tube must be capped when not in use.

Other Techniques for Nutritional Support

Gastrostomy and oesophagostomy tubes can be placed using special equipment. For example, *percutaneous endoscopic gastrostomy (PEG) tubes* can be placed endoscopically and special applicators can be used to facilitate both gastrostomy and oesophagostomy tube placement.

Other techniques may also be used to provide nutritional support but are generally reserved for specialist practices. *Enterostomy tubes* are small-bore feeding tubes placed directly into the duodenum or proximal jejunum. They are used predominantly in animals with gastric disease or pancreatitis (their use is associated with less release of pancreatic enzymes than more proximal feeding tubes). As the tube is small and the jejunum cannot expand to accommodate large boluses of food, a liquid diet must be fed as a constant-rate infusion and this necessitates intensive nursing care and monitoring.

Parenteral nutrition delivers nutrition directly into the bloodstream usually through a central venous catheter (a catheter placed in a major vessel such as the jugular vein). The use of parenteral nutrition requires intensive nursing and medical care and is associated with a range of metabolic derangements and other complications that must be carefully monitored and managed. It is generally reserved for specialist practices where it may be selected for patients that cannot tolerate enteral feeding or that cannot be anaesthetized for feeding tube placement.

Bibliography

Abood, S.K. and Buffington, C.A. (1991) Improved nasogastric intubation technique for administration of nutritional support in dogs. *Journal of the American Veterinary Medical Association* 199, 577–579.

Armstrong, P.J. and Lippert, A.C. (1988) Selected aspects of enteral and parenteral nutritional support. *Seminars in Veterinary Medicine and Surgery (Small Animals)* 3, 216–226.

Armstrong, P.J., Hand, M.S. and Frederick, G.S. (1990) Enteral nutrition by tube. *Veterinary Clinics of North America Small Animal Practice* 20, 237–275.

Chan, D.L. (2004) Nutritional requirements of the critically ill patient. *Clinical Techniques in Small Animal Practice* 19, 1–5.

Glaus, T.M., Cornelius, L.M., Bartges, J.W. and Reusch, C. (1998) Complications with non-endoscopic percutaneous gastrostomy in 31 cats and 10 dogs: a retrospective study. *Journal of Small Animal Practice* 39, 218–222.

Han, E. (2004) Esophageal and gastric feeding tubes in ICU patients. *Clinical Techniques in Small Animal Practice* 19, 22–31.

Heuter, K. (2004) Placement of jejunal feeding tubes for post-gastric feeding. *Clinical Techniques in Small Animal Practice* 19, 32–42.

Kerl, M.E. and Johnson, P.A. (2004) Nutritional plan: matching diet to disease. *Clinical Techniques in Small Animal Practice* 19, 9–21.

Levine, P.B., Smallwood, L.J. and Buback, J.L. (1997) Esophagostomy tubes as a method of nutritional management in cats: a retrospective study. *Journal of the American Animal Hospital Association* 33, 405–410.

Lippert, A.C., Fulton, R.B. Jr and Parr, A.M. (1993) A retrospective study of the use of total parenteral nutrition in dogs and cats. *Journal of Veterinary Internal Medicine* 7, 52–64.

Marks, S.L. (1998) The principles and practical application of enteral nutrition. *Veterinary Clinics of North America Small Animal Practice* 28, 677–708.

Perea, S.C. (2008) Critical care nutrition for feline patients. *Topics in Companion Animal Medicine* 23, 207–215.

Prittie, J. and Barton, L. (2004) Route of nutrient delivery. *Clinical Techniques in Small Animal Practice* 19, 6–8.

Pyle, S.C., Marks, S.L. and Kass, P.H. (2004) Evaluation of complications and prognostic factors associated with administration of total parenteral nutrition in cats: 75 cases (1994–2001). *Journal of the American Veterinary Medical Association* 225, 242–250.

Von Werthern, C.J. and Wess, G. (2001) A new technique for insertion of esophagostomy tubes in cats. *Journal of the American Animal Hospital Association* 37, 140–144.

Waddell, L.S. and Michel, K.E. (1998) Critical care nutrition: routes of feeding. *Clinical Techniques in Small Animal Practice* 13, 197–203.

Williams, J.M. and White, R.A.S. (1993) Tube gastrostomy in dogs. *Journal of Small Animal Practice* 34, 59–64.

7 Wound Management

debridement: removal of devitalized tissue and debris from the wound
granulation tissue: well-vascularized connective tissue that forms in healing wounds
lavage: wound irrigation
primary closure: ('first intention healing') immediate closure of a wound
secondary closure: closure delayed until granulation tissue has formed
second intention healing: ('open wound management') healing by contraction and epithelialization

The reader should be able to:

- list the stages of wound healing
- identify the differences between adherent and non-adherent dressings and explain when adherent dressings might be used
- compare the different forms of wound debridement
- compare the different forms of non-adherent dressing for the management of a granulating wound
- compare the properties and uses of silver and honey dressings
- formulate a management plan for a cat that presents with an acute degloving injury of a paw
- apply a wet-to-dry dressing
- apply a three-layer bandage with a non-adherent contact layer and hydrogel
- recognize features of successful and unsuccessful wound management

Most surgical wounds are created by making sharp incisions into healthy tissues and can be closed immediately (primary closure). In contrast, many traumatic wounds have large skin defects, heavy contamination, and devitalized tissue that prevent them from being closed immediately. Traumatic wounds often require active wound management to control or prevent infection and to promote the generation of a healthy wound environment before they will heal. This chapter describes the basic principles of wound management, predominantly using traumatic wounds as examples. The end point of wound management used here is the generation of a healthy granulation bed because, at this stage, the wound should be free from infection, detritus, and devitalized tissue, and should be ready for closure. Reconstructive surgery is described in Chapter 8.

Stages of Wound Healing

All wounds heal by progressing through three stages of wound healing: the inflammatory, proliferative, and maturation phases.

Inflammatory phase

The inflammatory phase starts shortly after a wound is created. Initially, a blood clot forms in the base of the wound and the fibrin network acts as a framework for the subsequent events in wound healing. Neutrophils quickly invade the wound, phagocytose bacteria, and die. Macrophages invade a little later, phagocytose dead neutrophils and detritus, and excrete enzymes necessary for autolysis. Macrophages are critical for wound healing as they control the local cellular responses through the release of cytokines. This inflammatory phase of wound healing is characterized by the production of copious exudate composed of dead neutrophils and sloughing tissue.

Proliferative phase

The proliferative phase of wound healing starts when most of the necrotic debris and bacteria have been removed, and the level of exudate begins to reduce. Fibroblasts and blood vessels invade the wound and deposit collagen. Together these produce the pink, vascularized granulation tissue that is characteristic of this phase of wound healing. Once granulation tissue has formed, the surface of the wound epithelializes by proliferation of epithelial cells from the wound edge.

Maturation phase

Wound maturation involves reorganization of collagen and wound contraction. It overlaps with the proliferative phase of wound healing, starting once granulation tissue has formed. Initially, maturation causes contraction of the open wound area. Later this leads to contraction and strengthening of the scar after the wound has epithelialized. This process continues for several months and is beneficial as the reorganized collagen increases the strength of the regenerated tissues. However, wound contraction can lead to distortion of adjacent tissues and limit movement if it occurs near the eye, mouth, anus, or a joint.

Principles of Dressing Selection

Dressings have a range of roles in wound management:

- control the surface environment;
- remove necrotic debris;
- absorb exudate;
- provide physical protection against trauma;
- prevent contamination of the wound;
- deliver topical medications; and
- provide support and immobility.

Selecting the appropriate dressing and applying it properly are very important aspects of wound management. Poor dressing selection and management

have the potential to impede, rather than facilitate, wound healing. Dressings have three basic components: (i) the primary or contact layer that has most influence on the wound surface; (ii) the secondary layer that provides absorbent capacity and support; and (iii) the tertiary layer that holds the other layers in place (Fig. 7.1). These three elements will be discussed individually.

Primary (contact) layer

The contact layer covers the wound surface and has most influence over wound healing. Contact layers may be *adherent* or *non-adherent*.

Adherent contact layer

Adherent contact layers adhere to the surface of the wound and, when removed, peel the surface layer of tissue and debris away from the wound. These are used to physically debride the wound to remove necrotic tissue and detritus during the inflammatory phase of wound healing. However, adherent dressings are non-selective and will damage healthy tissues, impeding granulation tissue formation.

WET-TO-DRY DRESSING The *wet-to-dry* dressing is an example of an adherent dressing that is popular in veterinary wound management. It is built up using layers of lint-free, gauze swabs. The contact layer is applied wet. As it dries, it adheres to the wound surface leading to debridement when it is removed. The dressing is generally used only for the first few days of wound management to accelerate the inflammatory phase of wound healing. However, because of the injury to healthy tissues that these dressings can cause, their use is controversial. The application of wet-to-dry dressings and alternative approaches to wound debridement are described below.

Non-adherent contact layer

Most dressings used in veterinary medicine have a non-adherent contact layer that does not damage the wound surface. Many of these dressings are described as being semi-occlusive or occlusive. These trap a layer of moisture at the wound surface that promotes granulation tissue formation and speeds wound healing. They usually have some absorptive capacity to store excess exudate.

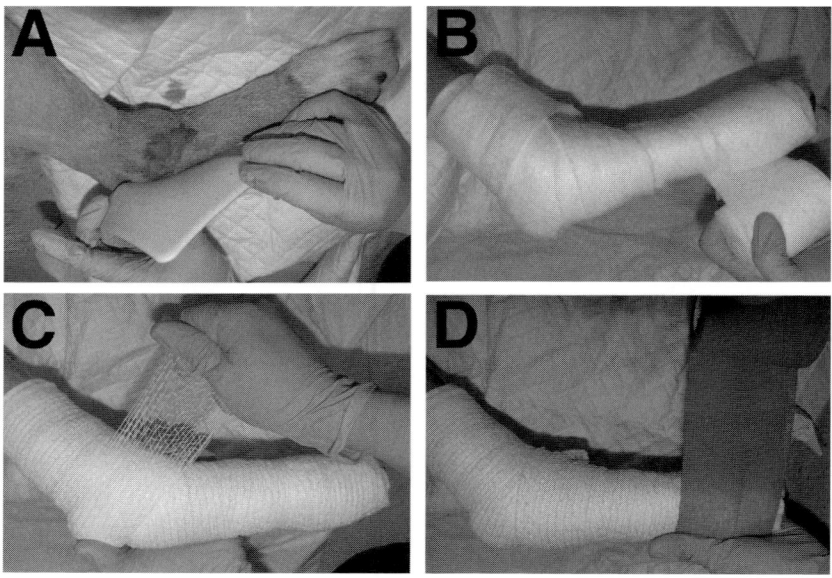

Fig. 7.1. Example of bandage layers: (A) primary (contact) layer – foam dressing; (B) secondary (padding) layer – polyester synthetic bandage; (C) tertiary layer (inner) – gauze bandage; (D) tertiary layer (outer) – cohesive, elastic bandage.

Semi-occlusive dressings allow some moisture to escape from the dressing but retain sufficient to maintain a moist wound environment. Occlusive dressings prevent any moisture from leaving the dressing. These forms of dressing are often used in combination with wound gels that provide further moisture to the wound surface. Although moisture at the wound surface promotes granulation tissue and epithelialization, saturation of the wound will lead to maceration and prevent wound healing. These dressings are managed to maintain moisture at the wound surface without leading to maceration.

Other forms of non-adherent dressing provide mainly physical protection and are more suited to management of wounds that have been closed or that are covered by epithelium.

HYDROGEL Hydrogels are polymer gels that are applied directly to the wound surface. They fill the contours of irregular wounds and provide even coverage. The gels have high water content and some absorptive capacity. They maintain a moist wound environment suitable for granulation tissue formation and epithelialization during the proliferative phase of wound healing. Hydrogels also maintain a local wound environment that is suitable for enzymatic action necessary for autolysis. In this way, they also encourage the sloughing of necrotic tissue during the inflammatory phase of wound healing. Hydrogels are applied to a depth of 5 mm over the wound surface and are held in place with additional dressings (typically foam dressings) (Fig. 7.2).

MANUKA HONEY Honey is a traditional wound therapy that is gaining in popularity because of its unique characteristics when used as a dressing. It has potent antibacterial properties effective against a range of organisms including antimicrobial-resistant bacterial strains. It provides a moist wound environment encouraging granulation tissue formation and epithelialization. Manuka honey also reduces wound inflammation and encourages natural sloughing of necrotic debris. Many of these properties are inherent to a wide range of honeys, but only medical grade Manuka honey can be recommended for wound treatment at this time. This is because Manuka honey, unlike other honeys, is not heat-treated (which destroys much of the antibacterial properties of honey). Instead, it has been gamma irradiated (to remove spore-forming bacteria, yeasts, and moulds) and assayed to provide a consistently high antibacterial effect.

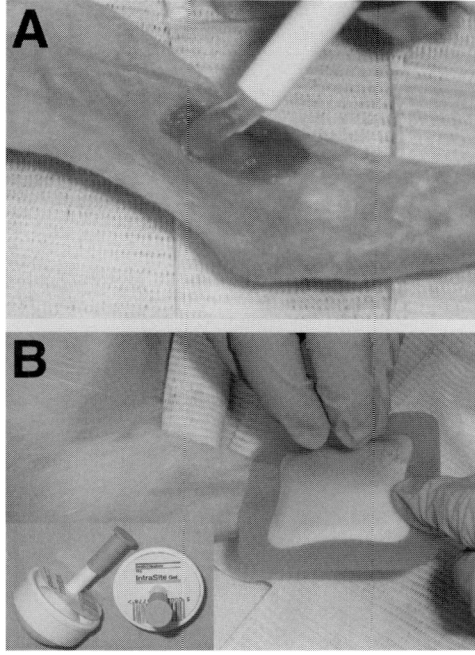

Fig. 7.2. Hydrogel: (A) applying hydrogel to the surface of a wound; (B) the hydrogel must be covered with a contact-layer dressing to keep it in place. Insert shows small tubes of hydrogels suitable for single use.

Manuka honey comes in a variety of formats for wound application. As well as tubes of Manuka honey for direct application to the wound, there is a range of Manuka honey-impregnated alginate, foam, and gauze dressings (see Fig. 7.3). Some studies demonstrate accelerated wound healing when Manuka honey is used in comparison to conventional wound dressings.

FOAM (HYDROCELLULAR) DRESSINGS Foam dressings are made from materials such as expanded polyurethane that act as sponges. They absorb wound fluid without adhering to the surface of the wound and provide a moist wound environment without causing surface trauma. They also provide padding for wounds. These dressings are extremely popular and are predominantly used for managing the proliferative phase of wound healing. They come in a range of sizes and thicknesses and are often used in combination with hydrogels (Figs 7.2 and 7.4).

Some confusion can arise over the classification and product labelling of foam dressings. Many of these have surface adhesives that allow them to stick to skin surrounding the wound. However, the adhesive is inactivated by moisture, which prevents it from adhering to the wound surface itself. As such, these dressings are non-adherent dressings but are labelled as being adhesive.

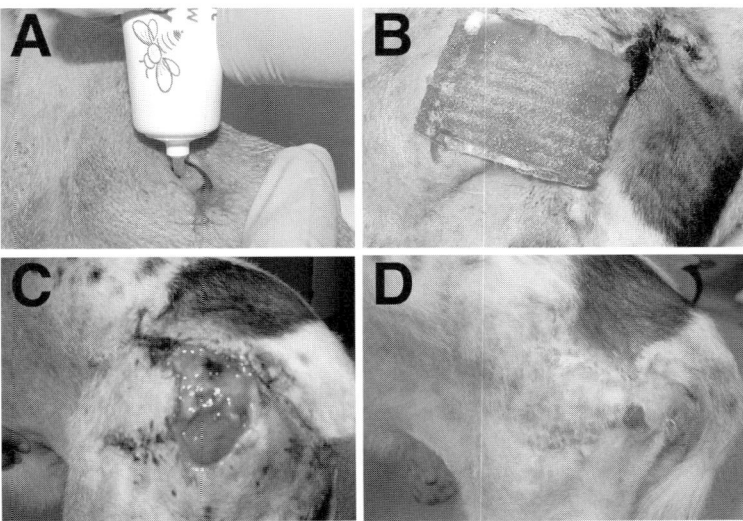

Fig. 7.3. Manuka honey formulations and uses: (A) tube of Manuka honey for wound management; (B) Manuka honey incorporated into an alginate dressing; (C) sloughing skin lesion managed with honey-impregnated alginate dressing; (D) this wound sloughed necrotic debris, developed granulation tissue, and contracted rapidly.

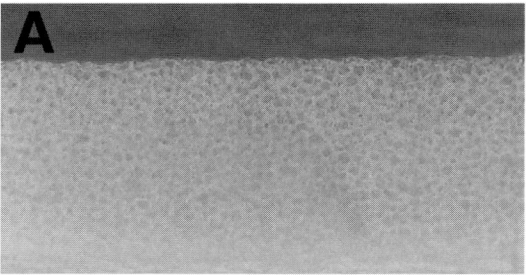

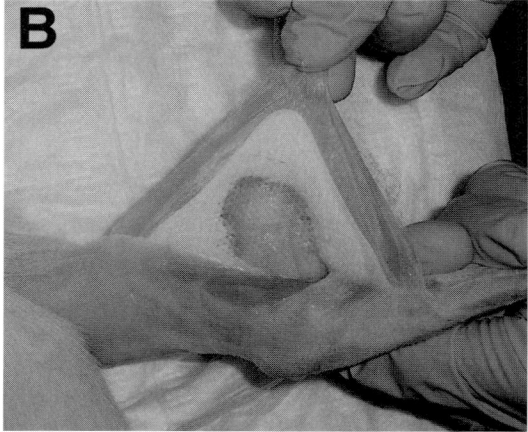

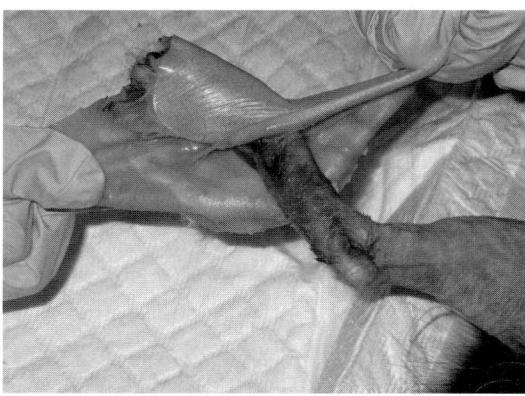

Fig. 7.5. Hydrocolloid dressing: this dressing is still quite tacky by the time of removal in this patient but provides a moist wound environment to promote healing.

Fig. 7.4. Foam dressing: (A) close-up view of the cut surface demonstrating the porous, foam structure of the dressing which makes it absorbent while still retaining some moisture at the wound surface; (B) removing a foam dressing – note the patch of exudate which has absorbed into the dressing preventing the wound from becoming macerated.

HYDROCOLLOID DRESSINGS Hydrocolloid dressings are composed of chemicals such as carboxymethy-lated cellulose that form gels as they absorb fluid. These dressings are quite absorbent, removing excess fluid, but also maintain a moist wound environment. The hydrocolloids have intrinsic adhesive properties that lessen as fluid is retained within the gel. These dressing should reach the stage of sticking only weakly to the wound surface by the time they are removed, minimizing surface trauma. However, they can cause some surface trauma when they are removed and are sometimes described as being 'low-adherent' dressings (Fig. 7.5).

ALGINATE DRESSINGS Calcium or sodium alginate dressings (from processed seaweed) are composed of pads of alginate fibres that are applied directly to the wound surface. The alginates transform into a highly absorbent gel when they come into contact with wound fluid. The gel is non-adherent and maintains a moist wound environment. Alginate dressings are among the most absorbent dressings and are good for highly exudative wounds. Due to their high absorbent capacity, they may be left for up to 7 days before being replaced but they must not be allowed to desiccate the wound surface. The calcium alginate dressings also confer the additional property of acting as local haemostatic agents through the release of calcium ions into the wound surface initiating the clotting cascade.

FILM DRESSINGS Film dressings are made from substances such as polyester that has no inherent absorptive capacity but which does not adhere to the wound. These are most suited to managing wounds with an intact epithelial surface (i.e. sutured incisions or epithelialized wounds). Two forms have become popular in veterinary medicine (see Fig. 7.6). Padded film dressings have a film contact layer that is perforated and backed with an absorbent pad. These dressings are used extensively to cover surgical wounds. The perforations allow small volumes of exudate to pass through the film into the padded layer. The padding provides additional protection against surface trauma. These dressings are comfortable, inexpensive, and effective at protecting surgical wounds. Spray-on film dressings are also popular. These can be sprayed over the surface of a closed surgical wound to provide a thin film that protects the wound from

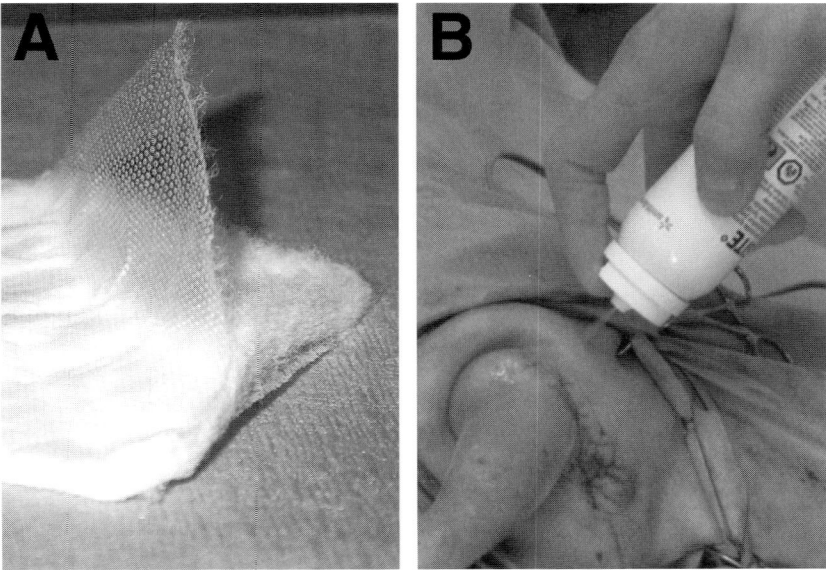

Fig. 7.6. Film dressings: (A) padded film dressing (perforated film peeled away from pad for demonstration); (B) spray-on film dressing being applied to a perineal wound.

surface contaminants and which does not require removal. These may be used in preference to padded film dressings in places that are awkward to dress (e.g. castration incision; perineum).

PARAFFIN GAUZE DRESSINGS Gauze impregnated with white paraffin gel provides an inert, non-adherent contact layer. This dressing is used predominantly to prevent contact between the wound surface and the secondary layers of dressing and probably does not accelerate wound progression in comparison to the other dressings discussed. The dressing can be used as a vehicle for topical wound products that are impregnated into the paraffin wax (e.g. chlorhexidine antiseptic).

NANOCRYSTALLINE SILVER DRESSINGS Dressings impregnated with microscopic deposits of silver are highly effective antibacterial dressings (Fig. 7.7). Silver ions are released from the dressing when the silver atoms come into contact with wound fluid or when the dressing is pre-moistened with water prior to being applied to the wound. Silver ions are cytotoxic, causing damage to the bacterial cell walls, enzymes, and DNA. These dressings are bactericidal and have a similar range of activity to medical-grade Manuka honey dressings. However,

the cytotoxic effect of silver ions is non-selective, and hence may cause some injury to the wound bed. When using these dressings, it is important to follow the manufacturer's guidelines carefully (particularly pre-soaking with water rather than saline) to ensure that they are effective.

Secondary layer

The secondary layer provides padding, support, and absorptive capacity. For many wound dressings, this layer is thin as it is only required to hold the contact layer in place. Natural, semi-synthetic, and synthetic materials are used (Fig. 7.8A).

Natural material

Cotton wool is popular because it is soft, highly absorbent, highly conformable, and inexpensive. The main disadvantages of cotton wool are that it forms lint that can contaminate the wound and that it flattens when it becomes wet, losing some of its padding features. Cotton wool is ideally suited to providing padding for heavy support dressings (e.g. the Robert Jones dressing) as its compressible and conformable characteristics make it easy to use to provide a thick, rigid dressing.

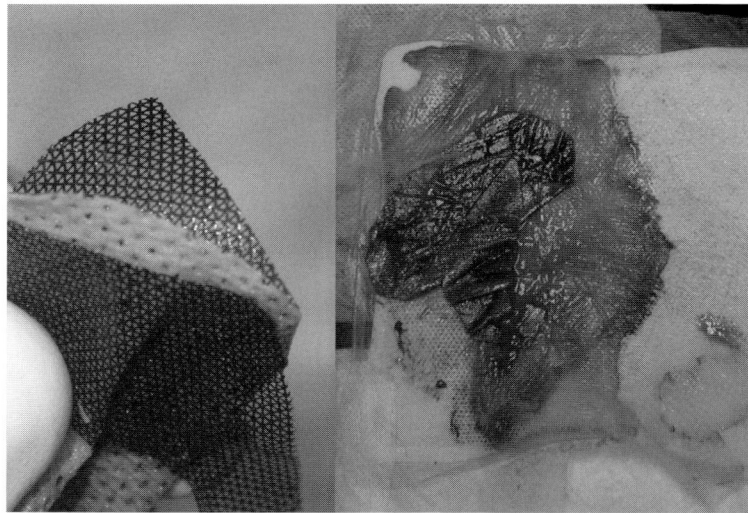

Fig. 7.7. Nanocrystalline silver dressing. There are different forms of sliver dressing. This one has a thin absorbent layer sandwiched between two outer layers of silver-coated polyethylene net and must be soaked in water prior to use. Nanocrystalline silver dressings are generally held in place by another contact dressing. In this case, a foam dressing has been used. The photograph demonstrates the dark wound fluid generated by the dressing as silver salts form.

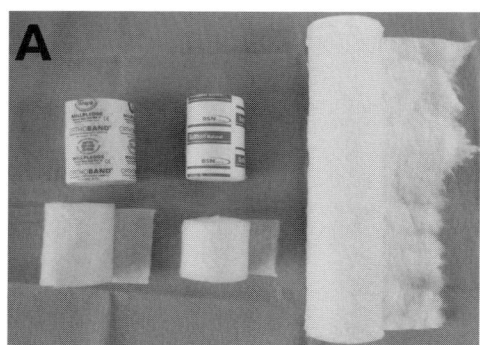

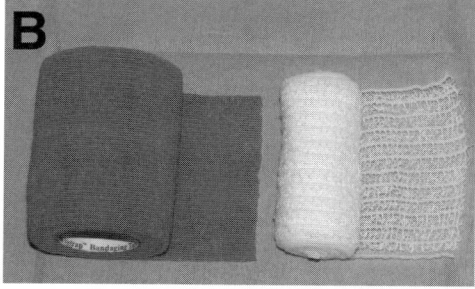

Fig. 7.8. Secondary and tertiary layers: (A) synthetic, semi-synthetic, and natural bandage materials for secondary layers; (B) cohesive elastic wrap, and gauze bandage, used for tertiary bandage layers.

Synthetic and semi-synthetic material

These dressings do not produce lint and provide comfortable padded support. They are popular as they are easy to apply and come in a range of convenient sizes. Synthetic dressings are made from materials such as polyester. They have little absorptive capacity but maintain their padded structure when exposed to moisture, and are good choices providing that wound exudate can be retained within the primary layer. The semi-synthetic materials are composed of cellulose and combine the properties of cotton wool and of the synthetic dressings. These dressings have more absorptive capacity than the synthetic dressings, retain their padded properties when wet, and do not form lint.

Tertiary layer

The tertiary layer fixes the rest of the dressing in place and provides compression (Fig. 7.8B). Conforming gauze bandages are knitted, stretchable bandages. These allow some air and moisture to move through the dressing to limit maceration of tissues. These are often used in conjunction with cohesive conforming bandages. Cohesive conforming bandages are elastic wraps that adhere to each other but not to skin. Following placement, the wrap clings to itself and contracts to hold the secondary layers firmly in place. This may be desirable in heavy support dressings but care is required to ensure that contraction of the wrap does not lead to compromise of the tissues.

Dressings on the flank and proximal limbs cannot be held in place easily with bandages. Adhesive strips can be used to fix dressings in place (Fig. 7.9). Dressings over larger wounds may be held in place with body wraps or tie-over bolus dressings (Fig. 7.10).

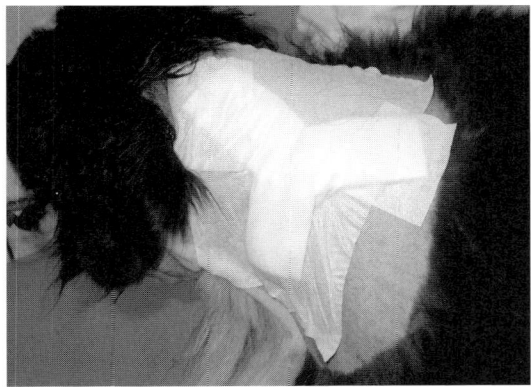

Fig. 7.9. Alternative ways of fixing dressings: adhesive tapes used to secure dressings over a neck wound.

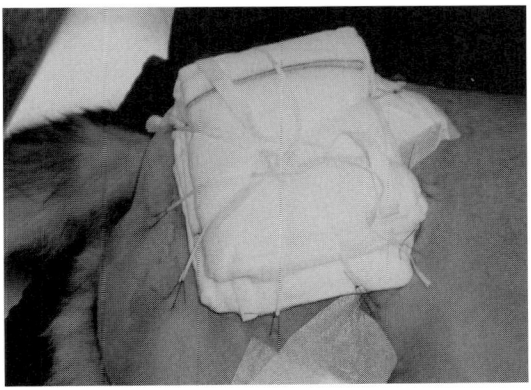

Fig. 7.10. Alternative ways of fixing dressings: tie-over 'bolus' dressing. The dressing is held in place using padding secured by tape threaded through suture anchors around the periphery of the wound.

Complications of dressing applications

Dressing-related complications include:

- *Contact dermatitis.*
- *Maceration*: this occurs when the wound surface or surrounding skin becomes saturated with sweat or exudate. To avoid this, dressings should be changed frequently to ensure that the wound surface remains moist but does not become saturated. Clipping fur from the interdigital spaces and ensuring the dressing does not become wet are also important.
- *Pressure sores*: these develop where dressings rub or compress the blood supply over bony prominences (e.g. olecranon). Pressure sores are often the result of poor bandaging techniques.

Managing Traumatic Wounds

Heavily contaminated and traumatized wounds require protracted wound management before they can be closed. Generally, they are managed as open wounds until granulation tissue forms as this is an indicator of a healthy wound environment. Other forms of traumatic wound (e.g. lacerations) may require much less wound management as they have less tissue trauma and contamination. Often, these are closed immediately or after only a short period of open wound management.

Regardless of the severity of the injury, general principles of wound management should be followed. Prevent further wound contamination by keeping the wound covered with a sterile dressing at all times. Use clean technique when performing dressing changes: (i) wash hands and wear examination gloves; (ii) wear suitable protective clothing; and (iii) work on clean surfaces and disinfect them after use. Do not share dressings or wound products between patients. Prevent further trauma to the wound as this causes inflammation, disrupts granulation tissue, and impedes wound healing. Stop the patient from interfering with the wound by applying suitable dressings and an Elizabethan collar. Ensure the dressing does not rub or move over the wound surface by applying it carefully. Restrict the patient's exercise to limit movement of the dressing over the wound: restrict dogs to lead-controlled exercise for toilet purposes only; confine cats inside and prevent them from jumping onto furniture.

Wound management is divided into three phases:

1. **initial wound assessment:** evaluating the severity of the wound and planning a course of treatment;
2. **managing the inflammatory phase of wound healing:** removing devitalized tissue and controlling infection; and
3. **managing the proliferative stage of wound healing:** providing a healthy environment to promote granulation tissue formation.

Stage 1: initial wound assessment

The goal of this initial assessment is to clean the wound and assess the severity of the injury. At this stage, the various options of immediate or delayed closure and methods of reconstruction can be considered, and a provisional plan for wound management can be established. It is important to assess the general health of the patient before assessing the wound. Traumatized patients may have concurrent injuries that require more urgent attention. If the wound cannot be assessed immediately, cover it with a lint-free, sterile dressing. Once the patient is stable, wound assessment and management can begin.

Restrain the patient to evaluate the wound

Initially, traumatic wounds can be difficult to assess because the patient is distressed or because the wound is obscured by necrotic tissue, exudate, and matted hair. It is often necessary to sedate or anaesthetize the patient to enable thorough initial wound evaluation.

Clip hair

Hair obscuring the wound is a source of contaminants, it prevents the wound from being cleaned and assessed easily, and it retains discharge and debris near the wound. Clip the hair coat widely around the wound and repeat this as the hair regrows. To prevent hair fragments from entering the wound during clipping, keep the wound covered with a lint-free, sterile dressing or pack the wound with water-soluble gel (e.g. Surgilube®, Nycomed US Inc., Melville, New Jersey, USA) before clipping. The gel acts as a barrier, catching fragments of hair, and can be removed by lavage.

Remove gross contaminants and necrotic tissue

During the initial assessment, gross contaminants such as plant material, hair, and grit are removed

using lavage (see below) or forceps. Remove tissues that are clearly non-viable as these will slough over the following few days if left *in situ* and this will contribute to inflammation delaying the onset of the proliferative phase of healing. Removing devitalized or compromised tissues is termed debridement (Fig. 7.11). Debridement during the initial assessment is performed by sharp surgical excision or by abrasion using the curved edge of a no. 10 scalpel blade. Sharp excision is preferred over abrasion as it causes less tissue trauma and inflammation. Debridement can be continued until capillary haemorrhage starts on the surface of the wound. However, indiscriminate debridement is likely to damage healthy tissues. If there is doubt about the viability of tissue, or if necrotic debris lies over delicate structures (e.g. nerve), the tissue can be left *in situ* and debridement can be repeated in 2 or 3 days if the necrotic tissue has not sloughed.

Devitalized tissue can be recognized by several features:

- temperature: necrotic tissue is cold;
- colour: necrotic tissue is pale, white, black, purple, or green;
- texture: skin becomes thin and loses its elasticity as it starts to slough; it may appear like cardboard or paper; as it sloughs, it begins to liquefy; and
- no bleeding when cut: necrotic tissue will not bleed actively when incised.

Perform wound lavage to remove contaminants including bacteria

Wound lavage (irrigation) is performed at all stages of wound management as it removes bacteria and microscopic contaminants from the wound surface. It also dislodges gross contaminants and exudate. Use isotonic saline or polyelectrolyte solution (e.g. 0.9% sodium chloride; Ringer's solution) in large volumes. Alternatively, dilute antiseptic solutions can be used but there is some risk that they will cause cytotoxic injury to fibroblasts and keratinocytes in the wound, and this might impede wound healing.

Lavage fluid is delivered under moderate pressure to dislodge surface contaminants without causing additional trauma or driving contaminants into the wound bed. To achieve a moderate pressure, fluid is delivered through a 19-gauge needle using a 35 ml syringe (Fig. 7.12).

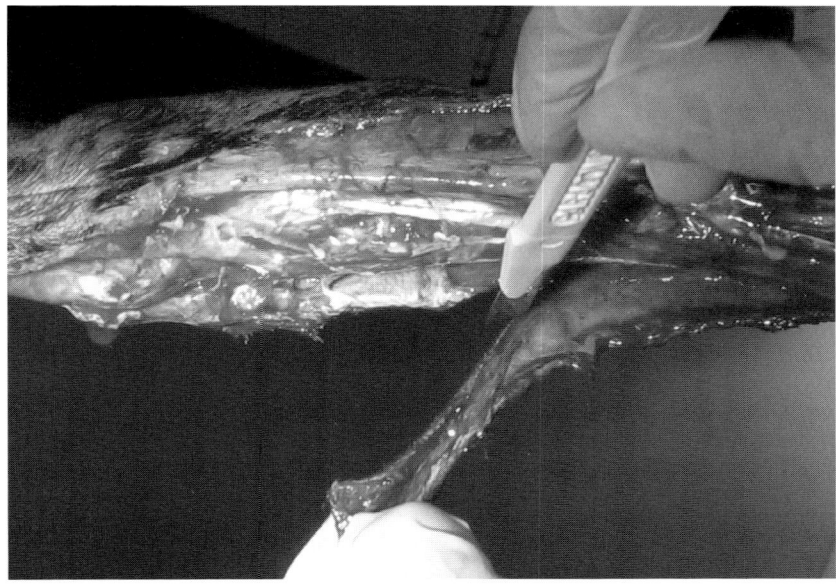

Fig. 7.11. Initial surgical debridement of a degloving injury on the foot of a dog.

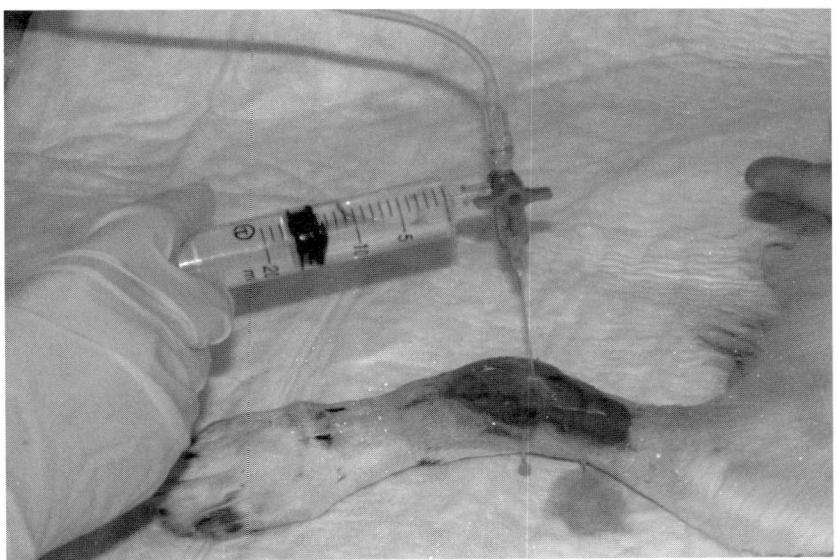

Fig. 7.12. Wound lavage: isotonic crystalloid solution, administration set, three-way tap, syringe, and needle used to deliver lavage fluid under moderate pressure (the operator is using clean technique to handle the wound).

Manage bacterial contamination

Traumatic wounds are classed as contaminated or dirty wounds depending on their level of contamination and whether or not they have become infected (see Chapter 2). Perioperative antimicrobial therapy is generally indicated and is often continued as a short therapeutic course at the onset of wound management. However, there is no evidence that open-ended antimicrobial therapy is of benefit and it is likely to promote the formation of resistant wound infections. Initially prescribe drugs that are active against a broad spectrum of Gram-positive and Gram-negative organisms, including the common commensal skin bacteria. Once the therapeutic course has been completed, further antimicrobial therapy should only be prescribed if there are clinical indicators of wound infection (e.g. exudate; inflammation; pyrexia) and drugs should be chosen based on the results of bacterial culture and sensitivity testing. Consider using Manuka honey or silver dressings for the long-term control of superficial wound infections during chronic wound management. There is much less risk of promoting the development of resistant bacterial strains using these dressings, and they are highly effective at controlling wound infection.

Stage 2: wound debridement

The initial wound debridement is unlikely to remove all contaminants and devitalized tissue from the wound. The inflammatory phase of wound healing will continue over the first few days while tissues slough and bacteria are destroyed.

This stage is associated with production of large volumes of purulent exudate. Dressings can be used to promote further debridement during this period, shortening the inflammatory phase of wound healing. Three methods of wound debridement are commonly used in veterinary surgery:

1. adherent dressing;
2. autolytic wound debridement; and
3. honey dressing.

Adherent wound dressings

The *wet-to-dry dressing* adheres to the surface of the wound and rips away necrotic tissue and contaminants at each dressing change. To apply a wet-to-dry dressing, sterile, lint-free gauze swabs are soaked in saline and thoroughly wrung out. These are moulded to the surface of the wound as a moist contact layer 2–4 swabs deep. A thick, dry, sterile absorbent layer (often more dry swabs) is laid on top and held in place with a bandage or tie-over dressing (Fig. 7.13). Fluid wicks through the dressing from the wound surface into the absorbent layer. As the contact layer dries, wound exudate and debris on the wound surface adhere to the open gauze network. If a wet-to-dry dressing is applied

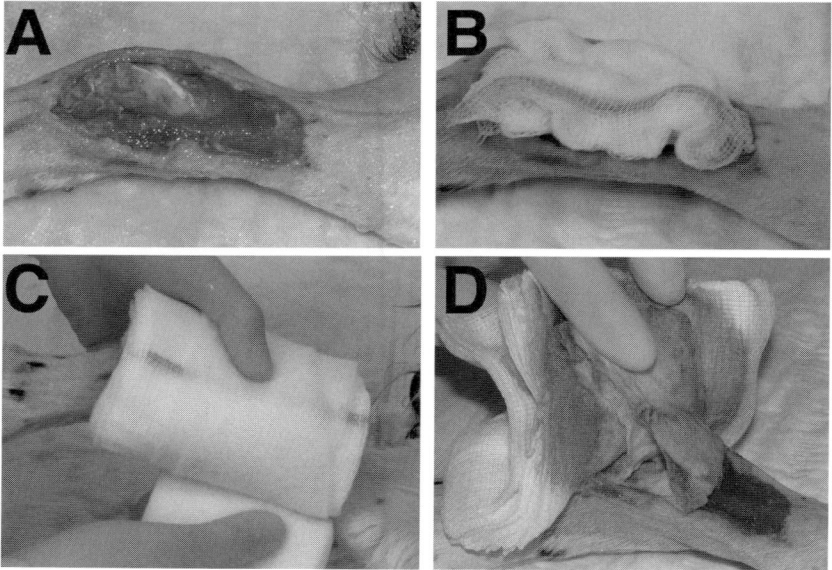

Fig. 7.13. Applying a wet-to-dry dressing: (A) shearing injury over the hock with exposed bone and torn muscle; (B) thin contact layer of moist swabs; (C) thick secondary layer of absorbent dressing; (D) dressing change 24 h later – the contact layer has adhered and is debriding the wound as it is removed.

effectively, at the time of dressing removal (usually 12–24 h), the contact layer will be firmly adhered to the wound. The contact layer must be removed without being loosened by pre-soaking so that the superficial layer of the wound is ripped away. Effective adherent dressings cause capillary haemorrhage and surface trauma when they are removed.

Wet-to-dry dressings must be changed at least once every 24 h. Dressing changes are painful and should be performed with the patient under general anaesthesia. If excessive exudate is produced and the absorbent layer becomes saturated, the dressing will be ineffective. If this occurs, the dressing should be changed more frequently. Lavage is performed at each dressing change to dislodge exudate and contaminants.

The wet-to-dry dressing is popular as it is perceived to be effective, easy to apply, and inexpensive. However, this form of wound debridement is non-selective, and healthy tissues will also be damaged during dressing changes. Persisting with this form of dressing once granulation tissue has begun to form may delay wound healing, inhibit granulation tissue formation, and prevent epithelialization. Alternative approaches that are less traumatic are gaining in popularity.

Autolytic wound debridement

Autolytic wound debridement utilizes gels and dressings to create an optimum environment for natural autolysis and sloughing of necrotic tissue. Hydrogels are commonly used in combination with other dressings (e.g. foam or hydrocolloid dressings) as they provide a moist environment conducive to enzymatic activity necessary for autolysis. Hydrogels also hydrate desiccated tissue making removal easier. Daily dressing changes are recommended for at least the first few days of wound management to allow inspection of the wound.

Lavage is performed at each dressing change to dislodge exudate and contaminants. Hydrogels opacify as they absorb fluid and can begin to resemble purulent discharge. When evaluating the wound after using a hydrogel, lavage the gel from the wound before making judgements about the health of the underlying tissue.

Manuka honey dressings

Manuka honey dressings provide an alternative method of wound debridement through selective sloughing of necrotic tissue while preserving healthy tissue. The mechanism of action is uncertain but an osmotic effect predominantly affecting damaged cells is thought to account for this process. This form of wound debridement appears to be very effective and may even replace initial surgical debridement (Fig. 7.3). The dressings also reduce local inflammation and pain, and may accelerate wound healing in comparison to other techniques. Honey can be applied directly to the wound surface and held in place with another dressing (e.g. foam dressing) or it can be applied in a honey-impregnated alginate or foam dressing. Wound lavage is performed at each dressing change to dislodge exudate and contaminants.

Recognizing the end point of the debridement phase

As bacteria and devitalized tissues are removed from the wound, the level of exudate drops, marking the start of the proliferative phase of wound healing. During dressing changes, the level of exudate will reduce substantially and buds of granulation tissue may be seen forming on the surface of the wound. The exudate becomes less viscous and less purulent. There should be no more evidence of devitalized tissues within the wound. If wet-to-dry dressings are used, active haemorrhage is seen throughout the wound bed when the contact layer is removed. These features signal the end of this phase of wound management. If the wound does not progress to this stage within 3 or 4 days, it may be because it has become infected or there is still devitalized tissue or detritus.

Commentary

Early debridement remains a controversial area in both veterinary and human wound management. Currently there are few good studies comparing the different approaches. Many of the recommendations made for veterinary wound management are extrapolated from guidelines in man but this transfer of recommendations may be inappropriate. Wound studies in man often evaluate wounds rarely encountered in veterinary patients (such as chronic venous ulcers). Similarly, the definitions of acceptable outcomes between the species make direct comparison difficult. In veterinary patients, major problems with patient tolerance of long-term wound management, and of the financial restrictions that are encountered, must be taken into account. Ultimately, all of the techniques described appear to achieve the goals of encouraging removal of devitalized tissue from the wound. The author favours wet-to-dry dressings, particularly for heavily contaminated wounds, and Manuka honey dressings for less contaminated wounds that have necrotic tissues (e.g. ischaemic wound sloughs). However, evidence may emerge to discredit the wet-to-dry dressing in veterinary wounds. A major advantage of both the autolytic wound debridement and the Manuka honey protocols is that both can be continued into the next stage of wound management, removing the need to actively decide when to change to another form of wound dressing.

Stage 3: encouraging granulation tissue and epithelialization

Granulation tissue formation and epithelialization occur in healthy wounds that are free from infection and necrotic tissue, have a moist wound surface, and are not subject to surface trauma. Following sloughing of devitalized tissue and management of bacterial contamination, a wide range of dressings can be used to protect the surface of the wound and provide a moist wound environment.

Foam dressing with or without hydrogel

Foam dressings are extremely popular and are often used in combination with hydrogels to encourage granulation and epithelialization. Dressing changes are performed every 48–72 h.

Other dressings

Most of the semi-occlusive and occlusive dressings that maintain moisture at the wound surface without allowing skin maceration will encourage granulation and epithelialization. Manuka honey in combination with foam dressings or alginates is also effective. Ultimately, the choice of dressing comes down to personal preference and availability. Ensuring that the dressing is held securely in place without rubbing the surface of the wound, and that the wound is inspected regularly, are probably more important than the type of dressing used.

Monitoring progress

Granulation tissue will begin to form rapidly if the wound environment is conducive to healing. Once the wound is covered in granulation tissue, the edges will start to epithelialize. Healthy granulation tissue (Fig. 7.14A) is recognized as:

- being red;
- being moist;
- having a slightly irregular surface;
- bleeding actively when manipulated;
- producing a low volume of serous exudate; and
- having a rim of advancing epithelium at the edge.

At each dressing change, there should be obvious signs of progression. First, the granulation tissue will fill the wound surface, and then epithelium will migrate from the wound edges. Finally, wound contraction will start at about the time that epithelialization is seen.

In comparison, unhealthy wounds fail to progress and are recognized by the following features:

- pale, flat, dry granulation tissue that does not bleed when manipulated ('chronic granulation tissue') (Fig. 7.14B);
- increase in volume of exudate;
- purulent exudate;
- failure of progression of epithelialization; and
- failure of progression of contraction.

Managing problem wounds

Failure of progression during wound management may be due to a variety of local or systemic factors.

Local wound factors

- persistence of infection;
- retention of foreign debris within the wound bed;
- retention of devitalized tissue;
- surface trauma from poorly applied dressings; and
- wound desiccation through poor choice of dressing.

When assessing the impact of local factors in problem wounds, review the type and manner of application of the dressing. Consider biopsying the wound bed for culture and sensitivity testing. Often, the best course of action is to debride the unhealthy granulation tissue and start again.

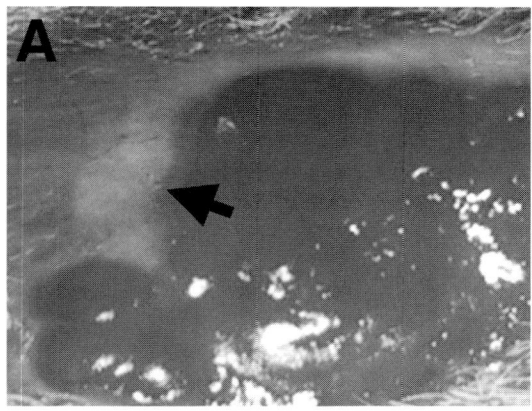

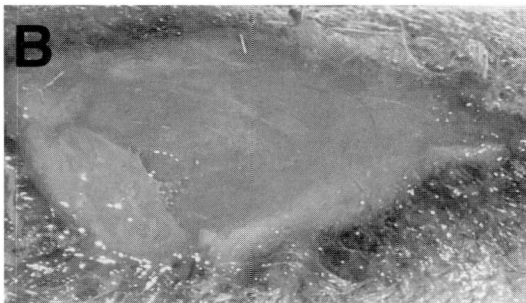

Fig. 7.14. Granulation tissue: (A) healthy wound with healthy granulation tissue (red, moist, uniform in appearance) with epithelialization (arrow); (B) unhealthy granulation bed (pale, dry, no epithelialization, no progression between dressing changes).

Systemic patient factors

A host of patient factors has been associated with delayed wound healing:

- hypoproteinaemia;
- uraemia;
- endocrinopathies;
- chronic debility;
- steroid therapy;
- concurrent disease; and
- states of negative nitrogen balance.

Although much has been made of the potential for these factors to adversely affect wound healing, it is difficult to demonstrate a direct effect of any of these unless extreme examples are evaluated. In reality, most wounds will heal in the face of such systemic problems, but these adverse factors, particularly if several are present in the same patient, may contribute to delayed wound healing.

Wound classification based on nature of injury

Lacerations

Lacerations are caused by sharp objects (e.g. glass; metal) and have less tissue trauma or contamination than other traumatic wounds. These may be amenable to early closure.

Puncture wounds

Puncture wounds are usually caused by bites. Typically, there is a small puncture wound in the skin but much more extensive injury to the underlying tissue. This is because the tooth penetrates skin and embeds in the deeper structures. As the victim moves away, the tooth tears through the underlying tissue causing extensive injury. The skin tends to be dragged over the underlying tissues and sustains less injury. These wounds are usually contaminated. *Pasteurella multocida*, a commensal organism of the feline oral cavity, is often cultured from cat bites. Other organisms include skin commensal bacteria and anaerobic bacteria.

Clip widely over the bite wound to evaluate the extent of the injury. Look for corresponding injuries on the other side of the patient's body. To fully evaluate the wound, incise and explore the bite track, debriding and lavaging the underlying tissues. Consider *en bloc* resection of the injured tissues or close the debrided wound having placed drains to remove any exudate that may form. Prescribe broad-spectrum antimicrobials that include agents with activity against anaerobic organisms, and modify treatment based on the results of culture and sensitivity testing.

Degloving and shearing injuries

Degloving and shearing injuries are associated with extensive tissue loss and contamination. Degloving injuries occur during vehicular trauma when a limb becomes trapped between the road and a wheel. Skin is stripped from the paw leaving a heavily traumatized wound with much devitalized tissue, heavy contamination, and no skin available for reconstruction (Fig. 7.11). Shearing injuries are similar but occur over joints. In addition to skin loss and contamination, ligament and joint capsule are ripped away and fragments are sheared from the bones of the joint (Fig. 7.13A). These injuries cause joint instability and long-term articular defects that will cause degenerative joint disease. Degloving and shearing injuries are always managed initially as open wounds, and many are left to heal by second intention.

Burns

Scalding is quite common in small animal patients and often occurs on the dorsum following spillage of hot drinks. The full extent of the injury takes up to 72 h to become apparent as it takes this period for severely injured skin to show signs of necrosis and sloughing. Initially, affected skin is erythematous and hair may begin to fall out. Lines of demarcation develop progressively and the devitalized skin becomes inelastic, starts to thin, and then sloughs. Burns may be managed as open wounds. Alternatively, many are amenable to *en bloc* resection and primary closure once the lines of demarcation have become apparent. Large burn wounds are prone to infection because commensal organisms on the skin of the patient can penetrate into the underlying tissues over areas where the skin has been lost.

Surgical incisions

Sutured surgical incisions heal rapidly because they have minimal tissue trauma or bacterial contamination. The gap between the apposed tissue edges is also small, so granulation tissue can quickly bridge it. The wound can be covered by a padded film dressing initially, to prevent bacterial contamination while a dry scab forms. Ideally, dressings will be maintained at least while the animal is hospitalized, as it is during this period that the patient is most likely to encounter significant wound pathogens from the environment.

Bibliography

Adams, D.C., Ramsey, M.L. and Marks, V.J. (2004) The running bolster suture for full-thickness skin grafts. *Dermatologic Surgery* 30, 92–94.

Anderson, D. (2003) Wound dressings unraveled. *In Practice* 25, 70–83.

Atiyeh, B.S., Dibo, S.A. and Hayek, S.N. (2009) Wound cleansing, topical antiseptics and wound healing. *International Wound Journal* 6, 420–430.

Bradley, M., Cullum, N., Nelson, E.A., Petticrew, M., Sheldon, T. and Torgerson, D. (1999a) Systematic reviews of wound care management: (2). Dressings and topical agents used in the healing of chronic wounds. *Health Technology Assessment* 3, 1–35.

Bradley, M., Cullum, N. and Sheldon, T. (1999b) The debridement of chronic wounds: a systematic review. *Health Technology Assessment* 3, iii–iv, 1–78.

Campbell, B.G. (2006) Dressings, bandages, and splints for wound management in dogs and cats. *Veterinary Clinics of North America Small Animal Practice* 36, 759–791.

Carville, K., Cuddigan, J., Fletcher, J., Fuchs, P., Harding, K., Ishikawa, O., Keast, D., *et al.* (2008) Wound infection in clinical practice. An international consensus. www.mepltd.co.uk, accessed 16 May 2010.

Dernell, W.S. (2006) Initial wound management. *Veterinary Clinics of North America Small Animal Practice* 36, 713–738.

Dryburgh, N., Smith, F., Donaldson, J. and Mitchell, M. (2008) Debridement for surgical wounds. *Cochrane Database Systematic Review* CD006214, DOI: 10.1002/14651858.CD006214.pub3.

Falabella, A.F. (2006) Debridement and wound bed preparation. *Dermatologic Therapy* 19, 317–325.

Fonder, M.A., Lazarus, G.S., Cowan, D.A., Aronson-Cook, B., Kohli, A.R. and Mamelak, A.J. (2008) Treating the chronic wound: a practical approach to the care of nonhealing wounds and wound care dressings. *Journal of the American Academy of Dermatology* 58, 185–206.

Griffin, G.M. and Holt, D.E. (2001) Dog-bite wounds: bacteriology and treatment outcome in 37 cases. *Journal of the American Animal Hospital Association* 37, 453–460.

Jones, A. and Vaughan, D. (2005) Hydrogel dressings in the management of a variety of wound types: a review. *Journal of Orthopaedic Nursing* 9, S1–11.

Lay-Flurrie, K. (2004) The properties of hydrogel dressings and their impact on wound healing. *Professional Nurse* 19, 269–273.

Lusby, P.E., Coombes, A. and Wilkinson, J.M. (2002) Honey: a potent agent for wound healing? *Journal of Wound Ostomy and Continence Nursing* 29, 295–300.

Meyers, B., Schoeman, J.P., Goddard, A. and Picard, J. (2008) The bacteriology and antimicrobial susceptibility of infected and non-infected dog bite wounds: fifty cases. *Veterinary Microbiology* 127, 360–368.

Mouro, S., Vilela, C.L. and Niza, M.M. (2010) Clinical and bacteriological assessment of dog-to-dog bite wounds. *Veterinary Microbiology* 144, 127–132.

Pavletic, M.M. (1993) Management of specific wounds. In: *Atlas of Small Animal Reconstructive Surgery*, 2nd edn. W.B. Saunders, Philadelphia, Pennsylvania, pp. 65–106.

Rippon, M., White, R. and Davies, P. (2007) Skin adhesives and their role in wound dressings. *Wounds UK* 3, 76–86.

8 Reconstructive Surgery

caudectomy: tail amputation
dehiscence: failure of wound healing leading to breakdown of a sutured wound
onychectomy: nail amputation
primary closure: 'first intention healing'; immediate closure of a wound
second intention healing: 'open wound management'; leaving a wound to close by wound contracture and epithelialization
skin flap: a flap of skin used for reconstruction that remains attached to the donor site by a pedicle from which it gets its blood supply
skin graft: a section of skin that is completely separated from its donor site and applied to a distant wound
tail docking: cosmetic tail amputation

The reader should be able to:

- list the different types of wound healing and when they might be selected for traumatic wounds on the flank and paw
- explain the importance of tension lines when planning wound closure and demonstrate where they run over the lateral neck and over the inguinal skin fold in a dog
- discuss the different methods of skin closure and summarize the advantages and disadvantages of each
- discuss the advantages and disadvantages of the methods of reconstructing large skin defects without generating tension using the terms undermining, walking suture, mattress suture, releasing incision, and advancement flap
- formulate a surgical plan for the excision of a 2 cm circular skin mass on the flank of a large dog with a 0.5 cm margin of normal tissue and without generating dog-ears or tension within the wound
- recognize patients that require advanced reconstructive surgery
- describe the key steps for digit amputation, hind limb amputation, and forequarter amputation in the dog

Types of Wound Closure

Wounds can be closed using a variety of reconstructive techniques, or left to heal by contraction and epithelialization. The principle forms of wound closure are shown below.

Primary closure

The wound is closed immediately after it is created, usually by direct apposition and suturing of its edges. Primary closure is performed on almost all surgical wounds (from coeliotomy incisions to tumour resections). It may also be considered for some traumatic wounds, particularly if there is minimal tissue compromise and very little contamination, or if all diseased tissues can be sharply debrided to leave a healthy wound bed.

Second intention healing

The wound is managed as an open wound until it closes by contraction and epithelialization. Initial wound management generates a healthy granulation bed. Wound management is extended using non-adherent dressings until the wound heals (see Chapter 7). This is an extremely versatile method of wound closure and is employed extensively in veterinary medicine, particularly for traumatic wounds on the distal limb where there is little free skin to facilitate surgical closure.

In comparison to primary closure, the advantages of second intention healing are that it:

- can be applied to most wounds;
- enables infection and devitalized tissue to be managed;
- overcomes problems of insufficient skin to perform primary closure; and
- does not require advanced surgical skills.

In comparison to primary closure, the disadvantages of second intention healing are that:

- it requires protracted wound management;
- it generates skin with thin epithelium and no hair, that is easily traumatized. As the wound matures, the epithelium thickens and the wound contracts, increasing the resistance to trauma;
- scarring near joints may limit movement;
- scarring near the eye or anus may cause distortion of the orifices; and
- large wounds may not close completely.

Delayed primary closure

The wound is managed for a few days until infection and devitalized tissue have been removed and is then closed (often at the time that granulation tissue has begun to form). This is underutilized in veterinary surgery but is very good for traumatic wounds with moderate tissue compromise or contamination. It has the advantage over primary closure that infection and devitalized tissue are managed prior to closure, reducing the risk of dehiscence. It has the advantage over second intention healing that it is quicker.

Application of wound closure methods

Most wounds in dogs and cats can be closed easily using either primary closure or second intention healing. Primary closure is usually simple to perform because the skin of dogs and cats is elastic, is abundant over areas such as the trunk, and has a vascular supply that supports undermining and advancement of the skin edges. When second intention healing is used, the results are generally good, as scarring is not excessive (in comparison to man) and the functional outcome, rather than the cosmetic one, is the primary concern. This chapter describes the principles of reconstructive surgery and how primary and second intention healing may be applied to veterinary wounds. More advanced reconstructive techniques and their applications are described in sufficient detail for the veterinarian to discuss the potential merits and disadvantages prior to referral.

Principles of Reconstructive Surgery

To perform successful reconstructive surgery, careful planning and meticulous attention to basic surgical principles are important. In particular, *careful tissue handling*, *control of dead space*, and *avoidance of tension* are critical.

Clip and drape widely

Clipping and draping widely around the area to be reconstructed ensures that there is adequate exposure to assess the wound intra-operatively and to perform key techniques such as undermining and advancement of the skin edges. It also reduces the risks of contamination of the wound.

Minimize tissue trauma

Minimizing tissue trauma when handling skin reduces inflammation and bruising and will help promote uncomplicated wound healing. Select the appropriate instruments to handle tissues (see Chapter 5). Consider using *stay sutures* as an alternative to forceps to manipulate skin as they cause less trauma over repeated manipulations (Fig. 8.1). Prevent tissues from desiccating. Use sharp cutting instruments (e.g. fresh scalpel blade) to make incisions.

Dissect under the panniculus muscle

The panniculus muscle (cutaneous trunci muscle; platysma) covers most of the trunk and much of the face. It lies in the subcutaneous fat and is identified as a thin layer of muscle just below the skin surface (Fig. 8.2). Direct cutaneous arteries run up to the panniculus muscle from the underlying tissues. From here, these vessels spread out to form the subdermal plexus of vessels that

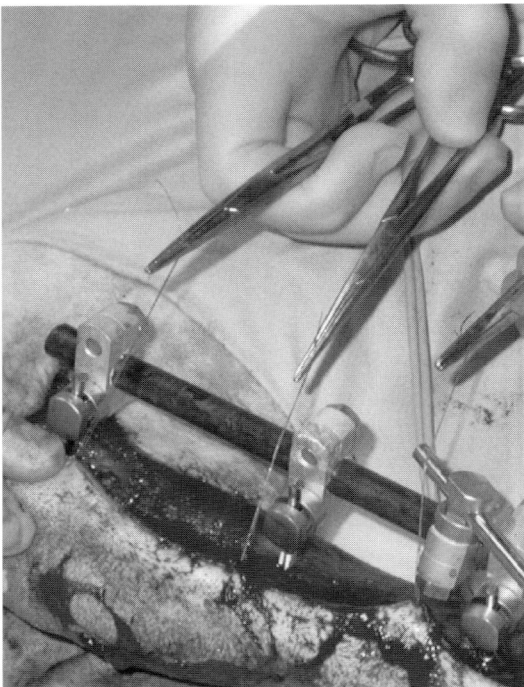

Fig. 8.1. Three stay sutures used to manipulate a skin edge during reconstructive surgery around this external fixator frame.

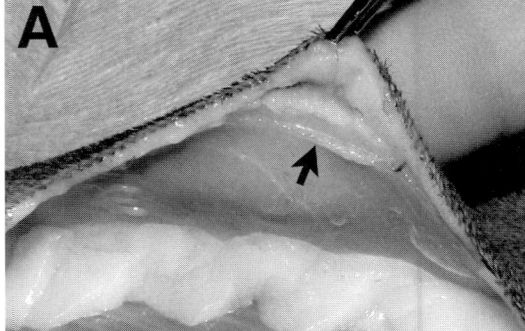

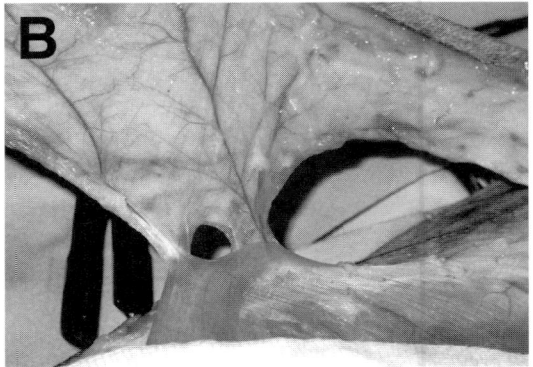

Fig. 8.2. Panniculus muscle and vascular supply to skin: (A) panniculus muscle just below the dermis in the subcutaneous fat (arrow); (B) direct cutaneous vessels running up from the underlying muscles to the level of the panniculus muscle before spreading out to supply the skin and plane of dissection to preserve this vascular supply.

provides the blood supply to the skin. The panniculus muscle serves as a useful landmark for skin dissection and reconstruction. *Dissect below the level of the panniculus muscle* as this causes minimal disruption to the skin's blood supply. In areas where there is no panniculus muscle (e.g. over the limbs, ventral midline, areas of the head), elevate tissues directly off the underlying musculoskeletal structures to preserve the more superficial subdermal plexus.

Avoid tension

Suturing wounds under tension inevitably leads to dehiscence. Tension across suture lines causes vascular compromise, inflammation, and necrosis of the skin edge and these predispose to infection and dehiscence. There are natural lines of tension running through the skin, and tension is also created when large skin defects are closed. Careful preoperative planning and application of simple principles help to overcome or avoid wound tension.

Orientate and close wounds parallel to tension lines

Tension lines run through the skin all over the body and are generated by the attachments of skin to the underlying tissues, by gravity, and by movement (particularly around joints). Tension lines have been mapped out in complex diagrams (Fig. 8.3) but are also easily assessed by skin manipulation. Manipulating skin in the same direction as the tension line demonstrates that there is no free skin in this orientation to close the wound. However, manipulating skin either side of the tension line demonstrates that there is mobile skin for reconstruction on either side of the tension line (Fig. 8.4). Make skin incisions *parallel to tension lines* to take advantage of this. Do not generate incisions that run perpendicular to tension lines as these are

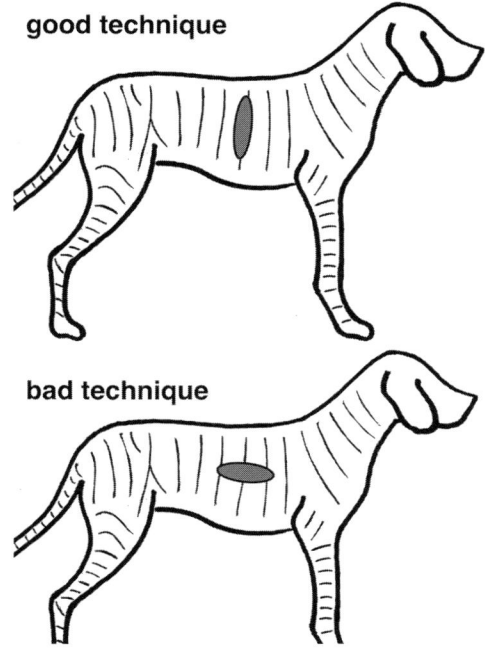

good technique

bad technique

Fig. 8.3. Tension line diagram used to plan incisions (shaded ovals represent elliptical incisions): make incisions parallel to tension lines, not perpendicular to them.

inevitably subjected to tension and are likely to dehisce.

Tension lines can be difficult to assess near areas of high motion (e.g. proximal limb) and may change with limb movement. When closing a wound in these regions, clip and drape the limb into the surgical field so that it can be manipulated during wound closure to assess how tension changes with limb movement.

Undermining and walking sutures

The techniques of undermining skin and placing walking sutures are highly effective at reducing and evenly distributing tension in the wound. Undermining involves freeing the edge of the skin wound from its underlying attachments by bluntly dissecting below the panniculus muscle. This increases the mobility of the skin edge bordering the wound and enables it to be moved further across the wound, reducing tension along the suture line. If large vessels are encountered during dissection coming from the deeper structures to the skin, try to preserve these to maintain the vascular supply to skin.

Walking sutures are placed after undermining to help distribute tension evenly through the wound

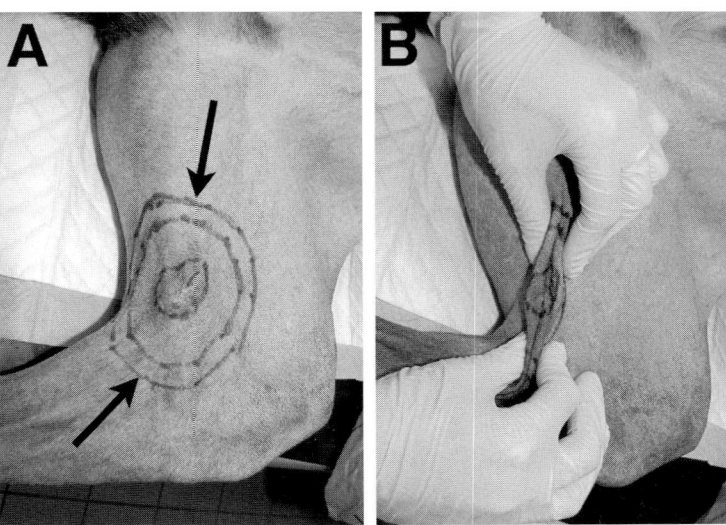

Fig. 8.4. Tension lines can be assessed by direct manipulation of skin. Figure shows preoperative view of sarcoma on the medial thigh. The lines represent the planned resection margins. (A) Manipulating the wound demonstrates that the tension line runs dorsoventrally through the planned incision site, as the edges of the marked area of skin cannot be drawn together in the direction of the arrows. (B) In contrast, the edges of the planned incision can be brought together orientated parallel to the tension line. The wound was closed in this orientation.

and to hold the undermined skin in its new position. The undermined skin is advanced towards the centre of the wound and anchored in place by suturing the subcutaneous fascia of the mobile skin to the fixed fascia of underlying muscle or fascia (Fig. 8.5). Place a row of walking sutures halfway from the edge of the incision to the depths of the undermined tissue plane. Place several walking sutures along this line, spaced approximately 2 cm apart to distribute the tension evenly at several points. Place a second line of walking sutures closer to the free edge of skin if further advancement is required (Fig. 8.6). Use monofilament, absorbable suture material (e.g. poli-glecaprone; polydioxanone II). It is important to ensure that the walking suture does not penetrate through the skin to the surface, as this acts as a route of bacterial contamination of the underlying tissues.

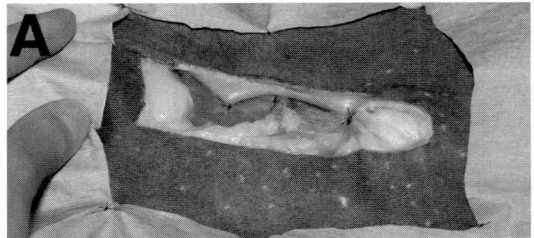
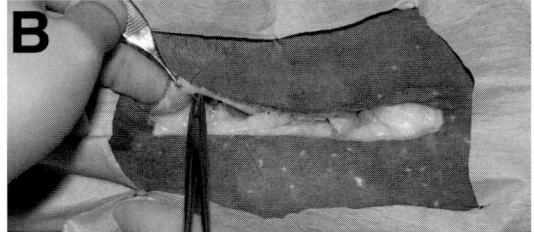
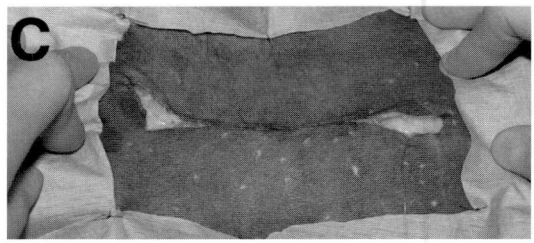

Fig. 8.6. Undermining and walking sutures 2: (A) the first layer of walking suture advances the skin edge towards the centre of the wound and distributes tension evenly between the walking sutures; (B and C) a second line of walking sutures is used to advance the skin edge over the entire wound.

Layered wound closure

Wounds that extend below the subcutaneous tissues into deeper fascial planes may benefit from layered closure (Fig. 8.7). Advancement and closure of each incised fascial plane helps to distribute tension throughout the deeper layers of the wound and to alleviate tension on the skin suture lines. As skin is intimately associated with the deeper tissues, advancing and closing the deeper layers helps advance the incised skin edge towards the centre of the wound.

Tension-relieving suture patterns

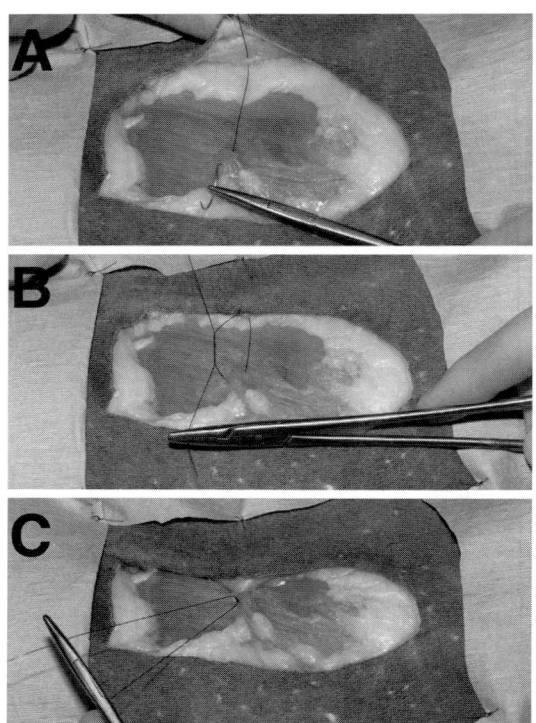

Fig. 8.5. Undermining and walking sutures 1. This skin defect has been undermined and is being closed using walking sutures: (A) take a bite of subcutaneous fascia (panniculus muscle in this case) and a bite of deeper fascia near to the centre of the wound; (B) tie a knot and tighten; (C) the skin edge advances towards the centre of the wound.

Tension-relieving suture patterns can be used to reconstruct deeper layers of a wound and to manage mild or moderate tension along the skin suture line (see p. 46). Continuous suture lines also relieve

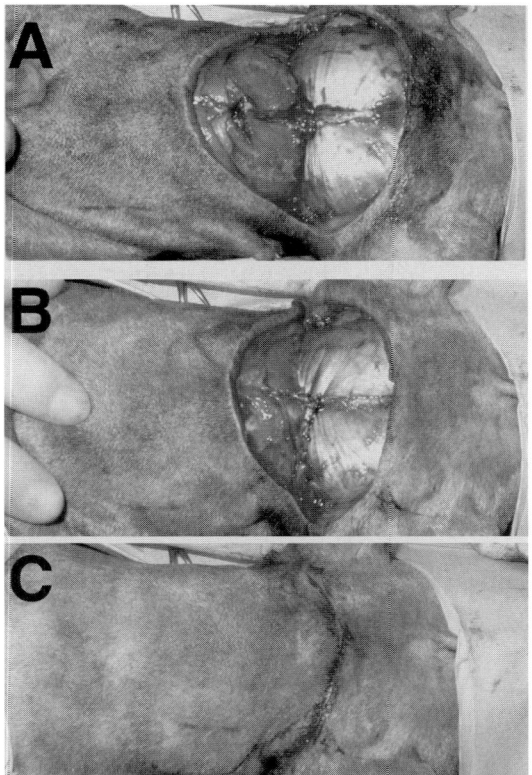

Fig. 8.7. Example of layered wound closure: the images demonstrate the effect of the first (deep) (A–B) and second (superficial) layer of closure (B–C) with progressive advancement of the skin edge.

tension by distributing tension along the entire suture line. These can be used to accommodate mild tension, particularly when used to close the panniculus muscle, the subcutaneous fat, and skin, separately.

Mattress sutures distribute tension over a wider area than other forms of interrupted suture and are classed as tension-relieving sutures. Popular forms of mattress suture include the horizontal, vertical, and cruciate patterns. However, when mattress sutures are used to reconstruct wounds with moderate or marked tension, ischaemia and necrosis may develop where the suture compresses skin, leading to wound complications. To reduce this effect, stents can be used to distribute pressure from the mattress suture over a wider footprint of skin (Fig. 4.18). Mattress sutures also tend to evert the wound edge and this impairs wound healing.

In general, it is best to avoid using mattress sutures and to deal with tension prior to closing skin using other techniques.

Releasing incisions

Releasing incisions are incisions made adjacent to a wound to allow further advancement of the wound edge to relieve tension. The major disadvantage of releasing incisions is that they generate new wounds to close the primary wound. Meshing the skin edge is an example of the use of releasing incision to relieve tension (Fig. 8.8). Although releasing incisions can be useful when reconstructing wounds, they are difficult to apply effectively and may cause wound healing complications, for example, by disrupting the vascular supply to the wound edge. Use other methods of dealing with tension in preference to releasing incisions.

Performing partial wound closure

An underutilized but effective method of avoiding tension is partial wound closure. If a wound cannot be closed completely without generating tension, partially close the wound and manage the remaining area by second intention healing (Fig. 8.9). This reduces the risk of dehiscence as the suture lines are

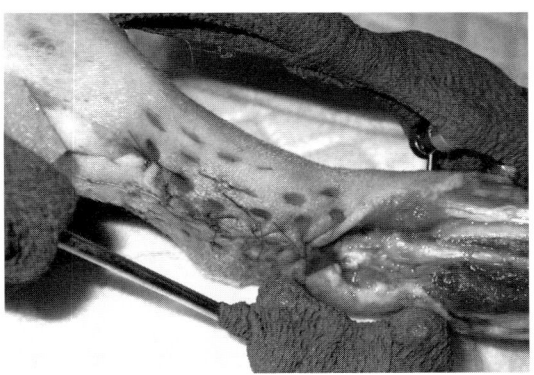

Fig. 8.8. Meshed skin incision: the meshed area of skin can be stretched and advanced. Make 2 or 3 staggered rows of releasing incisions. The incisions should be 5–10 mm in length and spaced 10 mm apart. This technique can work well and leaves a series of small wounds that quickly contract and heal by second intention. However, the incisions reduce the vascular supply to the skin edge (staggering the rows aims to overcome this).

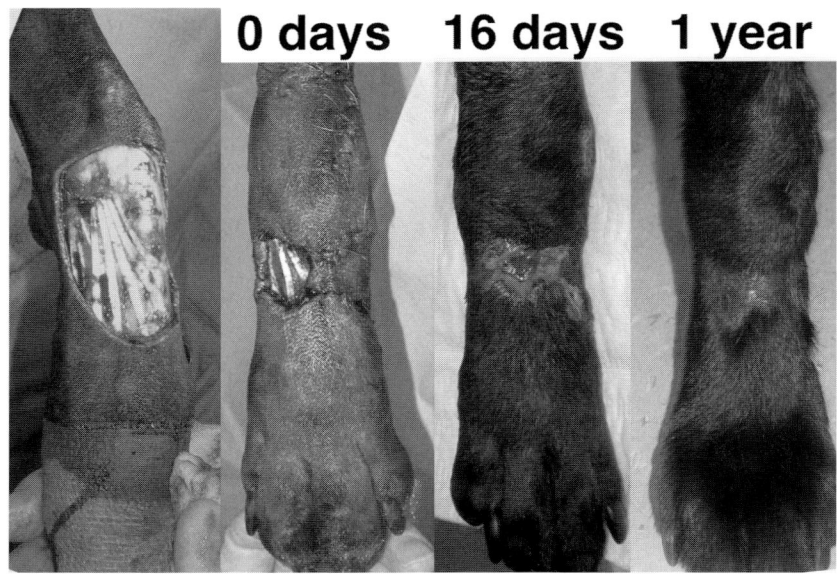

Fig. 8.9. Partial wound closure: mast cell tumour excision from carpus. The wound could be partly reconstructed using local flaps but attempting to appose the wound edges completely led to excessive tension. Instead, 80% of the wound was closed using local skin flaps and the remainder of the wound was left to heal by second intention. By 16 days post-operatively, the wound had developed a healthy granulation bed and had contracted dramatically. When re-evaluated 12 months later, the cosmetic and functional results were excellent and the wound was covered by normal skin.

not under tension, and accelerates the speed of second intention healing as the area of open wound is reduced.

Materials and patterns for skin closure

Several techniques can be used to appose the skin edges and the decision about which to use is based on a variety of patient, wound, and surgeon factors. The presence of subcutaneous fat is important for supporting wound healing, and subcutaneous fat is usually apposed using a simple continuous suture pattern. If the panniculus muscle is present, this should be incorporated into the subcutaneous closure as it provides further support to the wound. Use 2-0 to 4-0 monofilament, short-acting suture material (e.g. poliglecaprone).

Intradermal suture pattern

The intradermal suture pattern has become very popular for routine wound closure as it is quicker to place than simple interrupted sutures, suture

removal is not necessary, and patients cannot interfere with the suture line easily (see Chapter 4). The pattern also produces a very cosmetic wound closure when applied properly. It is particularly useful in sites where skin sutures will cause irritation (e.g. castration incision) or in patients who are fractious and will resent having stitches or staples removed. The pattern is easiest to place in patients that have quite thick skin. In thin-skinned animals, it is difficult to anchor the suture into the dermis without penetrating all the way through the skin. Use 3-0 or 4-0 short-acting, monofilament, synthetic material (e.g. poliglecaprone) on a swaged-on, reverse cutting, or taper-cut needle.

Appositional skin sutures

The simple interrupted pattern is the most versatile suture pattern for skin reconstruction and can be adapted to close any wound. It can be used to close two wound edges of unequal length (a common clinical scenario) by spacing sutures slightly wider apart on the longer side of the incision. Use 2-0 to

Chapter 8

4-0 non-absorbable, synthetic, monofilament suture material (e.g. polyamide; polypropylene). Sutures must be left in place for a minimum of 7 days. Routinely, they are removed 10–14 days post-operatively to give time for the wound to regain inherent strength.

Cruciate mattress sutures

Cruciate mattress sutures are popular for skin closure because they achieve a similar effect to simple interrupted sutures but are quicker to place. They are tightened only sufficiently to appose skin edges rather than to relieve tension, but may still cause some tissue eversion. Use the same range of suture materials and sizes described for simple interrupted skin sutures.

Skin staples

Skin staples are used to rapidly appose the skin edges. They are made of materials such as stainless steel and are applied using a multi-staple applicator (Fig. 8.10). However, for rapid, easy placement the subcutaneous tissues must have been reconstructed well and be holding the skin edges in reasonable apposition. The staples also tend to swivel round in the skin, making subsequent removal difficult. To place skin sutures, reconstruct the subcutaneous tissues so that the skin edges are sitting in close apposition. If the skin edges are gaping, use thumb forceps to hold them in apposition prior to applying the staple. Staple removers are required to remove staples.

Reconstructing circular wounds using elliptical incisions

Circular wounds are often generated following tumour removal and direct apposition of the edges of the incision is likely to generate 'dog-ears'. Dog-ears are proud folds of skin that form at the ends of sutured wounds where excess skin crumples. Converting circular wounds into long, elliptical incisions makes closure easier as the skin edges appose without forming dog-ears. If generating elliptical incisions, orientate the incision so that the long axis runs parallel to the tension line. Make the incision at least three times the width of the defect (Fig. 8.11).

The disadvantage of converting a circular incision into an elliptical one is that it generates a

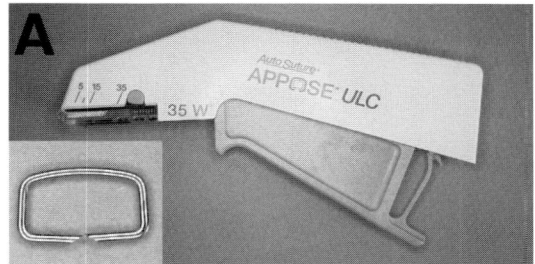
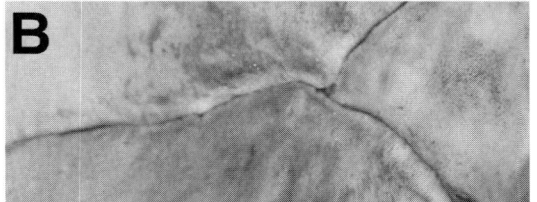
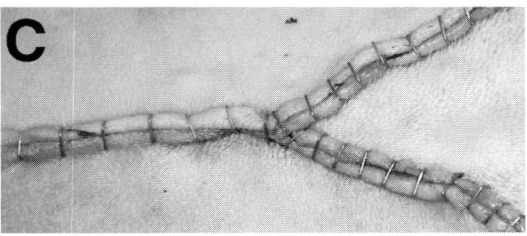

Fig. 8.10. Skin staples: (A) stapler and magnified view of staple. Applying staples: (B) reconstruct the subcutaneous tissues so that the skin edges lie in close apposition before (C) applying staples.

much bigger wound. Dog-ears are also of little clinical significance and remodel in the first few weeks following surgery. For inexperienced surgeons, creating elliptical wounds makes subsequent wound closure straightforward. More experienced surgeons may choose to just resect the tissue required to achieve the primary goal of surgery (e.g. tumour resection) and to reconstruct the wound using a combination of simple techniques without resorting to enlarging the wound into an elliptical incision.

Advanced reconstructive techniques

Advanced techniques used to manage large skin defects overcome tension by transferring skin from other parts of the body into the wound. Creating an advancement flap is a simple procedure but the other techniques described here require experience to plan and perform effectively.

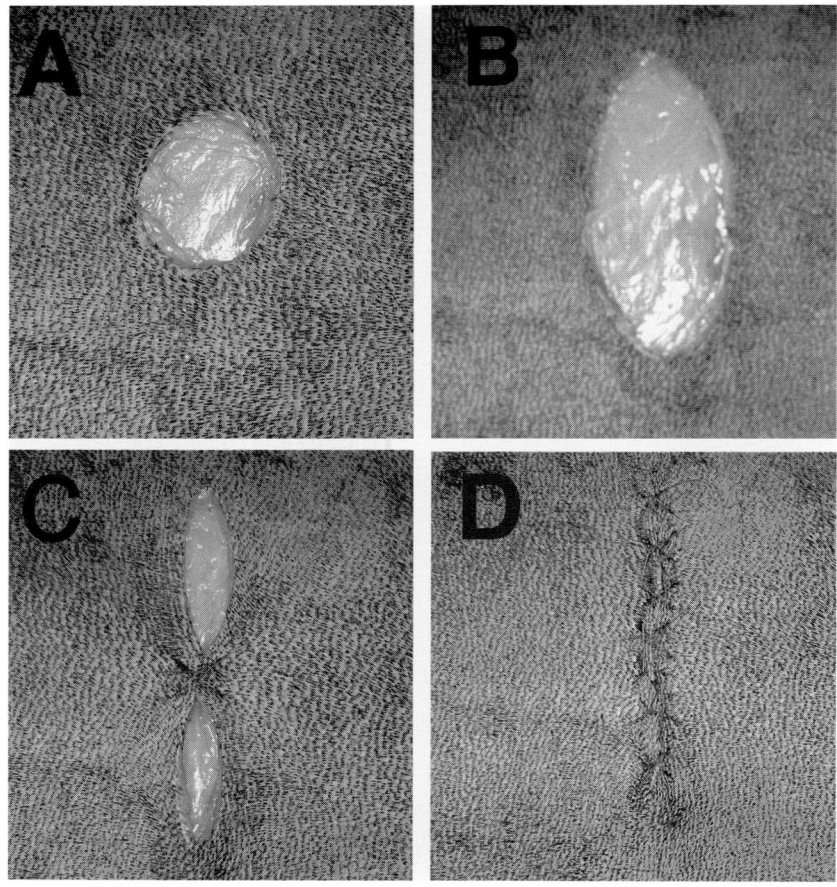

Fig. 8.11. Elliptical incision: (A) example of a circular wound; (B) convert the wound into an elliptical incision that is at least three times longer than the width of the wound; (C) start reconstructing the wound by apposing the skin in the centre of the incision; (D) completed closure without dog-ear formation.

Subdermal plexus flaps (simple flaps)

Subdermal plexus flaps mobilize skin adjacent to the wound and transfer it into the wound for closure. These can be used when there is abundant loose skin adjacent to the wound bed, but where simple undermining and advancement is insufficient to close the wound. The blood supply to the flap runs through the subdermal plexus entering the base of the flap (which remains attached to the donor site) and may be insufficient to ensure survival of the tip of the flap. These flaps are prone to vascular necrosis of their tips if excessive tissue is mobilized and this limits the length of flap that can be generated.

The *advancement flap* is the simplest of all skin flaps and is suitable for inexperienced clinicians to perform. A rectangle of skin is undermined and advanced from the wound edge into the skin defect (Figs 8.12 and 8.13). This flap has the advantage of not creating a wound at the donor site to close. However, the flap tends to recoil back towards its original position and this can lead to distortion of tissues (e.g. palpebral fissure when used to reconstruct the eyelid) (Fig. 8.14).

Other more complex forms of subdermal plexus flap include transposition, translation, and rotation flaps (see Fig. 8.15). These flaps generate a separate wound at the donor site where the flap is harvested but enable skin to be moved further than simple advancement flaps and do not suffer from elastic recoil.

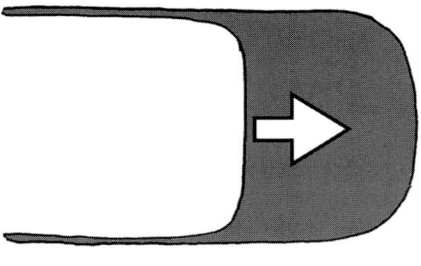

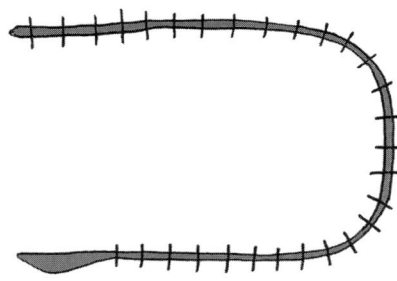

Fig. 8.12. Advancement flap diagram.

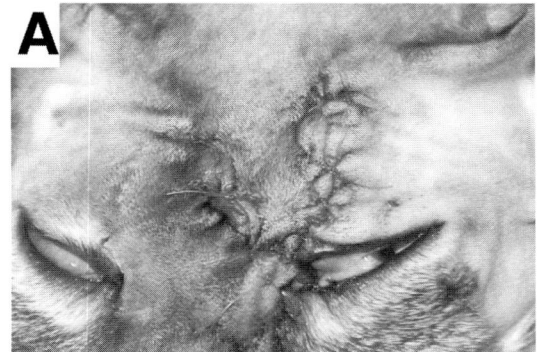

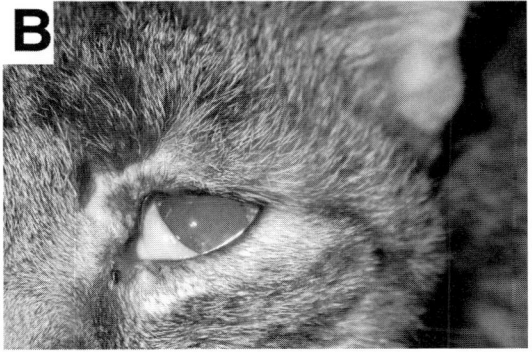

Fig. 8.14. Advancement flap with elastic recoil of edge: (A) advancement flap to reconstruct lid margin following mass removal; (B) elastic recoil led to distortion of the lid margin – a common complication of the advancement flap.

Axial pattern flaps (complex flaps)

Axial pattern flaps are large skin flaps that incorporate a large axial blood vessel to supply blood to the flap. These flaps are created over large subcutaneous blood vessels such as the caudal superficial epigastric artery. The skin flap and vessel are elevated together and the flap remains attached to the body where the blood vessel enters the base of the flap. Long skin flaps can be generated and moved over greater distances than subdermal plexus flaps because they receive a robust blood supply directly from the axial vessel (Fig. 8.16).

Free skin grafts

Skin grafting involves completely detaching a portion of skin from the flank and transferring it to another site, usually the distal limb (Fig. 8.17).

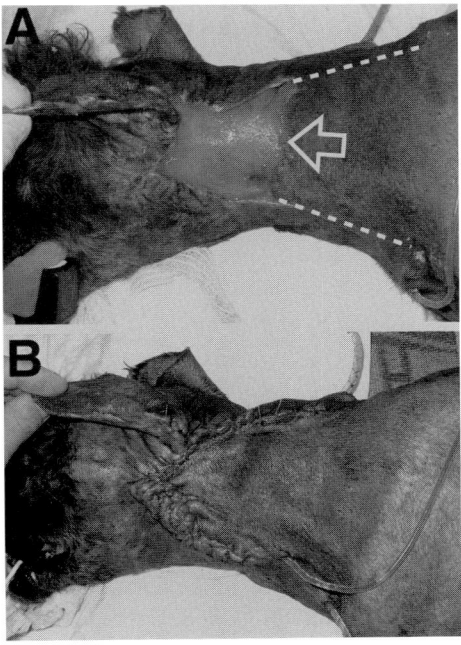

Fig. 8.13. Large advancement flap to close neck wound (lines delineate flap margin; arrow shows direction of advancement).

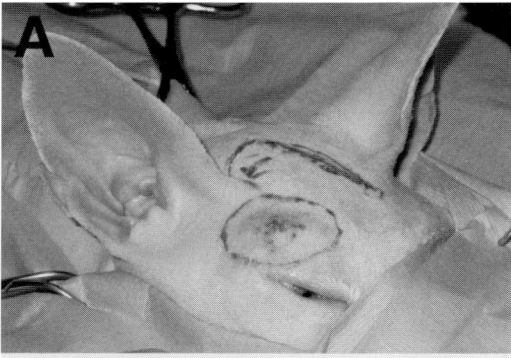

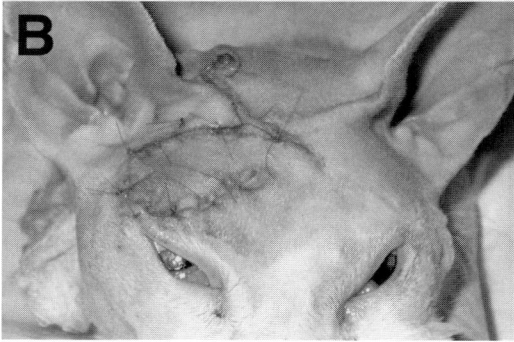

Fig. 8.15. Transposition flap: (A) actinic keratosis on the upper eyelid with resection line and skin flap mapped out. Transposition flaps share a common border with the skin defect that they fill; (B) flap in place following resection of the lesion.

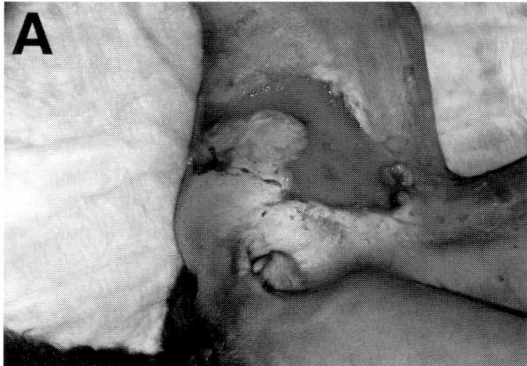

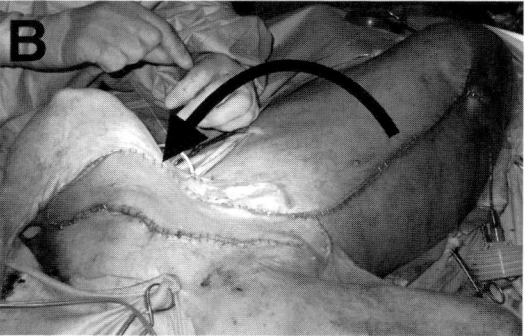

Fig. 8.16. Caudal superficial epigastric axial pattern flap: (A) large skin wound on the medial thigh; (B) axial pattern flap transposed to fill the medial thigh skin defect. The caudal superficial epigastric axial pattern flap mobilizes the skin of the caudal four mammary glands in the dog as a large flap with its base near the inguinal canal where the vessel originates. The flap has been rotated into the inguinal region (arrow) to fill the defect. The donor site has been closed by undermining and apposition of the wound edges.

The skin graft must re-establish a new blood supply from the wound bed by ingrowth of blood vessels before it undergoes ischaemic necrosis. Skin grafts are very effective at closing large skin defects but will fail: (i) if they are badly harvested; (ii) if there is movement between the graft and the wound bed; or (iii) if the wound bed is not healthy and well vascularized. Grafts are generally placed onto healthy granulation beds at the recipient site. The wound requires active management to generate a healthy granulation bed before the graft is placed and the graft requires three weeks of intensive dressing management to ensure survival. Skin grafting can become a protracted and expensive method of wound closure but has a high success rate in experienced hands.

Free meshed skin grafting is occasionally performed in general practice by experienced clinicians, and simpler graft techniques are technically less demanding. However, skin grafting should not be performed by inexperienced clinicians. Refer cases to an experienced colleague or specialist centre.

Reconstruction of Difficult Wounds

Large skin defects, wounds on the distal limb, and wounds near orifices are more difficult to manage than small wounds over the proximal limb or body.

Distal limb wounds

Wounds on the distal limb are difficult to manage because there is no spare skin for simple wound closure. The distal limb is, however, easily bandaged

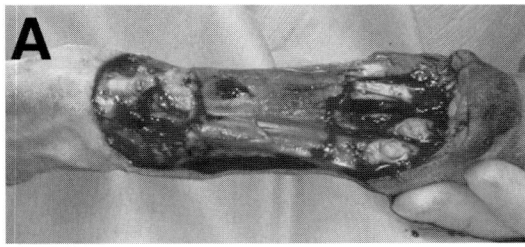

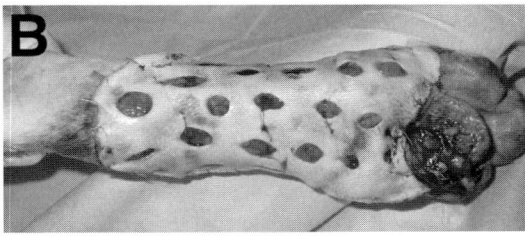

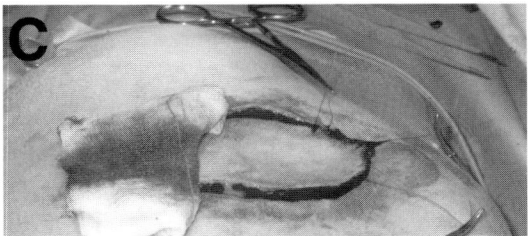

Fig. 8.17. Free meshed skin graft: (A) wound extending from below the tarsus to digits (plantar aspect); (B) free meshed skin graft in place; (C) harvesting the graft from the thoracic wall.

making wound management easier than at other sites. Two techniques are used extensively: (i) second intention healing; and (ii) free meshed skin grafting.

Second intention healing has the advantages that it requires no specialist skill or equipment and is an extension of basic wound management. However, the newly formed skin is thin and easily traumatized. Contraction of the scar may impair joint function but this is uncommon. Second intention healing remains a very good method of managing distal skin wounds in general practice but can become protracted and expensive.

Free meshed skin grafting is technically more demanding but provides a thicker covering of skin and a better hair coat than second intention healing, so ultimately resists trauma better. There is also less wound contraction. As skin grafts require complete immobility following placement to allow vessel ingrowth, the distal limb is ideally suited for their application as bandages can be applied easily.

Large defects over the trunk and proximal limb

Small- and medium-sized defects over the trunk are easily closed by simple apposition of wound edges as there is generally plenty of loose skin in the area to use for reconstruction. Large wounds can be managed by partial wound closure or using axial pattern flaps. Partial wound closure has similar advantages and disadvantages to second intention healing on the distal limb. One major issue is that the trunk and proximal limb are difficult to bandage. Tie-over bolus dressings are often used in preference to body wrap bandages in these areas. Axial pattern flaps, for example the caudal superficial epigastric and thoracodorsal flaps, are reliable and very effective but require careful planning and execution to be effective. These are generally not performed in general practice.

Wounds around the anus and over the face

Wounds near the anus and eyes are difficult to manage as, although there is free skin in the area, wound distortion can lead to functional problems. If simple closure is not possible, advancement and transposition flaps can be used but require careful planning.

Amputations: Limb, Digit, and Tail

Amputation is a 'salvage procedure' that is performed usually as a last resort when other treatments have failed. The advantages of amputation are that it is simple, quick, effective, inexpensive, and requires less aftercare than reconstructive surgeries. The disadvantages are that it is irreversible and affects mobility.

Indications for amputation include:

- primary bone tumour;
- malignant soft tissue tumour of the distal limb;
- large skin defects over the distal limb;
- complex fractures or luxations of the limb; and
- end-stage osteoarthritis affecting a single limb; and
- radial nerve, sciatic nerve, or brachial plexus injuries.

Before performing amputation, it is necessary to evaluate the patient for pre-existing neurological and orthopaedic diseases that may be exacerbated by loss of a digit or a limb. Small breed dogs and cats cope well with limb amputation and adapt quickly. Large breed dogs cope reasonably with limb amputation if they do not have pre-existing orthopaedic disease but are more likely to have ongoing mobility issues. Dogs and cats cope well with digit amputation providing that the main weight-bearing digits (digits 3 and 4 of each foot) are not removed. If digits 3 or 4 are removed, or if more than one weight-bearing digit is removed from a single foot, lameness may occur post-operatively.

Surgical techniques

There is a variety of methods for performing limb amputation. Forequarter amputation (removal of the forelimb with scapula) and mid-femoral hind limb amputation are described because these are simple and effective. For proximal limb tumours, more extensive hind limb amputation may be indicated, including removal of the entire femur and proximal hind limb muscles from the pelvis. This is a more demanding surgery that should be referred to an experienced colleague.

Forequarter amputation

Clip the forelimb from distal to the elbow up to the thoracic wall. Extend the clip from the sternum to the dorsum, and to several centimetres beyond the cranial and caudal edges of the scapula. Bandage the lower, unclipped limb and drape the limb into the surgical field.

Free the scapula dorsally

Make a skin incision along the scapula spine from dorsally to ventrally. When the acromion process is reached, extend the incision in a circular fashion around the proximal humerus (Fig. 8.18A). Sharply incise down onto the scapular spine and retract the skin and subcutaneous fat to expose the scapula and muscular attachments. Identify the most superficial layer muscle attached along the entire cranial edge of the scapular spine (omotransversarius and trapezius muscles) and the continuation of the insertion of the fan-shaped trapezius muscle as it runs dorsally around the top and onto the proximal third of the caudal edge of the scapula spine. Incise the insertion of the omotransversarius and trapezius muscles onto the scapula spine and bluntly dissect the muscles away from the scapula (Fig. 8.18B). Pull the dorsal scapula away from the thoracic wall to expose the rhomboideus muscle attaching along a broad insertion on the dorsal medial aspect of the scapula. Incise this with a scalpel as it inserts onto the scapula and use a

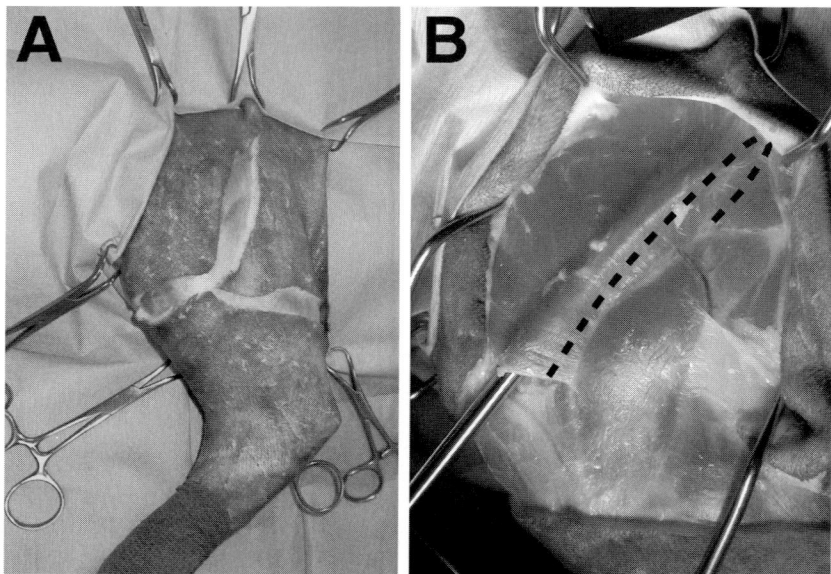

Fig. 8.18. Forequarter amputation 1: (A) make a skin incision along the scapula spine and encircling the proximal limb; (B) transect omotransversarius and trapezius muscles from their attachments to the scapula spine (dotted line).

periosteal elevator to remove the muscular insertion from the scapula. This mobilizes the scapula leaving it attached distally by the subcutaneous tissues, brachial plexus, axillary vessels, and some muscles (Fig. 8.19).

Ligate the vascular supply

Pull the dorsal scapula laterally and ventrally and bluntly dissect the medial fascia to expose the brachial plexus and axillary vessels. Identify the axillary vessels that are partly covered by nerve bundles of the caudal brachial plexus, and ligate the axillary artery and vein separately using the three-ligature technique (Fig. 4.9). Instill local anaesthetic into the brachial plexus nerve bundles and transect them one at a time (Fig. 8.20).

Complete the amputation

Continue to dissect the subcutaneous fat and skin away from the distal scapula and humerus. Work around the proximal humerus incising the brachiocephalicus cranially, the pectoral muscles medially, and the latissimus dorsi muscle caudally (Fig. 8.20). Ligate any large vessels as they are encountered. Once the soft tissues have been

resected from the humerus and scapula, the limb can be removed.

Reconstruct the wound

Suture the incised muscles to the deeper thoracic wall muscles and to each other, bringing the elevated insertions in towards the centre of the wound. Close the subcutaneous tissues and skin in an inverted 'Y' pattern (Fig. 8.20). Close dead space with tacking sutures as each layer of tissue is reconstructed. Consider placing a drain in the deeper layers of the wound.

Hind limb amputation

Position the patient in lateral recumbency. Clip the limb from distal to the stifle to the pelvis and extend the clip to the dorsal and ventral midlines. Extend the clip to the perineal fossa caudally and to include the flank skin fold medially.

Skin incision

Make a curvilinear skin incision from the cranial to the caudal aspect of the mid-lateral thigh to preserve a flap of skin from the lateral thigh for

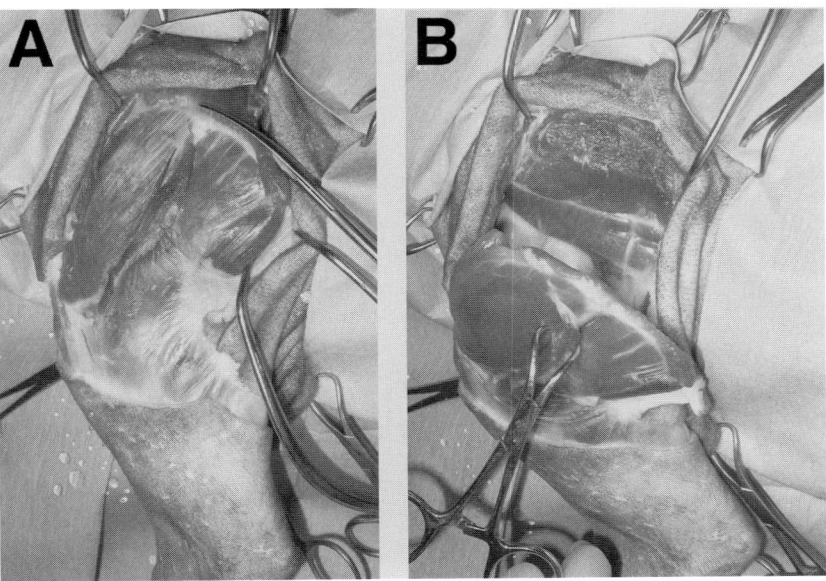

Fig. 8.19. Forequarter amputation 2: (A) elevate the rhomboideus muscle to free the scapula medially; (B) retract the scapula away from the body to expose the medial structures.

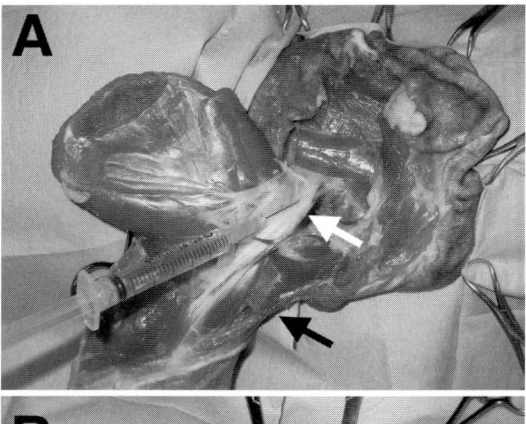

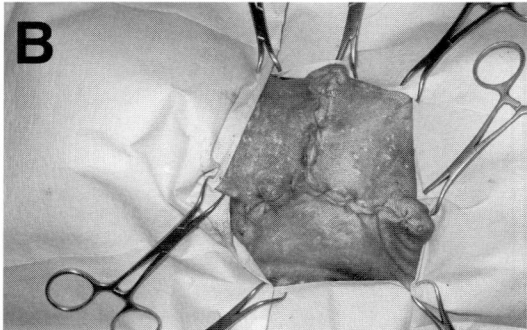

Fig. 8.20. Forequarter amputation 3: (A) instill local anaesthetic into the nerves of the brachial plexus and transect them; isolate the axillary vessels and double ligate and transect them (white arrow); incise the remaining muscular attachments to the forelimb (black arrow); (B) reconstruct the wound in an inverted 'Y' pattern.

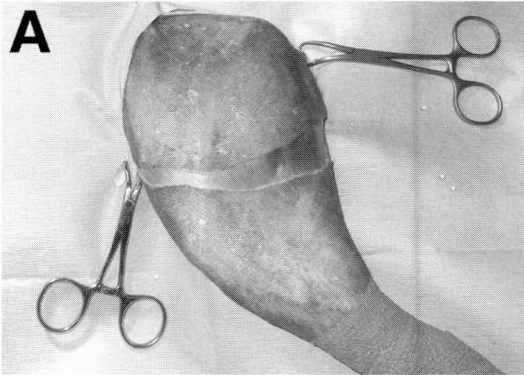

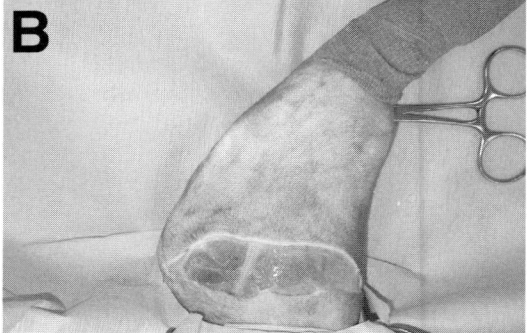

Fig. 8.21. Hind limb amputation 1: incise the skin around the thigh preserving more skin laterally (A) to facilitate reconstruction, and avoiding damage to the underlying femoral vessels medially (B).

closure. Extend this incision medially to encircle the proximal limb (Fig. 8.21).

Isolate the femoral vessels

Abduct the limb to expose the medial thigh. Feel for the femoral pulse within the femoral triangle just caudal to the pectineus muscle. Sectioning the pectineus muscle helps mobilize the limb but take care not to damage the adjacent femoral vessels. Bluntly dissect to expose the femoral artery vein and nerve (Fig. 8.22). Ligate the femoral artery and vein separately using the three-ligature technique (Fig. 4.9). Instill local anaesthetic into the femoral nerve before transecting it.

Transect the muscles of the medial thigh

Using a scalpel blade and diathermy, sharply transect the medial muscle bellies at the level of the

mid femur. Be careful not to damage the ligated stumps of the femoral vessels and ligate other vessels as they are encountered.

Transect the muscles of the lateral thigh

Reposition the limb in a neutral position and transect the tensor fascia lata and the muscles of the lateral thigh. Instill local anaesthetic into the sciatic nerve (between the femur and the biceps femoris muscle) before transecting it (Fig. 8.23).

Complete amputation by cutting the femur

Once the muscle attachments are transected, the femur should be exposed. Use a periosteal elevator to expose the femoral shaft and a hacksaw to transect it one-third of the way down the shaft.

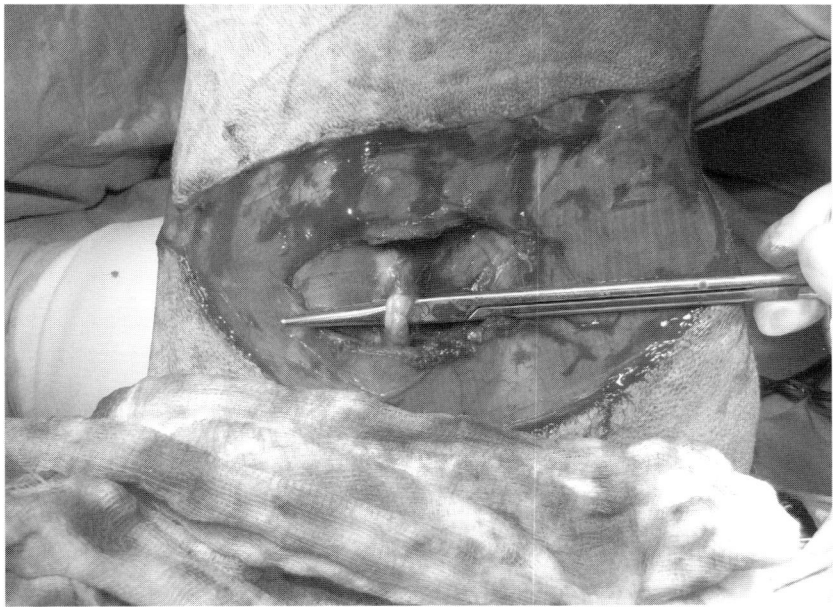

Fig. 8.22. Hind limb amputation 2: isolate the femoral vessels and ligate them – the pectineus muscle has been transected to improve exposure and facilitate this.

Reconstruct the wound

Close the wound in layers suturing the transected medial and lateral musculature together to cover the transected femur in two or three layers followed by reconstruction of the subcutaneous fat and skin (Fig. 8.24). Consider placing a drain in the deeper layers of the wound.

Digit amputation

The techniques for amputation of the central weight-bearing digits (3 and 4), of lateral and medial weight-bearing digits (2 and 5), and of the dewclaw (digit 1) all vary slightly. Amputation of the central weight-bearing digits is illustrated as this is the most complex. For simplicity, forelimb digit amputation is described but the techniques are identical on the hind limb (interchange metatarsal for metacarpal when reading these descriptions) (Fig. 8.25).

The digits are amputated just above the metacarpophalangeal joint. Amputation of the distal epiphysis leads to metacarpal atrophy over time causing the bone stump to retract from the soft tissues sutured over it. This limits post-operative complications associated with stump pain. If the distal epiphysis is left intact, no bone atrophy will occur and the end of the metacarpal bone may traumatize the overlying tissues.

Incise the skin

Make a linear incision along the dorsal aspect of the metacarpal bone from the distal third of the shaft to just proximal to the metacarpophalangeal joint. Extend the incision to encircle the digit to be amputated at the level of the metacarpophalangeal joint.

Expose the distal metacarpal bone and transect it

Continue the incision by combination of sharp dissection and elevation of the soft tissues from the underlying structures all the way around the digit to expose the distal metacarpal bone and joint capsule. Isolate and ligate large digital vessels as they are encountered. Elevate the soft tissues proximally to expose the distal metacarpal bone. Use a large pair of bone cutters to transect the distal shaft of the metacarpal bone to amputate the digit.

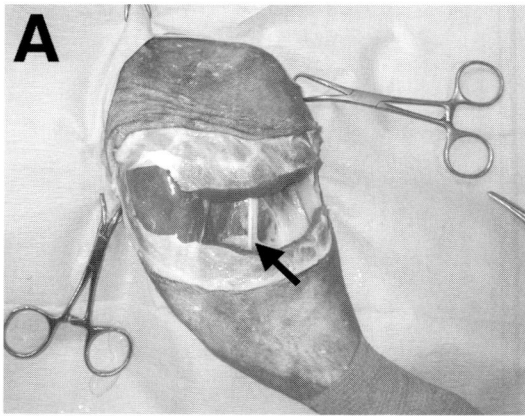

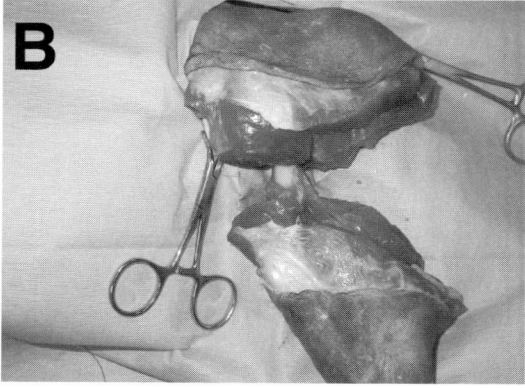

Fig. 8.23. Hind limb amputation 3: (A) transect the muscle of the lateral thigh to expose the sciatic nerve (arrow) and instill local anaesthetic into it before cutting; (B) transect the muscle circumferentially around the limb to expose the femoral shaft.

Reconstruct the wound

Appose the ligaments, tendons, and other soft tissue structures over the cut end of the bone. Suture the skin using an interrupted pattern. Apply and maintain a light dressing for several days and limit exercise until sutures are removed.

Cosmetic tail docking

In some countries, tail amputation has been performed for cosmetic reasons ('tail docking') in puppies. This is a highly controversial practice often regarded as unnecessary mutilation that has few health advantages for the dog. Originally, the

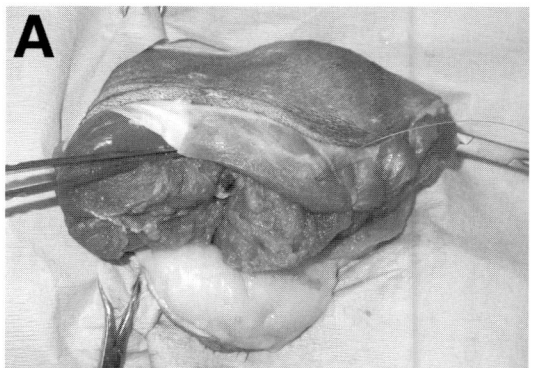

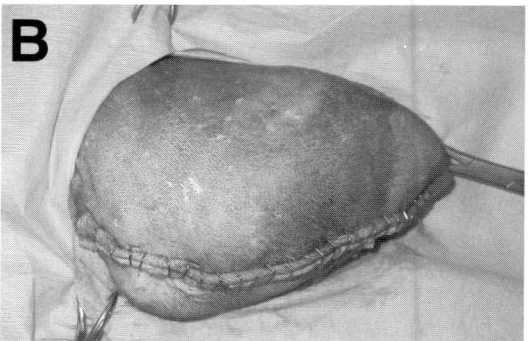

Fig. 8.24. Hind limb amputation 4: (A and B) reconstruct the wound using the transected muscles to cover the cut end of the femur.

practice was performed as it was thought to reduce the incidence of tail injuries in hunting dogs but it has been widely adopted within non-working lines of show dogs that are unlikely to sustain tail injury. Recent research has questioned if tail docking is justified, as the incidence of tail injuries in non-docked dogs remains low. In the UK, legislation has been introduced to outlaw amputation of dogs' tails for cosmetic reasons and the practice is considered to be unethical. However, amputation of an animal's tail for therapeutic reasons (i.e. the management of a current tail injury or disease) is considered to be ethical and uncontroversial.

Tail amputation (caudectomy)

Tail amputation (caudectomy) is also a salvage procedure reserved for intractable tail injuries or other diseases. Indications include neoplasia, trauma, and congenital deformity (screw tail). Once a tail injury

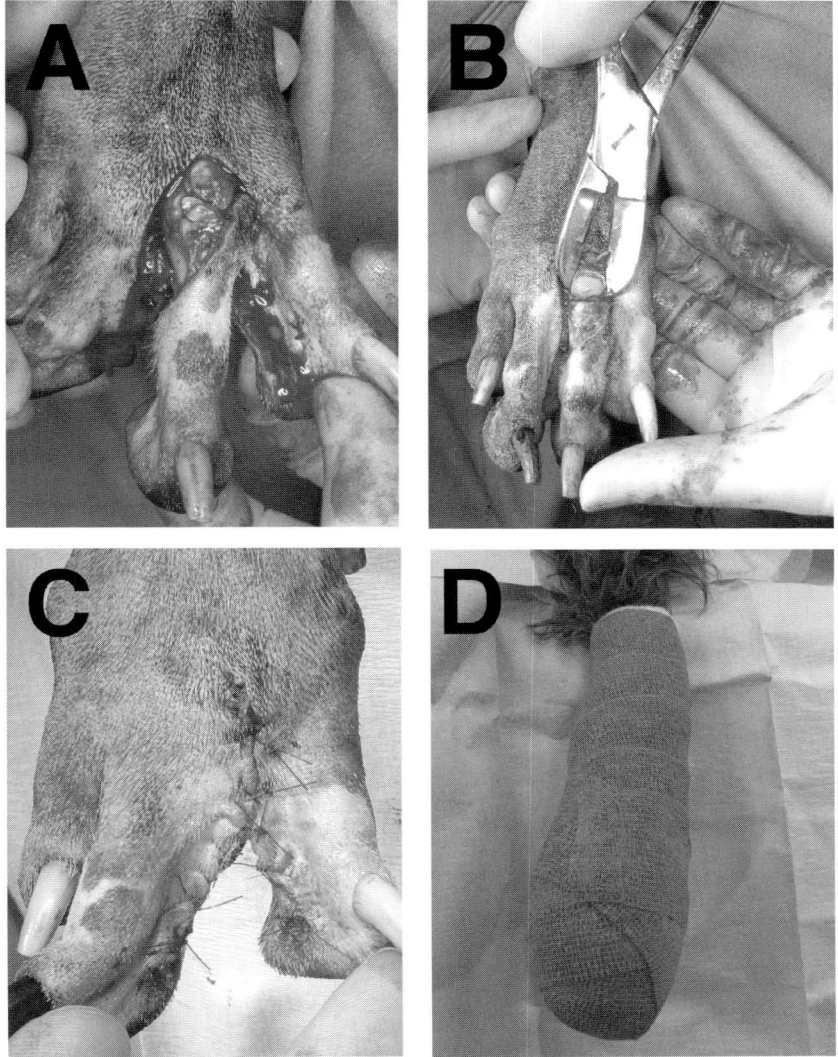

Fig. 8.25. Digit amputation: (A) incise the skin over the metacarpal bone and encircle the top of the digit; (B) expose the distal metacarpal bone and transect it; (C) reconstruct the wound; (D) protect the wound with a heavy support dressing.

is sustained, repeated trauma to the tail due to tail wagging may prevent healing, prompting amputation. Tail amputation is a simple procedure in most cases and requires no advanced surgical techniques or equipment. However, tail amputation to manage screw tail is challenging, and inexperienced clinicians should consider discussing management of these patients with an experienced clinician before proceeding.

Technique

Clip and prepare the tail for surgery. Position the patient in sternal recumbency with the tail suspended over the end of the table, and drape the surgical site. To prevent post-operative trauma, perform tail amputation high so that the tail does not get hit against objects when wagged, but avoid amputating at the tail base as this is technically challenging. A good compromise is to leave a short stump of tail that will not reach beyond the lateral thighs when the tail wags (Fig. 8.26).

Make a curvilinear incision on the dorsal aspect of the tail centred over the intervertebral joint immediately distal to the proposed resection site (this can be identified by palpation and manipulation of the tail). Make a corresponding curvilinear incision on the ventral aspect to complete the skin incision and encircle the tail. These incisions generate two semicircular flaps of skin that are sutured together following amputation to close the wound (Fig. 8.26).

Sharply excise soft tissues to the level of the vertebra, ligating vessels as they are encountered. Use a periosteal elevator to elevate soft tissue from the vertebral body. Use bone cutters to transect the mid-body of the vertebra, completing the amputation. Fold the two flaps of skin over the end of the cut vertebra. Suture the incised muscles and tendons together over the bone stump before suturing the subcutaneous tissues and skin (Fig. 8.26).

Screw tail

Screw tail is a congenital deformity common in bulldogs. The tail is misshapen and twisted from its base to produce a short, corkscrewing tail that becomes embedded within the perineal tissues. The deep folds of skin surrounding the tail become infected and this leads to irritation and distress for the patient (Fig. 8.27). If medical therapy fails (topical cleaning and systemic antibiotic therapy), high tail amputation to resect the deformed tail can be performed. This is a challenging surgery as the tail must be amputated close to its origin near the sacrum, risking injury to the sacral nerves, rectum, and pelvic diaphragm. Although this should not be undertaken by an inexperienced surgeon, surgery is highly effective at alleviating the clinical signs associated with this condition.

Declawing

Declawing (onychectomy) is removal of nails by amputation of the nail bed and part or all of the third phalanx to prevent regrowth. Generally, the

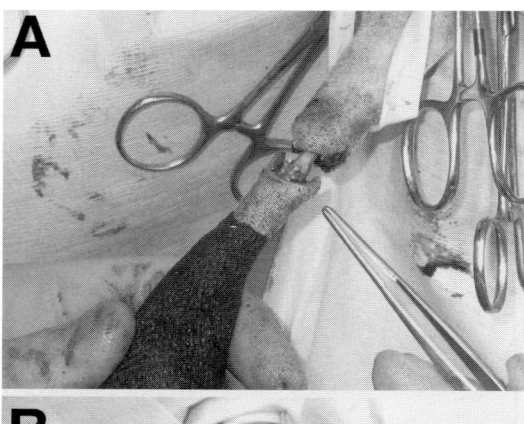
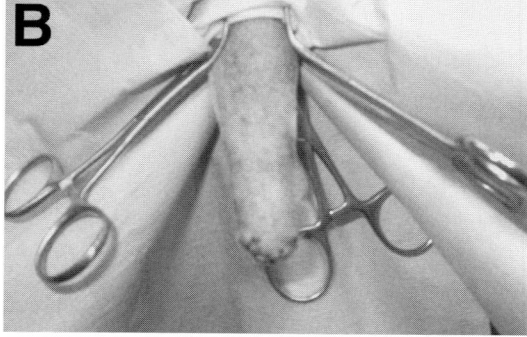

Fig. 8.26. Tail amputation: (A) coccygeal vertebra exposed prior to transection; (B) closure of the wound.

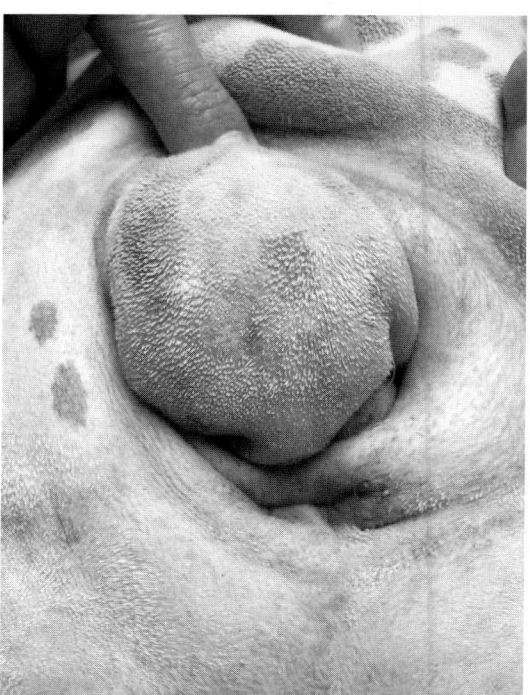

Fig. 8.27. Screw tail case.

term is used to describe removal of all of the nails of cats and is performed to prevent them from scratching furniture or fighting. This is a highly controversial practice. It is often regarded as an unnecessary mutilation that provides no health benefits and which prevents the cat from exhibiting normal behaviour, defending itself and being able to climb out of danger's way. It can also be difficult to provide adequate post-operative pain relief and to prevent wound infection and dehiscence. Numerous techniques have been described, of which those methods that amputate the distal portion of the third phalanx with the nail are preferred, as they are more effective. Declawing for non-therapeutic reasons is considered to be unethical and is outlawed in the UK. Welfare-orientated alternatives include the use of nail caps and pheromone sprays.

Bibliography

Anderson, D. (1997a) Practical approach to reconstruction of wounds in small animal practice: Part 1. *In Practice* 19 463–471.

Anderson, D. (1997b) Practical approach to reconstruction of wounds in small animal practice: Part 2. *In Practice* 19 537–545.

Boyer, J.D., Zitelli, J.A. and Brodland, D.G. (2001) Undermining in cutaneous surgery. *Dermatologic Surgery* 27, 75–78.

Degner, D.A. (2007) Facial reconstructive surgery. *Clinical Techniques in Small Animal Practice* 22, 82–88.

Diesel, G., Pfeiffer, D., Crispin, S. and Brodbelt, D. (2010) Risk factors for tail injuries in dogs in Great Britain. *Veterinary Record* 166, 812–817.

Fowler, D. (2006) Distal limb and paw injuries. *Veterinary Clinics of North America: Small Animal Practice* 36, 819–845.

Goldberg, L.H. and Alam, M. (2004) Elliptical excisions: variations and the eccentric parallelogram. *Archive of Dermatology* 140, 176–180.

Hedlund, C.S. (2006) Large trunk wounds. *Veterinary Clinics of North America: Small Animal Practice* 36, 847–872.

Irwin, D.H. (1966) Tension lines in the skin of the dog. *Journal of Small Animal Practice* 7, 593–598.

Johnston, D.E. (1990) Tension-relieving techniques. *Veterinary Clinics of North America: Small Animal Practice* 20, 67–80.

Mayhew, P. (2009) Tension-relieving techniques and local skin flaps. In: Williams, J.M. and Moores, A.L. (eds) *BSAVA Manual of Canine and Feline Wound Management and Reconstruction*, 2nd edn. BSAVA, Gloucester, UK, pp. 100–143.

Niles, J. and Williams, J. (1999) Suture materials and patterns. *In Practice* 21, 308–320.

Pavletic, M.M. (1999a) Local flaps. In: *Atlas of Small Animal Reconstructive Surgery*. W.B. Saunders Co., Philadelphia, Philadelphia, pp. 191–236.

Pavletic, M.M. (1999b) Tension-relieving techniques. In: *Atlas of Small Animal Reconstructive Surgery*. W.B. Saunders Co., Philadelphia, Pennsylvania, pp. 131–171.

Pope, E.R. (1990) Mesh skin grafting. *Veterinary Clinics of North America: Small Animal Practice* 20, 177–187.

Swaim, S.F. (1990) Skin grafts. *Veterinary Clinics of North America: Small Animal Practice* 20, 147–175.

Swiderski, J. (2002) Onychectomy and its alternatives in the feline patient. *Clinical Techniques in Small Animal Practice* 17, 158–161.

Tan, R.H., Bell, R.J., Dowling, B.A. and Dart, A.J. (2003) Suture materials: composition and applications in veterinary wound repair. *Australian Veterinary Journal* 81, 140–145.

9 Oncological Surgery and Skin Tumours

benign: a lesion that does not invade or spread aggressively
cancer staging: assessment of the extent and spread of a cancer
chemotherapy: use of drugs to treat cancer
grade of tumour: assessment of the degree of malignancy of a cancer
malignant: a tumour that invades locally and spreads to distant sites
metastasis: a secondary deposit of tumour that develops at a distant site following dissemination of cells from the primary tumour
oncology: the field of cancer management
paraneoplastic syndrome: a secondary syndrome caused by metabolically active products produced by a tumour
primary tumour: the original tumour
radiotherapy: use of radiation to treat cancer
secondary tumour: synonym for a metastatic lesion

The reader should be able to:

- describe the key components of cancer staging and explain the importance of this in the dog
- perform fine-needle aspirate, needle-core biopsy, and incisional biopsy of a small skin mass
- explain the advantages and disadvantages of the different methods of obtaining a biopsy and argue, with examples, when preoperative biopsy is not justified in the management of a patient with cancer
- formulate a treatment plan for the management of a cutaneous histiocytoma on the muzzle of a dog
- formulate a treatment plan for the management of a benign mammary tumour in the second mammary gland of a dog
- formulate a treatment plan for the investigation and management of a 1 cm grade II mast cell tumour on the flank of a dog
- compare and contrast the management of feline mammary tumour and canine mammary tumour

Surgery for the investigation and treatment of cancer (oncological surgery) is a major field. This chapter reviews the principles of cancer assessment and then applies these to the investigation and management of a range of common tumours. Cancer management is an ever-evolving field. Readers should consult current expert opinion for the most up-to-date recommendations for the management of cancers.

Cancer Staging

Cancer staging is the assessment of the type and extent of a cancer. It is a vital part of the preoperative assessment of a patient as it enables treatments to be planned and the outcomes of treatment to be predicted.

There are three steps to cancer staging:

1. assessing the primary tumour;
2. assessing spread to regional lymph nodes;
3. assessing spread to distant sites.

Primary tumour assessment

The goals of assessment of the primary tumour are to determine its histological type, grade, and relationship to surrounding tissues. Physical assessment of the tumour provides key information for planning treatment. For example, if the tumour is palpable, it can be assessed for its size and location, gross appearance, relationship to neighbouring structures, and adherence to deeper tissue planes. Imaging studies also provide useful information about the primary tumour. Radiography is most useful in assessing bone tumours and tumours located within the lung or thoracic cavity. Ultrasound provides much information about the interaction of soft-tissue masses with their neighbouring tissues and is invaluable in the assessment of abdominal cancers. Computed tomography (CT) and magnetic resonance imaging (MRI) provide more detailed studies of the interaction of the primary tumour

with the surrounding tissues, but access to these technologies is limited. Finally, tumour biopsy is a crucial part of the preoperative evaluation of most cancers. It is used to establish the origin and severity (or grade) of the tumour so that effective therapy can be planned. Several methods of tumour biopsy are used.

Fine-needle aspirate

Fine-needle aspirate (FNA) using a needle and syringe harvests small numbers of cells from the tumour for cytological assessment. Once the cells have been harvested into the needle, they are expelled onto a glass slide, spread into a monolayer, and air dried before being submitted for analysis (Fig. 9.1).

This is the simplest biopsy technique and is particularly easy to perform on cutaneous and subcutaneous masses. The procedure is quick, does not require anaesthesia, has a low complication rate, and is well tolerated. However, the aspirate may not collect a representative sample of the tumour and provides limited information, so misdiagnoses

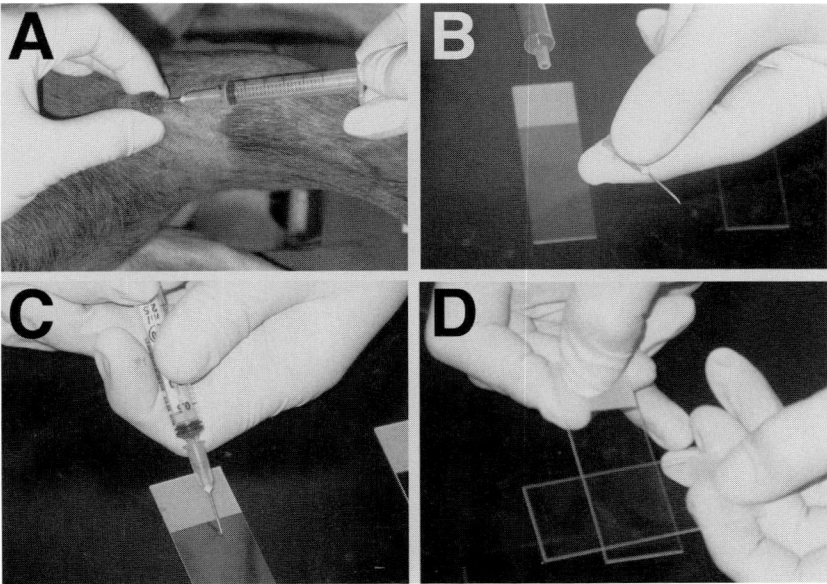

Fig. 9.1. Fine-needle aspirate: (A) use a 21–25 gauge needle and 2–5 ml syringe. Insert the needle into the centre of the mass and draw back on the plunger several times. Redirect the needle to increase the yield. Release the plunger before removing the needle from the mass so that cells in the hub of the needle are not sucked into the syringe barrel; (B) detach the syringe and fill it with air; (C) reattach the syringe to the needle and forcibly express the contents of the needle onto a glass slide; (D) make a smear by performing a squash-prep. Air-dry and stain the slide.

are common. FNA usually can identify the tissue of origin of the mass and whether or not the mass is likely to be cancerous but it is rarely possible to obtain a definitive diagnosis or grade of tumour. FNA is extremely useful as an early screening test but should, whenever possible, be supported by subsequent histopathological analysis of excised tissue.

Needle-core biopsy

The needle-core biopsy technique uses a large-gauge biopsy needle to collect a core of tissue from the tumour. The needle has a central biopsy channel and an outer cutting sheath. The needle is inserted into the tumour with the outer cutting sheath retracted (Fig. 9.2). Tissue fills the biopsy channel. The cutting sheath is advanced, amputating the portion of tumour sitting in the biopsy channel from the rest of the mass. The needle assembly is then removed from the tumour, retrieving the tissue sample within the biopsy channel. Once the core of tissue is collected, it is transferred into fixative (e.g. formalin) for preservation before being submitted for analysis.

A needle-core biopsy collects far more tissue than an FNA. An accurate diagnosis can usually be reached as the sample can be submitted for full histopathological analysis, although surgical biopsies will provide more information. The patient must be sedated or anaesthetized and the biopsy causes more trauma than an FNA.

Incisional biopsy

Incisional biopsy is a form of surgical biopsy usually performed under general anaesthesia. A wedge of tissue that preserves the tissue architecture is removed from the tumour for analysis. Incisional biopsy usually enables an accurate diagnosis and tumour grade to be established. The advantage of this technique is that as much information as possible can be gathered before treatment is attempted, but it is more invasive than the previous techniques.

To collect an incisional biopsy, excise a wedge of tissue from the mass using a scalpel. Ensure that the biopsy includes the boundary between the mass and surrounding tissues to establish how the tumour interacts with surrounding structures. Ensure that the sample is representative of the whole tumour by including tissue from deep within the mass. Plan the biopsy so that the biopsy tract

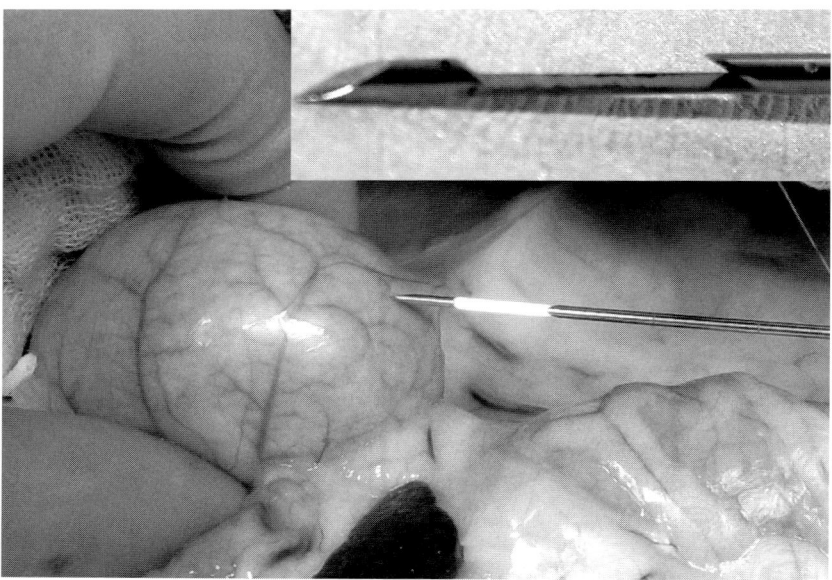

Fig. 9.2. Needle core biopsy of kidney: the needle about to be inserted with the outer sheath withdrawn (insert shows close-up of the biopsy channel and outer, cutting sheath).

can be resected easily with the primary mass as it may contain tumour cells. Suture the biopsy site closed using a series of simple appositional or mattress sutures (Fig. 9.3). Place the sample in at least ten times its volume of fixative (e.g. formalin) to ensure adequate tissue penetration, and submit it for analysis.

Excisional biopsy

Excisional biopsy is another form of surgical biopsy that involves removal of the entire mass for analysis. The advantages are that only one procedure is required to both reach a diagnosis and to remove the mass, and that the margins of excision can be evaluated. The disadvantage is that surgery is performed before the type and grade of tumour has been confirmed and this may mean that inadequate or inappropriate surgery is performed.

It is generally advisable to perform FNA, needle-core, or incisional biopsy in preference to excisional biopsy in the first instance. However, on occasion, excisional biopsy may be more appropriate, particularly if the results of incisional biopsy are unlikely to alter the surgery that is performed. Several examples of procedures where excisional biopsy may be preferred over other forms of biopsy are described:

- Example 1: castration to remove a testicular tumour; preoperative biopsy is unlikely to influence the recommendation to perform castration.
- Example 2: splenectomy to remove a bleeding splenic mass; preoperative biopsy will delay definitive management of haemoabdomen, and splenectomy will still be required.
- Example 3: lung lobectomy to remove a suspected primary lung tumour; the morbidity and risks associated with incisional biopsy are similar (or even higher) than those associated with lung lobectomy to remove the tumour.

Lymph node assessment

Lymph node assessment is a very important part of cancer staging. Many tumours metastasize through lymphatic vessels early in the course of disease, and tumour deposits within the regional lymph node may be the first indicators of extension of disease beyond the primary mass (Table 9.1). The regional lymph nodes draining the tumour can be assessed for enlargement, or tissue samples can be collected by FNA or surgical biopsy. Superficial lymph nodes are assessed for enlargement by palpation. Non-palpable nodes (e.g. medial iliac; sublumbar; presternal) can be assessed using radiography or

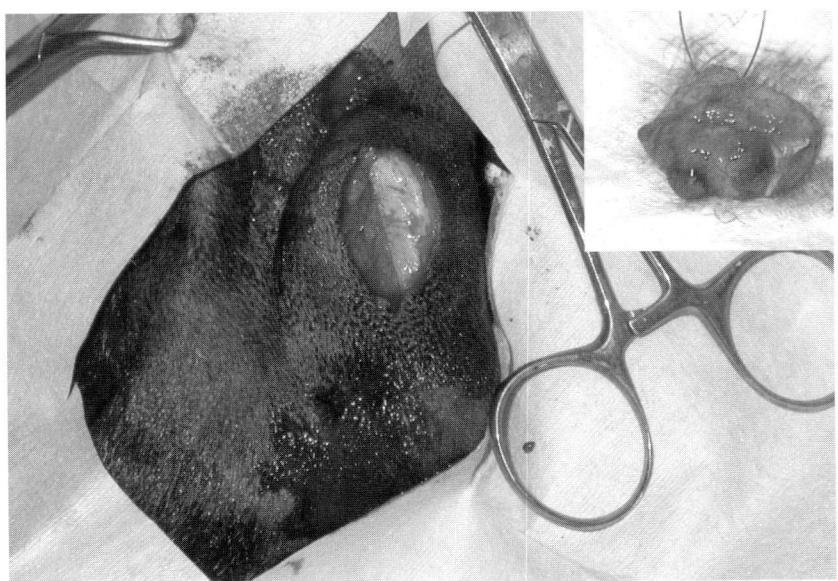

Fig. 9.3. Incisional biopsy site prior to closure (insert shows wedge of tissue removed for biopsy sample).

Table 9.1. Regional lymph nodes and the areas they drain.

Regional lymph node	Field of drainage
Mandibular; parotid; retropharyngeal	Head
Prescapular	Forelimb; neck
Axillary	Forelimb; cranial mammary glands
Inguinal	Hind limb; caudal mammary glands
Medial iliac	Hind limbs; prostate; perineum; bladder
Sternal	Cranial mammary glands; mediastinum
Tracheobronchial	Lung

ultrasound. Node enlargement often indicates metastatic spread but it is not always caused by tumour deposits developing within the node. Many tumours cause local tissue inflammation or develop secondary infection, both of which may cause regional lymph node enlargement. Similarly, not all cancerous lymph nodes are grossly enlarged, as nodes may only have microscopic deposits of tumour cells within them. Lymph node biopsy is a more accurate method of lymph node assessment.

Metastatic disease assessment

The final step of cancer staging is the assessment of distant metastatic disease. The sites of distant metastases depend on the type and location of the primary tumour, but many tumours metastasize through the bloodstream to well-vascularized organs such as the lungs, liver, and kidneys. Thoracic radiography and abdominal ultrasound are invaluable in assessing distant metastatic lesions. CT provides the most sensitive assessment for metastatic lesions to lung. Unfortunately, no imaging modality is sensitive enough to identify microscopic tumour deposits, and metastatic disease may be present despite no evidence being identified on imaging studies.

Principles of Cancer Surgery

Cancer surgery is performed for therapeutic, diagnostic, or palliative reasons. It can be extremely simple (e.g. the resection of a cutaneous histiocytoma) or extremely challenging (e.g. maxillectomy).

A common mantra is that the first surgery has the best chance of cure. Subsequent revision surgery is quite likely to fail, as an incompletely resected tumour disseminates into healthy tissues at the margins of the original resection. Surgery should never be attempted if the surgeon lacks the confidence or ability to perform the appropriate procedure, and the case should be referred. A set of key principles is adhered to in order to maximize the success of cancer surgery:

1. Do not undertake surgery which exceeds your ability or confidence.
2. Plan resection and reconstruction carefully.
3. Resect tumours with an appropriate margin of normal tissue.
4. Plan biopsy procedures so that the biopsy tract can be removed with the primary mass.
5. Consider scars from previous surgeries, biopsies, and drains to contain tumour deposits and include them with the primary tumour when planning margins of resection.
6. Ligate the blood supply to the tumour early during resection: cancer cells may shed into the bloodstream when the tumour is being manipulated intra-operatively.
7. Avoid contaminating unaffected tissues with cancer cells, by changing instruments and gloves between tumour resection and wound reconstruction.
8. Limit the use of drains as cancer cells may disseminate along the drain.

Skin and Subcutaneous Tumours

Skin tumours are the commonest form of cancer in dogs and cats and are usually managed by excision of the tumour.

Preoperative staging

Staging of skin tumours follows the principles of tumour staging discussed previously. FNA is often used to evaluate the tumour preoperatively as it is easy to perform on cutaneous and subcutaneous masses, and because FNA can usually distinguish mast cell tumours (the commonest malignant skin tumour of dogs) from other forms of cutaneous cancer. Incisional biopsy should be performed when FNA has provided little information or when major reconstructive surgery will be required.

Margins of excision

Tumours compress surrounding tissue as they enlarge, creating a pseudocapsule of compressed tumour cells and normal tissue. Invasive tumours (e.g. sarcomas) also extend microscopic tendrils into the surrounding tissue. For most tumours, resecting the tumour without a margin of grossly normal tissue is likely to leave tumour deposits in the margins of resection and lead to early recurrence. A key concept to successful oncological surgery is to resect the entire tumour including the pseudocapsule and any microscopic extensions of tumour. The margins of resection required to achieve this can be predicted from the type, stage, and location of the tumour established from preoperative staging. When planning margins of resection, it is important to appreciate that tumours invade into deeper tissues as well as laterally. Achieving a good margin of resection is often harder to achieve in the deeper tissues than it is in the skin surrounding the tumour.

The lateral margin of resection of a skin tumour is generally determined as a minimum distance of skin from the grossly visible tumour (e.g. 1 cm from the edge of the lesion). In deeper tissues, thick fascial planes act as good barriers to tumour extension (e.g. muscle, periosteum, bone). The association of the tumour to the next uninvolved fascial plane usually determines the deep margin of resection. Depending on the invasive potential of the tumour, the deep fascial plane may be left intact or removed. During tumour resection, the cutaneous trunci muscle is discounted as a deep fascial plane as it is too thin to act as a good barrier to tumour extension. To simplify the selection of appropriate margins of resection, the terms marginal resection, wide resection, and radical resection are often used.

Marginal resection

Marginal resection is resection of the tumour just outside its pseudocapsule. This almost always leaves tumour deposits within the resection margins and is generally not curative. The only tumours in which this is appropriate are completely benign tumours that do not invade into surrounding tissue, and the only common example in veterinary surgery is the lipoma (Fig. 9.4).

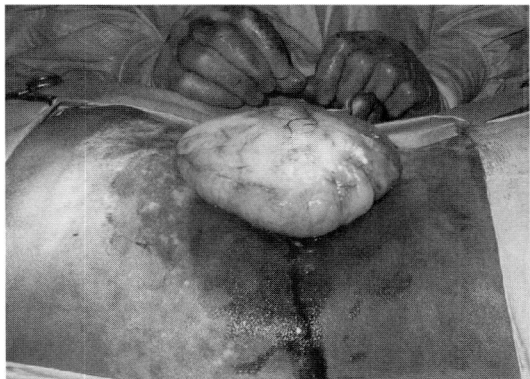

Fig. 9.4. Marginal resection of lipoma: a skin incision has been made directly over the tumour and it has been bluntly dissected from the surrounding tissues to remove it and its pseudocapsule.

Wide resection

Wide resection is removal of the mass with a margin of healthy tissue surrounding it. For most non-invasive cutaneous masses (e.g. mammary adenoma; cutaneous histiocytoma), a radial margin of resection of 1 cm of grossly normal skin around the tumour is adequate. The deep margin of resection should extend at least to the next deep fascial plane and, depending on the association with the base of the tumour, may involve resection of it (Fig. 9.5). For more invasive cutaneous tumours (e.g. mast cell tumour; soft-tissue sarcoma), a wider margin of resection is recommended. Resection of up to 3 cm of normal skin around the tumour, and a deep margin of resection that includes resection of the next unaffected deep fascial plane, is usually recommended (Fig. 9.6). When larger margins of resection are required (e.g. 3 cm lateral margin and the next fascial plane), a more aggressive approach to surgery is required and more advanced reconstructive techniques may be necessary. Many cases falling into this category are referred to specialist centres for surgery.

Radical resection

Radical resection is removal of the tumour including the tissue compartment within which it is located, and is performed for the management of highly invasive tumours. A common example is forequarter amputation for radial osteosarcoma.

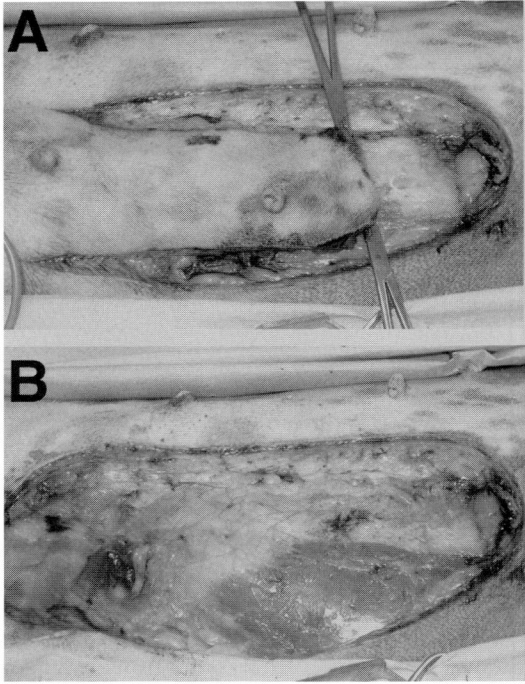

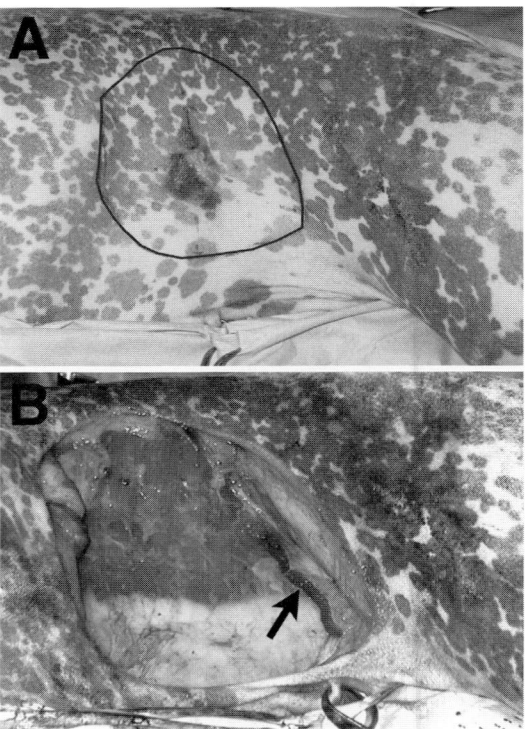

Fig. 9.5. Wide excision of a non-invasive tumour type. Mammary tumour: (A) a 1 cm radial margin of excision has been mapped around the tumours palpable within these two glands; (B) the deep margin of resection continues onto the next fascial plane (the external rectus fascia) but does not include it. This represents a standard example of mammary tumour excision that would be performed in general practice. The wound was easily reconstructed using undermining and walking sutures. (Images courtesy of E. Welsh.)

Fig. 9.6. Wide excision of an invasive tumour type. Mast cell tumour: (A) a 3 cm radial margin of excision has been mapped around the tumour; (B) the deep margin of excision extends to include the next deep, uninvolved fascial plane (external abdominal oblique muscle) and this has been resected (arrow). This wound was closed using layered wound closure and undermining and walking sutures, but several tension lines crossed this area necessitating a non-linear closure. This type of wound might have required an advanced reconstructive surgery to close and these cases are generally referred.

Reference Section – Common Skin Tumours

Cutaneous histiocytoma

Cutaneous histiocytomas are common in young dogs. Boxers, bulldogs, and shar peis are predisposed to developing them. Histiocytomas form alopecic, non-pruritic, raised nodules and are often found round the head, neck and perineum. These are benign tumours that do not invade into surrounding tissue and do not metastasize. They often regress spontaneously. Surgical excision is recommended for masses that do not regress within 3 months or which ulcerate. The prognosis is excellent but the condition must be distinguished from other, less common forms of histiocytic dis-

ease that include systemic histiocytosis and histiocytic sarcoma.

Canine mast cell tumour

Mast cell tumours are the commonest skin tumours in dogs. These are round cell tumours that are usually easily identified cytologically, as mast cells have a distinctive appearance with blue or purple cytoplasmic granules using standard stains. They form raised cutaneous or subcutaneous masses that are often hairless. Sometimes they release histamine that causes local oedema, erythema, pruritis, and ulceration. Handling the tumours may cause them to fluctuate in size rapidly due to the release of histamine and development of local oedema.

Biological behaviour

The majority of canine mast cell tumours do not metastasize and complete excision is generally curative. However, some mast cells tumours do metastasize to regional lymph nodes and parenchymatous organs including the spleen and liver. In widely disseminated cases, mast cells can also be identified in the peripheral blood smear.

The Patnaik grading system is commonly used to grade mast cell tumours:

- Grade I: least aggressive tumours that do not metastasize. Complete excision is curative.
- Grade II: intermediate grade tumours that rarely metastasize. Complete excision is generally curative if there is no evidence of lymph node involvement.
- Grade III: highly aggressive tumours that invade deeply into the surrounding tissues and usually metastasize. Complete excision is difficult to achieve and animals are likely to die of metastatic disease. Adjunctive therapy (chemotherapy or radiotherapy) is indicated to slow the progression.

Paraneoplastic syndrome

Histamine release, in addition to causing local oedema, increases gastric acidity leading to gastric ulceration and vomiting in some animals. Sudden histamine release may also cause systemic vasodilation and acute hypotension, causing shock.

Resection guidelines

Resection of grades I and II tumours with a 2 cm peripheral margin and resection including the next deep, unaffected fascial plane is recommended. For grade III mast cell tumours, 3 cm peripheral margins may be more appropriate. When mast cell tumours occur on limbs, it can be difficult to achieve a wide local excision given the paucity of skin for reconstruction and the proximity of the mass to bone or other vital structures for limb function. These cases may require advanced reconstructive surgery to achieve a local cure. Alternatives to consider include amputation or less aggressive resection to reduce tumour bulk before radiotherapy treatment.

Histamine released during manipulation of the tumours intra-operatively can cause severe hypotension and local oedema. Antihistamines against H1 receptors (e.g. chlorphenamine) and H2 receptors (e.g. cimetidine) are prescribed perioperatively and continued for several days post-operatively.

Adjunctive therapies

Mast cell tumours are relatively chemosensitive and radiosensitive. Radiotherapy following incomplete surgical excision may help reduce the local recurrence rate. Recently, a drug that inhibits key intracellular signalling pathways (Palladia™, Pfizer, New York USA) has shown promise in the management of canine mast cell tumours.

Prognosis

The prognosis for animals with completely resected grade I and II mast cell tumours without evidence of metastatic disease is excellent. The prognosis for grade III mast cell tumours is poor as most animals die of metastatic disease. Tumours located in the inguinal, preputial, muzzle, and perineal regions are associated with a worse prognosis.

Boxers, golden retriever, and shar peis are predisposed to developing multiple mast cell tumours. Although these are generally grade I or II tumours and can be managed by complete excision alone, some animals require numerous surgeries throughout their lives to remove tumours as they occur.

Feline mast cell tumour

Mast cell tumours are the second commonest form of cutaneous tumour in the cat. They form pale, alopecic nodules or plaques, often on the head and neck. They may be pruritic and be associated with erythema, oedema, and ulceration due to histamine release. Some animals have multiple cutaneous mast cell tumours.

Biological behaviour

The majority of feline cutaneous mast cell tumours are benign and less invasive than their canine counterparts, but they do occasionally metastasize. Correlating histological features with outcome in feline mast cell tumours is difficult, but pleomorphic, more invasive forms have a worse prognosis.

Resection guidelines

Local resection of feline mast cell tumours with a margin of normal tissue is often curative. Periocular mast cell tumours rarely recur, even following resection with minimal margins.

Prognosis

The prognosis for cats with completely resected tumours is generally good as the metastatic rate is low. A separate syndrome of visceral mastocytosis is also recognized, in which cats have systemic signs associated with mast cell infiltration of organs including the spleen and intestinal tract. Rarely, this has been described associated with concurrent cutaneous mast cell tumours, and carries a guarded prognosis.

Squamous cell carcinoma

Squamous cell carcinoma (SCC) is a common cutaneous tumour. There is a strong association between the development of SCC and exposure to ultraviolet light, and tumours are often found in sparsely haired areas for this reason. They form either proliferative, hairless masses, or ulcerative, indurated plaques. In dogs, the predilection sites are the nail bed, legs, nasal planum, scrotum, and anus. In cats, the tumours are most commonly identified in white-haired cats affecting the ear tips, upper eyelid, or nasal planum.

Biological behaviour

SCC may develop through progression from premalignant lesions confined to the superficial epithelium to more invasive SCC that invades into the underlying tissues. SCC located on the pinna, eyelids, and nasal planum tends to be locally invasive but rarely metastasizes. SCC located on the ventral abdomen of the dog is also usually locally invasive but slow to metastasize. However, multiple primary lesions may be present in any individual animal. SCC of the nail bed is locally invasive and usually causes destruction of the distal phalanx. Some reports suggest that digital SCC has a higher metastatic potential than other cutaneous SCC.

Resection guidelines

SCC of the face, leg, perineum, and abdominal wall requires wide local resection. SCC of the eyelid generally requires local skin flaps to reconstruct the lesion. SCC of the pinna and nail bed require radical resection involving partial pinnectomy (see Chapter 19) or digit amputation above the level of the metacarpophalangeal joint. Removal of SCC of the nasal planum involves extensive resection of the rhinarium. The long-term outcome can be good but owners require preparation for the cosmetic results of surgery.

Prognosis

The prognosis for completely excised cutaneous SCC in both dogs and cats is reasonable as the metastatic rate is low. However, due to the invasive nature of the primary tumour, local recurrence is common and late metastases can occur.

Cutaneous melanoma

Cutaneous melanomas are common in dogs but rare in cats. They develop in haired skin and form alopecic masses that may be heavily pigmented. The majority of cutaneous melanomas in dogs (85%) are benign. However, 50% of tumours affecting the non-haired skin of the mucocutaneous junctions and nail bed are malignant. Malignant melanoma has a high metastatic rate of 30–75%. The prognosis for benign cutaneous melanoma after complete excision is excellent but most animals with malignant melanoma succumb to metastatic disease.

Basal cell tumour

Basal cell tumours are very common. They originate from the basal layer of the epidermis and are usually benign and non-invasive. They rarely recur following complete resection. The prognosis is good but more aggressive forms are identified occasionally.

Sebaceous gland tumours

This group of tumours includes sebaceous adenoma, sebaceous hyperplasia, and sebaceous adenocarcinoma. The tumours appear as hard, greasy, proliferative, hairless, pale masses. Multiple masses are often identified in a single patient and they may become ulcerated and bleed. The majority are benign adenomas that are non-invasive. Occasionally, more invasive sebaceous adenocarcinomas develop but these rarely metastasize. Adenomas are resected with up to a 1 cm margin of normal tissue. Sebaceous adenocarcinomas require wider margins or resection including removal of the next deep, uninvolved fascial plane. The prognosis is good as most cause no clinical signs and resection is usually curative.

Perianal adenoma

Perianal adenomas (or hepatoid gland adenomas) are common benign tumours that do not metastasize. They affect predominantly older, male entire dogs and usually form in the skin around the anus. They can also develop on the tail or perineum. They form discrete, raised cutaneous masses that may become ulcerated. Their development appears to be androgen dependent as they rarely develop in castrated males or female dogs, and the tumours often regress following castration. Large or ulcerated tumours, and tumours that persist despite castration can be excised with up to 1 cm margin of normal tissue. They rarely recur and the prognosis is good.

Apocrine gland anal sac adenocarcinoma

See Chapter 12, p. 199 'Anal sacculectomy'.

Canine mammary tumours

Mammary tumours are very common in older, entire bitches and sex hormones appear to be involved in their development. They are less common in neutered bitches and are rare in male dogs. They may occur as single or multiple masses within the mammary glands and can become inflamed or ulcerated. Occasionally, extensive inflammation, induration, and oedema of the skin of the mammary chain and inner thigh develop, with extremely aggressive inflammatory mammary carcinoma.

Biological behaviour

Approximately half of mammary tumours in dogs are benign and the fibroadenoma is the commonest form. Malignant carcinomas may be classified as simple, mixed, or inflammatory. These have the potential to metastasize to the regional lymph nodes (axillary, inguinal, and medial iliac) or to the lungs. Mammary tumours rarely cause systemic signs of malaise until metastatic disease develops, but the inflammatory carcinoma is a notable exception.

Resection guidelines

A range of options for mastectomy is available:

- simple mastectomy: removal of the tumour and associated mammary gland;
- regional mastectomy: removal of the tumour and glands that share common lymphatic drainage. For glands 1, 2, or 3 this involves resection of the first three mammary glands and the axillary lymph node. For gland 4 or 5 this involves resection of the last two mammary glands; and
- radical mastectomy (mammary strip): removal of the entire mammary chain on the affected side (glands 1–5).

The type of surgery does not influence survival providing that the tumour is excised completely. However, 58% of dogs have development of further mammary tumours in adjacent glands following regional mastectomy, prompting some authors to recommend radical mastectomy (mammary strip) to reduce the requirement for further surgery.

Regardless of the number of glands removed, the recommendations are to resect the tumours with a minimum 1 cm margin of skin and to resect to the next deep fascial plane (generally the external rectus fascia). Incise the skin along the planned resection line. Ligate the vessels as they enter and exit the mammary gland cranially and caudally. Continue the resection on this line through the subcutaneous fat until the external rectus fascia is exposed. Dissect the subcutaneous fat away from the external rectus fascia to complete the dissection (Fig. 9.6). Reconstruct the site using undermining and walking sutures. Remove the inguinal or axillary lymph nodes if the caudal or cranial glands are removed to enable cancer staging.

If bilateral radical mastectomy is indicated (e.g. a dog with multiple tumours affecting both the left and right mammary chains), there is generally insufficient skin to enable reconstruction of the wound during a single surgery. For this reason, bilateral radical mastectomies should be staggered. Surgery is performed on one side first and, once this site has healed (e.g. 4–6 weeks later), surgery is repeated on the other side.

Adjunctive therapies

Ovariohysterectomy at the time of mastectomy does not appear to influence outcome in most dogs and hormone therapy is not recommended routinely.

Prognosis

The prognosis for dogs with completely excised benign mammary tumours is good. The prognosis for dogs with malignant mammary tumours is variable. Over 95% of dogs without lymph node or distant metastases at the time of surgery survive for more than 2 years. The proportion of dogs with lymph node involvement without distant metastases at the time of surgery is ~75% at 1 year and ~67% at 2 years. For animals with distant metastases the 1-year survival rate is only 13.6%. Complex carcinomas have a better prognosis than simple carcinomas, and inflammatory carcinomas have the worst prognosis (most animals are dead within 2 months).

Preventative therapy

Ovariohysterectomy (or ovariectomy) is extremely protective against the development of mammary tumours when it is performed in young animals. The incidence drops from 25% in entire dogs to less than 1% in bitches neutered before 6 months of age. The protective effect of neutering reduces as the age at neutering increases and the beneficial effect is largely lost after 2.5 years of age. The prophylactic effect of neutering is one of the main reasons to recommend early ovariectomy/ovariohysterectomy in bitches (see Chapter 14).

Feline mammary tumours

Mammary tumours are less common in cats than in dogs but sex hormones also appear to influence their development. Most mammary tumours are seen in female entire cats. Over 85% are malignant and metastasize early to regional lymph nodes and lungs. The commonest malignant tumour is the carcinoma and the commonest benign tumour is the fibroadenoma.

Resection guidelines

Radical mastectomy (mammary strip) is recommended because of the malignant and aggressive behaviour of most feline mammary tumours. In the cat, there is abundant loose skin on the ventral abdomen, and bilateral radical mastectomy can be performed during a single surgical procedure without compromising wound closure.

Prognosis

The prognosis for feline mammary carcinomas is poor with one report describing 1 and 2 year survival rates of ~32% and ~18%, respectively, and median survival time of 8 months given in another. Size has prognostic value as large tumours carry the worst prognosis.

Preventative therapy

Neutering before 1 year of age is very protective against the development of mammary tumours in female cats.

Fibroadenomatous hyperplasia

In the cat, benign fibroadenomatous hyperplasia is a syndrome that causes massive enlargement of one or all of the mammary glands due to hormone-induced hyperplasia of the tissue. It is important to differentiate this condition from mammary tumour. Fibroadenomatous hyperplasia affects pregnant cats, and young female cats around the time of the first oestrus. It may also develop in any cat treated with megestrol acetate or medoxyprogesterone acetate. In some animals, only a single gland is affected. In others, the entire mammary chain develops into a pendulous swelling that impedes walking. The glands are spongy and non-productive. They may become ulcerated or painful. Fibroadenomatous hyperplasia forms a distinct and readily recognized syndrome in most cases because of the young age and characteristic physical appearance in female, entire cats, or because of the history of administration of progestagens coupled with the clinical findings. Treatment includes ovariohysterectomy, discontinuing hormone therapies, and treatment with aglepristone. The diseased mammary tissue can also be resected if it does not regress with other treatments.

Lipoma

Lipomas are common, benign, mesenchymal tumours. They usually form mobile, large, globular, subcutaneous masses that have a soft texture consistent with fat. Occasionally, lipomas develop between layers of muscle and this reduces their mobility giving the impression that they are fixed in position. Lipomas rarely cause significant clinical signs but, as they enlarge, they may restrict movement.

The vast majority of lipomas are completely benign and not invasive. Marginal resection is generally curative (Fig. 9.4). Rarely, infiltrative lipomas form over the thoracic wall or in the perineal region. These invade into surrounding muscles and across the thoracic wall. Although these tumours are benign, they are challenging to resect and suspected cases should be referred.

Soft-tissue sarcomas

Soft-tissue sarcomas are a group of diverse mesenchymal tumours that affect the skin and subcutaneous tissues of dogs and cats. Their histological classification is complex but they share common features and are often considered together.

Biological behaviour

Soft-tissue sarcomas may be locally invasive but rarely metastasize. A series of grading systems is available that is used to predict response to surgery and required margins of resection. Grade I tumours

are less invasive and unlikely to metastasize in comparison to grade III tumours.

Resection guidelines

General guidance for resection of soft-tissue sarcomas is to assume that they are locally invasive and to remove them with a minimum of 3 cm of healthy skin and with resection of the next deep, unaffected fascial plane. However, when specific grading is available, more conservative resection may be successful. For example, resection of grade I soft-tissue sarcomas with small margins of healthy tissue is often curative. Radiotherapy has been described as a successful adjunctive therapy in combination with surgery.

Prognosis

The prognosis following complete excision of soft-tissue sarcomas is good as most will not have metastasized and surgery will be curative. However, local recurrence is a major cause of treatment failure due to their invasive nature.

Cutaneous haemangiosarcoma

Cutaneous haemangiosarcomas differ in their biological behaviour from visceral forms of haemangiosarcoma. The location of the tumour within the

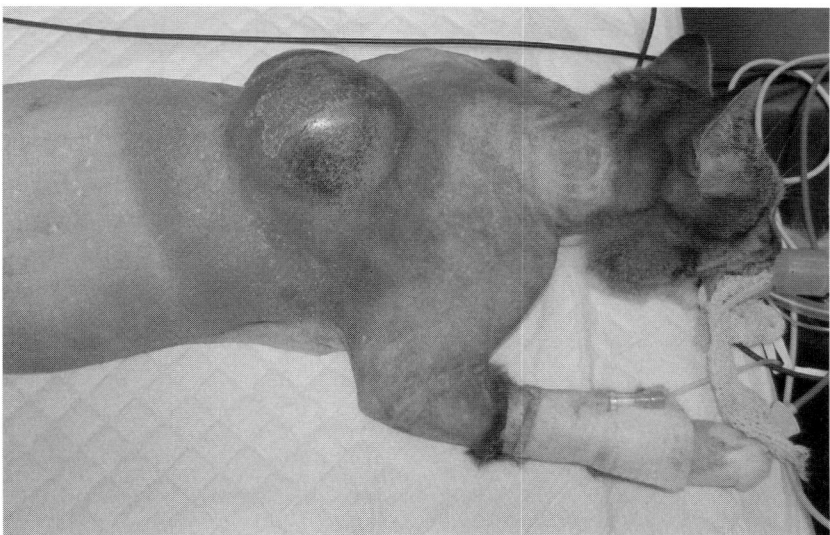

Fig. 9.7. Feline injection-site sarcoma: this tumour developed between the scapulae in this cat at the sites of previous vaccinations. Extensive resection and radiotherapy were required to resolve this lesion.

Oncological Surgery and Skin Tumours

layers of skin (i.e. cutaneous; subcutaneous; invading muscle) can be used to predict the prognosis. Both local recurrence and metastatic disease may develop, but many animals have reasonable long-term outcomes following complete, wide excision with or without chemotherapy.

Feline injection-site sarcoma

Feline injection-site sarcomas (also known as feline vaccine-associated sarcomas) are mesenchymal tumours that develop at injection sites, particularly following feline leukaemia virus and rabies vaccinations. The tumours may develop several years after the last injection and the cause is not clear, but the chronic inflammatory response to vaccine components at the site of injection has been implicated. Typically, they develop between the scapulae and may grow rapidly (Fig. 9.7). Feline injection-site sarcomas do not metastasize until late in the course of disease but they are extremely invasive locally. This makes effective treatment very difficult. Cases should be referred to a specialist veterinary oncologist.

Bibliography

Baez, J.L., Hendrick, M.J., Shofer, F.S., Goldkamp, C. and Sorenmo, K.U. (2004) Liposarcomas in dogs: 56 cases (1989–2000). *Journal of the American Veterinary Medical Association* 224, 887–891.

Berg, J. (2003) Surgical therapy. In: Slatter, D.H. (ed.) *Textbook of Small Animal Surgery*, 3rd edn. Saunders, Philadelphia, Pennsylvania, pp. 2324–2329.

Bergman, P.J., Withrow, S.J., Straw, R.C. and Powers, B.E. (1994) Infiltrative lipoma in dogs: 16 cases (1981–1992). *Journal of the American Veterinary Medical Association* 205, 322–324.

Bulakowski, E.J., Philibert, J.C., Siegel, S., Clifford, C.A., Risbon, R., Zivin, K. and Cronin, K.L. (2008) Evaluation of outcome associated with subcutaneous and intramuscular hemangiosarcoma treated with adjuvant doxorubicin in dogs: 21 cases (2001–2006). *Journal of the American Veterinary Medical Association* 233, 122–128.

Chang, S.C., Chang, C.C., Chang, T.J. and Wong, M.L. (2005) Prognostic factors associated with survival two years after surgery in dogs with malignant mammary tumors: 79 cases (1998–2002). *Journal of the American Veterinary Medical Association* 227, 1625–1629.

Clemente, M., De Andres, P.J., Pena, L. and Perez-Alenza, M.D. (2009) Survival time of dogs with inflammatory mammary cancer treated with palliative therapy alone or palliative therapy plus chemotherapy. *Veterinary Record* 165, 78–81.

Coomer, A.R. and Liptak, J.M. (2008) Canine histiocytic diseases. *Compendium of Continuing Education for the Practicing Veterinarian* 30, 202–204, 208–216; quiz 216–217.

Dennis, M.M., McSporran, K.D., Bacon, N.J., Schulman, F.Y., Foster, R.A. and Powers, B.E. (2011) Prognostic factors for cutaneous and subcutaneous soft tissue sarcomas in dogs. *Veterinary Pathology* 48, 73–84.

Dernell, W.S. and Withrow, S.J. (1998) Preoperative patient planning and margin evaluation. *Clinical Techniques in Small Animal Practice* 13, 17–21.

Dorn, C.R., Taylor, D.O., Schneider, R., Hibbard, H.H. and Klauber, M.R. (1968) Survey of animal neoplasms in Alameda and Contra Costa Counties, California. II. Cancer morbidity in dogs and cats from Alameda County. *Journal of the National Cancer Institute* 40, 307–318.

Ehrhart, E.J. and Withrow, S.J. (2007) Biopsy principles. In: Withrow, S.J. and Vail, D.M. (eds) *Withrow and MacEwen's Small Animal Clinical Oncology*. Saunders Elsevier, London, pp. 147–153.

Forrest, L.J. (2007) Diagnostic imaging in oncology. In: Withrow, S.J. and Vail, D.M. (eds) *Withrow and MacEwen's Small Animal Clinical Oncology*. Saunders Elsevier, London, pp. 97–111.

Fulcher, R.P., Ludwig, L.L., Bergman, P.J., Newman, S.J., Simpson, A.M. and Patnaik, A.K. (2006) Evaluation of a two-centimeter lateral surgical margin for excision of grade I and grade II cutaneous mast cell tumors in dogs. *Journal of the American Veterinary Medical Association* 228, 210–215.

Fulmer, A.K. and Mauldin, G.E. (2007) Canine histiocytic neoplasia: an overview. *Canadian Veterinary Journal* 48, 1041–1043, 1046–1050.

Gilson, S.D. (1995) Clinical management of the regional lymph node. *Veterinary Clinics of North America: Small Animal Practice* 25, 149–167.

Gimenez, F., Hecht, S., Craig, L.E. and Legendre, A.M. (2010) Early detection, aggressive therapy: optimizing the management of feline mammary masses. *Journal of Feline Medicine and Surgery* 12, 214–224.

Goldschmidt, M.H. (1984) Sebaceous and hepatoid gland neoplasms of dogs and cats. *American Journal of Dermatopathology* 6, 287–293.

Ito, T., Kadosawa, T., Mochizuki, M., Matsunaga, S., Nishimura, R. and Sasaki, N. (1996) Prognosis of malignant mammary tumor in 53 cats. *Journal of Veterinary Medical Science* 58, 723–726.

Lamm, C.G., Stern, A.W., Smith, A.J., Cooper, E.J., Ullom, S.W. and Campbell, G.A. (2009) Disseminated cutaneous mast cell tumors with epitheliotropism and systemic mastocytosis in a domestic cat. *Journal of Veterinary Diagnostic Investigation* 21, 710–715.

Lascelles, B.D., Parry, A.T., Stidworthy, M.F., Dobson, J.M. and White, R.A. (2000) Squamous cell carcinoma of the nasal planum in 17 dogs. *Veterinary Record* 147, 473–476.

Lepri, E., Ricci, G., Leonardi, L., Sforna, M. and Mechelli, L. (2003) Diagnostic and prognostic features of feline cutaneous mast cell tumours: a retrospective analysis of 40 cases. *Veterinary Research Communications* 27, 707–709.

Liptak, J.M. (2009a) The principles of surgical oncology: diagnosis and staging. *Compendium of Continuing Education for the Practicing Veterinarian* 31, E1–E13.

Liptak, J.M. (2009b) The principles of surgical oncology: surgery and multimodality therapy. *Compendium of Continuing Education for the Practicing Veterinarian* 31, E1–E14.

Litster, A.L. and Sorenmo, K.U. (2006) Characterisation of the signalment, clinical and survival characteristics of 41 cats with mast cell neoplasia. *Journal of Feline Medicine and Surgery* 8, 177–183.

London, C.A., Malpas, P.B., Wood-Follis, S.L., Boucher, J.F., Rusk, A.W., Rosenberg, M.P., Henry, C.J., *et al.* (2009) Multi-center, placebo-controlled, double-blind, randomized study of oral toceranib phosphate (SU11654), a receptor tyrosine kinase inhibitor, for the treatment of dogs with recurrent (either local or distant) mast cell tumor following surgical excision. *Clinical Cancer Research* 15, 3856–3865.

Marconato, L., Romanelli, G., Stefanello, D., Giacoboni, C., Bonfanti, U., Bettini, G., Finotello, R., *et al.* (2009) Prognostic factors for dogs with mammary inflammatory carcinoma: 43 cases (2003–2008). *Journal of the American Veterinary Medical Association* 235, 967–972.

Martano, M., Morello, E. and Buracco, P. (2011) Feline injection-site sarcoma: past, present and future perspectives. *Veterinary Journal* 188, 136–141.

Mayer, M.N. (2006) Radiation therapy for canine mast cell tumors. *Canadian Veterinary Journal* 47, 263–265.

McAbee, K.P., Ludwig, L.L., Bergman, P.J. and Newman, S.J. (2005) Feline cutaneous hemangiosarcoma: a retrospective study of 18 cases (1998–2003). *Journal of the American Animal Hospital Association* 41, 110–116.

Miller, M.A., Nelson, S.L., Turk, J.R., Pace, L.W., Brown, T.P., Shaw, D.P., Fischer, J.R., *et al.* (1991) Cutaneous neoplasia in 340 cats. *Veterinary Pathology* 28, 389–395.

Montgomery, K.W., Van Der Woerdt, A., Aquino, S.M., Sapienza, J.S. and Ledbetter, E.C. (2010) Periocular cutaneous mast cell tumors in cats: evaluation of surgical excision (33 cases). *Veterinary Ophthalmology* 13, 26–30.

Mullins, M.N., Dernell, W.S., Withrow, S.J., Ehrhart, E.J., Thamm, D.H. and Lana, S.E. (2006) Evaluation of prognostic factors associated with outcome in dogs with multiple cutaneous mast cell tumors treated with surgery with and without adjuvant treatment: 54 cases (1998–2004). *Journal of the American Veterinary Medical Association* 228, 91–95.

Murphy, S. (2006a) Skin neoplasia in small animals 2. Common feline tumours. *In Practice* 28, 320–325.

Murphy, S. (2006b) Skin neoplasia in small animals 3. Common canine tumours. *In Practice* 28, 398–402.

Novosad, C.A. (2003) Principles of treatment for mammary gland tumors. *Clinical Techniques in Small Animal Practice* 18, 107–109.

Overley, B., Shofer, F.S., Goldschmidt, M.H., Sherer, D. and Sorenmo, K.U. (2005) Association between ovarihysterectomy and feline mammary carcinoma. *Journal of Veterinary Internal Medicine* 19, 560–563.

Patnaik, A.K., Ehler, W.J. and MacEwen, E.G. (1984) Canine cutaneous mast cell tumor: morphologic grading and survival time in 83 dogs. *Veterinary Pathology* 21, 469–474.

Saba, C.F., Rogers, K.S., Newman, S.J., Mauldin, G.E. and Vail, D.M. (2007) Mammary gland tumors in male dogs. *Journal of Veterinary Internal Medicine* 21, 1056–1059.

Sabattini, S. and Bettini, G. (2010) Prognostic value of histologic and immunohistochemical features in feline cutaneous mast cell tumors. *Veterinary Pathology* 47, 643–653.

Schneider, R., Dorn, C.R. and Taylor, D.O. (1969) Factors influencing canine mammary cancer development and postsurgical survival. *Journal of the National Cancer Institute* 43, 1249–1261.

Seixas, F., Palmeira, C., Pires, M.A., Bento, M.J. and Lopes, C. (2011) Grade is an independent prognostic factor for feline mammary carcinomas: a clinicopathological and survival analysis. *Veterinary Journal* 187, 65–71.

Simpson, A.M., Ludwig, L.L., Newman, S.J., Bergman, P.J., Hottinger, H.A. and Patnaik, A.K. (2004) Evaluation of surgical margins required for complete excision of cutaneous mast cell tumors in dogs. *Journal of the American Veterinary Medical Association* 224, 236–240.

Soderstrom, M.J. and Gilson, S.D. (1995) Principles of surgical oncology. *Veterinary Clinics of North America: Small Animal Practice* 25, 97–110.

Sorenmo, K.U., Rasotto, R., Zappulli, V. and Goldschmidt, M.H. (2011) Development, anatomy, histology, lymphatic drainage, clinical features, and cell differentiation markers of canine mammary gland neoplasms. *Veterinary Pathology* 48, 85–97.

Strafuss, A.C., Smith, J.E., Kennedy, G.A. and Dennis, S.M. (1973) Lipomas in dogs. *Journal of the American Animal Hospital Association* 9, 555–561.

Stratmann, N., Failing, K., Richter, A. and Wehrend, A. (2008) Mammary tumor recurrence in bitches after regional mastectomy. *Veterinary Surgery* 37, 82–86.

Thamm, D.H. and Vail, D.M. (2007) Mast cell tumours. In: Withrow, S.J. and Vail, D.M. (eds) *Withrow and MacEwen's Small Animal Clinical Oncology*. Saunders Elsevier, London, pp. 402–424.

Thomson, M. (2007) Squamous cell carcinoma of the nasal planum in cats and dogs. *Clinical Techniques in Small Animal Practice* 22, 42–45.

Thomson, M.J., Withrow, S.J., Dernell, W.S. and Powers, B.E. (1999) Intermuscular lipomas of the thigh region in dogs: 11 cases. *Journal of the American Animal Hospital Association* 35, 165–167.

Vail, D.M. and Withrow, S.J. (2007) Tumors of the skin and subcutaneous tissues. In: Withrow, S.J. and Vail, D.M. (eds) *Withrow and MacEwen's Small Animal Clinical Oncology*. Saunders Elsevier, London, pp. 375–401.

Webb, J.L., Burns, R.E., Brown, H.M., Leroy, B.E. and Kosarek, C.E. (2009) Squamous cell carcinoma. *Compendium of Continuing Education for the Practicing Veterinarian* 31, 133–142.

Welle, M.M., Bley, C.R., Howard, J. and Rufenacht, S. (2008) Canine mast cell tumours: a review of the pathogenesis, clinical features, pathology and treatment. *Veterinary Dermatology* 19, 321–339.

Wilson, G.P. and Hayes, H.M. (1979) Castration for treatment of perianal gland neoplasms in the dog. *Journal of the American Veterinary Medical Association* 174, 1301–1303.

Withrow, S.J. (2007) Surgical oncology. In: Withrow, S.J. and Vail, D.M. (eds) *Withrow and MacEwen's Small Animal Clinical Oncology*. Saunders Elsevier, London, pp. 157–162.

Yamagami, T., Kobayashi, T., Takahashi, K. and Sugiyama, M. (1996a) Influence of ovariectomy at the time of mastectomy on the prognosis for canine malignant mammary tumours. *Journal of Small Animal Practice* 37, 462–464.

Yamagami, T., Kobayashi, T., Takahashi, K. and Sugiyama, M. (1996b) Prognosis for canine malignant mammary tumors based on TNM and histologic classification. *Journal of Veterinary Medical Science* 58, 1079–1083.

10 Principles of Abdominal Surgery

abdominal lavage: flushing the abdomen with saline
coeliotomy: entry into the abdominal cavity (generally through the linea alba)
incisional hernia: hernia caused by breakdown of an incision
laparotomy: entry into the abdominal cavity through the flank
serosal seal: seal produced by adhesions between damaged serosal surfaces

The reader should be able to:

- appreciate the importance of patient preparation for abdominal surgery and be able to implement this, placing emphasis on reducing the risk of contamination of the surgical site and ensuring adequate exposure during exploratory coeliotomy
- differentiate between the role of midline coeliotomy and flank laparotomy in veterinary surgery and discuss the merits of each approach in comparison to the other
- select appropriate landmarks for performing exploratory coeliotomy in a male dog and isolated cystotomy in a male cat
- explain and contrast the techniques for exploratory coeliotomy in the male cat and the male dog
- illustrate how to incise the linea alba without puncturing abdominal organs
- illustrate how to prevent desiccation of tissues during abdominal surgery
- illustrate how to limit contamination of the abdomen during enteric surgery
- describe how to close a midline coeliotomy incision and explain how this technique may affect the development of incisional hernia
- demonstrate on a cadaver how to perform a comprehensive exploration of the abdomen including evaluation of the left limb of the pancreas, the left adrenal gland, and the ductus deferentes

This chapter describes midline coeliotomy and abdominal exploration. It also describes techniques for preventing contamination and for encouraging an early serosal seal during hollow-organ surgery. These are the fundamental principles for successful abdominal surgery that will be referred to repeatedly in subsequent chapters dealing with specific abdominal procedures.

Surgical Anatomy

Each side of the abdominal wall (left and right) is composed of three layers of overlapping muscles:

- *external abdominal oblique* muscle (fibres run caudoventrally);
- *internal abdominal oblique* muscle (fibres run cranioventrally); and

- *transverse abdominis* muscle (fibres run dorso-ventrally).

The fasciae from these muscles coalesce into two thick sheets (aponeuroses) called the *external* and *internal rectus sheaths*. The rectus sheaths from the left and right sides of the abdomen coalesce to form the ventral, midline *linea alba*. The paired *rectus abdominis muscles* lie on either side of the linea alba. The internal and external rectus sheaths run over the inner and outer surfaces of these muscles before forming the linea alba.

In male dogs, the prepuce and penis extend along the caudal third of the ventral abdominal wall. Cranially, the prepuce is supported by paired *preputial muscles*. These muscles originate from cutaneous trunci muscle and run cranio-laterally from the prepuce. Blood is supplied to the prepuce through the *cranial preputial vessels* (branches of the caudal superficial epigastric vessels). The preputial vessels run parallel to the preputial muscles.

The *peritoneum* lies deep to the internal rectus sheath and is separated from it by loose fascia. The *falciform fat* is a large fat pad that lies immediately dorsal to the linea alba between the xiphisternum and the umbilicus. It obscures the cranial abdomen during surgery.

Route of Abdominal Entry

Coeliotomy (celiotomy) is a term used to describe incision into the abdominal cavity and usually refers to entry through the linea alba (midline coeliotomy). *Laparotomy* is a term used to describe incision into the abdomen through the flank muscles, although the term is now used extensively in place of coeliotomy when describing midline abdominal entry.

Midline coeliotomy is generally the best route of entry into the abdomen as it provides very good exposure to the entire abdominal cavity and is very versatile, enabling all abdominal procedures to be performed. In comparison, flank laparotomy provides limited exposure to a small area of the lateral abdomen. It enables only a limited number of procedures to be performed with little scope to deal with unexpected findings or intra-operative complications. Flank laparotomy is only used routinely to perform ovariohysterectomy in cats in some countries (e.g. the UK) and is described separately with this procedure in Chapter 14.

Midline Coeliotomy

Preparing for abdominal surgery

Patients undergoing abdominal surgery may contaminate the surgical site or operating theatre by defecating or urinating once anaesthetized. The bladder also obscures the caudal abdomen if it is full. Encourage the patient to urinate and defecate before surgery to avoid these problems. If this is not possible, the bladder can be manually expressed or catheterized once the patient is anaesthetized. However, patients that have a distended or friable abdominal organ should not have their bladders manually expressed because of the risk of rupturing the diseased organs. Examples include animals with urethral obstruction, intestinal obstruction, bleeding splenic tumour, pyometra, or pregnancy.

Clip and prepare the abdomen from cranial to the xiphisternum to caudal to the pubic brim, and from the midline to 2 cm lateral to the nipples on either side (Fig. 10.1). A large clip ensures that the whole abdomen can be explored during surgery and gives maximum flexibility if the abdominal incision needs to be extended quickly during surgery (e.g. to retrieve a bleeding ovarian pedicle during elective neutering).

Position the patient in dorsal recumbency. Many operating tables have adjustable sides that can be lifted to create a central trough to secure the patient in dorsal recumbency. Alternatively, tie the limbs to the table or use a positioning trough. Pack rolled towels or sandbags along the side of the patient for additional stability (Fig. 10.1).

Drape the surgical site. Abdominal surgery in male dogs is complicated by the presence of the penis and prepuce in the caudal surgical field. The preputial cavity is contaminated and difficult to clean. If it is left within the surgical field, there is also the risk that urine will leak into the surgical field. To overcome these problems, the penis and prepuce are usually deviated to one side (generally to the left side of the patient for right-handed surgeons) and restrained under the drapes using a towel clip (Fig. 10.2). If access to the penis is required intra-operatively (e.g. for urethral flushing during urolithiasis surgery), the prepuce can be prepared by flushing the cavity with dilute povidone-iodine solution. The penis can then be draped into the surgical field. Similarly, the nipples are secretory organs that may act as sources of contamination of the surgical field. These should be draped out of the surgical field unless there are specific reasons to incorporate them.

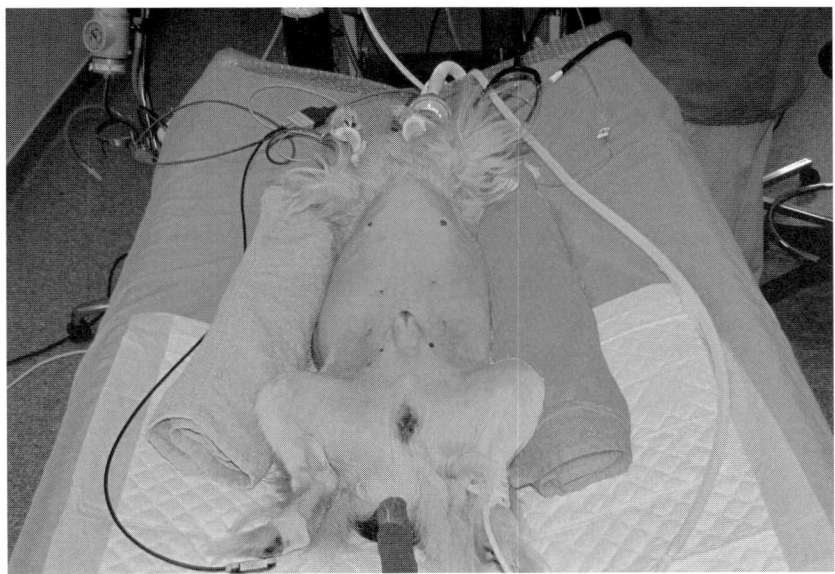

Fig. 10.1. Clip and positioning for abdominal surgery. A wide clip has been performed to ensure that the entire abdominal cavity (xiphisternum to pubis) can be evaluated. The sides of the operating table have been tilted to produce a trough and rolled towels have been packed along the flanks to provide further stability.

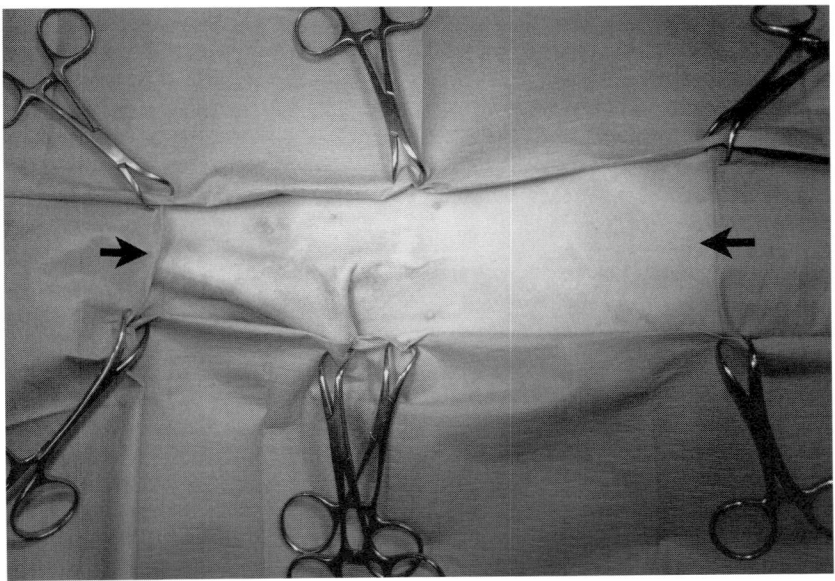

Fig. 10.2. Draping male dog for abdominal surgery: deviate the penis to one side and secure it under the drapes using a towel clip applied to the prepuce. Arrows indicate position of pubic brim and xiphisternum – the entire abdomen is included within the surgical field.

Principles of Abdominal Surgery

Length and positioning of the incision

The key to successful abdominal surgery is maximizing exposure to the abdomen. For exploratory coeliotomy, where all areas of the abdomen must be evaluated, a full abdominal incision extending from the xiphisternum to 1 cm cranial to the pubis is necessary to ensure that all areas can be explored. For more targeted surgeries (e.g. ovariohysterectomy; cystotomy; liver biopsy), the incision can be shorter and centred over the organs of interest. However, it is best practice to ensure the entire abdomen is clipped, prepared, and draped for surgery, even when a limited approach is planned, to enable the incision to be extended quickly if required (Fig. 10.3).

Perform swab and instrument counts

Swabs and instruments may be left in the abdomen at the end of surgery and will act as foreign bodies leading to serious complications (Fig. 10.4). Precautions should be taken to avoid this:

1. Count swabs at the start and end of surgery and ensure that the numbers tally.
2. Count small instruments (e.g. haemostats) at the start and the end of surgery and ensure that the numbers tally.
3. Use swabs with radiographic markers so that retained swabs can be detected easily (Fig. 10.4).

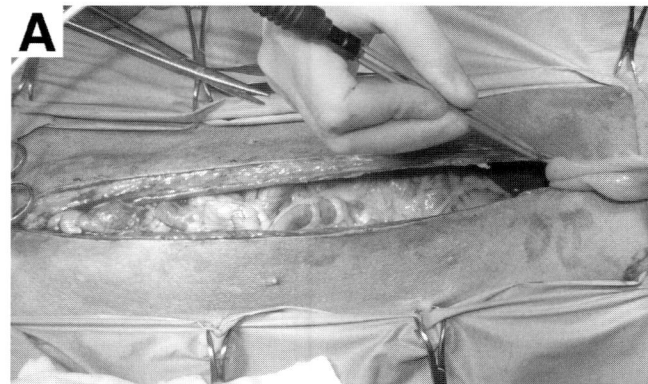

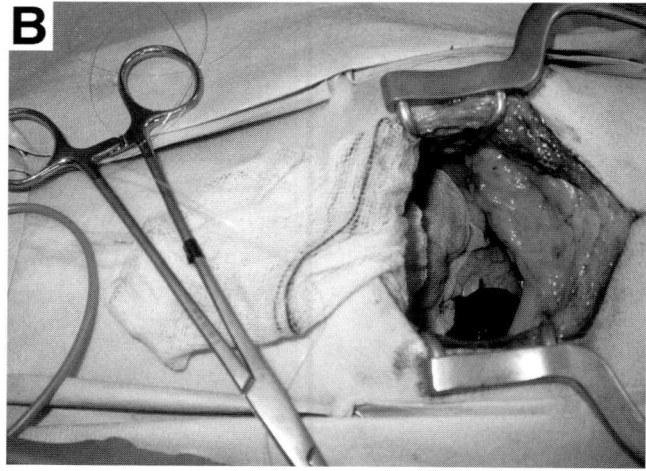

Fig. 10.3. Length of abdominal incision: (A) exploratory coeliotomy – incision from xiphisternum to pubis; (B) organ-centred coeliotomy – incision from xiphisternum to pubis to enable liver biopsy. In this case the entire abdomen has been clipped, prepared, and draped so the incision can be extended if required.

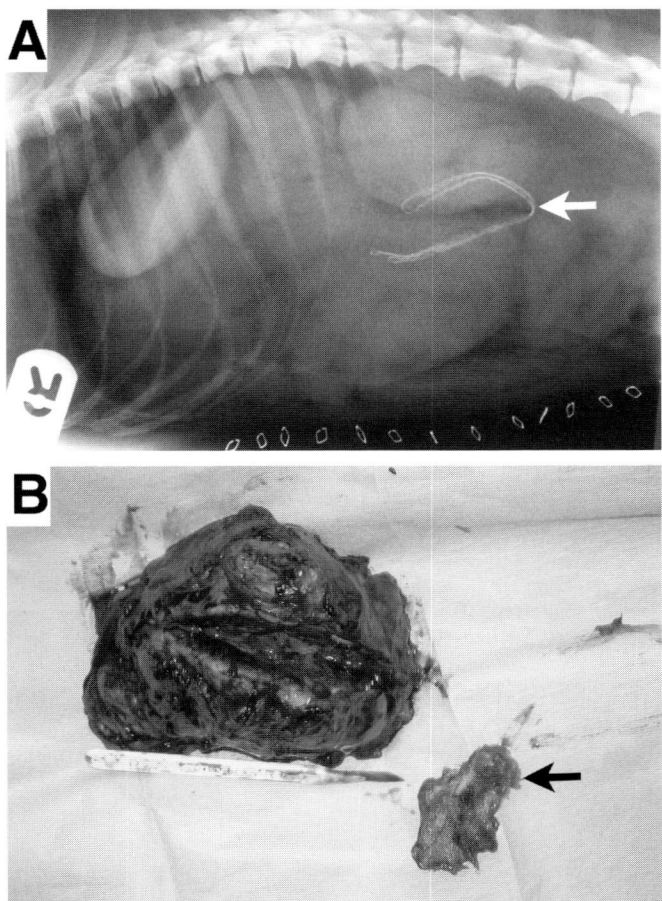

Fig. 10.4. (A) Radiograph of a retained swab identified by the radiographic marker (arrow). (B) A granuloma that formed around a swab left in the abdomen of a dog during elective surgery 9 months previously. The granuloma has been incised and the swab retrieved (arrow). This swab did not have a radiographic marker and the diagnosis was not confirmed until the swab was removed from the centre of the mass. This patient had life-threatening abdominal complications and was severely debilitated by the time that the swab was retrieved.

Skin and subcutaneous incision

Make a ventral midline skin incision along the proposed incision line and extend the incision into the subcutaneous tissues using a scalpel until the linea alba is exposed (Fig. 10.5). The linea alba is a thick, white, fibrous band located along the midline of the abdomen. On either side of the midline, the fibres of the external rectus sheath can be seen converging onto the linea alba, aiding its identification. Cranial to the umbilicus, the linea alba is easily identified as a palpable, thick band. It is less distinct caudal to the umbilicus, particularly in cats. Do not bluntly undermine fat

away from the linea alba to improve exposure. This is unnecessary and increases dead space and tissue trauma in comparison to sharp dissection as described above.

Extending the incision beyond the prepuce

In male dogs, the incision must deviate around the prepuce to extend caudally to the prepuce (Fig. 10.6). From 1 cm cranial to the prepuce, the midline skin incision is redirected to run lateral to the prepuce. It then continues parallel to the penis to the pubis. The preputial muscle is transected as

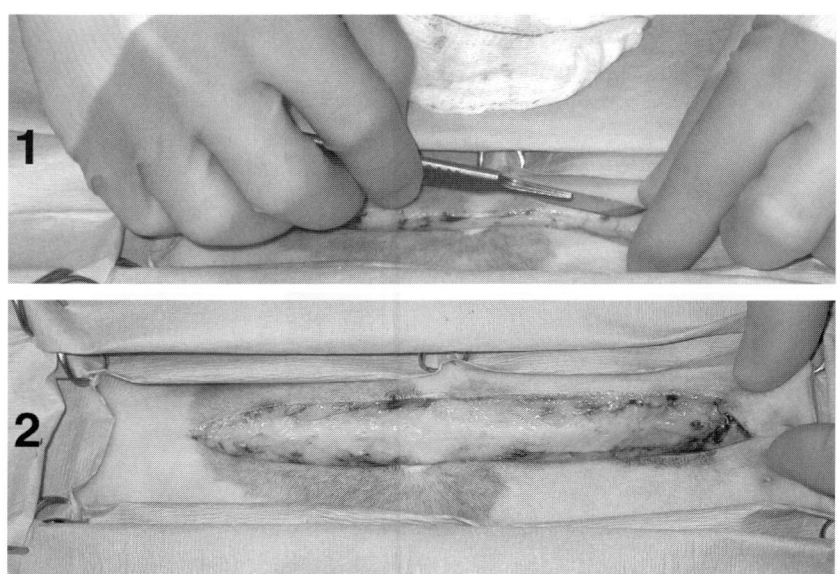

Fig. 10.5. Series demonstrating sharp incision through the skin and subcutaneous fat to expose the linea alba without performing blunt dissection: (1) incise through skin using the cutting edge of a no. 10 scalpel blade; (2) deepen the incision until the linea alba is reached.

it crosses the skin incision just cranial to the start of the prepuce, taking care not to cut the cranial preputial vessels that run deep to the muscle. The vessels are bluntly isolated from the subcutaneous fat, double ligated, and transected. The penis and prepuce are pushed away from the midline and sharp dissection is continued through the subcutaneous fat until the linea alba is exposed. The caudal superficial epigastric vessels run in line with the nipples just lateral to this incision. Take care to avoid lacerating them, particularly at the caudal end of the incision.

Incision through the linea alba – standard technique

Grasp the linea alba with rat-toothed thumb forceps in the centre of the incision and lift it to tent it up and away from the abdominal viscera. Make a stab incision into the linea alba without penetrating the abdominal viscera. To achieve this, use a no. 10 scalpel blade and hold it upside down so that the cutting edge points up away from the abdomen. Hold the blade parallel to the tabletop and introduce it through the linea alba 1 cm from the forceps. Push the scalpel through the linea alba towards the forceps creating a short incision (Fig. 10.7). By tenting the

abdominal wall up away from the underlying viscera and ensuring that the cutting edge of the scalpel faces away from the organs, the risks of inadvertent penetration of organs are minimized.

Once the initial incision has been made, insert the blade of a sharp pair of straight Mayo scissors into the abdomen through the incision and use it to lift the linea alba away from the underlying viscera. Having ensured that organs have not become trapped between the scissor blade and the linea alba, cut the linea alba to extend the initial incision. Palpate along the peritoneal surface of the linea alba with a finger to ensure that no organs are adhered to it before extending the incision further (Fig. 10.8). Repeat this process until the linea alba incision has been extended to the limits of the skin incision. Alternatively, a pair of closed thumb forceps may be used to lift the linea alba away from the underlying viscera so that the linea alba incision can be completed with the scalpel (Fig. 10.9).

Incising the linea alba – alternative method

Although spontaneous abdominal adhesions are rare in dogs and cats, organs occasionally adhere to the linea alba if previous surgery has been performed. In patients that have had previous

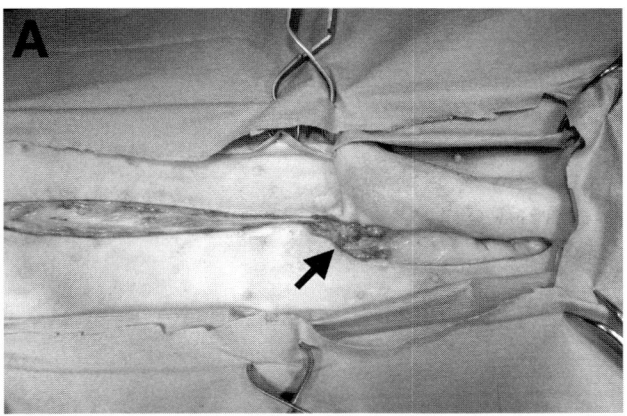

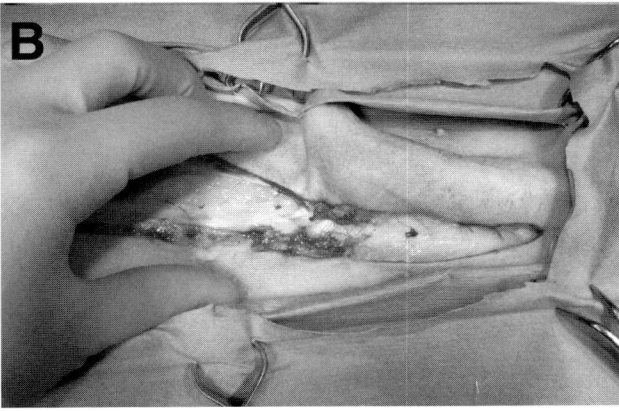

Fig. 10.6. Parapreputial incision: (A) the skin incision curves around the front of the prepuce and continues caudally, parallel to the penis. This exposes the preputial muscles and vessels (arrow); (B) the preputial muscle is incised and the vessels are ligated. The plane of dissection is redirected back towards the midline under the prepuce to expose the linea alba.

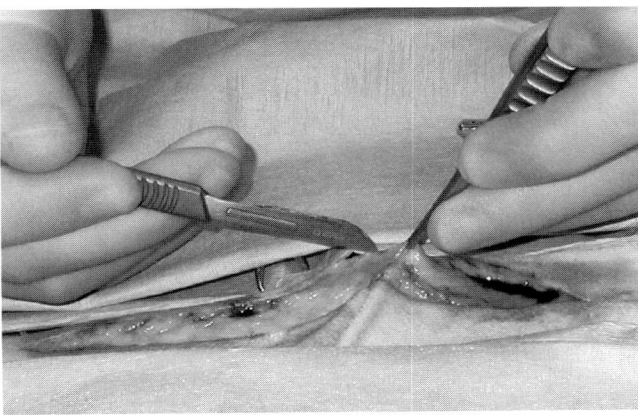

Fig. 10.7. Standard entry method: tent the linea alba away from the underlying viscera and make a stab incision using a reversed no. 10 scalpel blade.

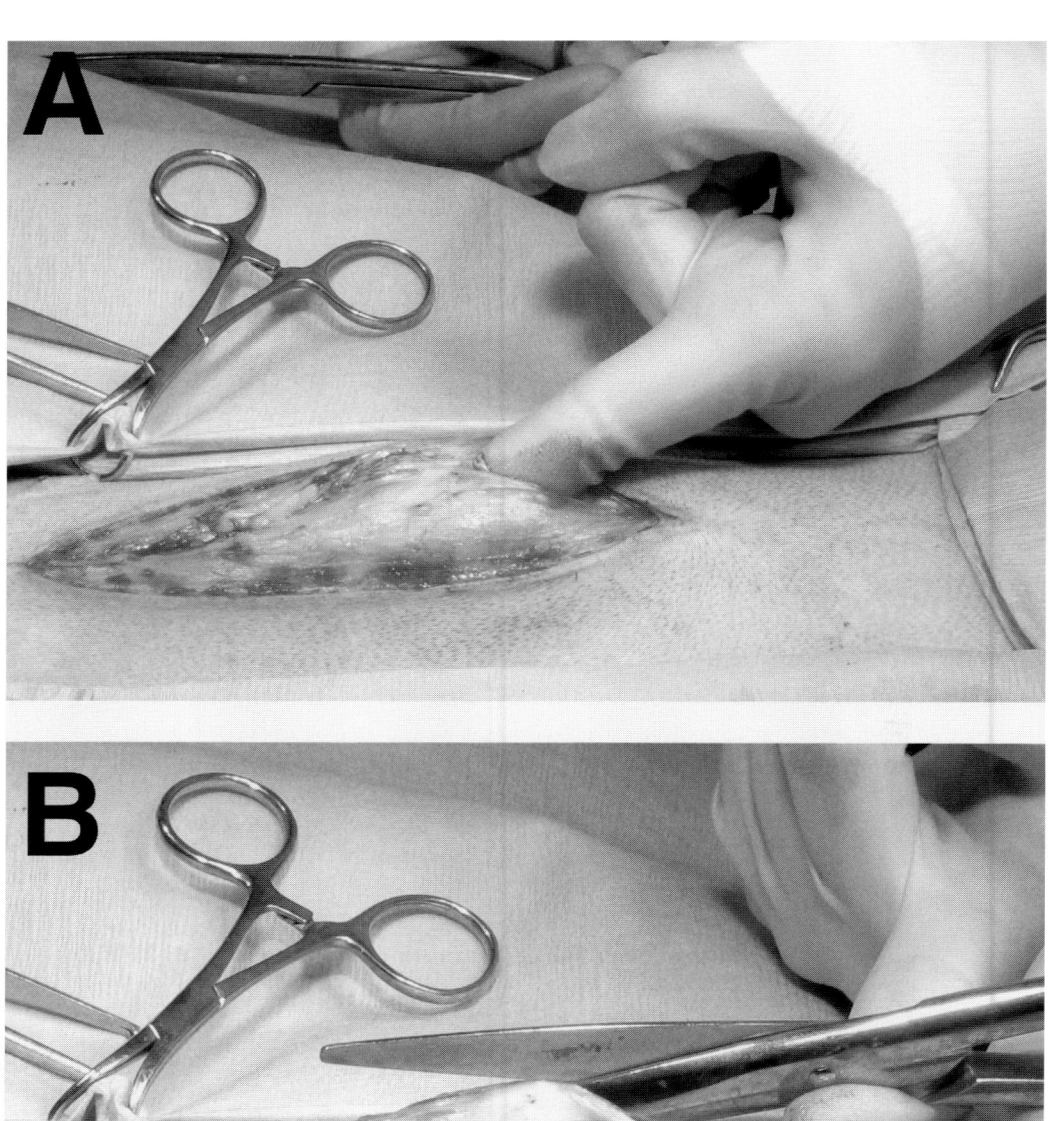

Fig. 10.8. Extending the incision with scissors: (A) feel along the peritoneal surface of the linea alba for adhesions; (B) use the blade of Mayo scissors to tent the linea alba and cut to extend the incision.

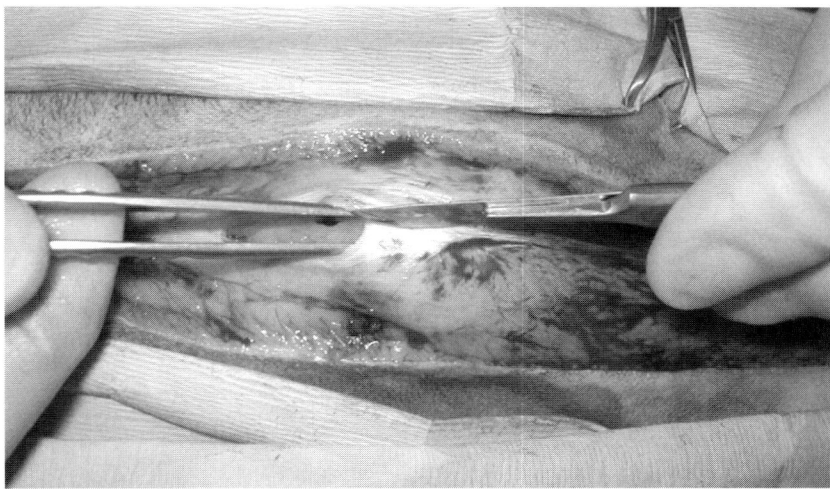

Fig. 10.9. Extending the incision with a scalpel.

abdominal surgery, start the abdominal incision cranial or caudal to the scar of the previous surgery in an uncompromised portion of linea alba where the risk of organ adhesion is minimal. Alternatively, a technique referred to as 'feathering' can be used to gain access to the abdomen. The curved portion of a no. 10 blade is used to make a shallow, partial-thickness incision through the linea alba over a 1–2 cm stretch in the centre of the incision site. This process is repeated until the linea alba has been incised through its full thickness at this point (Fig. 10.10). Once the linea alba has been penetrated, the incision is extended using standard techniques. This enables the abdomen to be penetrated in a controlled manner.

Maximizing Exposure

Abdominal surgery is greatly facilitated by maximizing the exposure to the abdominal organs. This helps identify pathology and provides room to manipulate the organs. Several simple steps can be taken to improve exposure.

Excise the falciform fat

The falciform fat attaches along the peritoneal surface of the linea alba from the xiphisternum to the umbilicus. It obscures the cranial abdomen. It can be reflected or removed to improve exposure during cranial abdominal surgery (e.g. gastrotomy;

liver biopsy; diaphragmatic rupture repair) (Fig. 10.11). The main blood supply to the falciform fat pad originates from dorsal to the xiphisternum and enters the fat pad cranially. Additional small vessels from the peritoneum extend into the pad laterally. To reflect the fat pad from one side, incise the lateral attachments to the linea alba with Metzenbaum scissors, ligating or cauterizing small vessels as required. For maximum exposure, remove the fat pad entirely. Detach it from both sides of the linea alba laterally, clamp and ligate the base of the pad at the xiphisternum, and excise it.

Positional changes

Tilting the patient so that its head is higher than its pelvis improves exposure of the cranial abdomen as the abdominal viscera fall away from the diaphragm and liver. Operating tables are often tiltable, or the patient can be propped up using a positioning cradle that is lifted on padding at one end.

Use abdominal retractors

Self-retaining abdominal retractors (e.g. Gosset; Balfour) greatly improve abdominal exposure (see p. 62). Protect the sides of the abdominal incision with moistened swabs before placing the retractors, to prevent desiccation of the incision margins (Fig. 10.12).

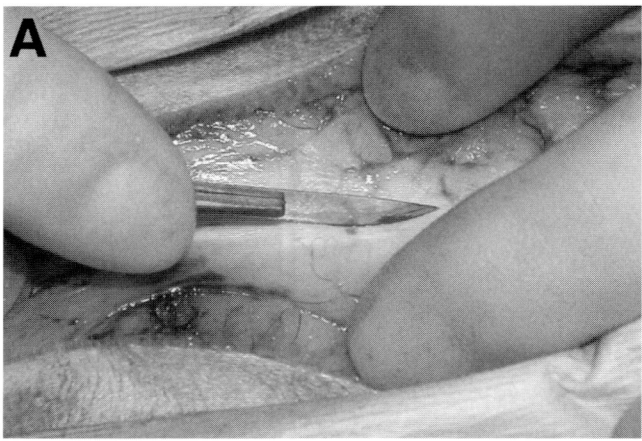

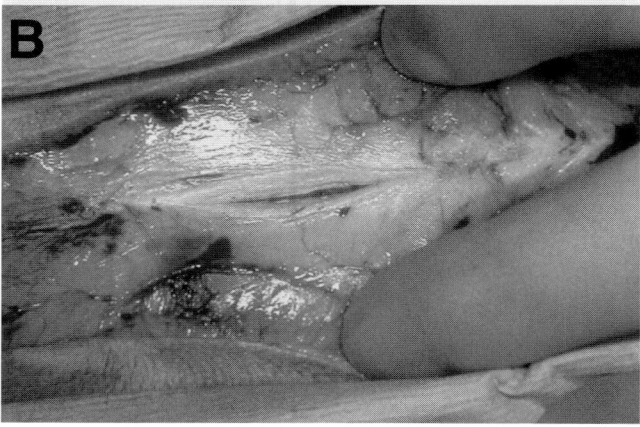

Fig. 10.10. Alternative 'feathering' method of abdominal entry: (A) make repeated partial thickness linea alba incisions over a short area using the curved edge of a no. 10 scalpel blade; (B) once the linea alba is penetrated, proceed as normal to extend the incision.

Prevent Tissue Desiccation

The surface of exposed tissues and organs may become desiccated during abdominal surgery, leading to inflammation. To prevent this, protect the edges of the abdominal incision with moistened swabs and keep the abdominal organs covered with more moistened swabs when possible. Lavage the exposed organs regularly with sterile saline during prolonged surgery (see p. 143).

Exploring the Abdomen

A systematic approach should be used to explore the abdomen. A popular method is to divide the abdomen into five regions (the four quadrants and the intestinal tract) and to examine each in turn.

Cranial quadrant

Assess the organs in the cranial quadrant (Fig. 10.13):

- **Diaphragm:** examine for defects.
- **Liver:** palpate each lobe gently. They should be of uniform colour and consistency with sharp edges. They should not extend beyond the costal arch. Round lobes or protrusion of the liver beyond the costal arch indicate hepatomegaly.
- **Gall bladder and biliary tree:** the gall bladder sits between the right-middle and quadrate liver

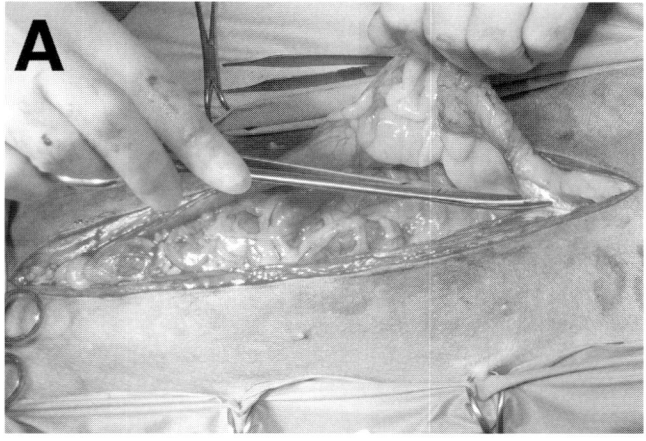

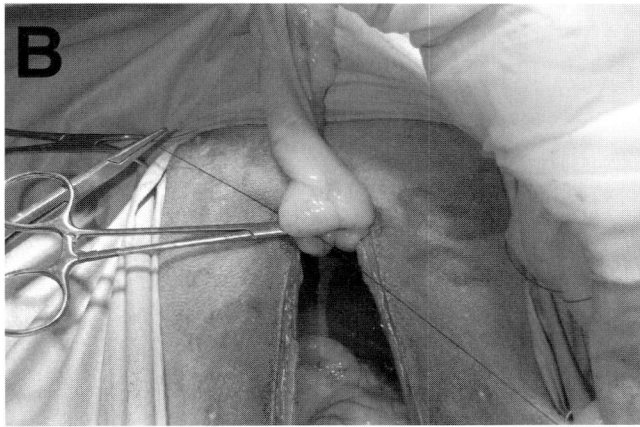

Fig. 10.11. Remove the falciform fat: (A) dissect the attachments to the linea alba on both sides of the abdominal incision; (B) ligate the base of the falciform fat pad as it emerges from under the xiphisternum before transecting it.

lobes. Gently squeeze the gall bladder to check that bile can be expressed into the duodenum. Trace from the gall bladder along the cystic duct and common bile duct to the duodenum.

- **Oesophageal cardia:** palpate for masses and hernias.
- **Stomach:** palpate for irregularities, masses, and foreign bodies (which often sink to the depths of the fundus where they are easily missed). Check the reflection of the omentum from the greater curvature. The visceral surface of the stomach is covered by the greater omentum and is completely enclosed within the omental bursa (lesser peritoneal cavity). The visceral surface of the stomach can be assessed by bluntly opening the omental bursa through an avascular portion of omentum if required.

- **Greater omentum, spleen, and left limb of pancreas:** carefully lift the spleen out of the abdomen and inspect it for masses (Fig. 10.14). Inspect the omentum and reflect it cranially to expose the deep leaf. The left limb of the pancreas and splenic artery can be seen running parallel to the greater curvature of the stomach within the deep leaf of the greater omentum (Fig. 10.15).

Right quadrant

Expose the right quadrant by performing the **duodenal sling** (Fig. 10.16). Locate the duodenum as it emerges from the stomach (confirm this by identifying the right limb of the pancreas in the mesoduodenum). Lift the duodenum up and pull it

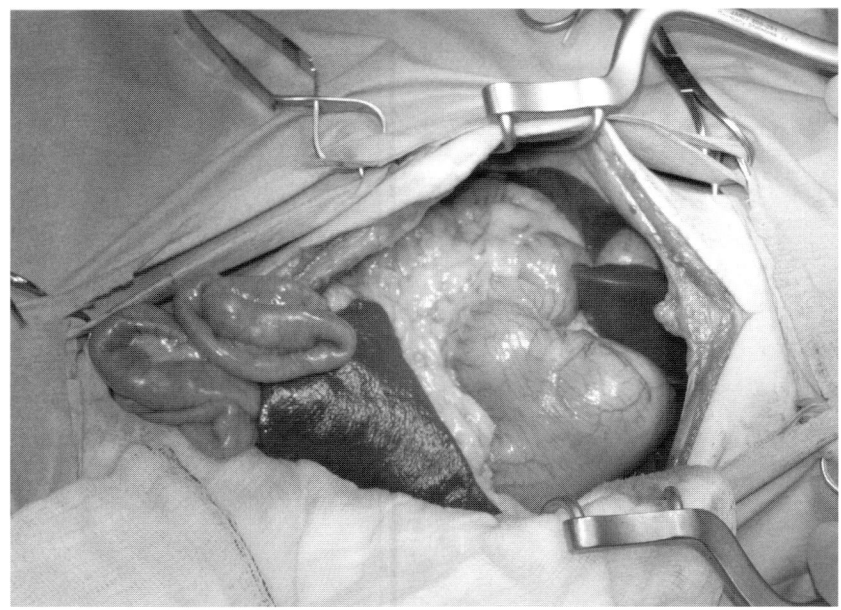

Fig. 10.12. Balfour retractors in position.

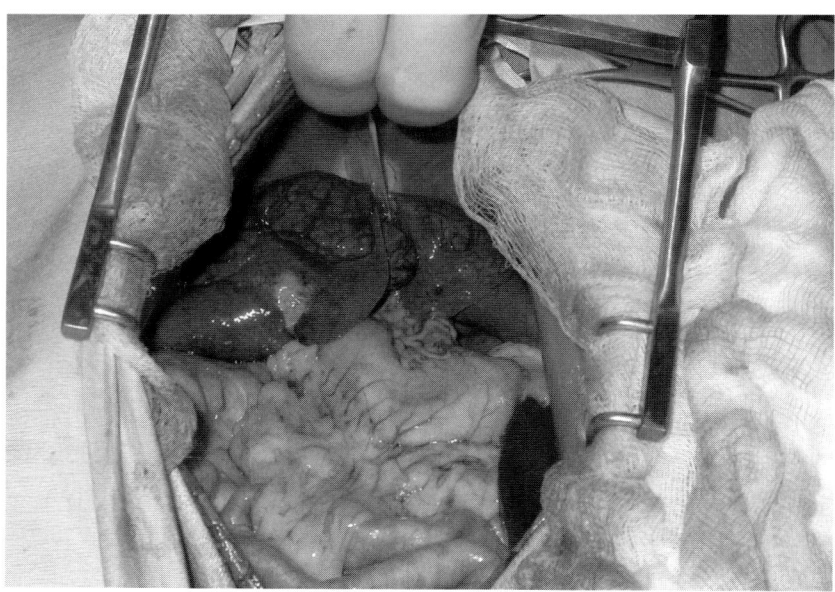

Fig. 10.13. Exposing the cranial quadrant: the liver, gall bladder, stomach, and omentum are visible. This cat has cancerous lesions in its liver.

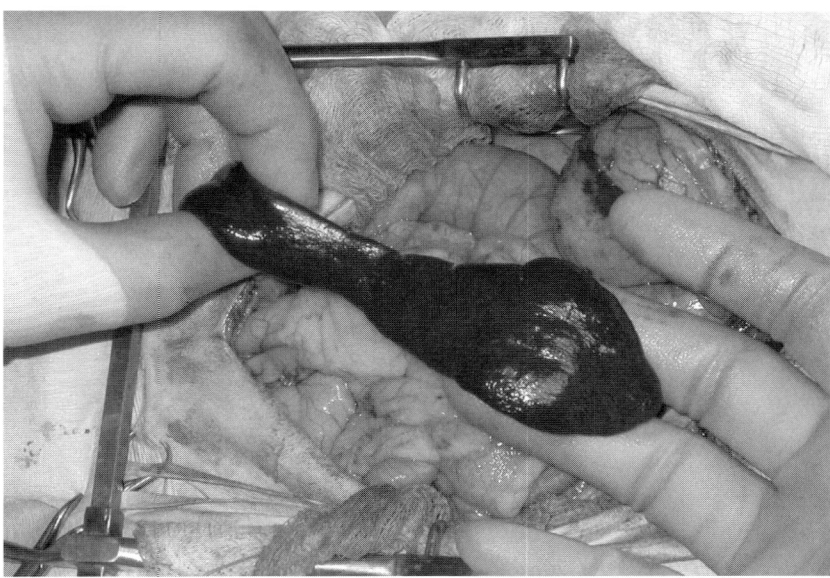

Fig. 10.14. Evaluating the spleen.

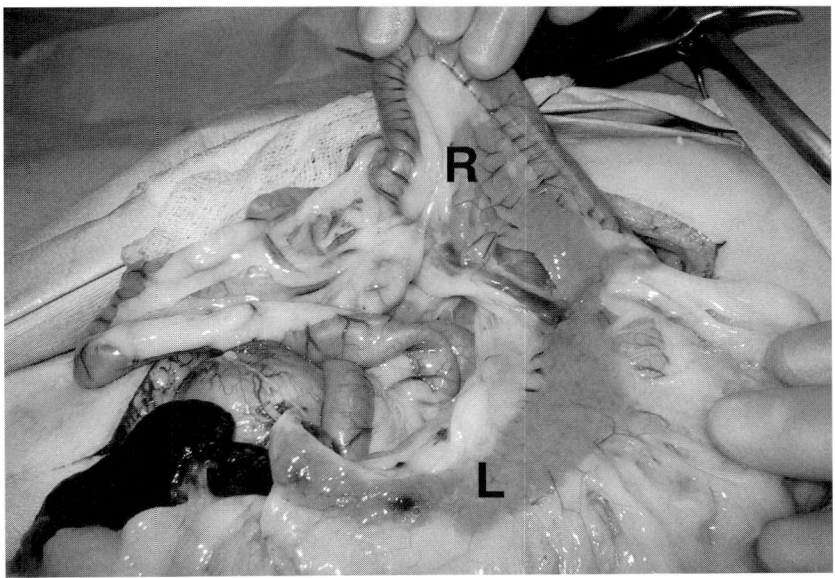

Fig. 10.15. Exposing the left limb of the pancreas: reflect the omentum cranially to reveal the left limb of the pancreas ('L'). The pancreas can be traced round to the right limb within the mesoduodenum in this view ('R').

towards the left side of the abdomen. This creates a sling of mesoduodenum behind which the small intestinal tract is held to expose the right paralumbar fossa:

- **Right limb of the pancreas:** this is located in the mesoduodenum abutting the duodenum. It should be salmon-pink with a finely lobulated surface.

Principles of Abdominal Surgery

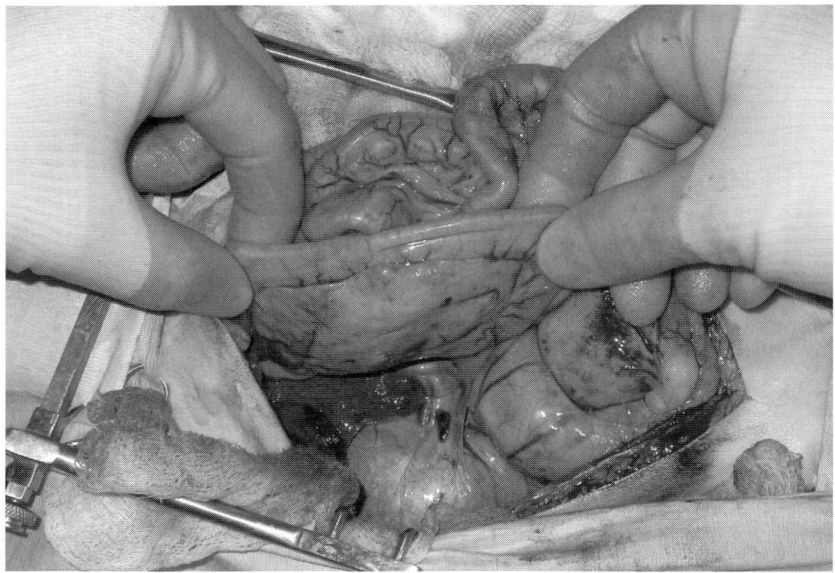

Fig. 10.16. Exploring the right quadrant: the duodenal sling has been used to expose the right kidney, right liver lobes, and the right paralumbar fossa. The right limb of the pancreas can be seen in the mesoduodenum.

- **Caudal vena cava:** this is the large vein running dorsally along the paralumbar fossa into the hepatic parenchyma. Ventral to this location, within the mesoduodenum, the **portal vein** can be seen running parallel to the caudal vena cava.
- **Kidney:** the cranial pole sits in the renal fossa within the caudate process of the liver. The kidney should be dark red, smooth, and regular. Inspect the renal vessels at the hilus.
- **Adrenal:** this is difficult to visualize as it sits cranial to the kidney and dorsal to the vena cava.
- **Ureter:** this runs from the hilus of the kidney, along the paralumbar fossa, to the bladder. It may be obscured by fat but should be assessed for dilation or other lesions.
- **Reproductive structures:** in females, the ovary and uterine horn are identified caudal to the kidney. The suspensory ligament runs laterally to the kidney to insert dorsally on the last rib. In males, the testicular artery and vein run from near the renal hilus to the inguinal canal. The ductus deferens courses from dorsal to the bladder (emerging from the prostatic parenchyma) and runs laterally through the inguinal canal. It loops around the ureter near the bladder neck.

- **Peritoneum:** assess the peritoneal surface for lesions.

Left quadrant

Expose the left quadrant by performing the **colonic sling** (Fig. 10.17). Lift the colon up and pull it to the right. The mesocolon is used to retract the intestines exposing the left paralumbar fossa.

- **Adrenal gland:** locate this on the dorsal abdominal wall cranial to the pole of the left kidney. Unlike the right adrenal, it is easy to identify and is not obscured by the aorta or vena cava.
- **Kidney:** the left kidney is positioned more caudally than the right. It is also more mobile.
- **Ureter.**
- **Reproductive structures.**
- **Peritoneum.**

Caudal quadrant

Push the intestinal tract cranially to expose the caudal quadrant (Fig. 10.18):

- **Inguinal canals:** check for hernias. The testicular vessels and ductus deferentes in males, and

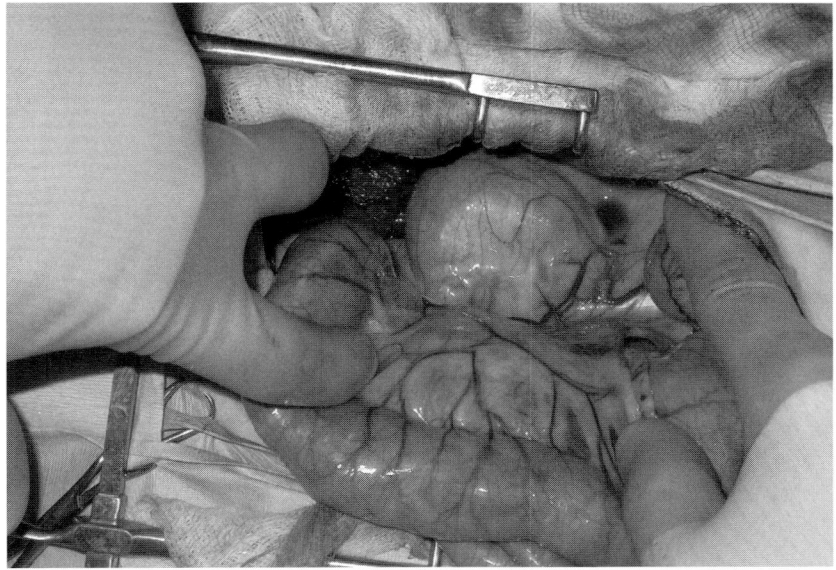

Fig. 10.17. Exploring the left quadrant: the colonic sling has been used to expose the left kidney and paralumbar fossa.

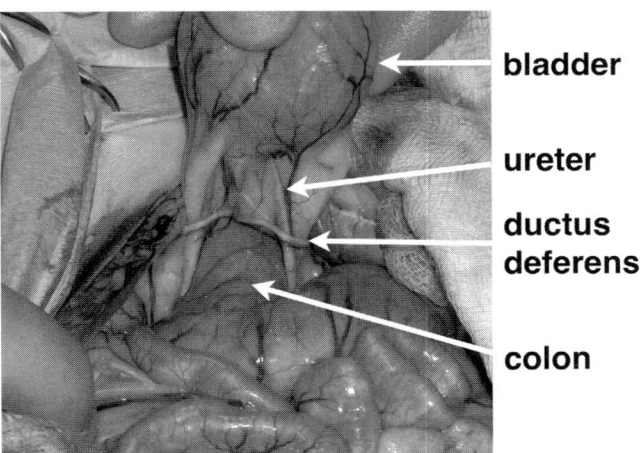

bladder

ureter

ductus
deferens

colon

Fig. 10.18. Exploring the caudal quadrant: the bladder has been reflected caudally to reveal the ureters and ductus deferens in this male cat.

the vaginal process of the round ligament in females, normally run into the inguinal canal.
- **Descending colon.**
- **Bladder:** inspect the bladder for masses and stones. Reflect the bladder caudally to expose its dorsal surface where the ureters enter the trigone.

- **Prostate:** in castrated or immature dogs, this may be very small. Pulling the bladder cranially may expose the prostate at the bladder neck. If it cannot be visualized, palpate dorsal to the bladder and urethra. The prostate should be smooth, bilobed, and symmetrical. In cats, the prostate is very small unless it is diseased.

Intestinal tract

Finally, carefully inspect the intestinal tract (Fig. 10.19). Start where the duodenum emerges from the pylorus. Work along the entire length of the small intestine and then the large intestine to ensure that the entire tract is evaluated. The intestinal wall is palpated for irregularities and is assessed for pinkness and peristalsis (both signs of intestinal health). The mesentery, mesenteric vessels, and mesenteric lymph nodes are also evaluated. The nodes are located close to the root of the mesentery and are checked for size and consistency. (NB: The mesenteric nodes are prominent in immature dogs and cats in comparison to adult animals and are often mistakenly considered to be enlarged.)

Limiting Contamination During Surgery

Abdominal lavage dilutes and removes contaminants (e.g. blood; bacteria, spilled intestinal contents; urine) from the abdomen. It is performed after prolonged abdominal surgery, hollow-organ surgery, or any surgery where there is contamination of the abdomen. Abdominal lavage is greatly facilitated by the use of suction with a Poole suction catheter (see p. 63). Use *isotonic, 0.9% sterile sodium chloride* that has been warmed to body temperature to prevent inducing hypothermia. As a guide, *200–300 ml/kg* of fluid are adequate for removing the majority of contaminants in a heavily contaminated abdomen (e.g. septic peritonitis). Alternatively, continue lavage until the fluid being removed runs clear.

There is a risk of contaminating the abdomen with urine or intestinal contents during bladder or gastrointestinal surgery. Several techniques should be employed to prevent contamination and to remove contaminants during surgery (Figs 10.20 and 10.21):

1. Isolate hollow organs from the rest of the abdomen with moistened swabs before cutting into them. Mobile organs (e.g. small intestine) can be exteriorized from the abdomen to further limit the risk of contamination of other organs.
2. Use bowel clamps (e.g. Doyen) to isolate the section of intestine being operated on and to prevent chyme from spilling into the abdomen.
3. Empty the bladder before incising into it, by urethral catheterization or intra-operative cystocentesis.
4. Perform regional lavage of the bladder or bowel after closing the incision in the organ but before removing the swabs used to isolate the organ from the rest of the abdomen. This removes contaminants

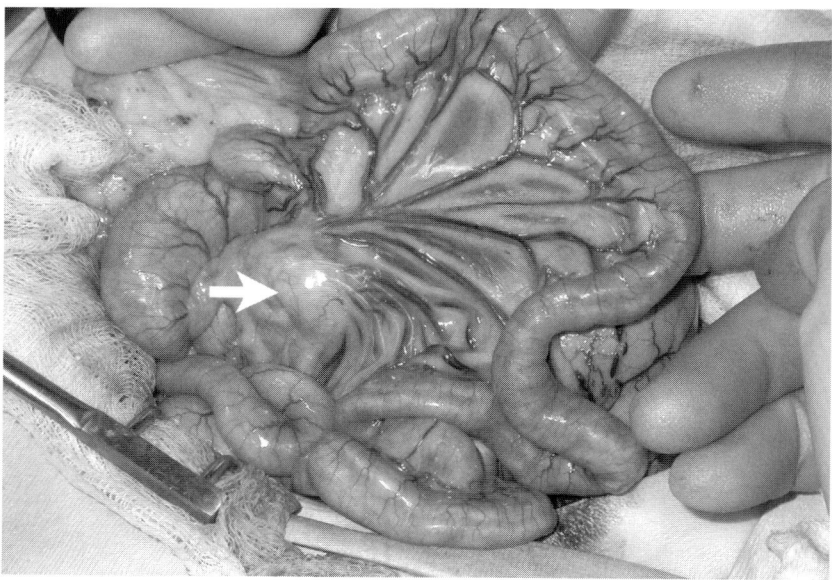

Fig. 10.19. Exploring the intestinal tract: arrow marks the mesenteric node draining this loop of intestine. Note the arcuate blood supply.

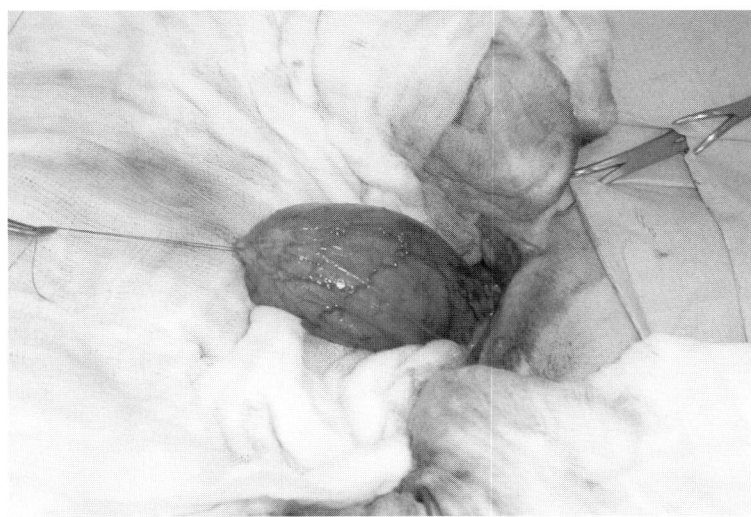

Fig. 10.20. Methods of limiting contamination during hollow organ surgery: isolate organs with moistened swabs before incising into them (e.g. bladder prior to cystotomy).

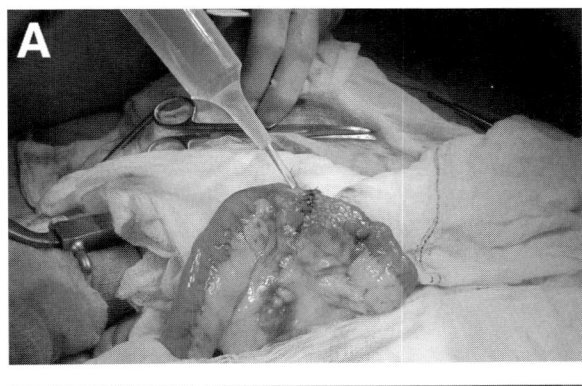

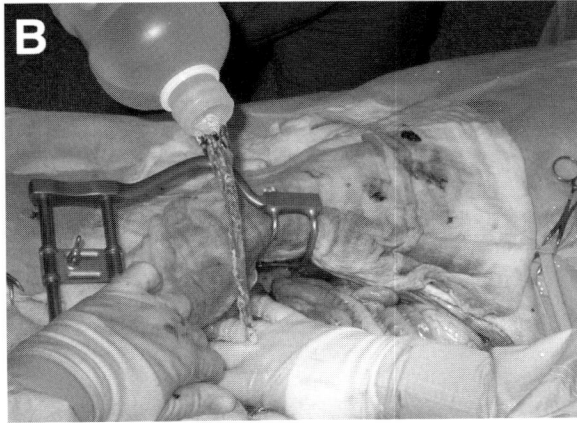

Fig. 10.21. Methods of removing contaminants: (A) regional lavage of a loop of intestine following foreign body removal and before returning it to the abdomen; (B) general abdominal lavage before abdominal closure.

Principles of Abdominal Surgery

before the organ is returned to the abdomen. After the organ has been returned to the abdomen, perform further abdominal lavage.

5. Discard swabs and instruments used to open hollow organs as they are likely to be contaminated.

Encouraging Early Serosal Seals

The mesothelial surface of the omentum readily adheres to traumatized serosa, sealing the surface and reducing leakage from hollow organs. The omentum also promotes local angiogenesis and provides lymphatic drainage away from the diseased area. These features can be harnessed to reduce leakage and improve healing of gastrotomy, enterotomy, and cystotomy incisions by performing a procedure called the *omental wrap*. The omentum, which is very mobile, is wrapped over the incision line and tacked in place with loose, absorbable sutures to produce an early serosal seal (Fig. 10.22). Omental wrapping is recommended following all hollow-organ surgery.

Closing the Abdomen

Return the abdominal organs to their original positions prior to closure. Ensure that the small intestinal tract is largely contained between the mesoduodenum and the mesocolon without being twisted. Replace the spleen along the left lateral abdominal wall. Finally, replace the omentum to cover the ventral surface of the intestinal tract.

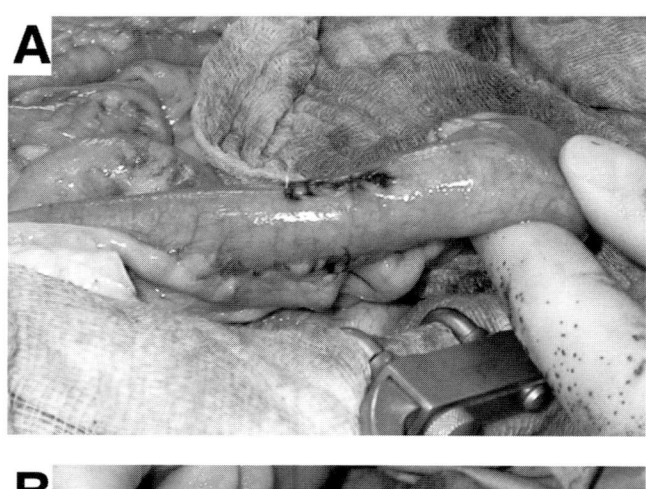

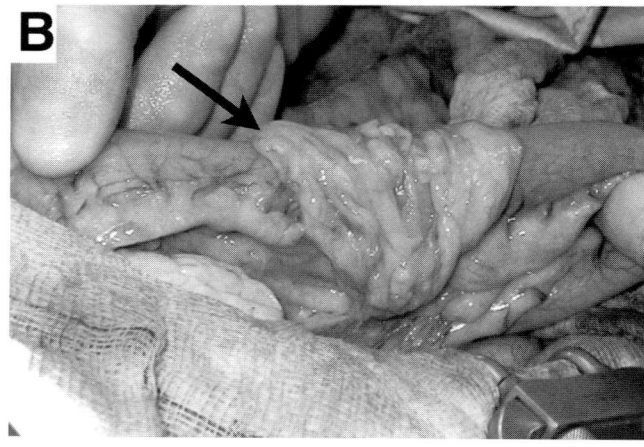

Fig. 10.22. Omental wrap: (A) intestinal biopsy site; (B) omentum laid over site (arrow) and tacked in place with one or two monofilament, short-lasting sutures.

The coeliotomy incision is closed by suturing the linea alba, subcutaneous fat, and skin separately. The suture line in the linea alba is critical as it prevents herniation post-operatively. The external rectus sheath provides most of the strength to the linea alba closure and must be included in every bite of suture. Including the rectus abdominis muscle or peritoneum is unnecessary and may lead to increased inflammation and adhesion formation.

Either simple continuous or simple interrupted suture patterns can be used to close the linea alba. Advantages of the simple continuous pattern are that less suture material is required and that it is faster. Concerns that the incidence of incisional herniation and other complications is higher when continuous suture patterns are used appear to be unfounded. For simple continuous closure, it is recommended that at least five throws are used to form the knot at the start of the suture line and that seven throws are used to form the knot at the end. Each piece of suture should include 4–7 mm of the external rectus sheath. The bites should be spaced 5–10 mm apart. Start at the caudal extent of the incision and work cranially (Fig. 10.23). For routine closure, use long-lasting, synthetic, absorbable, monofilament suture material (e.g. polydioxanone). If the patient is at increased risk of wound dehiscence, non-absorbable, synthetic, monofilament suture material (e.g. polypropylene) may be used. Select a suture size appropriate for the size of patient (<2.5 kg 3-0; 2.5–10 kg 2-0; 10–20 kg 0; >20 kg 1).

The subcutaneous fat and skin are closed routinely. In male dogs, suture the cut ends of the preputial muscle to restore cranial support to the prepuce.

Aftercare

Keep the incision covered with a non-adherent, light dressing for 48 h post-operatively. Restrict exercise for the first 14 days following surgery, by confining dogs to lead-controlled exercise for toilet purposes only and by keeping cats inside. Discourage animals from jumping on and off furniture during this period. Prevent self-inflicted trauma by keeping the wound covered with a dressing for longer or by using an Elizabethan collar if required.

Complications

Wound swelling, seroma, or infection may occur. In male dogs, swelling often occurs adjacent to the prepuce. Rarely, infection of the subcutaneous tissues extends through the incision into the abdomen

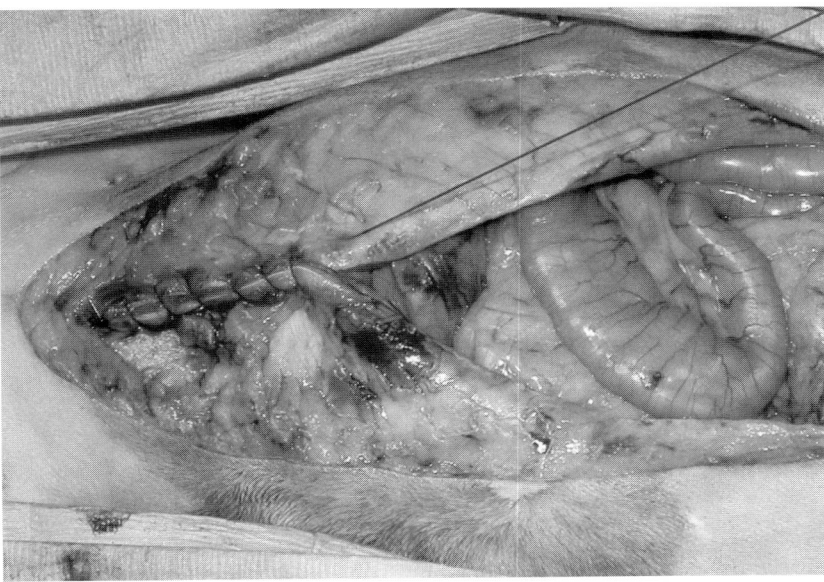

Fig. 10.23. Linea alba closure using simple continuous pattern ensuring that each suture engages the external rectus sheath. Start the suture line at the pubis and work cranially.

and causes septic peritonitis. Incisional hernia is a serious complication that may lead to evisceration. It probably results from technical failures during closure of the external rectus fascia. Failure to include the external rectus sheath in each suture bite during abdominal closure, and poor knotting, may both lead to incisional hernia.

Laparoscopic Surgery

Laparoscopic or 'keyhole' surgery is gaining in popularity in specialist veterinary practices. The basic technique involves inflating the abdomen with gas and inserting a rigid endoscope to evaluate the abdomen and perform a range of procedures (e.g. ovariectomy; liver biopsy; cryptorchid castration). Animals recover more rapidly than following conventional surgery but laparoscopy is probably no safer than conventional surgery, particularly when performed by surgeons with limited experience. Laparoscopic surgery carries a risk of iatrogenic organ injury during entry, and animals with respiratory or cardiac disease may be at increased risk of complications intra-operatively. This is an advanced technique that requires considerable investment in equipment and training

Bibliography

Adams, W., Ctercteko, G. and Bilous, M. (1992) Effect of an omental wrap on the healing and vascularity of compromised intestinal anastomoses. *Diseases of the Colon and Rectum* 35, 731–738.

Baines, S.J. (2001) Exploratory laparotomy. *UK Vet* 6, 59–71.

Bellenger, C.R. (2003) Abdominal wall. In: Slatter, D.H. (ed.) *Textbook of Small Animal Surgery*, 3rd edn. W.B. Saunders, Philadelphia, Pennsylvania, pp. 405–413.

Boothe, H.W. (1990) Exploratory laparotomy in small animals. *Compendium of Continuing Education for the Practicing Veterinarian* 12, 1057–1066.

Crowe, D.T. (1978) Closure of abdominal incisions using a continuous polypropylene suture: clinical experience in 550 dogs and cats. *Veterinary Surgery* 7, 74–77.

Crowe, D.T. (1990) The abdominal cavity: peritoneum, retroperitoneum, abdominal hernias and the adrenal glands. In: Harvey, C.E., Newton, C.D. and Schwartz, A. (eds) *Small Animal Surgery*. J.B. Lippincott Company, Philadelphia, Pennsylvania, pp. 279–322.

Evans, H.E. (1993) The liver. In: Evans, H.E. (ed.) *Miller's Anatomy of the Dog*, 3rd edn. W.B. Saunders, Philadelphia, Pennsylvania, pp. 451–462.

Gower, S.B., Weisse, C.W. and Brown, D.C. (2009) Major abdominal evisceration injuries in dogs and cats: 12 cases (1998–2008). *Journal of the American Veterinary Medical Association* 234, 1566–1572.

Heller, J. and Hunt, G.B. (2002) Clinical applications of the omentum in dogs and cats. *Australian Veterinary Practitioner* 32, 66–73.

Hermanson, J.W. and Evans, H.E. (1993) Muscles of the abdominal wall. In: Evans, H.E. (ed.) *Miller's Anatomy of the Dog*, 3rd edn. W.B. Saunders, Philadelphia, Pennsylvania, pp. 308–384.

Hosgood, G. (1990) The omentum – the forgotten organ: physiology and potential surgical applications in dogs and cats. *Compendium of Continuing Education for the Practicing Veterinarian* 12, 45–51.

Jobanputra, S. and Wexner, S.D. (2007) Systematic guide to complex cases from adhesive disease. *Colorectal Disease* 9, 54–59.

Kummeling, A. and Van Sluijs, F.J. (1998) Closure of the rectus sheath with a continuous looped suture and the skin with staples in dogs: speed, safety, and costs compared to closure of the rectus sheath with interrupted sutures and the skin with a continuous subdermal suture. *Veterinary Quarterly* 20, 126–130.

Rosin, E. and Richardson, S. (1987) Effect of fascial closure technique on strength of healing abdominal incision in the dog. A biomechanical study. *Veterinary Surgery* 16, 269–272.

Rosin, E. and Robinson, G.M. (1989) Knot security of suture materials. *Veterinary Surgery* 18, 269–273.

Seim, H.B. 3rd (1995) Management of peritonitis. In: Bonagura, E.D. (ed.) *Current Veterinary Therapy XII: Small Animal Practice*. W.B. Saunders, Philadelphia, Pennsylvania, pp. 764–772.

Welsh, E.M. (2005) Principles of abdominal surgery. In: Williams, J.M. and Niles, J.D. (eds) *BSAVA Manual of Canine and Feline Abdominal Surgery*, 1st edn. BSAVA, Gloucester, UK, pp. 1–22.

11 Hernias and Ruptures

centesis: drainage using a syringe and needle
dyschezia: difficulty defecating
dysuria: difficulty urinating
hernia: defect in the body wall allowing protrusion of organs
herniorrhaphy: repair of a hernia
incisional hernia: iatrogenic hernia through a coeliotomy incision
rupture: traumatic body wall defect
tenesmus: straining to defecate
thoracocentesis: drainage of fluid or air from the thorax using a needle and syringe

The reader should be able to:

- list the components of a hernia
- predict the historical and physical findings that might be seen with an incarcerated umbilical hernia that contains a strangulated loop of small intestine in a cat
- define the anatomic landmarks of umbilical, inguinal, scrotal, and perineal hernias
- describe how to close a small umbilical hernia
- classify the different forms of diaphragmatic defect
- identify the key radiographic findings of diaphragmatic hernia from representative abdominal and thoracic radiographs
- describe and appreciate the different presentations of perineal hernia
- illustrate the steps that might be required to safely anaesthetize and operate on a dog to repair an acute, traumatic diaphragmatic defect
- identify forms of hernia that an inexperienced veterinary surgeon should not attempt to repair

This chapter describes the principles of hernia classification and repair using the common abdominal hernias as examples. Particular emphasis is placed on the importance of a tension-free repair. Perineal hernia and diaphragmatic defects are considered individually, as their presentation, management, and repair differ from other abdominal hernias. The term rupture is often used to describe a traumatic body wall defect that allows herniation of abdominal organs but which lacks a hernia sac. The terms rupture and hernia are often used synonymously and can be considered together when discussing the principles of repair.

Principles of Herniorrhaphy

Hernia structure and classification

Hernias are abnormal body wall defects that may be congenital or acquired. The component parts of a hernia are:

1. hernia ring: edge of defect bordered by muscle or ligament;
2. hernia sac: out-pouching of peritoneum confining hernia contents;
3. hernia contents: abdominal organs that herniate through the hernia ring.

These are demonstrated in Fig. 11.1. 'True hernias' occur through natural body wall openings (e.g. inguinal hernia). 'False hernias' occur through muscular rents (e.g. perineal hernia).

Reducible versus irreducible hernias

Reducible hernias have contents that can be returned easily to the abdomen by gentle pressure (see Fig. 11.2). In contrast, the contents of irreducible hernias cannot be returned to the abdomen as they have become stuck. Hernias become irreducible for several reasons:

1. organ distension: herniated hollow organs (e.g. bladder; intestine) may become distended with urine, gas, or fluid preventing their return through the hernia ring. Alternatively organs may become congested and swollen because of compression or torsion of their vascular supply as it passes through the hernia ring;

2. contracture of the hernia ring;
3. incarceration: adhesions may form between the herniated organ and hernia ring, preventing reduction of the hernia contents.

Strangulated hernia

Compression or torsion of the vascular supply to a herniated organ may cause ischaemic necrosis, which is termed strangulation (Fig. 11.3). Organs in irreducible hernias are at risk of becoming strangulated.

Presenting signs

Most hernias cause subcutaneous swellings that characteristically disappear as the hernia contents are manipulated and returned to the abdomen. The hernia ring is usually palpable, confirming the presence of a body wall defect (Fig. 11.2). Irreducible hernias can be more difficult to diagnose as they are more likely to be mistaken for other causes of subcutaneous swelling. Hernias may also cause signs associated with dysfunction of herniated organs (e.g. vomiting if herniated small intestine becomes obstructed).

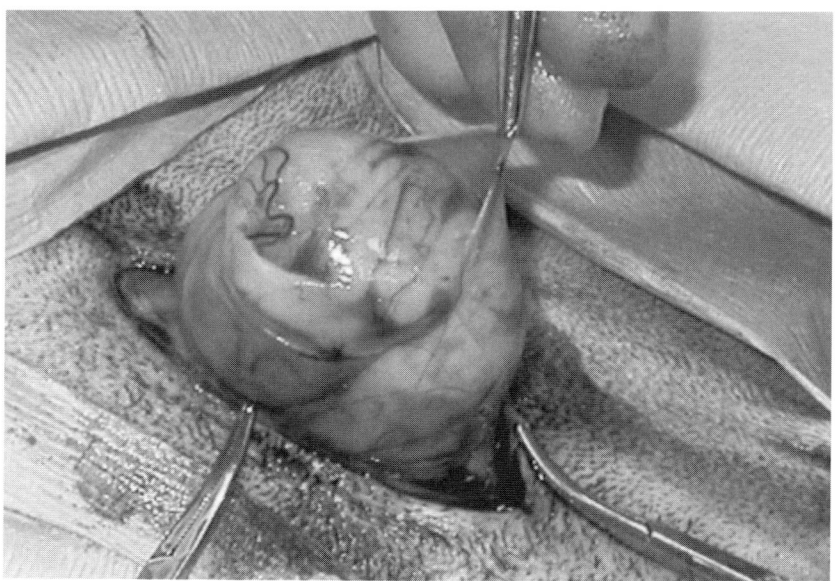

Fig. 11.1. Umbilical hernia demonstrating hernia sac and contents (omentum).

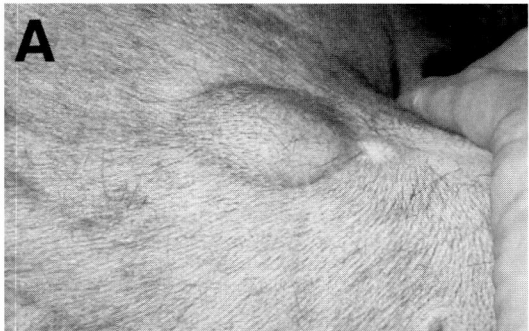

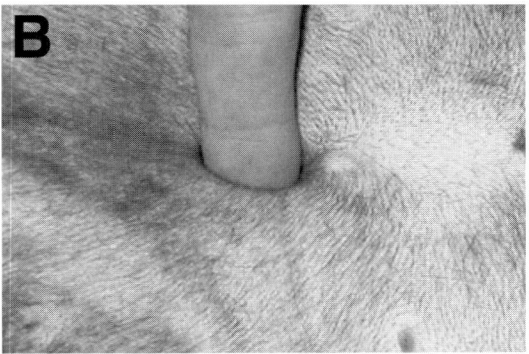

Fig. 11.2. Reducible umbilical hernia before (A) and after (B) the contents are reduced.

Investigation

The main differential diagnoses to consider for hernias are other causes of subcutaneous masses (e.g. tumour, abscess) and other causes of organ dysfunction (e.g. intestinal foreign body). Most hernias can be diagnosed from their clinical signs but additional imaging studies may be required. Ultrasound can be used to confirm loss of continuity of the body wall and the presence of misplaced abdominal organs within the hernia sac. Radiography is generally of little value in the assessment of umbilical, inguinal, and perineal hernias but remains the technique of choice for diagnosing diaphragmatic hernias (see below).

Timing of surgery

Most hernias do not cause severe organ dysfunction and can be repaired electively. However, hernias with obstructed or ischaemic contents and diaphragmatic hernias must be repaired urgently before life-threatening complications develop. Animals with irreducible hernias are at higher risk of developing severe organ dysfunction. These patients should be scheduled for surgery urgently, or monitored regularly for signs

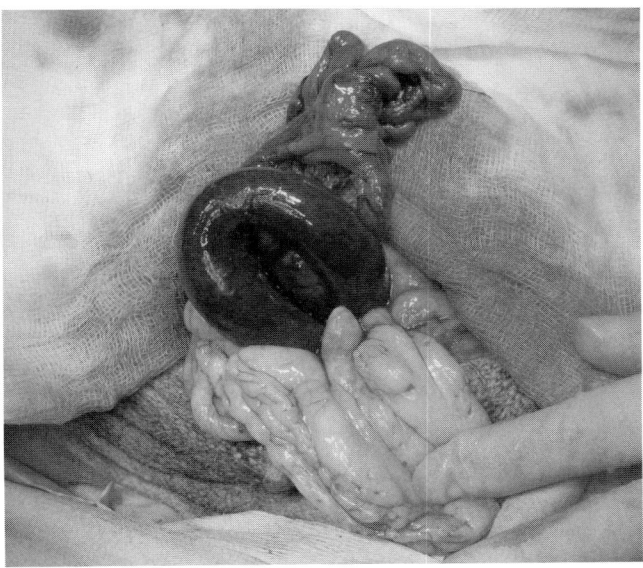

Fig. 11.3. Inguinal hernia with a strangulated loop of small intestine and necrotic omentum.

of deterioration. If a hernia becomes irreducible, firm, painful, red, or oedematous, or if the patient develops signs of organ obstruction (e.g. vomiting, dysuria), these are clear indicators that the herniated organs are becoming compromised and that emergency surgery should be performed.

Herniorrhaphy

The principles of hernia repair emphasize the importance of gentle tissue handling and closure without tension. The general application of these principles to hernia repair is described below, and modifications based on anatomic location and aetiology of the different forms of hernia are discussed separately.

Surgical approach

Incise the skin directly over the hernia. Use a combination of sharp and blunt dissection to expose the hernia sac. Incise the hernia sac taking care not to damage the hernia contents (Fig. 11.4).

Reduce the contents

Assess the contents of the hernia for organ compromise (see p. 181) and adhesions to the hernia ring. If the contents are not compromised and can be reduced easily, push them back into the abdomen and close the hernia ring.

If the hernia contents are not reducible:

1. break down adhesions to the ring using blunt dissection;

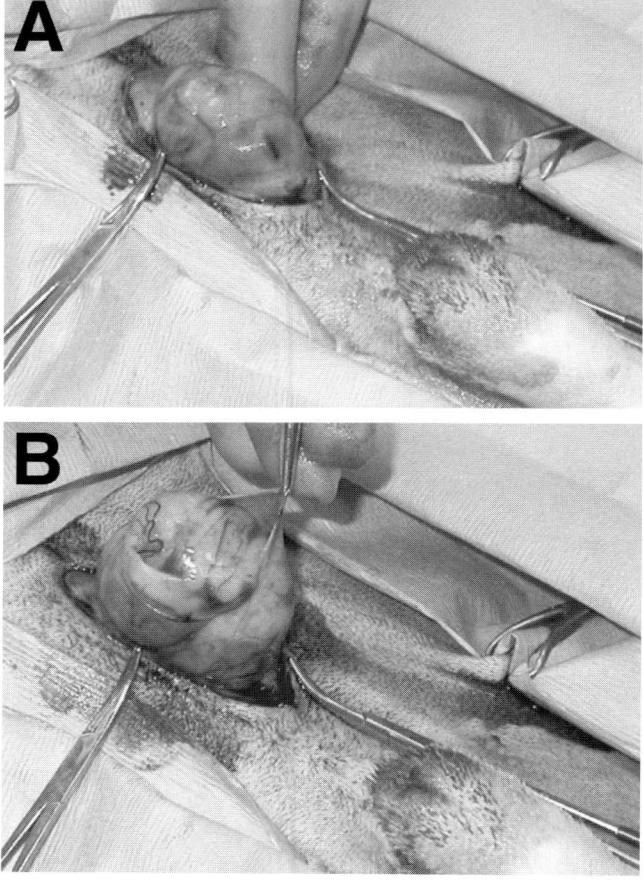

Fig. 11.4. Surgical approach to an umbilical hernia: (A) incise the skin directly over the hernia sac; (B) incise the sac to expose the contents.

2. decompress distended hollow organs by needle centesis;

3. enlarge the hernia ring by making an incision from the edge of the ring into the adjacent abdominal wall. Make the incision in an area that will be accessed easily for subsequent repair (Fig. 11.5).

It may be necessary to remove herniated organs that have become compromised. The limited access to the abdominal organs through the hernia ring is generally inadequate to fully evaluate and manage the diseased tissue. If the hernia contents are severely compromised, perform a separate midline coeliotomy to enable the compromised organs to be fully evaluated once they have been returned into the abdomen (Fig. 11.5).

Close the hernia ring

Two critical factors are required for successful hernia closure:

1. ensure that sutures engage healthy fascia;
2. ensure that the suture line has no tension.

The hernia sac can be resected or inverted into the abdomen before closing the ring. It is important to ensure that all sutures engage healthy tissue that has suitable strength to support abdominal closure (preferably external rectus fascia or abdominal ligaments). If there is devitalized or diseased muscle along the edge of the defect, this should be sharply resected. However, routine debridement of the hernia ring is unnecessary and may be detrimental if it

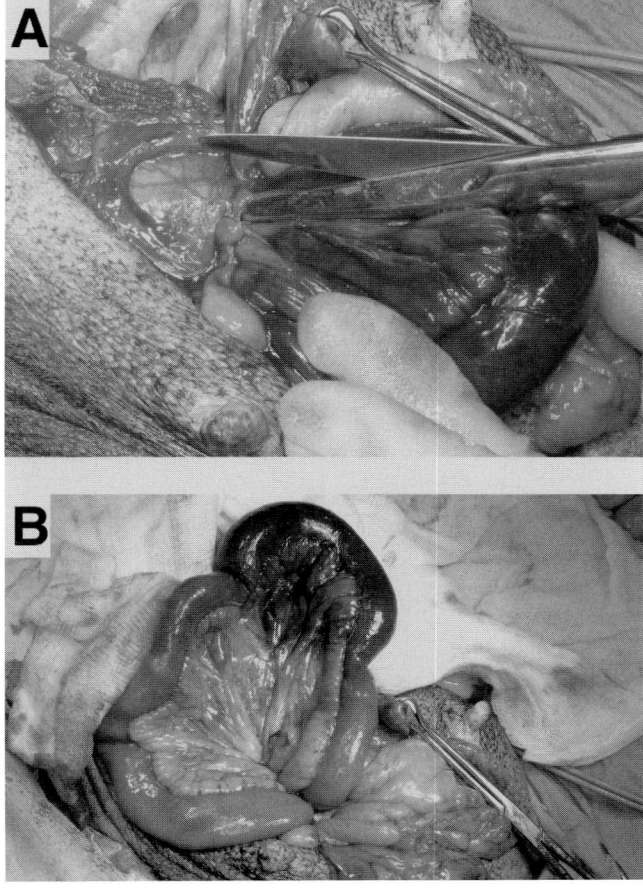

Fig. 11.5. Irreducible inguinal hernia with incarcerated, strangulated loop of small intestine: (A) enlarging the hernia ring by incising from its edge into surrounding healthy tissue enabled the contents to be reduced; (B) this was combined with ventral midline coeliotomy to facilitate reduction of the hernia contents into the abdomen where the necrotic loop of bowel could be resected easily.

is performed on healthy tissue, as it will cause inflammation and enlarge the defect.

Most hernias can be closed by simple apposition of the edges of the ring without placing tension along the suture line. Apply the same principles as those described for coeliotomy closure (see Chapter 10). Use a simple, appositional interrupted or continuous pattern. Select a suture size appropriate for the size of patient (e.g. <2.5 kg 3-0; 2.5–10 kg 2-0; 10–20 kg 0; >20 kg 1). Use monofilament, synthetic, long-lasting absorbable, or non-absorbable suture material (e.g. polydioxanone; polypropylene). For simple continuous closure, it is recommended that at least five throws are used to form the knot at the start of the suture line and that seven throws are used to form the knot at the end. If tension-free closure cannot be achieved using this simple approach, more advanced procedures, including the use of muscle flaps or meshes, are required.

Use of meshes, sheets, and muscle flaps

Synthetic meshes, collagen sheets, and muscle flaps can be used to repair hernias. These serve two functions: (i) they may be used to augment a simple herniorrhaphy; or (ii) they may be used to span a large hernia defect that cannot be closed by simple apposition. Patients that have large hernias requiring meshes or muscle flaps should be referred to an experienced colleague or specialist centre.

Synthetic meshes are manufactured from a range of absorbable and non-absorbable materials. Polypropylene mesh is a popular choice as it provides an inert and permanent barrier that can be used to span large defects. Its pores allow tissue to grow into and integrate with the mesh. The disadvantage is that if the mesh becomes contaminated, it will act as a nidus for infection, leading to sinus tract formation that will be difficult to treat.

Collagen sheets are manufactured from porcine small intestinal submucosa. They have low cellularity and antigenicity, limiting the inflammatory response that they induce when implanted into tissues. These sheets provide short-term physical support of the hernia but become fully incorporated into healing tissues over the first 12 weeks, ultimately generating a stronger scar. Collagen sheets may not be as strong as a polypropylene mesh initially, but they leave no permanent deposits to induce long-term foreign body reaction. Collagen sheets can be laid over existing hernia repairs to

augment them or they can be used to span defects that cannot be closed using simple techniques (Fig. 11.6).

Lastly, muscle flaps can be mobilized from surrounding tissues and moved into the hernia defect to repair it. The advantages of using a muscle flap over collagen sheets and synthetic meshes are that: (i) it will not induce a local foreign body reaction or act as nidus for infection; (ii) it repairs the hernia with well-vascularized tissue that should be of adequate strength; and (iii) it is inexpensive. The best example of this is the internal obturator muscle flap for perineal hernia repair. Muscle flaps are used in preference to synthetic meshes, which are reserved for cases where muscle flaps cannot be generated.

Prevent hernia recurrence and inheritance

Congenital hernias may have a genetic basis, and neutering is recommended to prevent transmission to subsequent generations. Neutering also reduces the rate of recurrence following repair of some hernias (e.g. perineal hernia).

Umbilical Hernia

Umbilical hernias are common congenital lesions that may be heritable. They cause subcutaneous swelling at the umbilicus and form from failure of the body wall to fuse around the umbilical vessels (Fig. 11.2). Usually, the hernia contains only falciform fat and it rarely causes significant clinical signs. Omentum, intestine, and other abdominal organs can herniate and, occasionally, very large umbilical hernias form. Umbilical hernias are usually easy to repair by making an incision directly over the hernia and simply apposing of the edges of the ring (Fig. 11.4). Alternatively, the hernia ring can be incorporated into the midline coeliotomy incision during other abdominal procedures (e.g. ovariohysterectomy), and repaired within the linea alba suture line.

Inguinal and Scrotal Hernias

The inguinal canal is an oblique channel running through the abdominal wall 2–4 cm lateral to the linea alba and just cranial to the pubis. Internally, it is bordered by the internal abdominal oblique muscle, the inguinal ligament, and the rectus abdominis muscle. Externally, it passes through the external rectus fascia. The external pudendal vessels

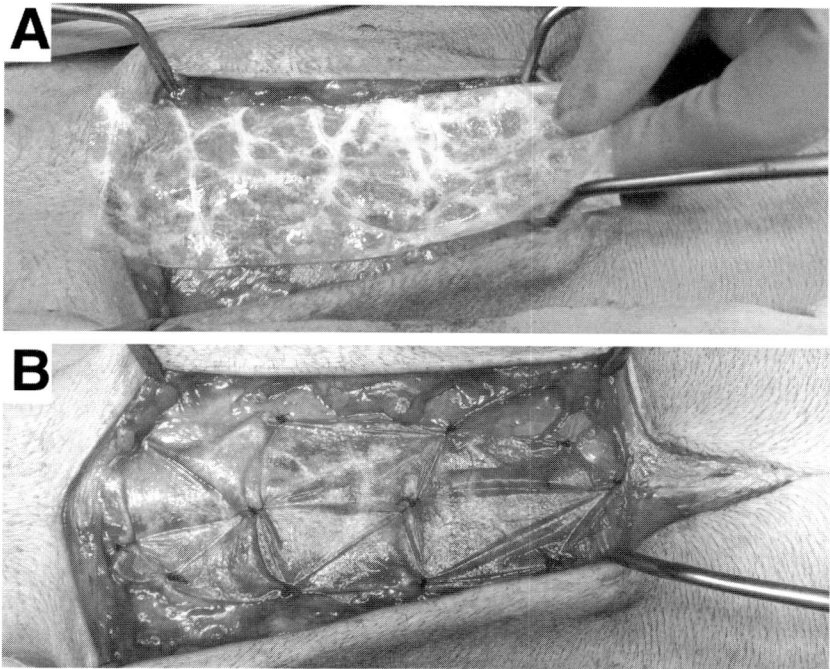

Fig. 11.6. Repair of a chronic, recurrent incisional hernia being augmented with a collagen sheet: (A) the sheet being positioned – it has been rehydrated in saline before being used; (B) the sheet sutured over the repair.

and, in males, the spermatic structures, pass through the inguinal canal. Hernias occur because the inguinal canal is too large, allowing abdominal organs to slip through. Organs may herniate into the subcutaneous inguinal region (*inguinal hernia*) or inside the parietal vaginal tunic into the scrotum (*scrotal hernia*).

Inguinal hernias

Inguinal hernias cause inguinal swelling. They can be unilateral or bilateral and are either congenital or acquired. Congenital inguinal hernias may be inherited and are more common in male dogs. Acquired, degenerate inguinal hernias are most common in entire, female dogs. Occasionally, traumatic inguinal hernias occur. Inguinal hernias are rare in cats.

Inguinal hernias can be challenging to repair because fat obscures the inguinal canal and because the canal runs obliquely through the abdominal wall and is difficult to assess. Various approaches can be used but a ventral midline approach to the body wall enables both inguinal canals to be assessed through a single incision.

Make a ventral midline abdominal skin incision level with, and between, the inguinal canals. Bluntly dissect between the subcutaneous fat and external rectus fascia to expose the inguinal canal and reduce the hernia contents. Alternatively, combine this approach with a caudal midline coeliotomy to facilitate assessment and reduction of the hernia contents from the peritoneal cavity (Fig. 11.7). Close the hernia ring leaving a gap for the pudendal vessels to pass through. Repairing inguinal hernias in uncastrated males is complicated because a large gap must be left in the suture line for the spermatic cord to pass through to prevent strangulation of the testicle. This compromises the efficacy of the repair. To overcome this, castrate males at the same time as repairing the hernia so that more of the inguinal canal can be sutured closed. Always check the contralateral inguinal canal to ensure that it is not enlarged, as bilateral hernias are easily missed.

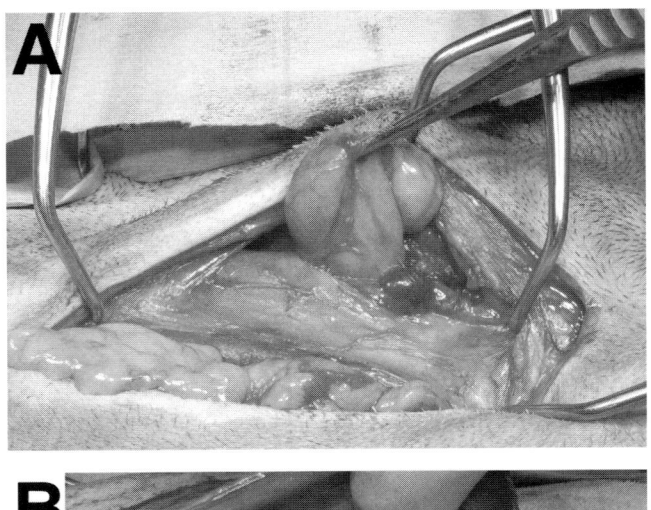

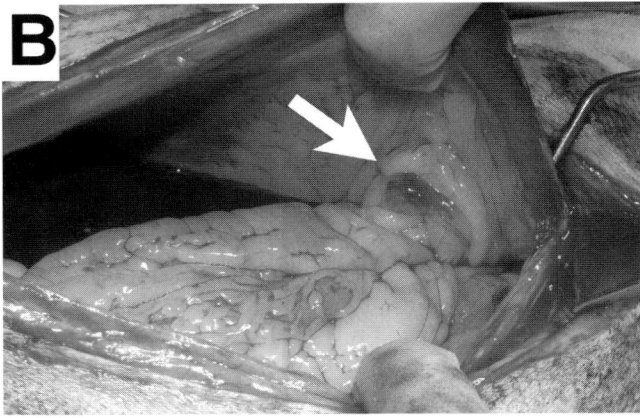

Fig. 11.7. Surgical approaches to inguinal hernia: (A) make a ventral midline skin incision and bluntly dissect between the external rectus sheath and subcutaneous fat to expose the inguinal canal; (B) perform a midline coeliotomy and assess the inguinal canals from the peritoneal surface (arrow shows omentum herniated through canal). These approaches are often combined.

Scrotal hernias

Scrotal hernias are uncommon congenital hernias that may be unilateral or bilateral. The hernias cause testicular swelling and organ obstruction. Sometimes scrotal hernias are only identified after castration because abdominal organs herniate through the skin incision. Scrotal hernia repair is more difficult than inguinal hernia repair.

In male cats, make a caudal midline skin incision from level with the inguinal canals extending back towards the perineum. Dissect laterally to expose the parietal tunic of the spermatic cord and also extend the incision into the abdomen through the linea alba. Incise the parietal tunic and inspect the

hernia contents. Reduce or resect the contents by a combination of gentle traction from the abdominal side with pushing from the testicular side. Evaluate the abdominal organs carefully for compromise. Perform castration and close the inguinal canal. In male dogs, make a parapreputial incision on the side of the hernia and proceed as described above.

Femoral Hernia

Femoral hernias occur through the femoral canal, the body wall opening in the most caudal aspect of the abdominal wall that allows the femoral vessels and nerve to leave the abdomen. The femoral canal is situated caudally and laterally to the inguinal canals and contains the femoral artery, vein, and nerve. Congenital femoral hernias are rare but traumatic femoral hernias are seen, often in combination with prepubic tendon avulsion (see below).

Femoral hernias are challenging to repair as the femoral nerve, artery, and vein run through the hernia, and because there are few suitable suture anchorage points on the caudal border of the defect. Potential complications of femoral hernia repair include femoral nerve damage and haemorrhage from the femoral artery. Femoral hernias should be referred to an experienced colleague or specialist centre for repair. Unfortunately, it is difficult to distinguish between femoral and inguinal hernias preoperatively.

Traumatic Abdominal Ruptures

Traumatic abdominal ruptures are caused by blunt abdominal trauma (e.g. falls; vehicular trauma) or penetrating abdominal injury (e.g. bites). Many animals with traumatic abdominal ruptures have concurrent abdominal injuries, so hernia repair should always be combined with exploratory coeliotomy. Consider referral to a specialist centre for all but the most simple of traumatic abdominal ruptures. Traumatic ruptures can occur at any point along the abdominal wall, and multiple defects may occur, but two common locations will be discussed.

Paralumbar and paracostal tears

Paralumbar and paracostal ruptures are often caused by bite wounds and are easily overlooked. The lateral abdominal muscles tear from the costal arch or lumbar fascia (Fig. 11.8). The rent in the muscle can be sutured or, if the muscle has avulsed directly from the lumbar fascia or costal arch, the edge can be anchored by suturing it to the ventral lumbar musculature or around the last rib.

Prepubic tendon avulsion

Avulsion of the rectus abdominis muscle from the pubis leads to ventral herniation of the bladder, colon, jejunum, or uterus (Fig. 11.9). The rupture may extend laterally through the femoral and inguinal canals. These ruptures present as bruising and subcutaneous swelling over the caudoventral abdominal wall, or with signs of organ compromise or obstruction (e.g. dysuria). Prepubic tendon avulsions are extremely difficult to repair and cases should be referred for specialist management.

Incisional Hernia

An incisional hernia develops when organs herniate through an abdominal incision (Fig. 11.10). Poor surgical technique (e.g. failure to include the external rectus sheath in the linea alba closure; poor suture selection; poor knot tying) is thought to

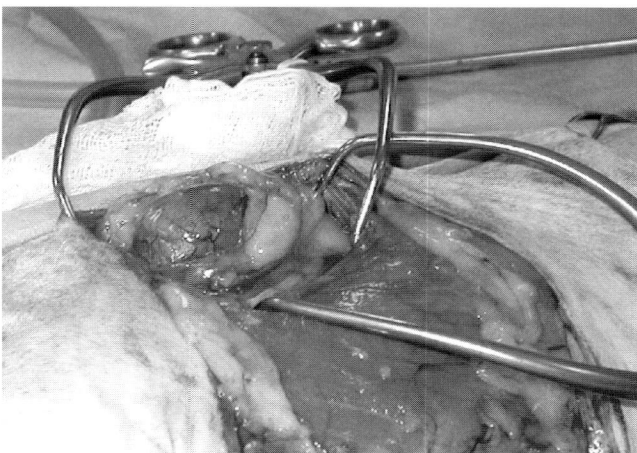

Fig. 11.8. Paracostal rupture following dog bite injury in a cat with herniation of the kidney and colon. The defect was repaired by suturing the torn muscle to the lumbar fascia.

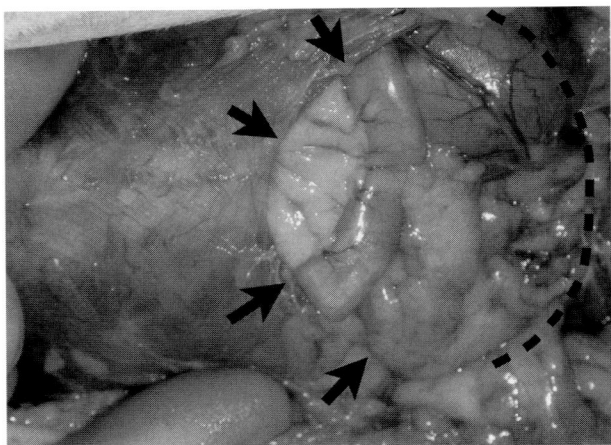

Fig. 11.9. Prepubic tendon avulsion: the edge of the defect (arrows) has avulsed from the pubis (dotted line), which is obscured by herniated organs (bladder and intestine).

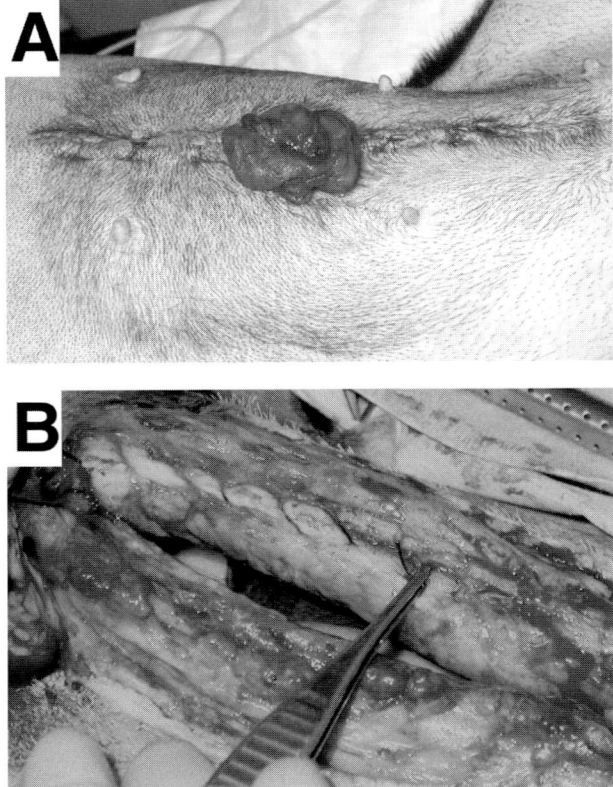

Fig. 11.10. Incisional hernias: (A) typical appearance of omentum protruding through the skin incision following ovariohysterectomy; (B) this hernia was caused by failure to include the external rectus sheath on one side of the linea alba suture line.

account for most incisional hernias. In the worst examples, incisional hernia combined with skin dehiscence leads to life-threatening evisceration. Features that should raise suspicion of incisional hernia are subcutaneous swelling over any abdominal incision line, fluid seepage through the skin incision (indicating organ strangulation and fluid transudation), and tissue protruding through the skin incision. The major differential diagnoses are seroma, abscess, wound infection, and suture line reaction. Incisional hernias are repaired by revision of the original incision, paying careful attention to suture placement. The repair usually requires that devitalized or infected tissue is debrided from the edge of the defect.

Perineal Hernia

Perineal hernia is an acquired defect of male, middle-aged dogs. It develops from degeneration of the muscles of the pelvic diaphragm. Most cases are idiopathic and result from atrophy of the levator ani muscle. Gender has a marked influence on the risk of developing perineal hernia. The majority of cases (93%) are uncastrated and this may indicate that androgens or prostatomegaly are involved in the pathogenesis of the condition. Occasionally, perineal hernia develops in castrated dogs, bitches, or cats. In these cases, perineal hernia may be secondary to diseases causing straining or perineal trauma (e.g. perineal urethrostomy; dystocia).

The pelvic diaphragm is composed of the external anal sphincter, the levator ani, and the coccygeus muscles. It provides lateral support to the rectum. Many of the signs associated with perineal hernia are caused by deviation of the rectum into the hernia leading to tenesmus, constipation, and faecal impaction. Abdominal organs including the prostate and bladder may also herniate, leading to signs of dysuria.

Presentation

Most dogs with perineal hernia are middle-aged, or old entire males. The Boston terrier, Pekingese, collie, and boxer are predisposed. Hernias may be unilateral or bilateral. Tenesmus, constipation, and perineal swelling are the commonest signs.

Approximately 20% of cases have a *retroflexed bladder*. The bladder is displaced caudally and flips backwards through 180° into the defect causing bladder neck obstruction. This leads to dysuria,

post-renal azotaemia, hyperkalaemia, shock, and other signs of acute urinary tract obstruction. The bladder may also become necrotic due to pressure necrosis of the wall.

Investigation

The diagnosis of perineal hernia can usually be confirmed by clinical examination. The presence of a large perineal swelling and the associated historical findings of dyschezia in an older, entire male dog are highly suggestive of the diagnosis (Fig. 11.11). Rectal examination allows direct palpation of the hernia ring and digital exploration of the deviated rectum in the subcutaneous space. Ultrasound can help to distinguish perineal hernia from other causes of perineal swelling and to identify involvement of the bladder or prostate.

Management of perineal hernia

Perineal hernia repair is technically demanding and cases should be referred to an experienced colleague or specialist centre.

Manage constipation

Digital evacuation of impacted faeces from the hernia may help to alleviate signs for a short period. Long-term use of bulk-forming laxatives (e.g. sterculia) helps prevent faecal impaction preoperatively and reduces tenesmus post-operatively.

Repair hernia

A range of surgical techniques has been used to repair perineal hernias. The walls of the defect cannot be apposed directly without tension so muscle flaps are often used to fill the defect. The internal obturator muscle flap is a comparatively simple technique that fills the defect with autogenous tissue.

Prevent recurrence

Castration is recommended as it reduces the incidence of recurrence to approximately a third of that in entire dogs.

Management of retroflexed bladder

Animals with retroflexed bladders deteriorate rapidly due to the effects of acute urinary tract

---

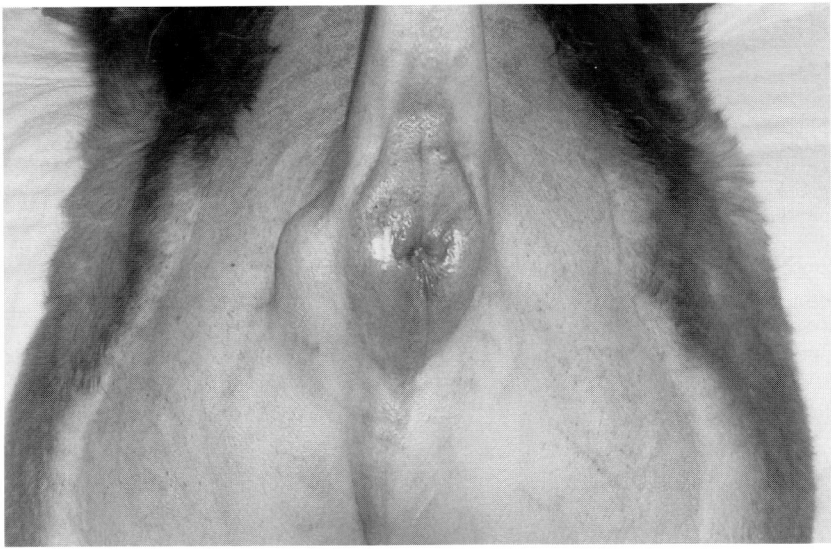

Fig. 11.11. Swelling of the left perineum in a dog with perineal hernia.

obstruction, and require emergency therapy to correct the problem.

Clip and prepare the skin over the perineal swelling. Perform cystocentesis through the perineal skin using a 23-gauge needle and syringe (see Fig. 11.12). Empty the bladder of urine and then apply digital pressure to the perineal hernia over the perineal fossa. These two steps should enable the bladder to flip back into position within the abdomen. Gently pass a rigid urinary catheter into the bladder and secure it to maintain the bladder in the abdomen. Connect the catheter to a collection system. The bladder can be kept in position for 2 or 3 days using the urinary catheter, enabling the patient to be stabilized and referred for surgery.

Complications and outcome

The prognosis following repair of perineal hernia is reasonable as tenesmus should be relieved and the bladder should not be able to retroflex. The major complications are infection of the incision and recurrence of the hernia. Clinical signs may recur because of breakdown of the original repair or because of development of a hernia on the contralateral side. Rectal prolapse may occur postoperatively but is usually temporary. Rarely, the sciatic nerve is damaged as it becomes trapped by sutures placed around the sacrotuberous ligament.

This causes hind limb paralysis and requires emergency surgery to release the trapped nerve before the damage becomes irreversible. Faecal incontinence is also sometimes reported post-operatively.

Diaphragmatic Defects

Diaphragmatic defects differ from the other forms of abdominal hernia because there are no external signs of herniation and because they often cause dyspnoea. There are two forms of diaphragmatic defect:

1. Pleuroperitoneal defects: these are common and allow direct communication between the abdomen and the pleural cavity. Herniated organs compress the lungs causing dyspnoea. These defects are usually referred to simply as 'diaphragmatic hernias or ruptures'.

2. Peritoneopericardial defects: these are uncommon congenital defects and allow the pericardial and peritoneal spaces to communicate. The pericardium and diaphragm are fused and a stoma allows organs to herniate into the pericardial sac. These hernias do not involve the pleural space and signs are usually associated with gastrointestinal obstruction or cardiac tamponade. These are always referred to by their full anatomic name of *peritoneopericardial diaphragmatic hernia* (PPDH).

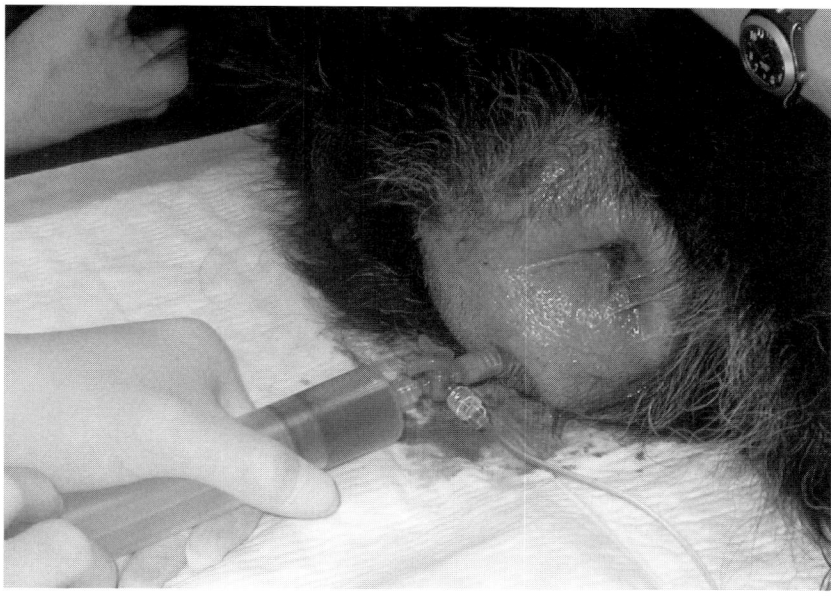

Fig. 11.12. Perineal hernia containing a retroflexed bladder: the bladder is being drained by cystocentesis through the perineal skin before being digitally manipulated into the abdomen and retained in position with a urinary catheter.

Anatomy

The diaphragm is a musculotendinous sheet. The two muscular crura originate from the ventral aspects of the lumbar vertebrae and run forward to form the dorsal portion of the diaphragm. The costal and sternal muscles form the lateral and ventral portions. Centrally, the diaphragm is composed of tendon. Three foramina allow passage of structures through the diaphragm. The aortic foramen sits dorsally on midline between the diaphragmatic crura and allows passage of the aorta, azygous vein, and thoracic duct. The oesophageal foramen lies ventral to the aortic foramen and allows passage of the oesophagus and vagus nerves. The caval foramen is the most ventral foramen and lies to the right of midline, allowing passage of the caudal vena cava.

Pleuroperitoneal hernias and ruptures (diaphragmatic rupture)

Pathophysiology

Most diaphragmatic defects are caused by blunt abdominal trauma (e.g. fall from height; hit by car). The sudden increase in intra-abdominal pressure causes tearing of the diaphragm and forces organs forward into the thorax. Most cases have single ruptures ventral to the oesophageal foramen, but dorsal defects and multiple defects can also occur. The organ that is herniated most often is liver followed by falciform fat, stomach, small intestine, spleen, omentum, and gall bladder. Rarely, kidney, uterus, or colon will herniate. A small number of diaphragmatic hernias (<10%) are congenital.

Herniated organs compress the lungs and cause dyspnoea. Pleural effusion may also accumulate from transudation of fluid from twisted, herniated liver lobes and will contribute to dyspnoea. Occasionally, dyspnoea is further compounded by herniation and gaseous distension of portions of the gastrointestinal tract within the thorax (e.g. stomach) (Fig. 11.13).

Presenting signs

Animals with diaphragmatic rupture typically present with acute-onset dyspnoea shortly following trauma. However, in some patients there is no apparent association between trauma and the development of signs because the traumatic event has not been witnessed or because the hernia is congenital. There may also be a delay (sometimes

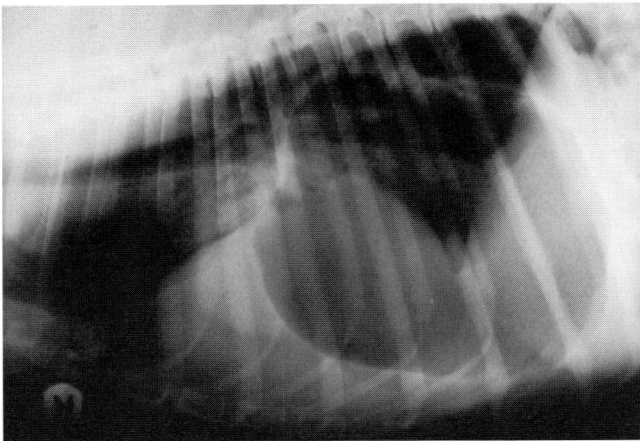

Fig. 11.13. Displacement and distension of the stomach into the thorax. The stomach is identified as a large, gas-filled viscus in the thorax. (Image courtesy of E. Welsh.)

of several weeks) between trauma and the onset of signs, because few organs herniate at the time of the original injury and signs only become apparent when more organs herniate at a later date. Occasionally, the main signs are of gastrointestinal obstruction rather than of dyspnoea.

Physical examination

Physical findings are suggestive of unilateral or bilateral pleural disease and respiratory compromise. Thoracic auscultation may reveal muffled or absent lung or heart sounds. Thoracic percussion is hyper-resonant over areas with herniated organs or pleural effusion, and hyporesonant over areas with gas-filled loops of intestine or stomach. Borborygmi from herniated intestine are sometimes heard on thoracic auscultation and are characteristic of diaphragmatic rupture. Sometimes, abdominal palpation reveals that the abdomen is comparatively empty of organs because they have become displaced into the thorax.

Differential diagnoses

The key differential diagnoses to consider of dyspnoea following trauma are pneumothorax, pulmonary contusions, and thoracic wall trauma (e.g. flail chest). Thoracic radiography quickly distinguishes between these injuries although diaphragmatic rupture is often seen in conjunction with other thoracic injuries. Pleural effusions caused by herniated organs must be distinguished from other causes of pleural effusion (e.g. congestive heart failure; pyothorax; chylothorax).

Diaphragmatic rupture should be suspected in any patient presenting with signs of dyspnoea following trauma but it also cannot be excluded simply because of a lack of history of trauma. It should be considered as a possible differential diagnosis in any case with pleural effusion.

Investigation

Confirming the diagnosis of diaphragmatic rupture relies on demonstrating abdominal organs within the thoracic cavity radiographically. It is very difficult to diagnose diaphragmatic rupture in patients that do not have herniated abdominal organs in the thorax at the time of investigation. Several key radiographic features can be used to help reach a diagnosis (Figs 11.14–11.17):

1. loss of diaphragmatic continuity;
2. presence of gas-filled or ingesta-filled intestine or stomach in the thorax;
3. delineation of parenchymatous organs within the thorax.

If pleural effusion is present, draining this may help identify these characteristic features.

Abdominal radiographs may also help to confirm the diagnosis. When liver lobes herniate, the gastric axis adopts an upright position similar to that seen with microhepatica (Fig. 11.18). Herniated organs

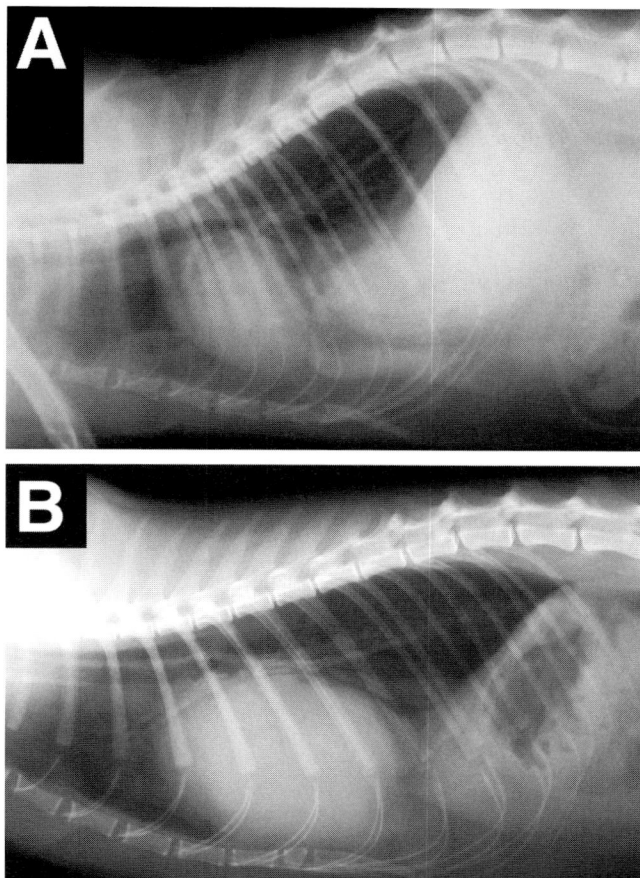

Fig. 11.14. Comparison of radiographic features of pleuroperitoneal defects and PPDH – lateral projection: (A) diaphragmatic rupture with loss of diaphragmatic definition ventrally; (B) PPDH with loss of diaphragmatic definition only at the cupula of the diaphragm.

(e.g. spleen; stomach; small intestine) may also be identified by their absence on abdominal radiographs. Abdominal ultrasound can be used to confirm the diagnosis but the interpretation is difficult.

Preoperative management

The main cause of death perioperatively is respiratory compromise, which is exacerbated by anaesthesia and stress. Providing supportive care for up to 24 h before surgery reduces the risks and improves survival. Supportive care is reviewed in Chapter 13 and includes:

1. *Oxygen therapy*.
2. *Intravenous fluid therapy*.

3. *Pain relief*: thoracic pain associated with trauma may lead to a shallow, rapid respiratory pattern that is inefficient. Appropriate analgesia reduces discomfort and can improve ventilation, helping to stabilize the patient.
4. *Cage-rest with minimal handling*: this reduces the oxygen requirements of the body and promotes a more controlled and effective respiratory pattern.
5. *Thoracocentesis*: if a pleural effusion is present, thoracocentesis will be beneficial providing that the patient does not become distressed by the procedure (see Chapter 23).

Once the patient's respiratory function has improved and it is stable, surgery should be performed

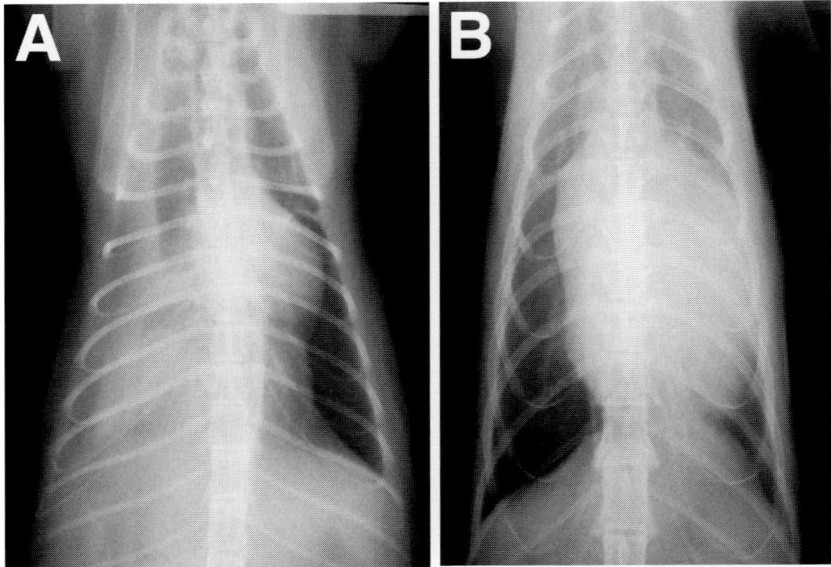

Fig. 11.15. Comparison of radiographic features of pleuroperitoneal defects and PPDH – dorsoventral projection: (A) diaphragmatic rupture with complete loss of diaphragmatic definition unilaterally; (B) PPDH with loss of diaphragmatic definition at the cupula of the diaphragm but preservation laterally.

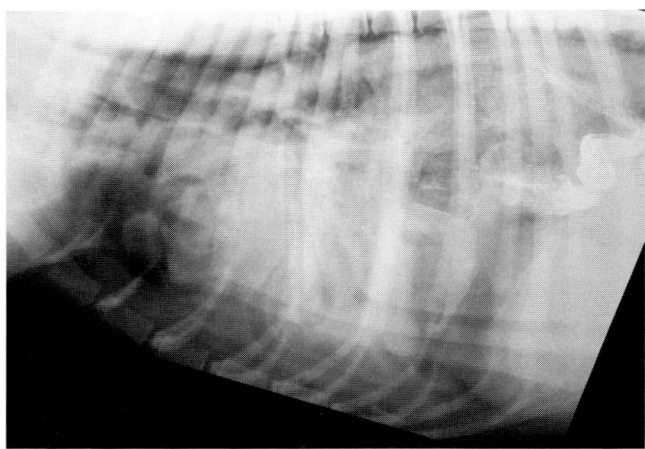

Fig. 11.16. Gas-filled loops of small intestine in the thorax.

without further delay. Monitor the response to supportive care frequently (e.g. every 5 min initially) while avoiding unnecessary handling of the patient. If the patient deteriorates despite supportive care, either surgery should be performed urgently before the patient deteriorates further, or the supportive care should be altered to improve the response of the patient. Clear indicators that rapid surgical intervention should be prioritized over further supportive care include displacement of the stomach into the thorax and identification of other abdominal injuries such as a gastrointestinal tract rupture.

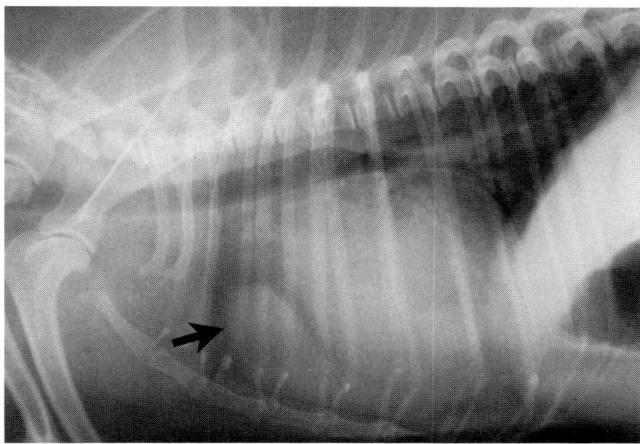

Fig. 11.17. Displacement of parenchymatous organs into the thorax: liver (arrow) is displaced into the thorax.

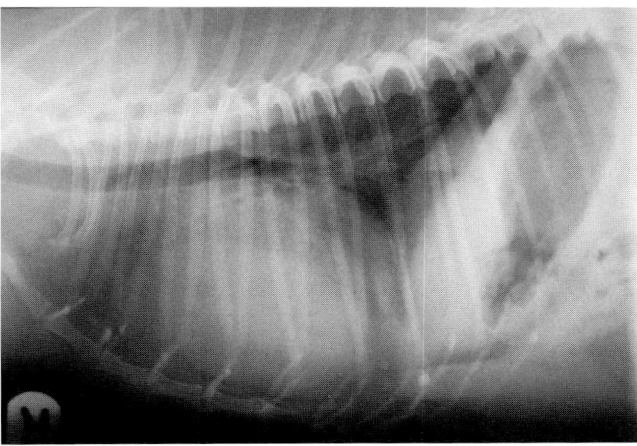

Fig. 11.18. Apparent microhepatica: the gastric axis slopes cranioventrally due to herniation of a large portion of liver. Normally, the gastric axis lies parallel to the intercostal spaces.

Herniorrhaphy

Most acute traumatic diaphragmatic ruptures are easily diagnosed and managed in general practice. However, some cases are more difficult to manage and may require referral for specialist management. Animals with long-standing diaphragmatic defects should be referred as these defects can be very difficult to repair. Chronically herniated organs may form adhesions to the lungs and can be severely compromised. Median sternotomy, lung lobectomy, or muscle flaps and meshes may be required to repair the hernia. Closing the abdominal wall after reduction of the hernia can also be difficult, as the abdominal wall contracts due to the reduction in the volume of intra-abdominal organs while organs are displaced into the chest.

ANAESTHESIA Effective anaesthesia is as important as effective surgery in managing patients with diaphragmatic rupture. It is important to separate these roles whenever possible so that one veterinary surgeon performs surgery while another manages the patient's anaesthetic. The period from induction of anaesthesia to reduction of the hernia is a major risk period and should be shortened as much as possible. Several steps can be taken to reduce the risk during this period:

1. **Clip the abdomen before anaesthesia if this does not distress the patient.**
2. **Induce anaesthesia rapidly using intravenous agents:** this allows rapid intubation and mechanical ventilation.
3. **Start intermittent positive pressure ventilation (IPPV) immediately:** large respiratory effort may not be matched by effective lung inflation in animals with diaphragmatic rupture. The physiological dead space is increased in compressed lungs, limiting gas exchange, and large respiratory effort may only serve to move organs in and out of the thorax through the defect rather than to inflate the lungs. IPPV helps to overcome these problems. Review anaesthesia texts for details of technique. In brief, select an anaesthetic system suitable for prolonged IPPV (T-piece; Bain; circle), deliver IPPV at around 20 breaths/min. Aim for a longer expiratory than inspiratory phase (2:1). Do not over-inflate the lungs.
4. **Elevate the thorax in relation to the abdomen:** abdominal organs will fall away from the diaphragm.
5. **Position the worse affected side of the thorax towards the table** so that the less compromised lung is uppermost and able to expand fully.

SURGICAL APPROACH Most diaphragmatic ruptures can be repaired through a ventral midline coeliotomy incision. Extend the incision to the xiphisternum and excise the falciform fat (see Chapter 10).

IDENTIFY THE DEFECT AND REDUCE CONTENTS There is usually a single defect located ventral to the oesophageal foramen that is easy to find. However, some cases have dorsal, less accessible ruptures. If the rupture cannot be easily identified, trace the herniated organs forward into the defect (Fig. 11.19 A–B). Always check for multiple defects.

Start to reduce the hernia contents by applying gentle traction to herniated small intestine, omentum, or spleen (Fig. 11.19 C–F). Reduce organs one at a time starting with the most mobile (usually small intestine or omentum). Leave reduction of herniated liver lobes until last as these are often friable. Do not apply traction to a herniated liver lobe as it may fragment. Instead, hook a finger around the tip of the herniated liver lobe within the thorax and push it back into the abdominal cavity. Assess the herniated organs and resect non-viable portions. Assess the lungs for injury through the diaphragmatic defect.

If the hernia cannot be reduced, enlarge the hernia ring by incising it from the ventral border of the defect towards the costal attachment to the diaphragm. Extending the defect in a ventral direction (rather than dorsally) ensures that the extended area is easily accessible for repair.

Sharply dissect devitalized tissues from the edge of the defect. Ensure that all sutures engage healthy muscle or tendon. The easiest suture pattern to use to close a diaphragmatic defect is a continuous one. Start the suture line at the most dorsal (least accessible) portion of the defect and work ventrally towards the more accessible area of diaphragm. If the diaphragm has avulsed from the costal attachments laterally, anchor the edge of the diaphragmatic muscle by passing suture around the rib adjacent to the defect (Fig. 11.19 G–H).

RE-ESTABLISH NEGATIVE PRESSURE IN THE THORAX Once the diaphragmatic defect is closed, perform needle thoracocentesis through the diaphragm to drain most of the air from the thoracic cavity (see p. 353). Do not perform forced lung inflation to expel air as the last suture of the diaphragmatic repair is tied, as this is highly dangerous. Forced inflation of collapsed lung induces trauma to the alveoli through over-inflation and leads to alveolar inflammation and flooding (*re-expansion pulmonary oedema*). This is thought to have accounted for the high rate of perioperative mortality associated with diaphragmatic rupture repair before this practice was stopped.

Post-operative management

The commonest major post-operative complication is dyspnoea caused by pneumothorax, pleural effusion, or re-expansion pulmonary oedema. Patients must be carefully monitored for signs of dyspnoea and provided with appropriate support in the first 48 h post-operatively. Animals that have had chronic diaphragmatic ruptures repaired may require intensive and specialist therapy in the post-operative period to deal with severe complications caused by thoracic and abdominal organ injuries.

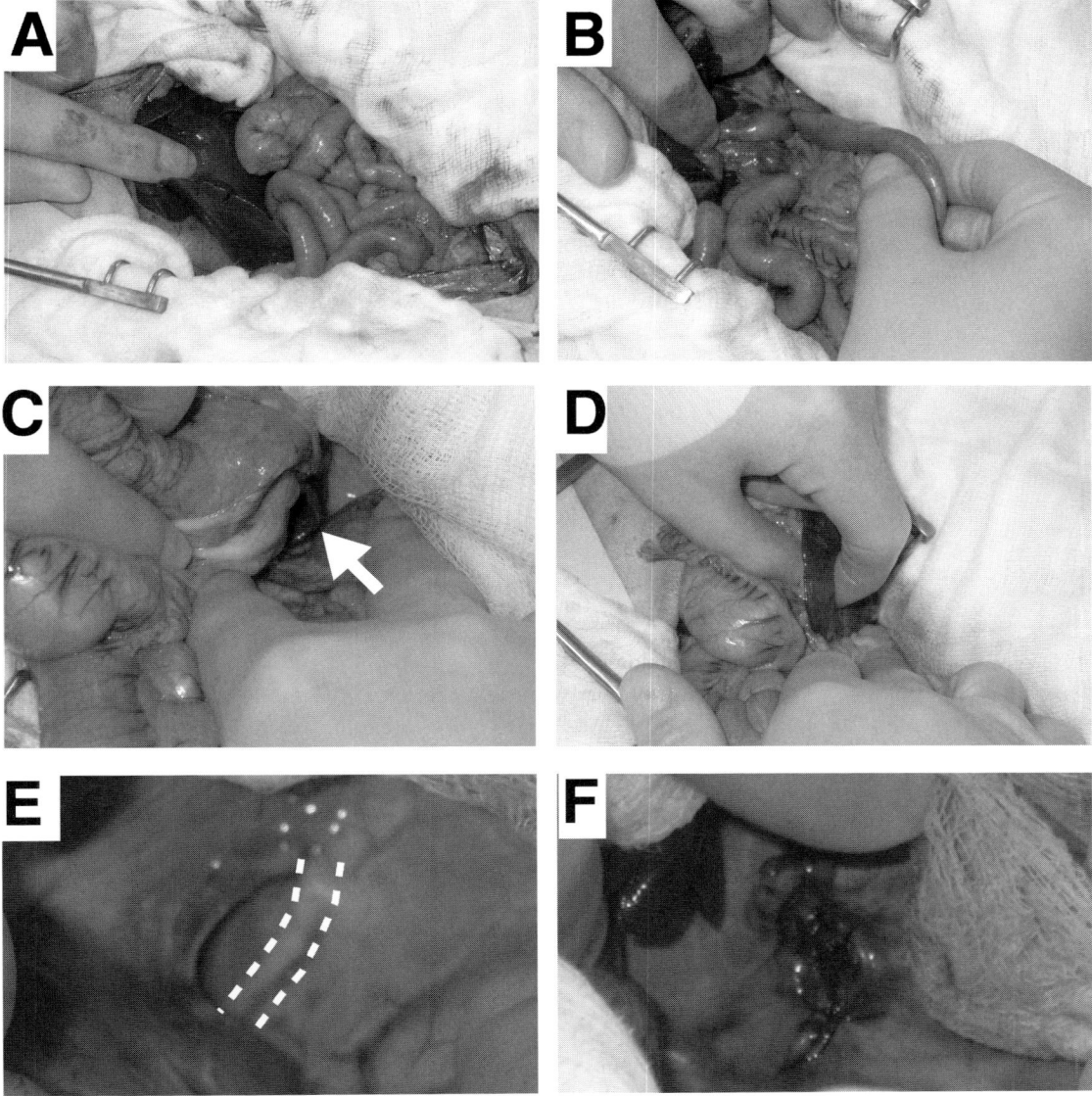

Fig. 11.19. Congenital diaphragmatic hernia repair in a 13-week-old Staffordshire bull terrier: (A) the omentum, stomach and spleen are missing from the abdomen (finger pointing to liver); (B) the hernia is identified by tracing the small intestine forward to the defect. The contents are reduced by first applying gentle traction to the small intestine which reduces the duodenum and right limb of the pancreas; (C) the stomach and tip of the spleen (arrow) are identified emerging from the hernia; (D) the spleen is grasped and gently removed from the thorax. This action also reduces the remaining hernia contents (omentum) in this case; (E) the defect is a right-sided, dorsal defect between the right crus of the diaphragm and the thoracic wall. There is no lateral edge of the defect to suture to as it has formed where the muscle normally attaches onto the costal arch. However, sutures can be anchored around the adjacent rib (dotted lines); (F) successful closure of the defect by suturing the defect to the adjacent rib using circumcostal sutures.

Prognosis

The majority of animals that undergo surgical correction for diaphragmatic rupture survive and recover completely. Recurrence is uncommon but may occur if the original repair breaks down or if a second diaphragmatic defect has been missed during surgery. Animals that develop re-expansion pulmonary oedema generally die within 24 h of surgery but the incidence should be very low providing that the lungs are not over-inflated during surgery.

Peritoneopericardial diaphragmatic hernias (PPDHs)

PPDHs are congenital hernias that allow the pericardial and peritoneal spaces to communicate and abdominal organs to herniate into the pericardial sac. They do not involve the pleural space and often have mild signs. Clinical signs usually relate to dysfunction of herniated gastrointestinal tract rather than to dyspnoea. Falciform fat, liver, gall bladder, and small intestine herniate most frequently and organs often move freely in and out of the hernia. Concurrent ventral body wall hernias and sternal defects may also be seen.

Presenting signs

PPDH may account for some perinatal deaths but the condition can be clinically silent for many years and most patients are diagnosed for the first time in adulthood. PPDH is often identified as an incidental finding during evaluation of other thoracic diseases. Some patients present with signs relating to gastrointestinal obstruction (e.g. chronic vomiting). Others become dyspnoeic. Occasionally, PPDH will cause cardiac tamponade through direct pressure of herniated organs on the heart leading to signs of right-sided heart failure.

Clinical findings

There may be few clinical findings to support the diagnosis. Cardiac auscultation may reveal muffling of the heart or borborygmi over the cardiac region. PPDH may extend to include malformation of the xiphisternum and caudal sternebrae leading to the formation of a concurrent ventral body wall hernia.

Investigation

PPDH share many of the radiographic features of pleuroperitoneal defects. They may be distinguished from pleuroperitoneal defects as all of the herniated organs are centred around the heart and because only the cupula of the diaphragm is effaced on dorsoventral thoracic radiographs (the lateral diaphragmatic contours can still be seen) (Figs 11.14B and 11.15B). PPDH is easily mistaken for generalized cardiomegaly or pericardial effusion if individual abdominal organs cannot be identified within the hernia. Cardiac ultrasound is useful for confirming the diagnosis by identifying abdominal organs within the pericardial sac.

Conservative management

As PPDH may be clinically silent and is often diagnosed as an incidental finding, conservative management can be considered. No specific action is required but patients should be monitored for signs of cardiac dysfunction and organ compromise. The disadvantages of conservative management are that the patient may deteriorate rapidly and that it is not suitable for patients with signs of organ dysfunction or cardiac tamponade.

Surgical management

Most PPDH cases are referred for surgical management as they are sporadically identified in general practice and it is, therefore, difficult for general practitioners to gain experience in their management. Uncomplicated cases are usually simple to manage but concurrent ventral body wall hernias and sternal defects may complicate the repair. Although the pleural cavity is usually intact at the start of surgery, it is easy to penetrate it during surgery, causing pneumothorax.

Complications and prognosis

The prognosis following repair of PPDH is reasonable. Most patients survive and have resolution of their signs. Pneumothorax may develop if the pleural cavities are punctured during hernia repair.

Bibliography

Beittenmiller, M.R., Mann, F.A., Constantinescu, G.M. and Luther, J.K. (2009) Clinical anatomy and surgical repair of prepubic hernia in dogs and cats. *Journal of the American Animal Hospital Association* 45, 284–290.

Bilbrey, S.A., Smeak, D.D. and Dehoff, W. (1990) Fixation of the deferent ducts for retrodisplacement of the urinary bladder and prostate in canine perineal hernia. *Veterinary Surgery* 19, 24–27.

Brown, C.N. and Finch, J.G. (2010) Which mesh for hernia repair? *Annals of the Royal College of Surgeons of England* 92, 272–278.

Clarke, K.M., Lantz, G.C., Salisbury, S.K., Badylak, S.F., Hiles, M.C. and Voytik, S.L. (1996) Intestine submucosa and polypropylene mesh for abdominal wall repair in dogs. *Journal of Surgical Research* 60, 107–114.

Formaggini, L., Schmidt, K. and De Lorenzi, D. (2008) Gastric dilatation-volvulus associated with diaphragmatic hernia in three cats: clinical presentation, surgical treatment and presumptive aetiology. *Journal of Feline Medicine and Surgery* 10, 198–201.

Fossum, T.W. (2007) Surgery of the lower respiratory system: pleural cavity and diaphragm. In: Fossum, T.W. (ed.) *Small Animal Surgery*, 3rd edn. Mosby Elsevier, St Louis, Missouri, pp. 896–929.

Fox, M.W. (1963) Inherited inguinal hernia and midline defects in the dog. *Journal of the American Veterinary Medical Association* 143, 602–604.

Gibson, T.W., Brisson, B.A. and Sears, W. (2005) Perioperative survival rates after surgery for diaphragmatic hernia in dogs and cats: 92 cases (1990–2002). *Journal of the American Veterinary Medical Association* 227, 105–109.

Gower, S.B., Weisse, C.W. and Brown, D.C. (2009) Major abdominal evisceration injuries in dogs and cats: 12 cases (1998–2008). *Journal of the American Veterinary Medical Association* 234, 1566–1572.

Hayes, H.M., Jr, Wilson, G.P. and Tarone, R.E. (1978) The epidemiological features of perineal hernia in 771 dogs. *Journal of the American Animal Hospital Association* 14, 703–707.

Hermanson, J.W. and Evans, H.E. (1993) Muscles of the abdominal wall. In: Evans, H.E. (ed.) *Miller's Anatomy of the Dog*, 3rd edn. W.B. Saunders, Philadelphia, Pennsylvania, pp. 308–384.

Holt, D.E. (2004) Perineal hernias in dogs. *Standards of Care Emergency and Critical Care Medicine: VetLearn.com* 6, 1–5.

Hosgood, G. (1990) The omentum – the forgotten organ: physiology and potential surgical applications in dogs and cats. *Compendium of Continuing Education for the Practicing Veterinarian* 12, 45–51.

Hosgood, G., Hedlund, C.S., Pechman, R.D. and Dean, P.W. (1995) Perineal herniorrhaphy: perioperative data from 100 dogs. *Journal of the American Animal Hospital Association* 31, 331–342.

Hunt, G.B. and Johnson, K.A. (2003) Diaphragmatic, pericardial, and hiatal hernia. In: Slatter, D.H. (ed.) *Textbook of Small Animal Surgery*, 3rd edn. Saunders, Philadelphia, Pennsylvania, pp. 471–487.

Minihan, A.C., Berg, J. and Evans, K.L. (2004) Chronic diaphragmatic hernia in 34 dogs and 16 cats. *Journal of the American Animal Hospital Association* 40, 51–63.

Neiger, R. (1996) Peritoneopericardial diaphragmatic hernia in cats. *Compendium of Continuing Education for the Practicing Veterinarian* 18, 461–479.

Niles, J.D. and Williams, J.M. (1999) Perineal hernia with bladder retroflexion in a female cocker spaniel. *Journal of Small Animal Practice* 40, 92–94.

Pavletic, M.M. (2005) Abdominal wall hernias. *Standards of Care Emergency and Critical Care Medicine: VetLearn.com* 7, 1–7.

Reimer, S.B., Kyles, A.E., Filipowicz, D.E. and Gregory, C.R. (2004) Long-term outcome of cats treated conservatively or surgically for peritoneopericardial diaphragmatic hernia: 66 cases (1987–2002). *Journal of the American Veterinary Medical Association* 224, 728–732.

Robinson, R. (1977) Genetic aspects of umbilical hernia incidence in cats and dogs. *Veterinary Record* 100, 9–10.

Schmiedt, C.W., Tobias, K.M. and Stevenson, M.A. (2003) Traumatic diaphragmatic hernia in cats: 34 cases (1991–2001). *Journal of the American Veterinary Medical Association* 222, 1237–1240.

Shaw, S.R., Rozanski, E.A. and Rush, J.E. (2003) Traumatic body wall herniation in 36 dogs and cats. *Journal of the American Animal Hospital Association* 39, 35–46.

Smeak, D.D. (2003) Abdominal hernias. In: Slatter, D.H. (ed.) *Textbook of Small Animal Surgery*, 3rd edn. Saunders, Philadelphia, Pennsylvania, pp. 449–470.

Spattini, G., Rossi, F., Vignoli, M. and Lamb, C.R. (2003) Use of ultrasound to diagnose diaphragmatic rupture in dogs and cats. *Veterinary Radiology and Ultrasound* 44, 226–230.

Stampley, A.R. and Waldron, D.R. (1993) Re-expansion pulmonary edema after surgery to repair a diaphragmatic hernia in a cat. *Journal of the American Veterinary Medical Association* 203, 1699–1701.

Strande, A. (1989) Inguinal hernia in dogs. *Journal of Small Animal Practice* 30, 520–521.

Sullivan, M. and Lee, R. (1989) Radiological features of 80 cases of diaphragmatic rupture. *Journal of Small Animal Practice* 30, 561–566.

Sullivan, M. and Reid, J. (1990) Management of 60 cases of diaphragmatic rupture. *Journal of Small Animal Practice* 31, 425–430.

Van Sluijs, F.J. and Sjollema, B.E. (1989) Perineal hernia repair in the dog by transposition of the internal obturator muscle. I. Surgical technique. *Veterinary Quarterly* 11, 12–17.

Waldron, D.R., Hedlund, C.S. and Pecham, R. (1986) Abdominal hernias in dogs and cats: a review of 24 cases. *Journal of the American Animal Hospital Association* 22, 817–823.

Waters, D.J., Roy, R.G. and Stone, E.A. (1993) A retrospective study of inguinal hernia in 35 dogs. *Veterinary Surgery* 22, 44–49.

Welches, C.D., Scavelli, T.D., Aronsohn, M.G. and Matthiesen, D.T. (1992) Perineal hernia in the cat: a retrospective study of 40 cases. *Journal of the American Animal Hospital Association* 28, 431–438.

Wilson, G.P. 3rd, Newton, C.D. and Burt, J.K. (1971) A review of 116 diaphragmatic hernias in dogs and cats. *Journal of the American Veterinary Medical Association* 159, 1142–1145.

Wilson G.P. 3rd and Hayes, H.M., Jr (1986) Diaphragmatic hernia in the dog and cat: a 25-year overview. *Seminars in Veterinary Medicine and Surgery (Small Animal)* 1, 318–326.

Worth, A.J. and Machon, R.G. (2005) Traumatic diaphragmatic herniation: pathophysiology and management. *Compendium of Continuing Education for the Practicing Veterinarian* 27, 178–191.

12 Gastrointestinal Surgery

anal sacculectomy: removal of an anal sac
colopexy: anchoring the colon to the abdominal wall
enterectomy: removal of a portion of the intestine
enteroplication: anchoring adjacent loops of intestine together to prevent intussusception
enterotomy: incision into the intestine
gastropexy: anchoring the stomach to the abdominal wall
gastrotomy: incision into the stomach
intussusception: invagination of one section of intestine inside another
melaena: altered blood in stool (appears tarry and black)

The reader should be able to:

- explain how the site and degree of obstruction influences the severity of signs in a cat with intestinal foreign body
- explain the differences in pathogenesis between a linear foreign body and a focal foreign body in the intestinal tract of a dog
- list the key radiographic features of intestinal obstruction in the dog or cat
- illustrate how to perform gastrotomy and enterotomy for retrieval of a focal foreign body
- illustrate how to remove a linear foreign body that is tethered at the base of the tongue and that extends to the distal small intestine in a kitten
- illustrate with the aid of a diagram what an intussusception is and describe how to reduce it
- explain how a dog might present with gastric dilatation and volvulus syndrome (GDV) and illustrate how the dog may be successfully treated
- describe how to perform enterectomy to remove an intestinal adenocarcinoma from the mid-jejunum of a cat
- list the common causes and treatment of megacolon in the cat
- list the common causes and treatment of rectal prolapse in the cat

In this chapter, conditions causing gastrointestinal obstruction and vomiting (foreign body ingestion, intussusception, and neoplasia) are described first, followed by the key surgical procedures. Gastric dilatation and volvulus syndrome (GDV) is considered separately as it requires very specific management. Finally, rectal and anal diseases that may require surgery are discussed at the end of the chapter.

Foreign Body Ingestion

Gastrointestinal foreign body ingestion is very common, particularly in young animals. Linear foreign bodies (ingested string or thread) cause particularly severe intestinal obstruction and secondary damage.

Pathophysiology

Foreign bodies may cause obstruction or perforation of the gastrointestinal tract. Occasionally, they may also lead to poisoning.

Obstruction

Gastrointestinal obstruction is the most common consequence of foreign body ingestion and usually leads to vomiting. Foreign bodies can also cause diarrhoea in combination with vomiting, as they cause general disruption of intestinal function. Some foreign bodies sit in the fundus of the stomach where they do not interfere with gastric emptying and cause few signs. Eventually, these may move on and cause obstruction. Intestinal foreign bodies generally are associated with signs of obstruction and vomiting. However, some reach the large intestine without causing obstruction and pass in the faeces.

The severity of signs relates to the degree of obstruction. Foreign bodies may cause *complete* or *partial obstruction*. Complete obstruction rapidly causes vomiting and quickly leads to dehydration and metabolic disturbances. Partial obstruction may have a more insidious onset of signs leading to intermittent vomiting, chronic inappetence, and weight loss.

The location of the obstruction also influences the severity of signs. *High gastrointestinal obstructions* (pylorus; duodenum) cause severe, acute-onset signs characterized by persistent vomiting of partly digested food. Obstructions above the entry of the common bile duct into the duodenum lead to non-bilious vomiting while obstructions below the common bile duct often lead to vomit containing bile. *Low intestinal obstructions* (jejunum; ileum; colon) have a slower onset of signs and vomiting is likely to be intermittent. Dehydration and metabolic disturbances take longer to develop but, ultimately, patients can become severely debilitated and malnourished.

Perforation

Sharp foreign bodies can penetrate through the gastrointestinal wall. More commonly, perforation occurs through pressure necrosis. The intestinal wall becomes stretched over the foreign body, preventing blood flow into the area and causing ischaemic necrosis. Perforation leads to peritonitis and septicaemia.

Toxicity

Rarely, metallic foreign bodies cause toxicity through absorption of metals. For example, zinc from coins and galvanized items can cause vomiting, severe haemolytic anaemia, pancreatitis, and acute renal failure.

Linear foreign body

Linear foreign bodies (ingested string or thread) lead to a specific syndrome of severe intestinal compromise with multiple points of perforation. One end of the foreign body becomes snared, usually around the base of the tongue or in the pylorus. The free end continues to pass along the alimentary tract with peristalsis (Fig. 12.1). This continued peristaltic action against the linear foreign body causes the intestinal tract to concertina along the foreign body. As the end of the foreign body passes distally, it becomes stretched taut, leading to pressure necrosis along the mesenteric border of the intestinal mucosa. Initially, these cases present with signs of partial obstruction but the intestinal injury progresses rapidly leading to multiple points of perforation and secondary peritonitis (Fig. 12.5)

Historical and clinical findings

Vomiting may be acute or chronic in onset and may be intermittent or continuous. The signs are dependent on the site and degree of obstruction. Diarrhoea is also frequently reported in animals with partial intestinal obstruction, so the presence of diarrhoea cannot be used to exclude the diagnosis of foreign body obstruction.

Depending on the severity of signs, patients may be systemically well or severely shocked. Although animals with acute-onset, continuous vomiting become dehydrated rapidly, those with chronic intermittent signs may be severely debilitated and malnourished by the time the diagnosis is reached. Rapid deterioration of animals with either acute or chronic vomiting must be identified as a possible indicator of perforation and peritonitis. Unfortunately, there may be few specific historical or physical findings to indicate that foreign body ingestion has occurred. However, some historical and clinical findings are clear indicators that further investigation is required. Historical findings that support a diagnosis of foreign body ingestion include:

- known foreign body ingestion/history of vomiting foreign material recently;
- prior history of foreign body ingestion;
- very frequent vomiting (e.g. every few minutes);
- vomiting which does not resolve within 48 h;
- vomiting which does not respond to symptomatic treatment; and
- vomiting large quantities of food more than 4 h after eating or vomiting food at times completely dissociated from feeding (indicates delayed gastric emptying).

Physical findings that support a diagnosis of foreign body ingestion (or other significant abdominal disease) include:

- pain on abdominal palpation;
- palpation of an intestinal mass;
- palpation of distended loops of small intestine;
- detection of free abdominal fluid;
- palpation of bunched intestinal tract (indicating linear foreign body); and
- string snared around the base of the tongue or protruding from the anus (indicating linear foreign body) (Fig. 12.1).

Differential diagnoses of vomiting

A wide range of alimentary and non-alimentary conditions cause vomiting (Table 12.1) and distinguishing gastrointestinal obstruction from other causes of vomiting is critical. Most patients that present with acute-onset vomiting have idiopathic, self-limiting gastroenteritis and require, at most, symptomatic therapy until the problem resolves (usually within 24 or 48 h). However, failing to identify foreign body obstruction or other major abdominal disease may quickly lead to devastating gastrointestinal injury, perforation, and peritonitis.

Investigation

The investigation of acute vomiting aims to identify indicators of gastrointestinal obstruction or evidence of other diseases that may lead to vomiting.

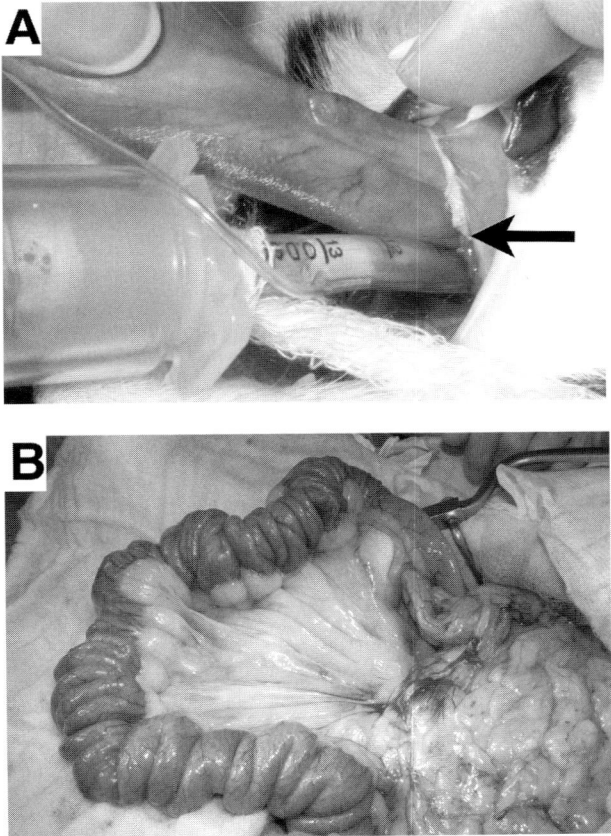

Fig. 12.1. Linear foreign body: (A) thread (arrow) snared round base of tongue; (B) concertinaed intestinal tract around linear foreign body.

Table 12.1. Differential diagnoses for vomiting.

ABDOMINAL, ALIMENTARY	**METABOLIC**
Dietary + idiopathic self-limiting vomiting	Disrupted calcium homeostasis
Foreign body obstruction	Hypoadrenocorticism
Gastric ulcer (secondary to uraemia, hepatic disease, drugs, neoplasia)	Hypokalaemia
Gastritis	Ketoacidosis
Gastrointestinal neoplasia	Uraemia
GDV	
Infection or infestation	**DRUG INDUCED**
Inflammatory bowel disease	Chemotherapeutic agents
Intestinal entrapment (e.g. hernia)	Cyclosporine
Mesenteric volvulus	Digoxin
Ileus	Erythromycin
ABDOMINAL, NON-ALIMENTARY	**TOXIN INDUCED**
Pancreatitis	Ethanol
Peritoneal tumour	Ethylene glycol
Peritonitis	Lead
Pyelonephritis	
Pyometra	**CENTRAL NERVOUS SYSTEM**
	Cerebellar disease
	Meningitis
	Vestibular disease

Serum biochemistry haematology, and urinalysis

Blood and urine analyses are used to evaluate general organ dysfunction that may cause vomiting (e.g. renal failure; hepatitis) and to test specifically for pancreatitis (e.g. canine pancreatic lipase immunoreactivity (cPLI); lipase; amylase). These tests are also used to measure the severity of hypovolaemia, electrolyte imbalances, and other secondary problems.

Abdominal radiography

Some foreign bodies are radio-opaque and are easily identified (Fig. 12.2A) but, as many foreign bodies are radiolucent, other criteria must be assessed before the diagnosis is excluded. Signs of gastrointestinal obstruction are often the clearest indicators of foreign body ingestion.

Gastric distension with food, fluid, or gas may indicate obstruction, particularly if the patient has not been fed in several hours (Fig. 12.2B). Normally, the stomach empties completely within 4 h. Food retained for greater than 8 h is suggestive of significantly delayed gastric emptying.

Small intestinal obstruction is generally significant. If loops of small intestine exceed two times the height of the mid-body of the fifth lumbar vertebra (dogs) or three times the height of the vertebral end plate of the second lumbar vertebra (cats), this is highly suggestive of intestinal obstruction (Fig. 12.3). Be cautious not to mistake normal large intestine for distended small intestine. Linear foreign bodies produce distinctive radiographic hallmarks that include a pleated appearance to the small intestine and curvilinear gas shadows in the intestinal lumen delineating individual pleats (Fig. 12.4).

Radiographic findings of free abdominal fluid and pneumoperitoneum are suggestive of intestinal perforation and peritonitis (see p. 211).

Abdominal ultrasound

For experienced operators, abdominal ultrasound is more sensitive than radiography for diagnosing gastrointestinal foreign body. Foreign bodies cause acoustic shadowing within the intestinal tract. The loops of intestine proximal to the foreign body become distended and have reduced peristalsis. However, it is important to distinguish distended small intestinal from normal large intestine.

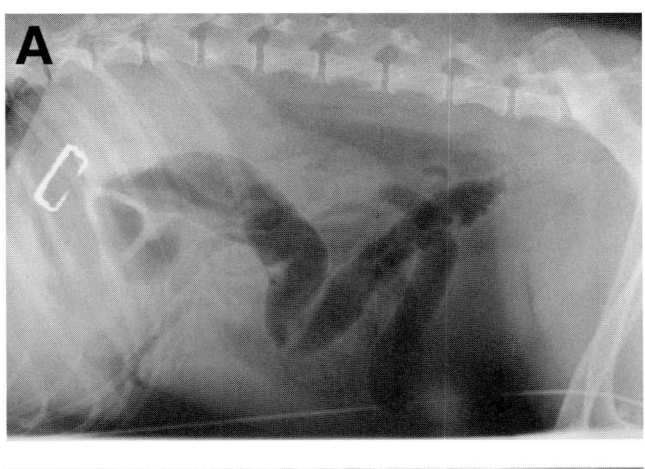

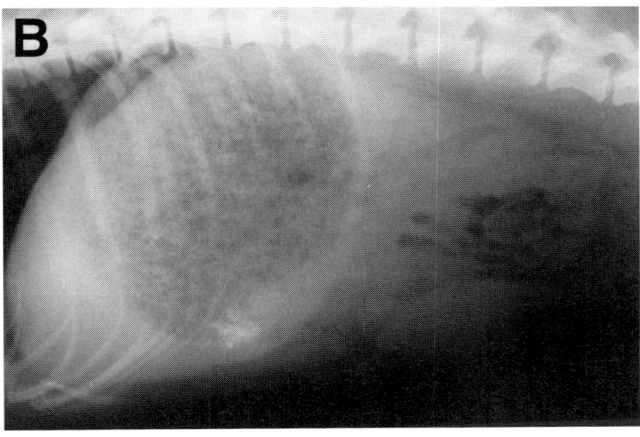

Fig. 12.2. Radiographs of gastric foreign bodies: (A) radio-opaque foreign body (belt buckle); (B) gastric distension several hours after being fed, indicating delayed gastric emptying.

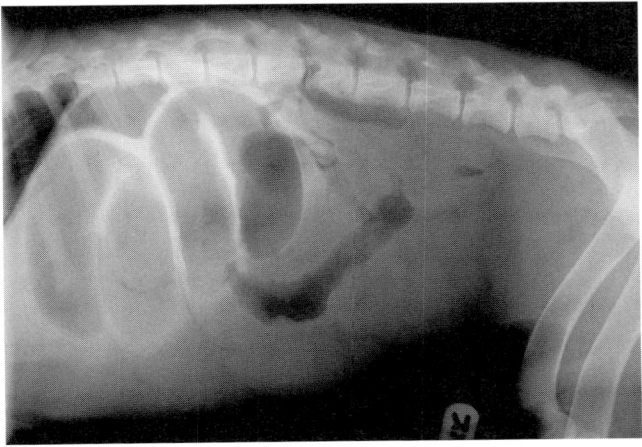

Fig. 12.3. Distended intestinal loops indicating intestinal obstruction.

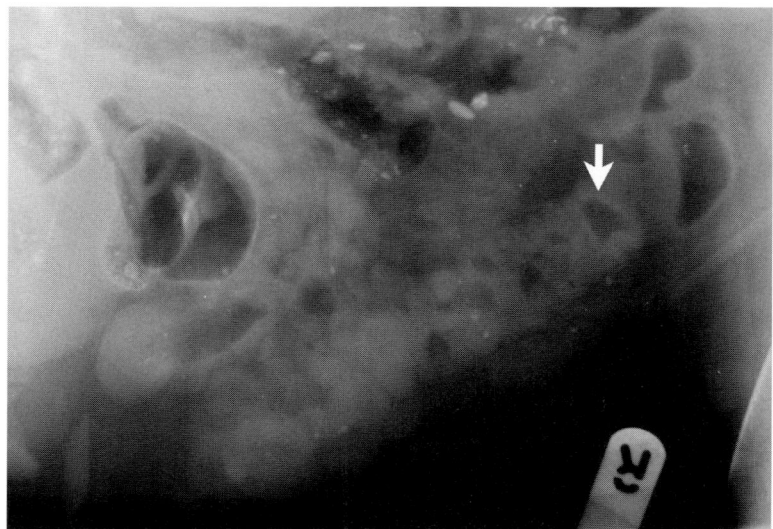

Fig. 12.4. Radiographic appearance of a linear foreign body: the small intestine has a concertinaed appearance and curvilinear gas shadows (arrow) are present within the lumen.

Management

Foreign bodies must be removed before severe intestinal compromise occurs and this requires emergency surgery. Animals should receive supportive care, including fluid therapy to correct fluid deficits and electrolyte imbalances, before being anaesthetized for surgery. Foreign body removal is usually performed in general practice but cases with chronic foreign bodies or with peritonitis are challenging and should be referred to an experienced colleague or specialist centre.

Induce vomiting

Some gastric foreign bodies in dogs can be retrieved by inducing vomiting. This should only be considered for patients that have ingested smooth, small foreign bodies that are not causing obstruction. It is contraindicated in animals that have swallowed caustic or abrasive substances, or in animals with signs of intestinal obstruction. The practice carries the risks of inducing severe oesophagitis and of inhalation of vomit. It is also often unsuccessful. Apomorphine administered by injection or conjunctivally induces emesis although it is also associated with adverse effects such as hypotension, ocular irritation, and respiratory depression.

Consider endoscopic retrieval in preference to inducing vomiting.

Endoscopic retrieval

Endoscopic removal is the treatment of choice for gastric foreign bodies as it does not have the risks associated with abdominal surgery. It also has the advantage that it can be attempted immediately before surgery. It is not suitable for intestinal foreign bodies.

Surgical removal

Most gastrointestinal foreign bodies are removed surgically. They may be located anywhere in the gastrointestinal tract and may move from the stomach into more distal areas between the time of investigation and surgery, even if this is only a few minutes. Always perform a full exploratory coeliotomy and work consistently along the entire tract checking for distension and luminal masses. Pay particular attention to the stomach. Foreign bodies that are free in the gastric lumen tend to sink to the dependent portion and are easily missed. Foreign bodies can be removed surgically by performing gastrotomy (stomach) or enterotomy (small intestine). If the intestinal tract becomes severely compromised over the area of obstruction, enterectomy will be necessary. These techniques are described in detail below.

Manage peritonitis

Animals with perforation and peritonitis require specific therapy and have a guarded prognosis (see Chapter 13).

Linear foreign bodies

Linear foreign bodies must be removed as soon as possible to minimize intestinal injury. When the foreign body is visible in the mouth or at the anus, do not apply traction as this is likely to cause severe intestinal trauma. Release the foreign body from around the base of the tongue (if present) by cutting it before surgery.

The foreign body is removed by performing a series of small enterotomies (Fig. 12.5). First, perform a gastrotomy and retrieve the proximal foreign body from the stomach or oesophagus by gentle traction. Transect the foreign body distally and close the gastrotomy site. Perform an enterotomy in the distal duodenum and retrieve the proximal portion of the remaining foreign body by gentle

traction. Again, transect the foreign body distally, close the enterotomy site, and repeat this process in a step-wise fashion until all of the foreign material has been removed. This may necessitate five or six separate incisions. When applying gentle traction, ensure that the foreign body does not cut further through the intestinal wall.

Patients with severe intestinal compromise or intestinal perforation may require enterectomy and management of peritonitis but their prognosis is likely to be poor. Consider euthanasia of patients with severe secondary intestinal injury.

Prognosis

The prognosis following removal of discrete foreign bodies is good. Over 90% of patients recover completely. However, delay between the onset of signs and intervention is associated with a worse outcome. The prognosis for patients following removal of linear foreign bodies is worse and this may be due to the increased rate of intestinal perforation and the necessity for multiple enterotomies for retrieval. The most common serious complication of gastrointestinal surgery is dehiscence, which leads to peritonitis. This occurs in up to 7% of cases and is often fatal.

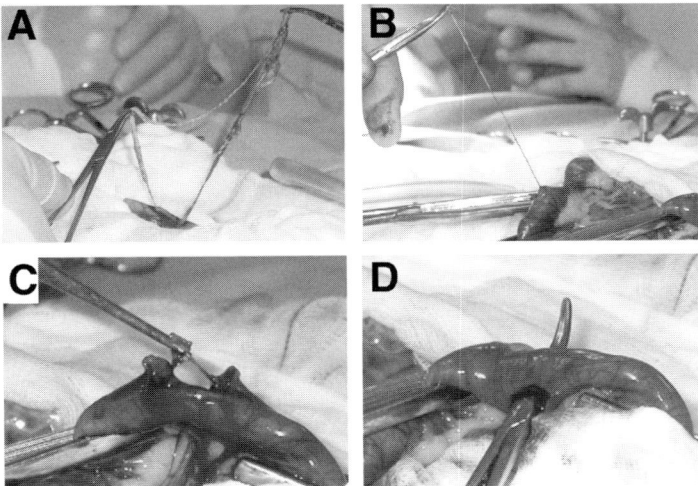

Fig. 12.5. Multiple enterotomies to remove linear foreign body: (A) having released the proximal point of obstruction, perform an enterotomy in the proximal intestine to retrieve part of the foreign body; (B) cut the foreign body and retrieve the proximal section by gentle traction; (C) repeat this sequentially, progressing distally along the intestinal tract until all the foreign body has been removed; (D) perforation of the mesenteric surface of the intestinal tract due to pressure necrosis caused by the linear foreign body. This section was excised by performing an enterectomy.

Intussusception

Intussusception occurs when a section of intestine invaginates inside itself, allowing the distal portion of intestine to envelop the proximal segment (Fig. 12.6).

Aetiopathogenesis

Intussusception is often classified as being idiopathic, particularly in young animals, but pre-existing intestinal disease may also precipitate the problem. It may be caused by exaggerated peristaltic motion. Intussusception is often associated with heavy worm burdens in young animals and can be associated with inflammatory bowel disease. In older animals, intestinal tumours may act as a nidus for intussusception to form around. Intussusception causes complete or partial intestinal obstruction. The intussuscepted portion of intestine may become ischaemic and perforate.

Historical and clinical findings

The signs associated with intussusception range from acute-onset, persistent vomiting to chronic, intermittent vomiting associated with diarrhoea.

The intussusception may be palpable as a firm, tubular structure in the abdomen, and other clinical findings consistent with intestinal obstruction will be found. Occasionally, the invaginated proximal loop of small intestine is long enough to pass through the rectum and out of the anus where it can be mistaken for a rectal prolapse (see p. 197).

Investigation

Radiographic and ultrasonographic features include evidence of small intestinal distension (see above). Ultrasound often provides a definitive diagnosis as the intussusception has a distinctive, multi-layered appearance compared with normal bowel.

Management

Surgery to correct intussusception should be performed as soon as possible to reduce the risk of ischaemic necrosis and perforation.

Reduction

The intussuscepted portion of bowel may be reduced if no adhesions have formed between the

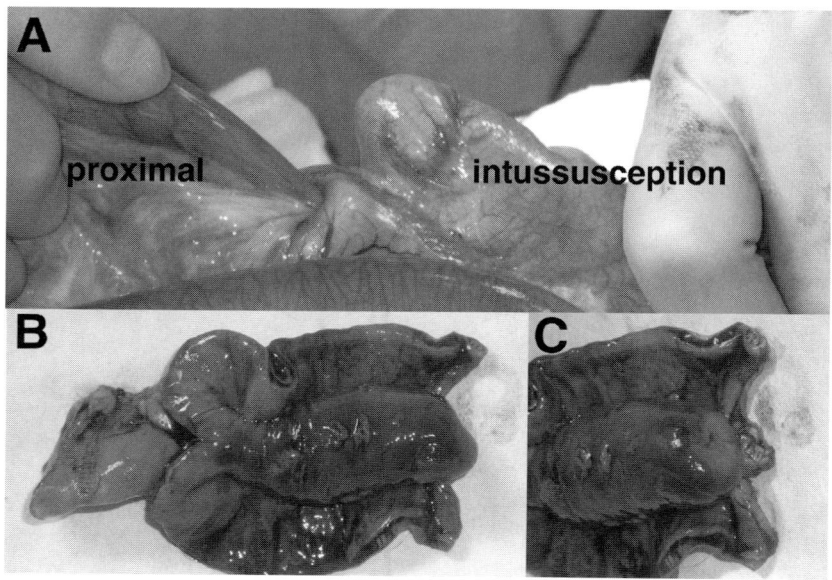

Fig. 12.6. Intussusception: (A) proximal small intestine invaginated into distal intestine at the ileocaecocolic junction to create an intussusception; (B and C) intussusception opened longitudinally to show proximal loop of intestine invaginated inside with adhesions.

inner and outer segments. Apply gentle traction to the proximal loop of intestine while squeezing the distal end of the intussusception (Fig. 12.7). Ensure that the loop of bowel is isolated from the rest of the abdomen as the intussusception may rupture during reduction.

Resection

Perform an enterectomy if the intussusception cannot be reduced or has become necrotic, or if the intussusception is associated with an intestinal tumour.

Enteroplication

The intussusception may recur soon after being reduced. Enteroplication is a procedure that reduces the risk of recurrence by fixing loops of small intestine to each other to prevent them from becoming

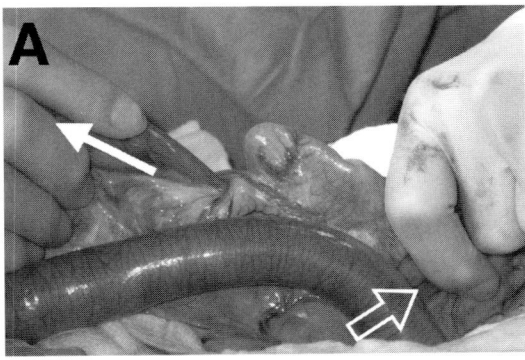

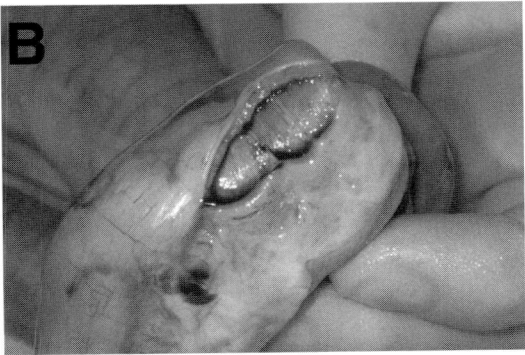

Fig. 12.7. Manual reduction of intussusception: (A) apply traction to the proximal intestine (closed arrow) at the same time as squeezing the base of the intussusception (open arrow); (B) the intussusception may tear during manual reduction.

invaginated inside their neighbouring sections (see p. 187). This is a controversial procedure, as complications, including perforation and peritonitis, have been reported and the risks of complications may outweigh the benefits of the procedure. If a primary cause for the intussusception can be identified and treated at the time of surgery (e.g. intestinal tumour), there may be little benefit in performing enteroplication.

Manage underlying disease process

Treat underlying intestinal disease (e.g. endoparasites; inflammatory bowel disease; neoplasia). Submit resected tissues for analysis to help identify undiagnosed intestinal disease.

Prognosis

Post-operative complications including peritonitis and recurrence of intussusception may occur. Mortality rates of up to 25% have been reported.

Gastrointestinal Neoplasia

Gastrointestinal tumours may develop as discrete masses (e.g. adenocarcinoma) or infiltrative diseases (e.g. lymphosarcoma) and are often malignant. Clinical signs include vomiting, diarrhoea, weight loss, and melaena. Animals with bleeding intestinal masses may develop non-regenerative anaemias.

Focal intestinal masses can be removed by performing an enterectomy including 3–5 cm margins of grossly healthy intestine on either side of the tumour. Remove the local mesenteric lymph node to aid tumour staging by bluntly dissecting it from the surrounding mesentery, being careful not to traumatize the vascular supply to the intestinal tract. Infiltrative tumours can be diagnosed from intestinal biopsies. The prognosis is dependent on the tumour type and stage, but most intestinal tumours in dogs and cats are malignant.

Inflammatory Bowel Disease

Inflammatory bowel disease commonly causes chronic vomiting or diarrhoea. A range of investigative steps is described (consult appropriate texts). Mucosal biopsies can be collected from the stomach, proximal small intestine, and colon by endoscopy and may provide sufficient information to reach a diagnosis. However, endoscopic biopsies do not include the submucosa or muscularis and cannot be collected from the mid and distal jejunum or ileum. An alternative to endoscopic biopsy is full-thickness surgical biopsy (see p. 183). Samples should be collected from the stomach, duodenum, jejunum, and ileum. Colonic samples may also be collected if signs indicate a large-intestinal component to the disease.

Pyloric Outflow Obstruction

Pyloric outflow obstruction (POO) is a syndrome caused by a group of chronic diseases. Pyloric pathology inhibits gastric emptying and this leads to gastric distension and vomiting that becomes dissociated from feeding. Over time, weight loss, debility, and chronic electrolyte and acid–base disturbances develop. POO may be secondary to neoplasia, inflammatory bowel disease, or gastric foreign body. It can also be a primary problem caused by mucosal or muscular hypertrophy of the pylorus. Primary POO is classed as congenital (onset less than 1 year of age) or acquired (later onset of signs) and may be linked to hyperacidity of the stomach. Primary POO is seen most frequently in small breed, brachycephalic dogs. With the exception of POO secondary to gastric foreign body, the management of POO requires careful investigation and advanced surgical techniques. Cases are best referred to a specialist centre. Among other treatment options, surgery to widen the pyloric outflow tract (pyloroplasty) or to remove the diseased pylorus (pylorectomy or 'Billroth' procedures) can be considered. The prognosis is guarded.

Feline Megacolon

Constipation is common in cats and may lead to megacolon. The colon becomes grossly distended with hard, impacted faeces and the cat is unable to defecate normally. The colonic wall becomes irreversibly stretched and loses normal contractile function creating an incurable problem. Megacolon is classified on the basis of its aetiology, which is complex.

Congenital megacolon is extremely uncommon. Primary congenital megacolon results from failure of development of normal colonic innervation. Secondary congenital megacolon is associated with atresia ani and other conditions that cause colonic obstruction.

Most cases of megacolon in cats are acquired. *Feline idiopathic megacolon* is the commonest form affecting over 60% of cases. The aetiology is unknown but factors that disrupt the normal defecatory pattern or lead to primary colonic smooth muscle dysfunction may contribute to the disease. *Secondary acquired megacolon* occurs secondary to conditions impeding defecation such as sacral nerve injury (sacral and tail injuries), rectal tumours, and pelvic fracture. *Feline dysautonomia* also causes megacolon along with a range of other symptoms.

Historical and clinical findings

Cases with megacolon present with unproductive straining to defecate, pain on defecation, and abdominal distension because of massive colonic enlargement and impaction with faeces. Megacolon can become debilitating leading to weight loss, inappetence, and occasional vomiting.

Investigation

History and clinical findings are highly suggestive of megacolon. Abdominal radiographs confirm the presence of massive colonic enlargement and impaction with faecaliths (Fig. 12.8). Pelvic radiographs and rectal examination (under general anaesthesia) identify whether or not pelvic narrowing or other forms of colonic obstruction have contributed to megacolon. Neurological examination, including careful assessment of sacral nerve function, helps identify neurological injury that may have contributed.

Medical management

Both medical and surgical management can be considered. The goals of medical management are to relieve faecal impaction and to achieve semi-regular defecation. Under general anaesthesia, faecaliths can be removed by administering enemas and digitally breaking down the faecaliths *per rectum*. Animals should be rehydrated before attempting to remove faecaliths as this helps to lubricate the stool. To prevent ongoing impaction with faeces, prokinetic agents (cisapride) and laxatives (lactulose) are prescribed. High-fibre diets can also be used to keep stools soft. Many cats tolerate regular micro-laxative administration. A reasonable goal

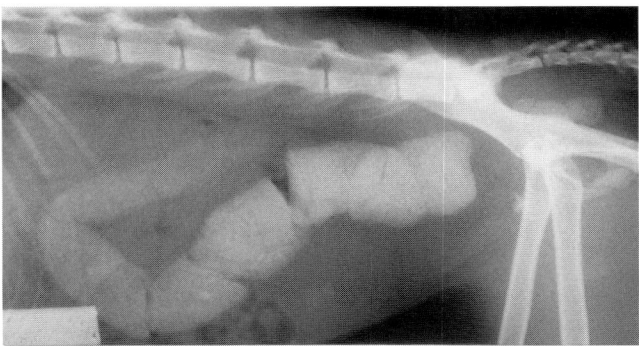

Fig. 12.8. Radiograph of cat with feline idiopathic megacolon demonstrating massive enlargement of the colon with impacted faeces.

of medical management is to enable the patient to defecate at least every 48 h.

Surgical management

Surgery to manage feline megacolon should not be attempted by inexperienced surgeons. Cases should be referred to an experienced colleague or specialist centre for management. Most patients benefit from *subtotal colectomy* in which 90–95% of the colon is removed, and this is the preferred surgical treatment. Subtotal colectomy leads to the passage of extremely soft stools as the absorptive capacity of the colon is lost. This prevents faecal consolidation and impaction. Although this surgery is generally well tolerated, patients are likely to have watery diarrhoea post-operatively and this may be difficult for owners to manage. Over time, the intestinal tract adapts and the stool will begin to solidify. By 3 months post-operatively, most patients will have soft, formed stools often likened to cowpats in their consistency. Faecal incontinence and recurrence of constipation in the small portion of remaining colon are potential long-term complications.

Animals with pelvic narrowing may respond to widening of the pelvic canal but this is an aggressive surgery and there is no guarantee that normal colonic function will return. Subtotal colectomy is usually performed in preference.

Please note that these recommendations apply to cats and not to dogs. Radical colonic surgery may be very poorly tolerated in the dog. Consult a specialist for advice when dealing with intractable canine megacolon.

Surgical Techniques

The principles of abdominal surgery should be reviewed before undertaking gastrointestinal surgery (see Chapter 11).

General principles of gastrointestinal surgery

Perform a full ventral midline coeliotomy incision from the xiphisternum to just cranial to the pubis. Patients often have multiple lesions along their gastrointestinal tract that may not be identified preoperatively and it is important to ensure that the entire gastrointestinal tract can be evaluated fully.

Prevent cross-contamination

- Isolate the affected portion of the gastrointestinal tract from the rest of the abdomen by exteriorizing it and using moistened swabs.
- Perform local lavage and discard the swabs before returning the tissue to the abdomen.
- Dedicate one area of the instrument tray to contaminated instruments to avoid cross-contamination of clean instruments.
- Handle foreign bodies with instruments and discard them from the surgical field immediately.
- Change gloves after closing the gastrointestinal tract but before closing the abdomen.
- Use fresh forceps, scissors, and needle-holders to complete the abdominal surgery following closure of the gastrointestinal tract.
- Place omental wraps around incision lines to promote the formation of an early serosal seal.

Prevent spillage of luminal contents

Take steps to prevent spillage of luminal contents before incising into the stomach or intestine:

1. Apply bowel clamps: squeeze the intestine between two fingers and push the intestinal contents away from the proposed incision site ('milking the intestinal contents'); then apply non-crushing bowel clamps (e.g. Doyen's) to stop the contents flowing back (Fig. 12.9).

2. Use stay sutures to elevate the proposed gastric incision site away from the luminal contents: it is difficult to apply bowel clamps to isolate an area of the stomach. Instead, stay sutures can be used to elevate the proposed incision site (Fig. 12.10). As the gastric contents pool in the dependent portion of the stomach, this prevents spillage when the lumen is incised.

Assessing gastrointestinal viability

The viability of the gastrointestinal tract must be assessed and non-viable portions should be removed. Areas of uncertain viability should also be resected as they may become ischaemic and perforate. Several key features can be used to assess gastrointestinal viability:

- **Colour:** viable bowel is pink. When pressed, the bowel should blanch but rapidly recolour as blood flows back into the area. Red bowel is compromised but may remain viable. Blue, purple, black, or green bowel is non-viable and should be excised. The mucosa may show signs of compromise before the serosa does. Evaluate the mucosal colour from the incision site and resect tissue if the mucosa is not pink.
- **Bleeding from incision site:** viable bowel should bleed profusely when incised. Continue to resect bowel until active bleeding is seen from the incised mucosa.
- **Palpation:** areas of bowel with palpable thinning are likely to be necrotic and should be excised.
- **Peristalsis:** peristaltic waves migrating along a loop of bowel indicate that it is likely to be viable. However, some degree of ileus is common in the intestinal tract during surgery, so peristalsis is not always seen, even in healthy bowel.
- **Mesenteric blood supply:** assess the mesenteric vessels for active pulsation and ensure that they are not thrombosed.

Suture materials and patterns

Monofilament, synthetic, absorbable suture material (e.g. Glycomer™ 631; polydioxanone II) is suitable for gastrointestinal surgery. Sizes 2-0 and 3-0 may be used for gastric surgery; sizes 3-0 and 4-0 may be used for small intestinal surgery. Use suture attached to swaged-on, tapercut, or taperpoint needles as these penetrate the gastrointestinal wall easily without creating large needle tracts.

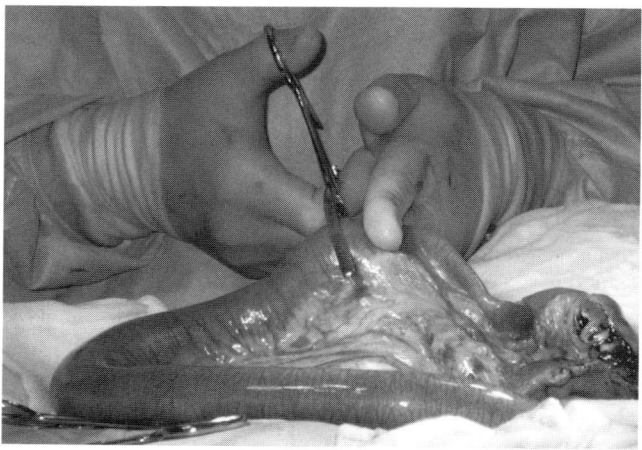

Fig. 12.9. Prevent spillage by milking luminal contents away from the planned incision site and applying non-crushing intestinal clamps.

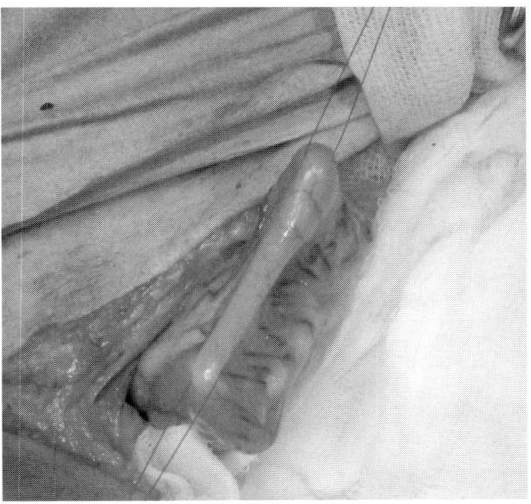

Fig. 12.10. Prevent spillage of gastric contents by using stay sutures to elevate the incision site away from the pool of fluid in the gastric lumen.

Simple appositional (continuous or interrupted) patterns are suitable for all gastrointestinal surgery (Fig. 12.11). They cause less luminal narrowing than inverting and everting patterns and promote rapid healing. Simple continuous patterns are quick to place and use less suture material than interrupted patterns. However, they can be awkward to place without an assistant. The simple interrupted pattern is easier to place but takes more time and uses more suture material. Take 3–4mm bites of tissue and space sutures up to 3mm apart. Ensure that the *submucosa* is included in every bite as this is the main suture-holding layer of the gastrointestinal tract.

In the intestinal tract, single-layered appositional patterns should always be used. In the stomach, an inverting pattern (e.g. Cushing) may be used in the outer layer of a two-layer closure as this promotes an early serosal seal. As the stomach is so large, luminal narrowing caused by the inverting pattern is not of concern. Do not use crushing or everting patterns as they are associated with delayed wound healing and luminal narrowing.

Do not resect more than 50% of the small intestine

Resections of large portions of the small intestine lead to *short bowel syndrome*. In this syndrome, intestinal transit time is very fast, malabsorption

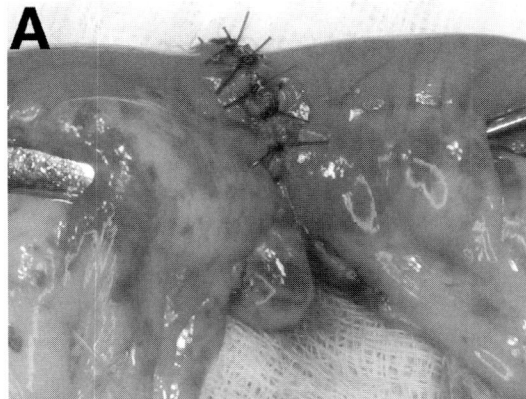

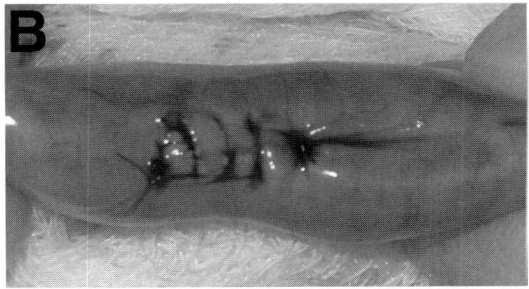

Fig. 12.11. Gastrointestinal suture patterns: (A) simple, interrupted pattern (enterectomy); (B) simple, continuous pattern (enterotomy).

occurs, and animals rapidly become malnourished because of the paucity of functional small intestine. The prognosis is poor.

Gastrotomy

Select the incision site

Pick a site on the parietal surface of the stomach midway between the lesser and greater curvatures, and midway between the pylorus and fundus. This area is accessible and has a good blood supply. Incisions near the pylorus may cause pyloric obstruction due to post-operative scarring.

Incise into the lumen

Elevate the incision site between two stay sutures. Make a stab incision into the stomach using a no. 11 scalpel blade. Extend the incision using the scalpel or Metzenbaum scissors. The incision should run parallel to the curvatures of the stomach (Fig. 12.12).

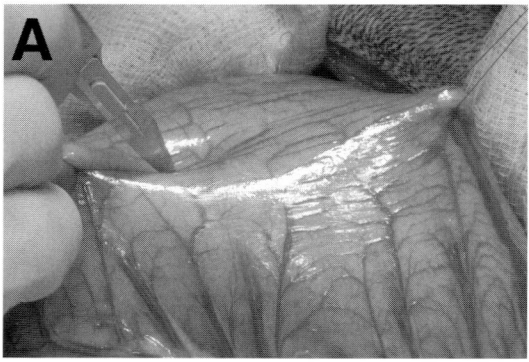

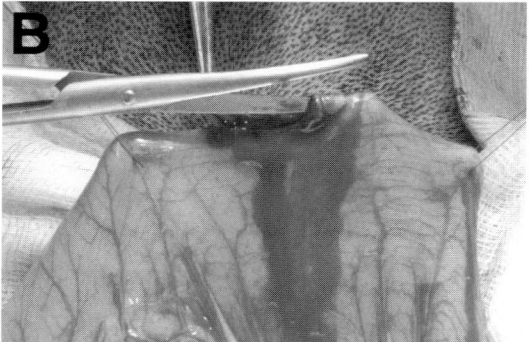

Fig. 12.12. Gastrotomy: (A) incise with a scalpel; (B) extend the incision with Metzenbaum scissors.

The mucosa and submucosa tend to fall away from the seromuscular layers as they are separated by loose fascia. Ensure that all layers of the stomach are incised.

Close the incision

A single-layered, full-thickness simple appositional suture pattern is adequate. Alternatively, in larger cats and adult dogs, a two-layered closure can be performed to generate an early serosal seal. Close the submucosa and mucosa together with a simple appositional continuous pattern (promoting rapid healing of these layers). Close the seromuscular layer with an inverting Cushing pattern to provide an early serosal seal (Fig. 12.13).

Enterotomy (small intestine)

Select the incision site

The incision should be made along the anti-mesenteric border in a healthy area of the intestine.

This causes less compromise to both sides of the incision line than incisions closer to the mesenteric border. Milk the intestinal contents away from the planned incision site and isolate it using non-crushing bowel clamps.

When performing enterotomy to remove a foreign body, do not make the incision directly over the foreign body as this area is compromised and more likely to undergo suture line dehiscence. Locate the incision in a site proximal or distal to the point of obstruction in an area of healthy intestine. The foreign body can be milked to the incision and retrieved.

Incise into the lumen

Make a stab incision into the lumen on the anti-mesenteric border with a no. 11 scalpel blade. Extend the incision longitudinally using the scalpel or Metzenbaum scissors. Ensure that the incision is long enough to allow removal of the foreign body without stretching or tearing of the edges of the incision (Fig. 12.14). Push the foreign body along to the incision site, grasp it with instruments, and remove it.

Close the incision and perform a leak test

Close the enterotomy incision using a single layer, simple appositional pattern. Before removing the bowel clamps, instill up to 5 ml of sterile saline into the intestinal lumen using a 25-gauge needle and syringe inserted through the anti-mesenteric surface of the intestine just distal to the enterotomy site. Gently squeeze the fluid backwards and forwards across the enterotomy site to check for leakage (Fig. 12.15). Place additional sutures as required or remove the suture line and start again if leakage is seen.

Intestinal biopsy

Intestinal biopsy is performed by modifying the basic enterotomy technique. Make a small enterotomy incision (5–10 mm long) along the anti-mesenteric border of the intestine. Make a second incision parallel to the first, and 2–3 mm lateral to it. Remove the sliver of intestine isolated between the two incisions (ensure that all four layers of the intestinal wall are included). Close the biopsy site with a simple appositional suture pattern. Place the biopsy in fixative. Gastric biopsy can be performed

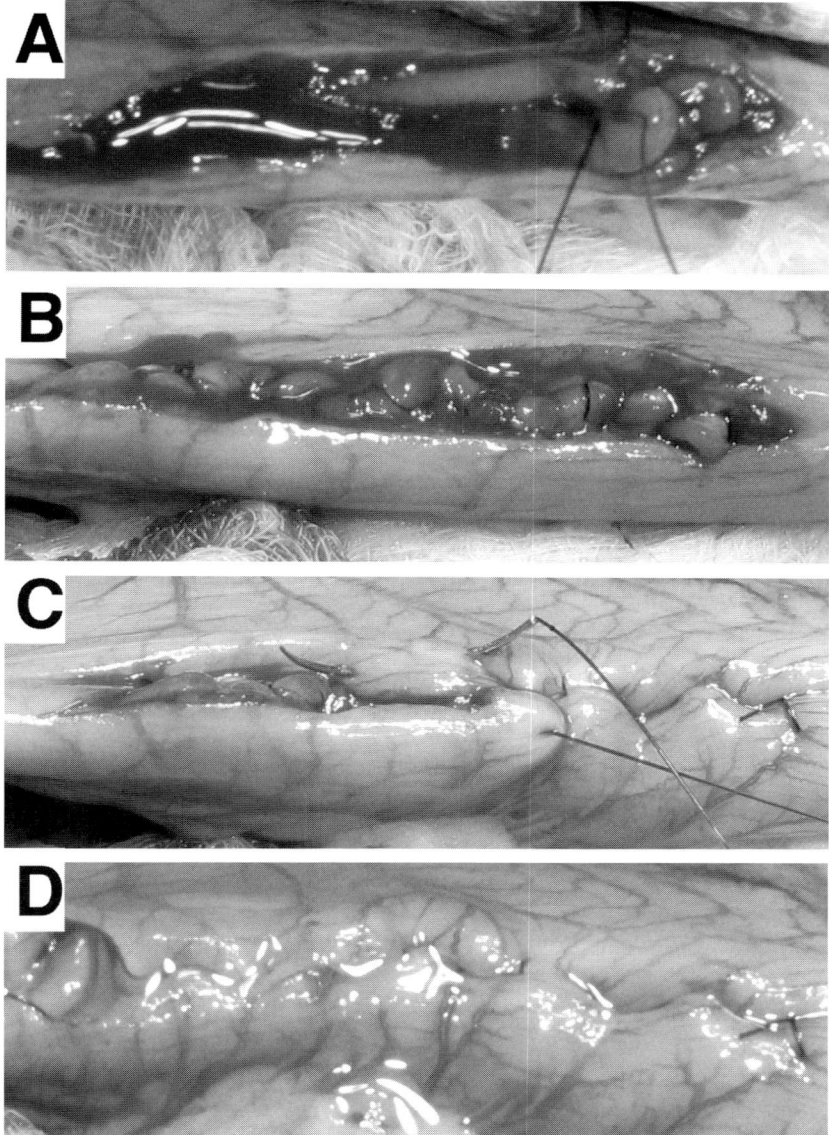

Fig. 12.13. Gastrotomy two-layered closure: (A and B) simple appositional suture pattern to close the mucosa and submucosa; (C and D) Cushing (inverting) pattern to close the seromuscular layer.

by making similar modifications of the gastrotomy technique.

Enterectomy (small intestine)

Enterectomy is indicated for removal of non-viable segments of intestine and for management of intestinal masses.

Select enterectomy sites and transect the vessels and mesentery supplying the area

Select sites proximal and distal to the compromised area of intestine to act as margins of resection. All of the compromised intestine must be removed so ensure the resection sites are in healthy tissue. Exteriorize the portion of intestine to be resected

---

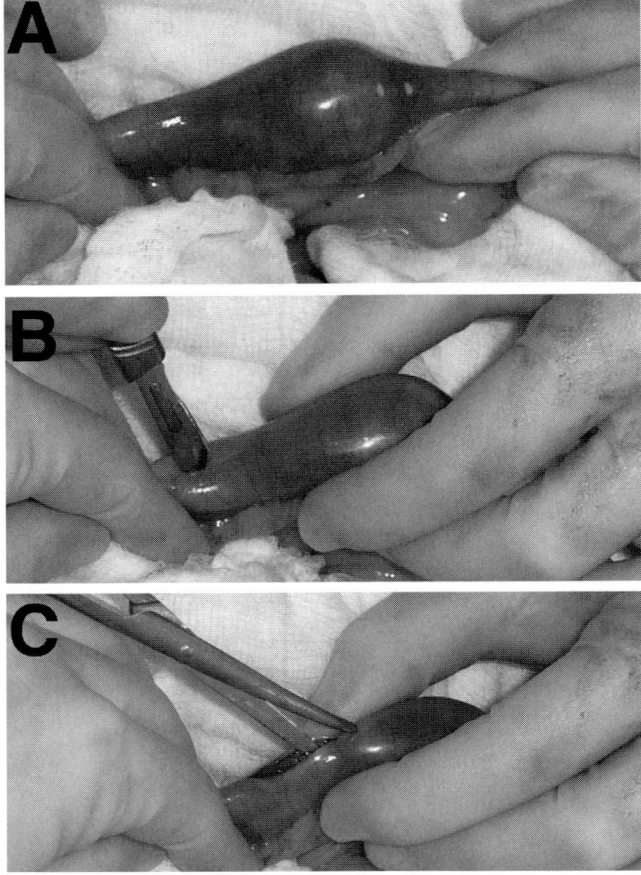

Fig. 12.14. Enterotomy: (A) isolate the portion of intestine to be incised; (B) incise into the anti-mesenteric surface with a scalpel; (C) extend the incision with Metzenbaum scissors. In this example, an assistant is occluding the intestine with her fingers instead of using intestinal clamps. This is extremely effective but impractical in most veterinary practices, as it necessitates having a sterile surgical assistant.

and isolate it using moistened swabs. Identify the blood vessels running through the mesentery to supply the portion of bowel to be resected. Double ligate and divide these vessels. Incise the mesentery to isolate the affected loop of intestine (Fig. 12.16).

Prevent contamination by occluding the bowel

Milk the intestinal contents away from the planned resection sites. At the proximal resection site, apply non-crushing bowel clamps (Doyen) to the bowel proximal to the planned incision line. Then place crushing forceps (e.g. haemostats) on the bowel just distal to the intended incision site (in the

portion of bowel to be resected) to prevent leakage when the resected section of intestine is removed. Repeat this at the distal resection site placing non-crushing forceps distally and crushing forceps just inside the resection line in the portion of bowel to be resected (Fig. 12.17).

Excise the affected portion of intestine

Transect the intestine between the proximal pair of clamps (proximal resection site). Repeat this between the distal pair of clamps (distal resection site) and remove the excised portion of intestine. If the two loops of intestine are of different diameter, modify the smaller end before proceeding (see below).

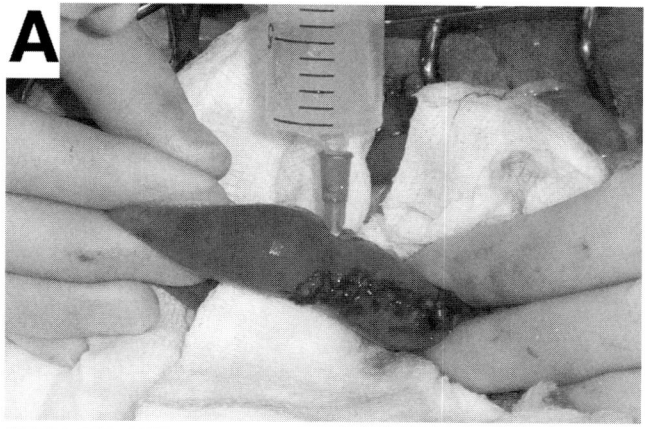

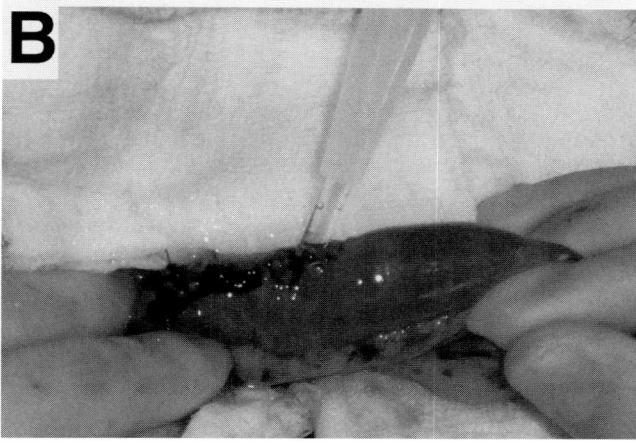

Fig 12.15. Enterotomy: (A) perform a leak test; (B) perform local lavage of the enterotomy site before returning it to the abdomen.

Anastomose the transected ends of intestine

Align the cut ends of intestine matching the mesenteric borders, ensuring that neither is rotated. Place one suture to appose the resection sites at the mesenteric borders. Place a second suture to appose the anti-mesenteric borders (Fig. 12.18). These sutures maintain orientation of the two loops of intestine while the anastomosis is completed. Lay the intestine on a swab and complete the suture line on one side between the mesenteric and anti-mesenteric sutures with a series of simple interrupted sutures placed 3–4 mm apart. Turn the intestine over and repeat this process on the second side (Fig. 12.19). Perform a leak test to ensure that the anastomosis is complete and perform local lavage (Fig. 12.15).

Close the mesentery

Appose the edges of the incised mesentery below the anastomosis site with a simple continuous suture pattern to prevent intestine becoming entrapped in the mesenteric rent (Fig. 12.20).

Anastomosing sections of intestine of different diameter

The proximal loop of intestine may have a distended lumen due to obstruction. To accommodate differences in luminal diameter, incise from the edge of the resected bowel along the anti-mesenteric border of the smaller portion of intestine until the circumference of both transection sites is equal. Then complete the anastomosis (Fig. 12.21).

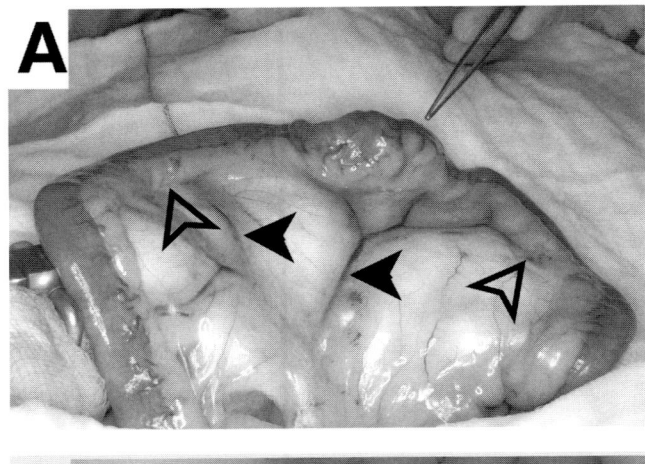

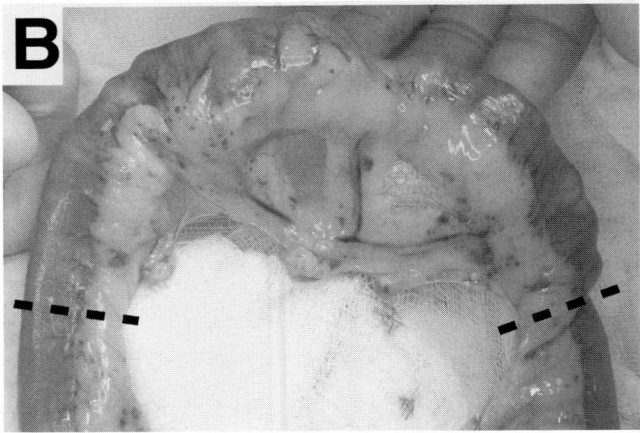

Fig. 12.16. Identify the area of intestine to be removed and isolate the blood supply: (A) this intestinal tumour (forceps) will be resected with 5 cm margins of healthy intestine. Closed arrowheads indicate arcuate mesenteric vessels that will be ligated. Open arrowheads indicate collateral vessels on the mesenteric surface which must be ligated; (B) the vessels have been double ligated and transected and the mesentery has been incised to isolate the portion of intestine to be resected. Dotted lines indicate proposed resection sites.

Colotomy and colectomy

There are few indications for colotomy or colectomy in general practice. Colotomy can be performed in a similar manner to enterotomy. Colectomy is more technically demanding than small intestinal enterectomy and should not be performed by inexperienced surgeons. The colonic blood supply is linear rather than arcuate and the blood supply to the descending colon also supplies the rectum and must be preserved. The colon is also less mobile than the small intestine making it difficult to manipulate. The main modification of small intestinal enterectomy technique required to perform colectomy is to isolate the vasa recta at the mesenteric border (to preserve as much of the longitudinal blood supply to the colon as possible).

Enteroplication

Lay the small intestinal tract out in large loops. Suture each loop to its neighbour using three or four sutures anchored through the seromuscular layer along the anti-mesenteric borders and spaced 2–4 cm apart. Avoid creating sharp, hairpin bends by not placing sutures near the turns of each loop, to prevent kinking and obstruction (Fig. 12.22).

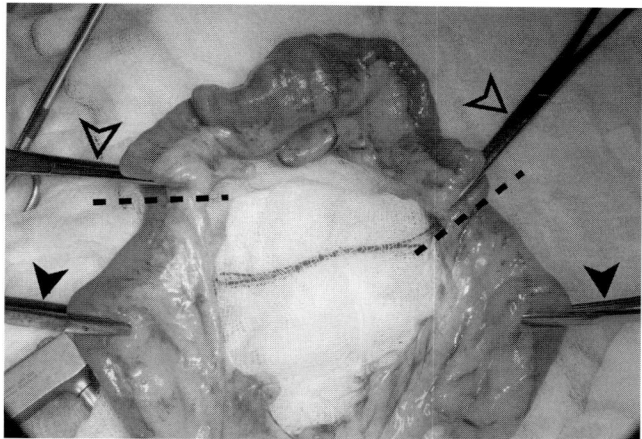

Fig. 12.17. Prevent contamination: open arrowheads – crushing forceps; closed arrowheads – non-crushing intestina clamps (Doyen's); dotted lines – resection lines.

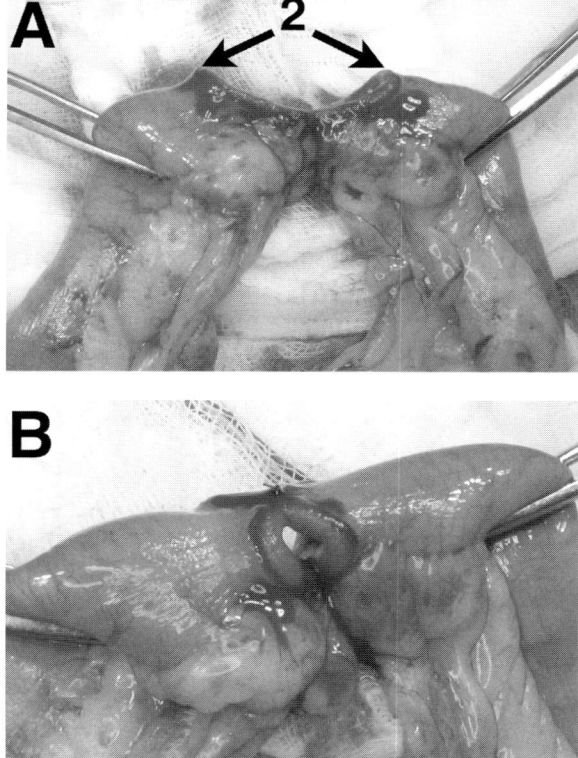

Fig. 12.18. Enterectomy: (A) align the cut ends of intestine and place a suture to appose the resection sites at the mesenteric border (the first suture has been placed; the arrows indicate points of placement of the second suture in the anti-mesenteric border); (B) following placement of the second suture to align the anti-mesenteric borders.

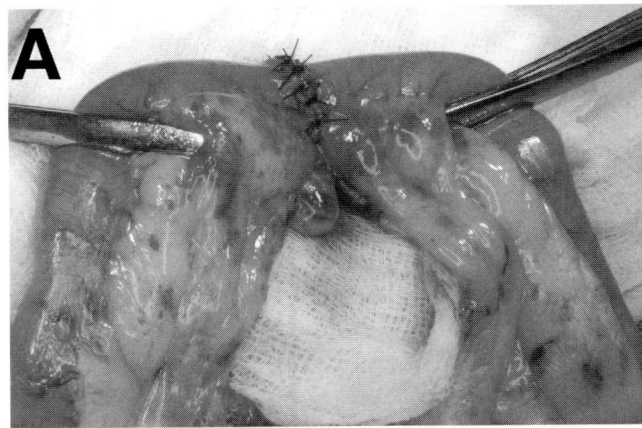

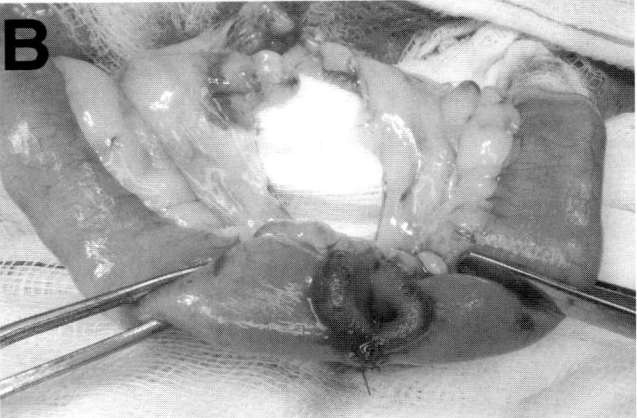

Fig. 12.19. Enterectomy: (A) close one side of the enterectomy site with a series of interrupted sutures; (B) turn the loop of intestine over and complete the enterectomy closure.

Post-operative care

Animals that have undergone gastrointestinal surgery require similar post-operative management to those undergoing any abdominal procedure (see Chapter 11). Non-steroidal anti-inflammatory drugs should not be administered as they are contraindicated in animals with intestinal disease and have been associated with spontaneous gastrointestinal perforation. There is no evidence that early enteral feeding increases the risk of leakage and animals can be fed within the first 24 h of surgery.

Gastric Dilatation and Volvulus Syndrome

Gastric dilatation and volvulus syndrome (GDV) is a life-threatening condition that develops over a period of a few hours. The stomach dilates and rotates along its long axis leading to hypovolaemic shock, dyspnoea, and gastric necrosis.

Aetiology

The aetiology of GDV is unknown but several risk factors have been identified:

- **Body conformation:** large breed, deep-chested dogs are predisposed to GDV. Breeds include the Great Dane, Irish Wolfhound, St Bernard, Newfoundland, bloodhound, Akita, Rottweiler, German Shepherd, standard poodle, Weimaraner, setters and collies.
- **Familial risk:** dogs with a close relative that has had GDV are at increased risk of developing the condition.

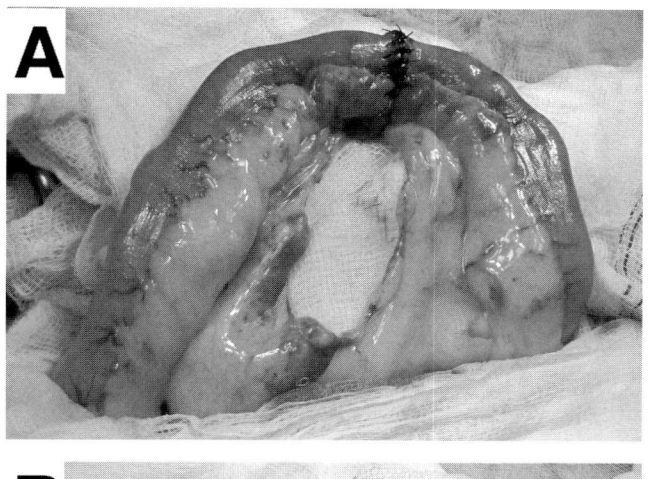

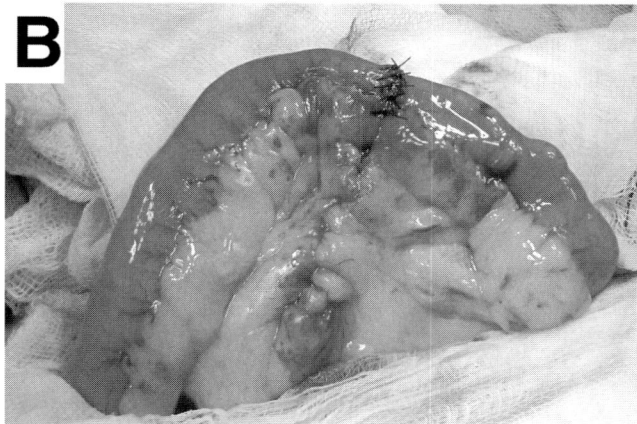

Fig. 12.20. Enterectomy: suture the rent in the mesentery: (A) before suturing; (B) after suturing.

- **Previous episode of GDV:** there is a high risk of recurrence unless gastropexy has been performed (see p. 194).
- **Diet and stress:** feeding a single large meal once a day, feeding particular diets, feeding from a height, and stress have all been implicated in the development of GDV.

GDV rarely affects small breed dogs and is very uncommon in cats. When GDV occurs in cats, it is usually secondary to herniation of part of the stomach into the thorax following diaphragmatic rupture.

Pathogenesis

GDV is characterized by distension of the stomach with fluid and gas, and by rotation of the stomach. However, it is unknown which occurs first. Fluid may come from ingesta or from transudation from the wall of the stomach. Gas may accumulate from aerophagia or from fermentation of gastric contents. The stomach usually rotates in a clockwise direction (i.e. the pylorus moves from the right-hand side of the abdomen, ventrally and to the left, displacing the fundus to the right). It may rotate through 360° or more. Occasionally the stomach will rotate in the opposite direction (anticlockwise). GDV causes a series of secondary problems that rapidly become life-threatening.

Gastric obstruction

Rotation of the cardia prevents eructation and displacement of the pylorus prevents emptying. These lead to persistent vomiting of small volumes of fluid and food.

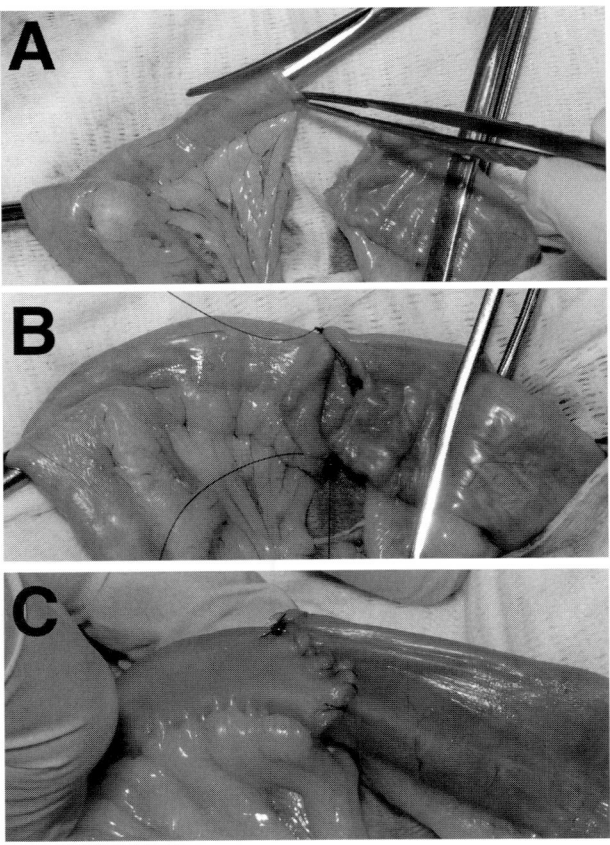

Fig. 12.21. Addressing luminal disparity: (A) incise the anti-mesenteric border of the smaller loop of intestine; (B and C) this extends the circumference of the resection site to match that of the larger loop of intestine, enabling the anastomosis to be completed.

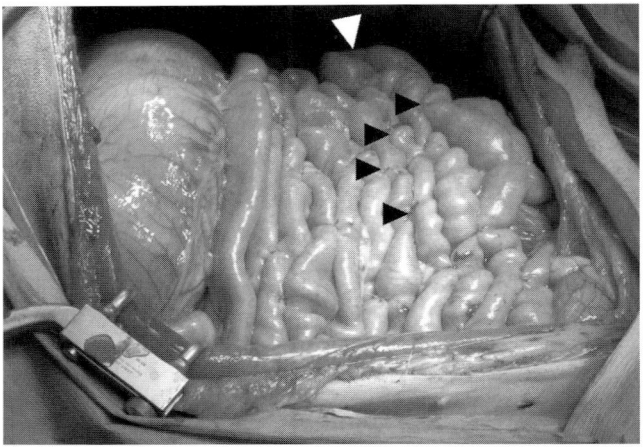

Fig. 12.22. Enteroplication: sutures are placed between adjacent loops of intestine (black arrowheads) while ensuring that the bends at the end of each loop are not so tight as to cause obstruction (white arrowhead).

Gastric wall necrosis

As the stomach distends, intragastric pressure builds and the blood vessels running through the gastric wall become compressed. This leads to gastric wall ischaemia, ulceration, and, eventually, perforation.

Cardiovascular compromise and shock

The distending stomach pushes against the adjacent viscera causing compression of the caudal vena cava and portal vein. This reduces venous return to the heart and causes blood to pool in the gastrointestinal tract. Toxins released from compromised abdominal organs depress cardiac function. Cardiac arrhythmias affect 10% of cases at presentation. These factors all contribute to reducing cardiac output and rapidly cause severe shock.

Dyspnoea

The distended stomach pushes against the diaphragm preventing chest expansion leading to dyspnoea and hypoxia.

Electrolytes and acid–base disturbances

A complex range of electrolyte and acid–base disturbances is caused by tissue hypoxia, dyspnoea, vomiting, and pooling of fluid and electrolytes in the gastrointestinal tract. Hypokalaemia and metabolic acidosis are the commonest abnormalities detected.

Splenic congestion and necrosis

The spleen moves with the stomach as it is attached by the gastrosplenic ligament. It often becomes displaced and lies along the right body wall. The splenic vessels become stretched and occluded leading to congestion and splenic enlargement.

Historical and clinical findings

Presenting signs are characteristic and develop over a period of a few hours:

- **persistent vomiting** of small volumes of fluid every few minutes;
- **abdominal distension and tympany** due to gastric dilation with gas. The abdomen becomes hyper-resonant on percussion;

- **dyspnoea**;
- **abdominal pain**; and
- **shock:** collapse, pale mucous membranes, prolonged capillary refill time, loss of peripheral pulses, weak femoral pulses, cold extremities, and tachycardia.

Investigation and diagnosis

Acute-onset vomiting, dullness, and abdominal distension in a large breed dog should generate a high index of suspicion that GDV has occurred. The diagnosis can be confirmed radiographically from the right lateral abdominal view (Fig. 12.23). The key features used to confirm the diagnosis are:

- absence of fluid-filled pylorus in the cranioventral abdomen;
- a large, gas-filled viscus in the cranial abdomen replacing normal stomach; and
- compartmentalization lines within the gas viscus.

Additional findings may include free gas in the abdominal cavity (indicative of gastric perforation) and loss of serosal detail (indicative of peritoneal effusion).

The diagnosis can also be confirmed intra-operatively: the stomach is grossly distended; the pylorus is not located in the right ventral abdomen; the oesophageal cardia is twisted; the ventral surface of the stomach may be covered by omentum as the parietal surface (normally seen in healthy dogs) is displaced.

Initial stabilization

Patients with GDV suffer from severe shock and are at increased risk from general anaesthesia. However, if surgery is delayed for several hours while their condition is stabilized, the risk of devastating secondary problems, such as gastric necrosis, increases. Surgical correction of the problem is prioritized early in the management of the patient. It not only prevents further gastric deterioration, but it also has a dramatic effect on improving venous return to the heart and relieving dyspnoea. Most animals receive only a short period of initial stabilization, and surgery is undertaken within the first hour following presentation. The cornerstones of initial stabilization are gastric decompression and shock therapy (see Chapter 13). In addition, perioperative antimicrobial therapy and pain relief are indicated.

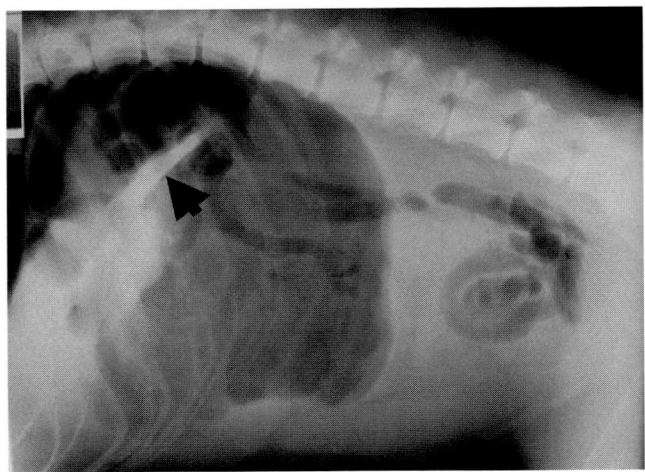

Fig. 12.23. Radiograph of dog with GDV: compartmentalization lines (arrow) formed by folds of the wall of the stomach indicate gastric torsion.

Gastric decompression

Gastric decompression has a dramatic effect on improving peripheral perfusion and reversing signs of shock because it relieves pressure that has contributed to dyspnoea and reduced venous return to the heart. It should be prioritized early during stabilization and repeated as necessary. Gastric decompression is achieved by orogastric intubation or paracentesis.

OROGASTRIC INTUBATION Orogastric intubation (passing a stomach tube) can be performed in unsedated patients. Pre-measure and mark a large-bore stomach tube from the tip of the nose to the 13th rib. Pre-measuring the tube ensures it reaches the gastric lumen without being pushed distally through the stomach wall. Position the dog in a sitting position, if possible, and get an assistant to restrain it. Place a gag in the mouth that will allow the tube to be passed (e.g. a roll of bandage). Lubricate the tip of the tube. Pass it through the centre of the gag and feed it down the oesophagus until the pre-measured point is reached (Fig. 12.24). Gas may be heard escaping from the tube as it enters the stomach, and gastric tympany should resolve immediately. Sometimes the tube cannot be passed through the oesophageal cardia. Do not force the tube. Repositioning the patient (e.g. from lying to sitting) may relieve pressure on the cardia and allow the tube to pass. The ability or inability to pass a stomach tube cannot be used to establish whether or not volvulus is present.

PARACENTESIS Paracentesis (needle drainage of the stomach through the body wall) can be performed if orogastric intubation fails. Clip and prepare the left lateral abdominal wall just caudal to the costal arch. Percuss the area to confirm that it is over the stomach and that the spleen is not trapped between the stomach and body wall (the area should be hyper-resonant rather than dull on percussion). Insert a large-bore needle through the body wall into the stomach to relieve gas (Fig. 12.25).

Surgical management

The goals of surgery are to:

1. reposition the stomach;
2. assess organ viability;
3. perform gastropexy (i.e. prevent recurrence).

Reposition the stomach

Locate the pylorus by tracing the duodenum forwards. Check the direction of rotation by assessing twisting at the cardia and the position of the pylorus in relation to the rest of the stomach.

CLOCKWISE ROTATION Pull the pylorus ventrally and to the right while pushing the body of the stomach (distended viscus) dorsally and to the left.

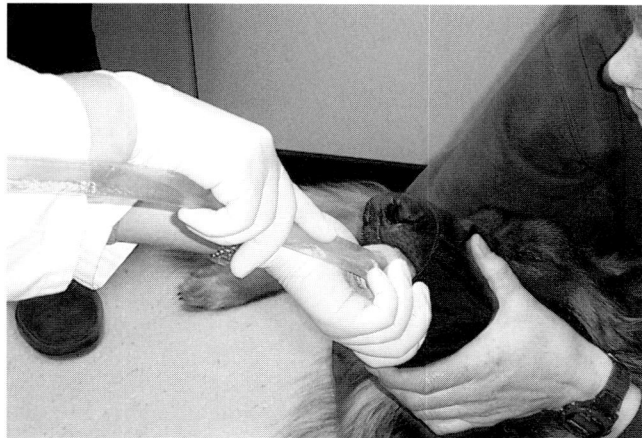

Fig. 12.24. Orogastric intubation to relieve tympany using a roll of bandage as a gag.

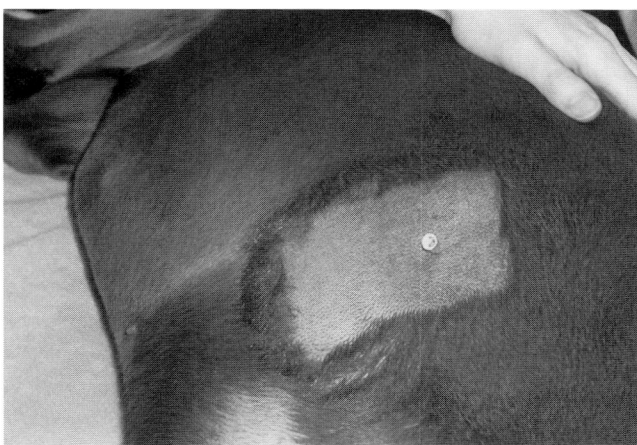

Fig. 12.25. Paracentesis to relieve tympany.

ANTICLOCKWISE ROTATION (LESS COMMON) The pylorus lodges dorsal to the fundus. Pull the pylorus from dorsally towards the right as the fundus is pushed towards the left.

Ensure that the stomach is repositioned properly. The pylorus will lie next to the right abdominal wall, the ventral surface of the stomach will not be covered with omentum, and the cardia will be untwisted.

Assess organ viability

Assess the stomach and resect devitalized areas. The spleen will be congested but splenectomy is rarely necessary. Perform splenectomy only if the spleen appears to be necrotic or if it remains congested and enlarged after it has been repositioned for 10 min.

Perform incisional gastropexy

GDV recurs following derotation in over 75% of cases that do not have gastropexy performed. Gastropexy markedly reduces the risks of recurrence to <10% and should be performed in all cases. A wide range of techniques has been described but two features should be incorporated:

- the pylorus should be anchored to the right body wall; and
- the muscular layers of the pylorus and the abdominal wall should be incised to ensure that adequate scar tissue forms at the pexy site.

Incisional gastropexy is quick, easy, and effective and is recommended for inexperienced surgeons.

SELECT SITE FOR GASTROPEXY Once the stomach is repositioned normally, pull the pylorus up to the right body wall behind the costal arch. Select an area of the right body wall at least 4 cm from the linea alba, and behind the last rib, which the pylorus reaches easily (Fig. 12.26).

INCISE BODY WALL AND STOMACH At the selected gastropexy site, make a 3–6 cm dorsoventral, linear incision through the peritoneum and first layer of abdominal wall muscle. The incision should be parallel to, and behind, the last rib. Make a corresponding incision in the seromuscular layer of the stomach over the pyloric antrum without penetrating the submucosa or mucosa (Fig. 12.27). This is simple as the submucosa and mucosa are loosely attached to the seromuscular layer and fall away as the incision is made. If the mucosa is inadvertently penetrated, suture it closed before proceeding.

SUTURE THE TWO INCISION LINES TOGETHER Suture the cranial edges of the gastric and abdominal incisions together using a continuous suture pattern

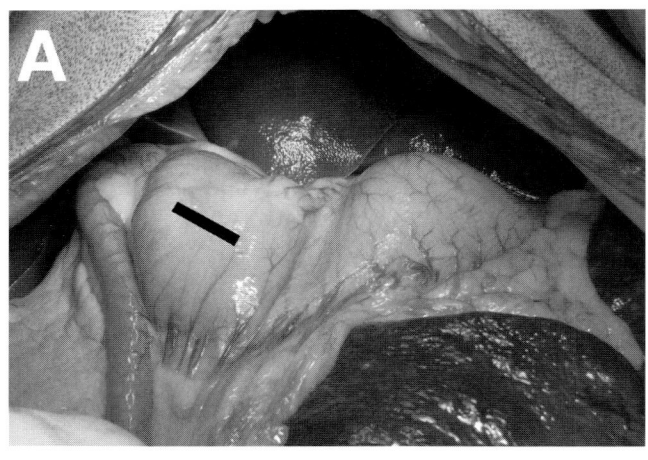

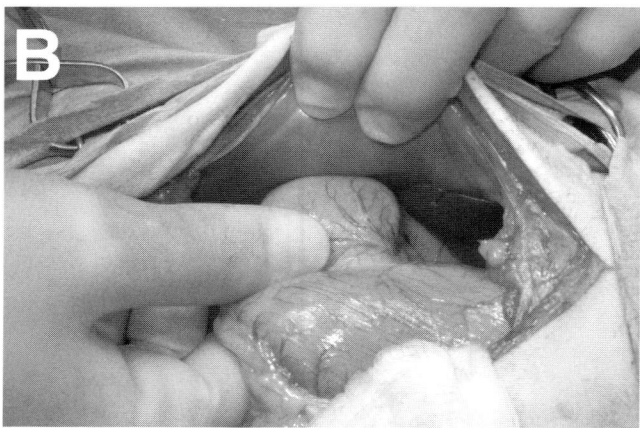

Fig. 12.26. Gastropexy: (A) anatomy demonstrating pyloric antrum and position of gastropexy incision (line); (B) push the pyloric antrum to the right body wall to determine the gastropexy position.

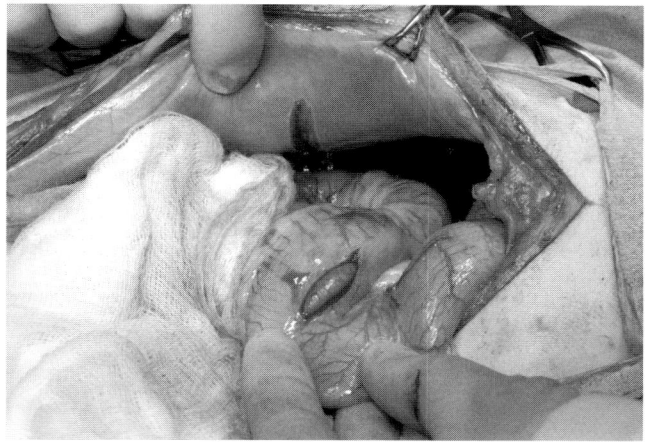

Fig. 12.27. Gastropexy: incisions in the right body wall and the pyloric seromuscular layer.

of 2-0, long-lasting or permanent suture material (e.g. polydioxanone; polypropylene). Start the continuous suture line by suturing the dorsal (deepest) apex of the gastric incision to the dorsal apex of the abdominal wall incision. Continue the suture line to appose the cranial edges of the incisions until the ventral apices are reached, and tie off the suture line (Fig. 12.28). Repeat the process to appose the caudal edges of the two incisions (Fig. 12.29).

Post-operative care

Patients require post-operative monitoring and supportive care until their physiological parameters return to normal. In addition to management of shock, routine post-operative care for coeliotomy should be instigated. Cardiac arrhythmias continue to develop post-operatively and may require treatment.

Complications

Major post-operative complications include the progression of shock and the development of gastric perforation and peritonitis. GDV can recur if the gastropexy breaks down but the incidence is less than 5%.

Some patients have recurrent episodes of gastric dilatation. The aetiopathogenesis is unknown but both primary gastric hypomotility, and secondary gastric wall injury due to stretching caused by GDV, have been proposed. Although gastropexy should prevent volvulus, recurrent gastric dilatation can be

debilitating as it causes intermittent clinical signs of abdominal discomfort, vomiting, dyspnoea, and cardiovascular compromise. Treatment with prokinetic agents and metoclopramide has been described but cases may not respond to therapy.

Prognosis

The mortality rate of dogs with GDV is greater than 15%. A range of factors associated with a worse outcome has been identified, including clinical signs lasting for greater than 6h prior to presentation, and the development of peritonitis or sepsis. Euthanasia should be considered intra-operatively if there is gastric wall necrosis or peritonitis.

Prophylactic gastropexy

Owners of predisposed breeds of dog sometimes request prophylactic gastropexy at the time of neutering. As gastropexy is effective at preventing recurrence after an episode of GDV, this seems rational. However, no studies have demonstrated the effectiveness of elective gastropexy or that the risks of the procedure do not outweigh the benefits. Incisional or other forms of right-sided gastropexy can be performed. Laparoscopic prophylactic gastropexy has also been described. Prophylactic surgery of this nature may be considered to be unethical in some countries (see discussion of neutering, p. 211) and prophylactic gastropexy may disqualify dogs from being shown.

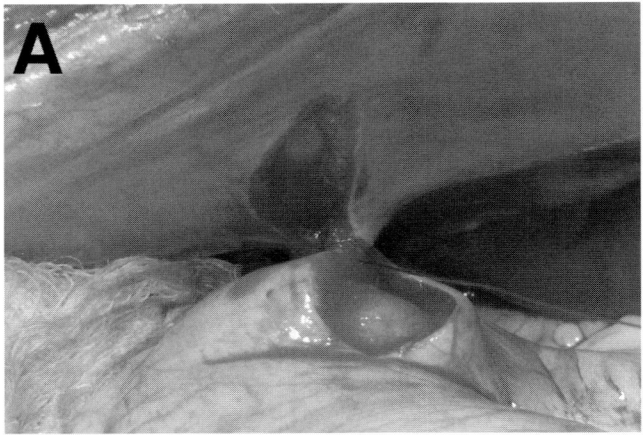

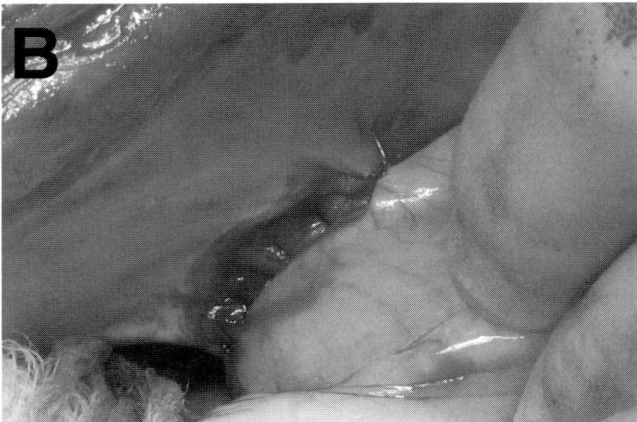

Fig. 12.28. Gastropexy: start to suture from the deepest (dorsal) aspect of the two incisions (A) and appose the cranial edges of the two incisions (B).

Related syndromes

GDV generally presents as an acute, life-threatening condition but both recurrent gastric dilatation without volvulus and gastric volvulus without dilatation have been reported. These syndromes may present with low-grade clinical signs or may be identified incidentally, but it seems likely that both could precipitate an acute episode of GDV. Surgery at an early stage following diagnosis is prudent, to reposition the stomach and perform gastropexy.

Rectal Prolapse

Rectal prolapse is quite uncommon. It usually occurs secondary to conditions that cause straining such as endoparasitism, colitis, rectal mass, perineal hernia, dystocia, and dysuria. Initially, only the mucosa prolapses but, as the condition progresses, the muscular layers also prolapse.

Historical and clinical findings

Rectal prolapse forms an annular mass protruding from the anus. Initially, the prolapsed tissue will be red and may bleed. As more tissue prolapses and the vascular supply becomes compromised, the tissue may become cyanotic or black, indicating ischaemic necrosis.

Investigation

The main differential diagnoses for rectal prolapse are rectal tumour and intussusception that has

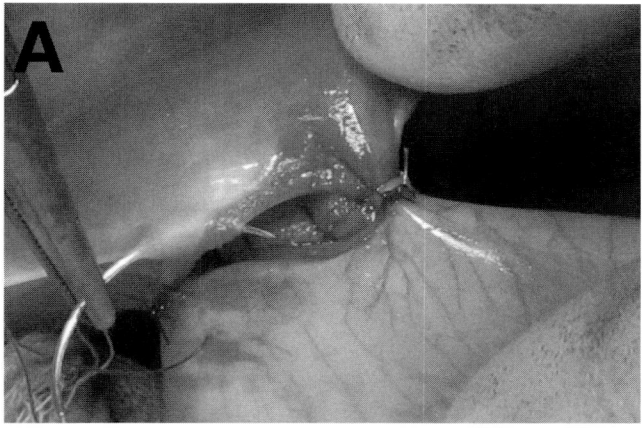

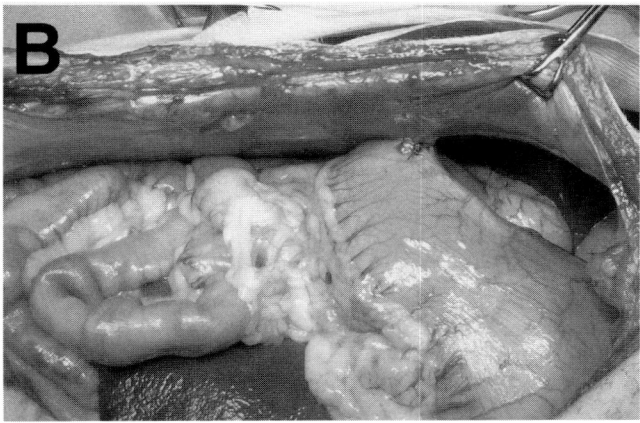

Fig. 12.29. Gastropexy: (A) complete the gastropexy by apposing the caudal edges of the body wall and pyloric incisions with a continuous suture pattern; (B) the completed gastropexy anchoring the pylorus to the right body wall.

protruded through the anus. Rectal masses can easily be differentiated from rectal prolapse. Intussusception protruding through the anus is very rare but appears identical to rectal prolapse on external appearance. To distinguish between the two, insert a lubricated probe (e.g. thermometer) between the anal orifice and wall of the protruding tissue. The probe will stop after a few millimetres if the mass is a rectal prolapse but will continue into the colon if the mass is an intussusception (Fig. 12.30). Abdominal palpation and imaging may help distinguish between these diseases.

Management

Rectal prolapses must be replaced quickly as they become more oedematous and compromised the longer that they are left. Most can be replaced manually but those that have become necrotic must be resected. For treatment to be effective, it is important to address the underlying problem that led initially to straining.

Manual reduction

Anaesthetize the patient. Lubricate the prolapse and gently push it back into the anal orifice. The prolapse may not return easily but steady, continuous pressure applied to it is usually sufficient. Once the prolapse is reduced, place a loose purse-string suture in the anal orifice. The suture should be tight enough to prevent the prolapse from recurring but still allow defecation. To gauge how tight to place the suture, place a rectal probe of a

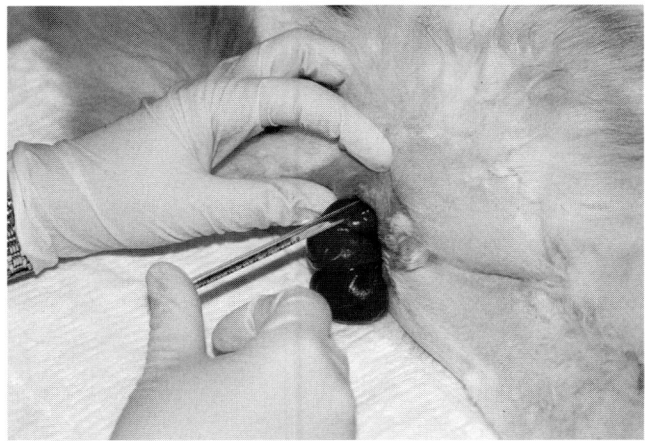

Fig. 12.30. Use a probe to distinguish between rectal prolapse and intussusception (image courtesy of E. Welsh).

diameter equivalent to a small stool (e.g. in a kitten use a thermometer or 1 ml syringe barrel; in a large breed dog use a 10 ml syringe barrel) and then tie the purse-string suture (Fig. 12.31). Leave the purse-string suture in place for 3–5 days. Prescribe bulk-forming laxatives (e.g. sterculia) so that soft, formed stools are produced that will pass easily through the purse string without inducing straining.

Colopexy

Colopexy can be performed for recurrent rectal prolapse. The goal of colopexy is to pull the colon forward into the abdomen and fix it to the body. This maintains traction on the rectum preventing further prolapse.

Reduce the prolapse. Perform a caudal midline coeliotomy, identify the descending colon, and apply cranial traction. Anchor 3–6 cm of the colon to the left body wall by placing the sutures through the anti-mesenteric surface of the colon. Ensure that they engage the muscular layers without penetrating the colonic lumen (Fig. 12.32). Use 2-0 to 3-0 polypropylene and place sutures in a simple interrupted or continuous pattern.

Resection of the prolapsed tissue

If prolapsed tissue becomes necrotic or cannot be reduced, it must be resected. Refer cases to an experienced colleague or specialist centre as this surgery is technically demanding.

Anal Sacculectomy

Anal sac disease is common in dogs but rare in cats (Fig. 12.33). The main indications for anal sac removal (anal sacculectomy) are for management of recurrent or persistent anal sacculitis and for management of anal sac tumours. Perianal gland adenocarcinoma is the commonest anal sac tumour and is frequently associated with the paraneoplastic syndrome, *pseudohyperparathyroidism*. In this condition, patients may present because of signs relating to hypercalcaemia rather than anal sac disease.

Anal sacculectomy is a simple procedure but complications associated with poor technique and incomplete resection can be devastating. Surgery should only be performed by a veterinary surgeon who is confident in their ability. Surgery can be performed unilaterally or bilaterally.

Anatomy

The anal sacs are located at 4 o'clock and 8 o'clock positions around the anus, approximately 1 cm from the mucocutaneous junction. The medial edge of each sac and its duct run between the external and internal anal sphincters. The ducts are easily visualized and catheterized at the anal orifice. The caudal rectal nerve, innervating the external anal sphincter, runs close to the anal sac.

Technique

Position the patient in sternal recumbency with the tail pulled and tied dorsally. Express the anal sacs, clip

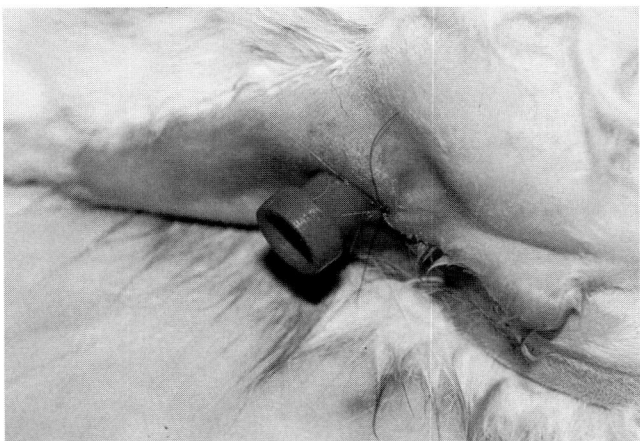

Fig. 12.31. Placing a loose purse-string suture to prevent recurrence of the prolapse using a blood collection tube as a guide (image courtesy of E. Welsh).

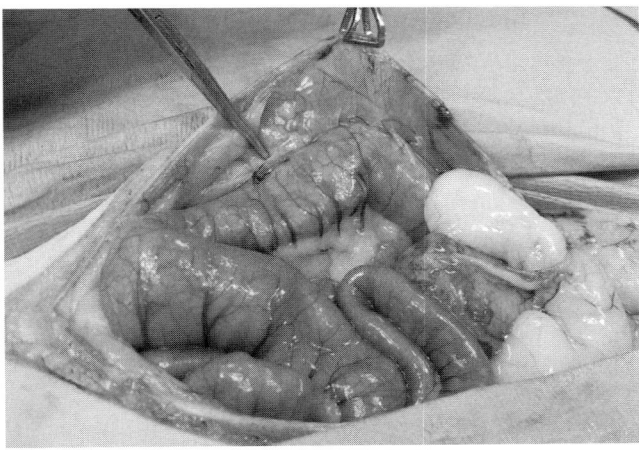

Fig. 12.32. Colopexy (image courtesy of E. Welsh).

the skin around the anus, and place a purse-string suture ensuring that the anal sac orifices remain accessible. Packing the anal sac with wax using injection cartridges greatly facilitates removal. Once the wax has set, prepare the skin for aseptic surgery.

Palpate the anal sac subcutaneously. If wax has not been used, insert a blunt probe (e.g. a small haemostat) into the anal sac via the duct to act as a guide. Make a linear skin incision directly over the anal sac, approximately 1 cm from the anal orifice. Expose the sac by bluntly dissecting through the subcutaneous fat. Dissect the sac free from the surrounding tissue. Start at the lateral tip of the sac and continue the dissection all around the sac working towards the duct. Continue the blunt dissection close to the duct to dissect it from between the internal and external anal sphincters. Ligate and transect the duct and remove the anal sac. Repeat on the other side if required. Self-retaining retractors (e.g. Gelpi retractors) greatly facilitate dissection.

Problems with dissection include difficulty in freeing the anal sac from its deep attachments, and rupture of the sac during dissection. If the sac ruptures during dissection, ensure that all of the sac

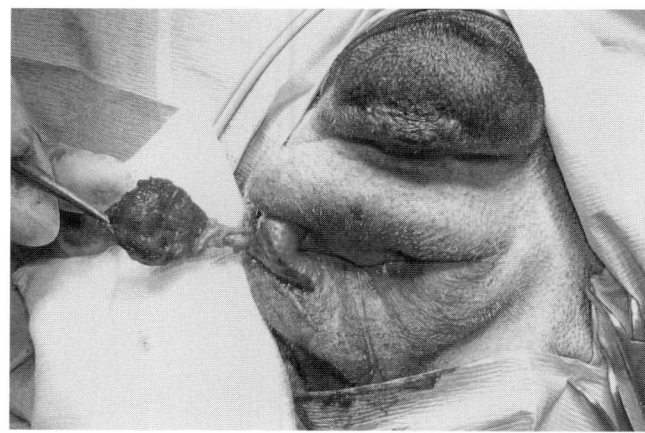

Fig. 12.33. Closed anal sacculectomy (this dog had a hyperplastic anus and screw tail hence the unusual appearance of its perineum).

and duct are removed. Anal sacs that have been ruptured or that contain large masses may be challenging to remove.

Complications

Complications include dehiscence, infection and, rarely, faecal incontinence. Chronic discharging sinuses will develop if anal sac material is left *in situ*, and are difficult to treat.

Prognosis

The prognosis for anal sacculectomy for management of anal sacculitis is good providing that no anal sac remnants are left. Most anal sac tumours are malignant and have metastasized by the time of diagnosis. The prognosis for patients with anal sac tumours is guarded, but anal sacculectomy can help relieve signs of dyschezia and of hypercalcaemia.

Bibliography

Adams, W.M., Sisterman, L.A., Klauer, J.M., Kirby, B.M. and Lin, T.L. (2010) Association of intestinal disorders in cats with findings of abdominal radiography. *Journal of the American Veterinary Medical Association* 236, 880–886.

Applewhite, A.A., Hawthorne, J.C. and Cornell, K.K. (2001) Complications of enteroplication for the prevention of intussusception recurrence in dogs: 35 cases (1989–1999). *Journal of the American Veterinary Medical Association* 219, 1415–1418.

Aronson, L.R., Brockman, D.J. and Brown, D.C. (2000) Gastrointestinal emergencies. *Veterinary Clinics of North America Small Animal Practice* 30, 555–579.

Bebchuk, T.N. (2002) Feline gastrointestinal foreign bodies. *Veterinary Clinics of North America Small Animal Practice* 32 (4), 861–880.

Beck, J.J., Staatz, A.J., Pelsue, D.H., Kudnig, S.T., MacPhail, C.M., Seim III, H.B. and Monnet, E. (2006) Risk factors associated with short-term outcome and development of perioperative complications in dogs undergoing surgery because of gastric dilatation-volvulus: 166 cases (1992–2003). *Journal of the American Veterinary Medical Association* 229, 1934–1939.

Bennett, P.F., Denicola, D.B., Bonney, P., Glickman, N.W. and Knapp, D.W. (2002) Canine anal sac adenocarcinomas: clinical presentation and response to therapy. *Journal of Veterinary Internal Medicine* 16, 100–104.

Bennett, R.R. and Zydeck, F.A. (1970) A comparison of single layer suture patterns for intestinal anastomosis. *Journal of the American Veterinary Medical Association* 157, 2075–2080.

Boag, A.K., Coe, R.J., Martinez, T.A. and Hughes, D. (2005) Acid-base and electrolyte abnormalities in dogs with gastrointestinal foreign bodies. *Journal of Veterinary Internal Medicine* 19, 816–821.

Brockman, D.J., Washabau, R.J. and Drobatz, K.J. (1995) Canine gastric dilatation/volvulus syndrome in a veterinary critical care unit: 295 cases (1986–1992). *Journal of the American Veterinary Medical Association* 207, 460–464.

Burkitt, J.M., Drobatz, K.J., Saunders, H.M. and Washabau, R.J. (2009) Signalment, history, and outcome of cats with gastrointestinal tract intussusception: 20 cases (1986–2000). *Journal of the American Veterinary Medical Association* 234, 771–776.

Cote, D.D., Collins, D.M. and Burczynski, F.J. (2008) Safety and efficacy of an ocular insert for apomorphine-induced emesis in dogs. *American Journal of Veterinary Research* 69, 1360–1365.

Crawshaw, J., Berg, J., Sardinas, J.C., Engler, S.J., Rand, W.M., Ogilvie, G.K., Spodnick, G.J., *et al.* (1998) Prognosis for dogs with nonlymphomatous, small intestinal tumors treated by surgical excision. *Journal of the American Animal Hospital Association* 34, 451–456.

Dyess, D.L., Bruner, B.W., Donnell, C.A., Ferrara, J.J. and Powell, R.W. (1991) Intraoperative evaluation of intestinal ischemia: a comparison of methods. *Southern Medical Journal* 84, 966–969, 974.

Ellison, G.W. (1989) Wound healing in the gastrointestinal tract. *Seminars in Veterinary Medicine and Surgery (Small Animal)* 4, 287–293.

Ellison, G.W. (1993) Gastric dilatation volvulus. *Veterinary Clinics of North America Small Animal Practice* 23, 513–530.

Elwood, C., Devauchelle, P., Elliott, J., Freiche, V., German, A.J., Gualtieri, M., Hall, E., *et al.* (2010) Emesis in dogs: a review. *Journal of Small Animal Practice* 51, 4–22.

Felts, J.F., Fox, P.R. and Burk, R.L. (1984) Thread and sewing needles as gastrointestinal foreign bodies in the cat: a review of 64 cases. *Journal of the American Veterinary Medical Association* 184, 56–59.

Formaggini, L., Schmidt, K. and De Lorenzi, D. (2008) Gastric dilatation-volvulus associated with diaphragmatic hernia in three cats: clinical presentation, surgical treatment and presumptive aetiology. *Journal of Feline Medicine and Surgery* 10, 198–201.

Fossum, T.W. and Hedlund, C.S. (2003) Gastric and intestinal surgery. *Veterinary Clinics of North America Small Animal Practice* 33 (5), 1117–1145.

Fossum, T.W., Rohn, D.A. and Willard, M.D. (1995) Presumptive, iatrogenic gastric outflow obstruction associated with prior gastric surgery. *Journal of the American Animal Hospital Association* 31, 391–395.

Gianella, P., Pfammatter, N.S. and Burgener, I.A. (2009) Oesophageal and gastric endoscopic foreign body removal: complications and follow-up of 102 dogs. *Journal of Small Animal Practice* 50, 649–654.

Glickman, L.T., Glickman, N.W., Perez, C.M., Schellenberg, D.B. and Lantz, G.C. (1994) Analysis of risk factors for gastric dilatation and dilatation-volvulus in dogs. *Journal of the American Veterinary Medical Association* 204, 1465–1471.

Glickman, L.T., Glickman, N.W., Schellenberg, D.B., Simpson, K. and Lantz, G.C. (1997) Multiple risk factors for the gastric dilatation-volvulus syndrome in dogs: a practitioner/owner case-control study. *Journal of the American Animal Hospital Association* 33, 197–204.

Glickman, L.T., Lantz, G.C., Schellenberg, D.B. and Glickman, N.W. (1998) A prospective study of survival and recurrence following the acute gastric dilatation-volvulus syndrome in 136 dogs. *Journal of the American Animal Hospital Association* 34, 253–259.

Glickman, L.T., Glickman, N.W., Schellenberg, D.B., Raghavan, M. and Lee, T. (2000a) Non-dietary risk factors for gastric dilatation-volvulus in large and giant breed dogs. *Journal of the American Veterinary Medical Association* 217, 1492–1499.

Glickman, L.T., Glickman, N.W., Schellenberg, D.B., Raghavan, M. and Lee, T.L. (2000b) Incidence of and breed-related risk factors for gastric dilatation-volvulus in dogs. *Journal of the American Veterinary Medical Association* 216, 40–45.

Goldsmid, S.E., Bellenger, C.R., Hopwood, P.R. and Rothwell, J.T. (1993) Colorectal blood supply in dogs. *American Journal of Veterinary Research* 54, 1948–1953.

Gomez, J.A. (1974) The gastrointestinal contrast study. Methods and interpretation. *Veterinary Clinics of North America* 4, 805–842.

Graham, J.P., Lord, P.F. and Harrison, J.M. (1998) Quantitative estimation of intestinal dilation as a predictor of obstruction in the dog. *Journal of Small Animal Practice* 39, 521–524.

Gurnee, C.M. and Drobatz, K.J. (2007) Zinc intoxication in dogs: 19 cases (1991–2003). *Journal of the American Veterinary Medical Association* 230, 1174–1179.

Hayes, G. (2009) Gastrointestinal foreign bodies in dogs and cats: a retrospective study of 208 cases. *Journal of Small Animal Practice* 50, 576–583.

Hill, L.N. and Smeak, D.D. (2002) Open versus closed bilateral anal sacculectomy for treatment of non-neoplastic anal sac disease in dogs: 95 cases (1969–1994). *Journal of the American Veterinary Medical Association* 221, 662–665.

Hill, P.B., Lo, A., Eden, C.A., Huntley, S., Morey, V., Ramsey, S., Richardson, C., *et al.* (2006) Survey of the prevalence, diagnosis and treatment of dermatological conditions in small animals in general practice. *Veterinary Record* 158, 533–539.

Hoffmann, K.L. (2003) Sonographic signs of gastroduodenal linear foreign body in 3 dogs. *Veterinary Radiology and Ultrasound* 44, 466–469.

Kirpensteijn, J., Maarschalkerweerd, R.J., Van Der Gaag, I., Kooistra, H.S. and Van Sluijs, F.J. (2001) Comparison of three closure methods and two absorbable suture materials for closure of jejunal enterotomy incisions in healthy dogs. *Veterinary Quarterly* 23, 67–70.

Leib, M.S., Monroe, W.E. and Martin, R.A. (1987) Suspected chronic gastric volvulus in a dog with normal gastric emptying of liquids. *Journal of the American Veterinary Medical Association* 191, 699–700.

Lewis, S.J., Andersen, H.K. and Thomas, S. (2009) Early enteral nutrition within 24 h of intestinal surgery versus later commencement of feeding: a systematic review and meta-analysis. *Journal of Gastrointestinal Surgery* 13, 569–575.

Macphail, C. (2002) Gastrointestinal obstruction. *Clinical Techniques in Small Animal Practice* 17, 178–183.

Macphail, C. (2008) Surgical views: anal sacculectomy. *Compendium of Continuing Education for the Practicing Veterinarian* 30, 530–535.

Mayhew, P.D. and Brown, D.C. (2009) Prospective evaluation of two intracorporeally sutured prophylactic laparoscopic gastropexy techniques compared with laparoscopic-assisted gastropexy in dogs. *Veterinary Surgery* 38, 738–746.

Meyer-Lindenberg, A., Harder, A., Fehr, M., Luerssen, D. and Brunnberg, L. (1993) Treatment of gastric dilatation-volvulus and a rapid method for prevention of relapse in dogs: 134 cases (1988–1991). *Journal of the American Veterinary Medical Association* 203, 1303–1307.

Monnet, E. (2003) Gastric dilatation-volvulus syndrome in dogs. *Veterinary Clinics of North America Small Animal Practice* 33, 987–1005, vi.

Muir, W.W. (1982) Acid-base and electrolyte disturbances in dogs with gastric dilatation-volvulus. *Journal of the American Veterinary Medical Association* 181, 229–231.

Oakes, M.G., Lewis, D.D., Hosgood, G. and Beale, B.S. (1994) Enteroplication for the prevention of intussusception recurrence in dogs: 31 cases (1978–1992). *Journal of the American Veterinary Medical Association* 205, 72–75.

Popovitch, C.A., Holt, D. and Bright, R. (1994) Colopexy as a treatment for rectal prolapse in dogs and cats: a retrospective study of 14 cases. *Veterinary Surgery* 23, 115–118.

Raghavan, M., Glickman, N.W. and Glickman, L.T. (2006) The effects of ingredients in dry dog foods on the risk of gastric dilatation-volvulus in dogs. *Journal of the American Animal Hospital Association* 42, 28–36.

Rasmussen, L. (2003) Stomach. In: Slatter, D.H. (ed.) *Textbook of Small Animal Surgery*, 3rd edn. Saunders, Philadelphia, Pennsylvania, pp. 592–640.

Rosin, E., Walshaw, R., Mehlhaff, C., Matthiesen, D., Orsher, R. and Kusba, J. (1988) Subtotal colectomy for treatment of chronic constipation associated with idiopathic megacolon in cats: 38 cases (1979–1985). *Journal of the American Veterinary Medical Association* 193, 850–853.

Scherkl, R., Hashem, A. and Frey, H.H. (1990) Apomorphine-induced emesis in the dog – routes of administration, efficacy and synergism by naloxone. *Journal of Veterinary Pharmacology and Therapeutics* 13, 154–158.

Schrader, S.C. (1992) Pelvic osteotomy as a treatment for obstipation in cats with acquired stenosis of the pelvic canal: six cases (1978–1989). *Journal of the American Veterinary Medical Association* 200, 208–213.

Schwandt, C.S. (2008) Low-grade or benign intestinal tumours contribute to intussusception: a report on one feline and two canine cases. *Journal of Small Animal Practice* 49, 651–654.

Shoieb, A.M. and Hanshaw, D.M. (2009) Anal sac gland carcinoma in 64 cats in the United Kingdom (1995–2007). *Veterinary Pathology* 46, 677–683.

Tyrrell, D. and Beck, C. (2006) Survey of the use of radiography vs. ultrasonography in the investigation of gastrointestinal foreign bodies in small animals. *Veterinary Radiology and Ultrasound* 47, 404–408.

Ward, M.P., Patronek, G.J. and Glickman, L.T. (2003) Benefits of prophylactic gastropexy for dogs at risk of gastric dilatation-volvulus. *Preventative Veterinary Medicine* 60, 319–329.

Washabau, R.J. and Holt, D. (1999) Pathogenesis, diagnosis, and therapy of feline idiopathic megacolon. *Veterinary Clinics of North America Small Animal Practice* 29, 589–603.

Weaver, A.D. (1977) Canine intestinal intussusception. *Veterinary Record* 100, 524–527.

Weisman, D.L., Smeak, D.D., Birchard, S.J. and Zweigart, S.L. (1999) Comparison of a continuous suture pattern with a simple interrupted pattern for enteric closure in dogs and cats: 83 cases (1991–1997). *Journal of the American Veterinary Medical Association* 214, 1507–1510.

Williams, L.E., Gliatto, J.M., Dodge, R.K., Johnson, J.L., Gamblin, R.M., Thamm, D.H., Lana, S.E., *et al.* (2003) Carcinoma of the apocrine glands of the anal sac in dogs: 113 cases (1985–1995). *Journal of the American Veterinary Medical Association* 223, 825–831.

Wilson, G.P. and Burt, J.K. (1974) Intussusception in the dog and cat: a review of 45 cases. *Journal of the American Veterinary Medical Association* 164, 515–518.

Wylie, K.B. and Hosgood, G. (1994) Mortality and morbidity of small and large intestinal surgery in dogs and cats: 74 cases (1980–1992). *Journal of the American Animal Hospital Association* 30, 469–474.

Yanoff, S.R., Willard, M.D., Boothe, H.W. and Walker, M. (1992) Short-bowel syndrome in four dogs. *Veterinary Surgery* 21, 217–222.

Chapter 12

13 Peritonitis Management and the 'Acute Abdomen'

abdominocentesis: needle drainage of abdominal effusion

acute abdomen: syndrome of rapid-onset abdominal pain and shock

ascites: peritoneal effusion

effusion: accumulation of fluid in a body cavity

exudate: inflammatory fluid

haemoabdomen: blood in the peritoneal cavity

hypovolaemia: reduced blood volume

peritonitis: inflammation of the peritoneum

shock: a life-threatening syndrome, common to a variety of different disease processes, that is characterized by cellular hypoxia usually due to poor tissue perfusion

transudate: non-inflammatory fluid

The reader should be able to:

- describe the pathogenesis of acute haemorrhagic shock in a dog and its clinical progression from health to death
- describe the pathogenesis of acute septic shock in a dog caused by Gram-negative infection and its clinical progression from health to death
- formulate a treatment plan for a dog with hypovolaemic shock caused by acute vomiting (assuming that the dog has no other medical problems and vomiting has resolved)
- describe end points for resuscitation of a shocked patient
- compare and contrast the safety of whole blood transfusion in a male dog and in a male cat, neither of which has received previous transfusion
- describe hypotensive resuscitation and illustrate when it might be used
- define what the acute abdomen syndrome is and illustrate, with examples, conditions that may cause it
- list the different classifications of peritonitis
- list the basic elements of treatment of acute, septic peritonitis caused by intestinal perforation in a dog
- formulate an antimicrobial treatment plan based on the results of abdominocentesis and Gram-staining in an adult dog with peritonitis
- describe how to collect a sample of abdominal fluid by abdominocentesis

The '*acute abdomen*' is a term used to describe a range of life-threatening abdominal diseases that develop rapidly over the course of a few hours and that are characterized by sudden-onset abdominal pain. The acute abdomen syndrome typically leads to hypovolaemic or septic shock necessitating intensive management. Many causes of the acute abdomen require early surgical interventions but a host of medical conditions can also lead to the syndrome. Distinguishing between surgical and non-surgical causes requires careful evaluation and integration of clinical findings, clinical pathology, and diagnostic imaging. As the underlying disease may progress rapidly, frequent patient re-evaluation is necessary until a diagnosis is reached or the problem is resolved.

Examples of common surgical causes of the acute abdomen:

- gastric dilatation and volvulus (GDV);
- septic peritonitis;
- intestinal volvulus;
- ruptured pyometra;
- linear foreign body; and
- bleeding splenic tumour.

Examples of medical conditions that may cause or be mistaken for the acute abdomen:

- acute pancreatitis;
- viral enteritis (e.g. parvovirus);
- feline infectious peritonitis;
- diabetic ketoacidosis; and
- acute liver failure.

This chapter describes managing shock and recognizing and investigating the acute abdomen, peritonitis and haemoabdomen.

Diagnosing and Managing Shock

Shock is a complex syndrome resulting in cellular hypoxia usually as a result of poor tissue perfusion. Most patients with shock suffer from a complex array of interconnected problems but, to simplify this topic, shock can be classified into the common syndromes of *hypovolaemic, haemorrhagic, septic,* and *cardiogenic shock.* Hypovolaemic, haemorrhagic, and septic shock are common in patients suffering from the acute abdomen syndrome.

Hypovolaemic and haemorrhagic shock

Hypovolaemic shock results from an absolute or a relative decrease in circulating blood volume. It is the commonest form of shock and leads to poor tissue perfusion through the effects of compensatory vasoconstriction, hypotension, and reduced cardiac output.

Hypovolaemic shock is caused by a variety of mechanisms:

- increased loss of body fluid (e.g. vomiting; diarrhoea; polyuria; acute blood loss);
- failure to replace fluid losses (e.g. dehydration);

- sequestration of body fluid in a compartment that does not contribute to circulation (e.g. abdominal effusion); this is often referred to as accumulation of fluid in a 'third space'; and
- sequestration of blood in vasodilated capillary beds or congested organs (e.g. splenic torsion).

Haemorrhagic shock is a specific form of hypovolaemic shock in which hypovolaemia is compounded by anaemia due to the loss of red blood cells through haemorrhage.

In the early stages of hypovolaemic shock, compensatory mechanisms may maintain peripheral perfusion for a short period. These patients may have pink mucous membranes and strong peripheral pulses but will demonstrate tachycardia and tachypnoea. Within a short period, compensatory mechanisms will fail and more overt signs of shock will develop. The key clinical features of hypovolaemic shock are:

Signs of poor peripheral perfusion

- Pallor.
- Poor peripheral pulse quality.
- Prolonged capillary refill time.
- Cold periphery.
- Weakness.
- Hypotension.

Compensatory cardio-respiratory changes

- Tachycardia.
- Tachypnoea.
- Cats, unlike dogs, may not become tachycardic.

Altered mentation

- Reduced level of consciousness.

Septic shock

Septic shock is usually caused by overwhelming bacterial infection. It is mediated through the release of a host of cytokines which leads to altered vascular tone, increased vascular permeability, and occlusion of small vessels within capillary beds. In addition, degenerating Gram-negative bacteria release endotoxic lipopolysaccharides from their cell walls that accelerate the systemic inflammatory response and contribute to shock. Septic shock has an early hyperdynamic phase followed by a late hypodynamic phase.

Hyperdynamic shock is characterized by reduced vascular tone caused by toxin-induced dilation of capillary beds, pooling of blood in the periphery, and compensatory increased cardiac output. This leads to:

- congested mucous membranes;
- slow capillary refill time;
- hyperdynamic (bounding) pulses;
- tachycardia;
- tachypnoea;
- dullness and collapse; and
- pyrexia.

Hypodynamic shock eventually follows from hyperdynamic shock as cardiac output, which cannot be maintained in the face of hypoxia and toxins, drops leading to the classic signs of shock:

- pale mucous membranes;
- slow capillary refill time;
- cold extremities;
- weak peripheral pulses; and
- hypotension.

Decompensatory (terminal) shock

Decompensatory shock is the common outcome of progressive hypovolaemic or septic shock in which the compensatory mechanisms attempting to maintain peripheral perfusion fail completely. The brain and heart begin to suffer from severe hypoxia leading to respiratory and cardiac depression. Peripheral vasodilation occurs leading to massive blood pooling in the periphery. Clinical signs of bradycardia, severe hypotension, extreme pallor, cyanosis, loss of peripheral pulses, hypothermia, and stupor occur. This is generally irreversible leading to anuric renal failure, coma, pulmonary oedema, cardiopulmonary arrest, and death.

Gastrointestinal ulceration and acute renal failure are common sequelae to advanced stages of shock.

Treating Shock

The mainstays of shock therapy are oxygen supplementation to compensate for cellular hypoxia, and fluid therapy to improve peripheral perfusion.

Oxygen therapy

Supplemental inspired oxygen should be given to all patients in shock from the outset of treatment (Fig. 13.1). Several techniques can be used but, if the method used causes distress to the patient, it can become counterproductive.

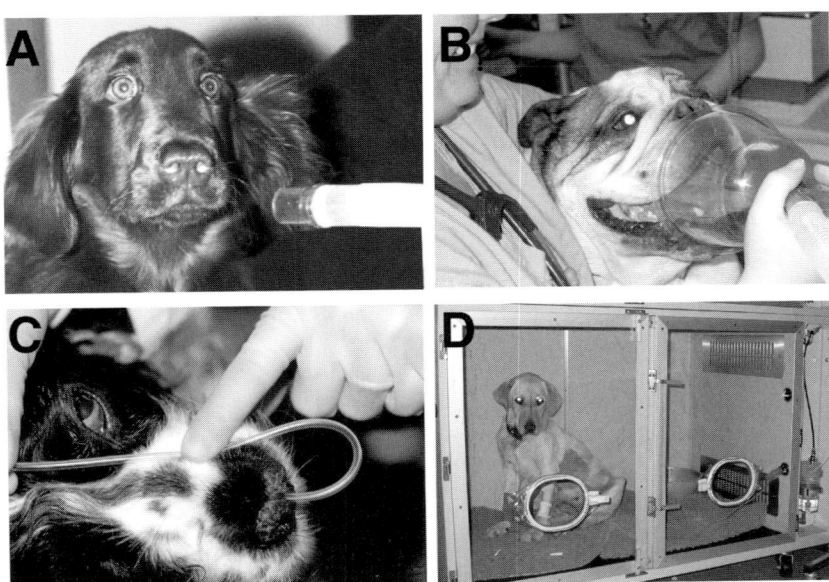

Fig. 13.1. Examples of oxygen supplementation: (A) flow-by; (B) mask; (C) nasal catheter; (D) oxygen cage.

Peritonitis Management and the 'Acute Abdomen'

- **Flow-by:** oxygen is delivered at 6–8 l/min through an anaesthetic system held close to the nostrils or mouth. This is very well tolerated but it is the least efficient method of supplementing oxygen.
- **Mask:** oxygen is delivered at 6–8 l/min through an anaesthetic system attached to a facemask. This is more efficient than flow-by supplementation but may not be tolerated.
- **Nasal catheters:** a small-bore, pliable catheter is inserted into each nostril (having pre-measured it to the medial canthus of the eye to determine length) using the same technique as naso-oesophageal tube placement (see p. 67). Oxygen is delivered at 1–6 l/min. Nasal catheters are effective but can be uncomfortable and are often removed by the patient.
- **Oxygen cage:** this is effective but patients can overheat easily. The inspired oxygen concentration drops each time the door is opened, reducing the efficiency when animals are receiving frequent evaluations and treatments.

Fluid therapy – intravenous access

Good intravenous access is required to provide effective fluid therapy. A large-bore intravenous catheter placed in the cephalic or saphenous vein is adequate for most patients. However, using a single catheter will limit the rate at which fluid therapy can be administered, particularly in giant breed dogs. Consider placing two intravenous catheters to maximize peripheral venous access in larger dogs.

Intravenous access can also be achieved using *intra-osseous needles* and *jugular catheters*. Intra-osseous needles are very effective as the medullary cavity provides a direct route to deliver large volumes of fluid quickly into the venous system, and remains patent, even during severe hypovolaemic shock. This method is generally reserved for paediatric patients that are too small for intravenous catheterization. The intra-osseous needle is introduced into the greater trochanter of the femur. Use a veterinary intra-osseous needle and follow the manufacturer's placement guidelines.

Jugular catheters can be used to deliver large volumes of fluid quickly and can be left in place for up to 7 days. Multi-lumen catheters enable co-administration of a range of products and blood sampling through a single catheter. Placement of jugular catheters is technically challenging. They must be placed under aseptic conditions and managed carefully to prevent infection. Jugular catheters are used in some general practices and most referral centres, but inexperienced operators should not use them without specific training.

Fluid resuscitation – choice of fluid

The administration of crystalloids and colloids in combination has become the mainstay of shock therapy.

Crystalloids

Crystalloids can be used to expand the circulating blood volume rapidly during treatment of shock, but the fluid rapidly moves from plasma to equilibrate with the interstitial fluid. In fact, a bolus of crystalloids provides only short-term support of the circulation as less than 20% of the fluid administered will remain in the intravascular space after 1 h. To extend the period that the fluid remains in the circulation, crystalloids are often used with colloids (see below). From the range of crystalloids available, the balanced polyionic replacement solutions, which are buffered to near physiological pH and approximate the electrolyte concentrations of plasma, are good initial choices. These solutions include compound sodium lactate (Hartmann's), Plasma-Lyte® A (Baxter International Inc., Deerfield, Illinois, USA), and Normosol™-R (Hospira Inc., Lake Forest, Illinois, USA).

Colloids

Colloids are high molecular weight molecules that increase the oncotic pressure of plasma. Colloids provide more effective expansion of intravascular volume than crystalloids, as they remain in the intravascular space for much longer and increase oncotic pressure, helping to retain fluid in the vascular space. A combination of colloids and crystalloids provides the most rapid and sustained expansion of the vascular space. The starch-based synthetic colloids (e.g. hydroxyethyl starch; pentastarch) have long plasma half-lives and will have a significant effect in plasma for up to 24 h. These are good choices for combined use with crystalloids to manage hypovolaemic shock, as they will help maintain perfusion for longer and reduce the risk of tissue and pulmonary oedema. Colloids may interfere with the coagulation cascade and the manufacturer's recommendations for use should be followed to limit the risk of this complication. Other fluids that have potent colloid properties include plasma and haemoglobin-based oxygen-carrying solutions (see below).

Fluid resuscitation – rate of administration

The guidelines for fluid therapy for shock given below assume that the patient does not have concurrent conditions that increase the risk of complications such as primary heart disease, oliguric renal failure, pulmonary contusion, cerebral contusion, or ongoing haemorrhage. If these or similar conditions are present, fluid therapy must be altered accordingly.

Initially, large volumes of crystalloid are administered rapidly to restore circulating volume. A total of up to 55 ml/kg in cats and 90 ml/kg in dogs is given within a short period (e.g. 60 min). A quarter of the calculated total volume of crystalloid is given as a bolus or a rapid infusion and the patient is monitored for evidence of improving peripheral circulation. This is repeated until signs of peripheral perfusion improve or the total calculated dose is given. Although this produces rapid re-expansion of vascular volume, the effects may not be sustained as most of the fluid will redistribute into the interstitial space within the first hour. More effective fluid resuscitation is achieved by concurrent administration of colloids using an initial bolus of 10–20 ml/kg in dogs (as a rapid bolus) or 10–15 ml/kg in cats (given over 15 min to prevent nausea). Using crystalloid and colloid together reduces the total dose of crystalloid required to restore the circulating volume by up to 40%.

Once the vascular space has been re-expanded and peripheral perfusion is improving, fluid therapy is administered to replace ongoing losses and body deficits, and to correct underlying metabolic derangements. Colloids may be continued as infusions (e.g. 20 ml/kg/day) and crystalloids are selected and administered depending on the individual requirements of the patient.

Monitoring response to therapy

Patients being treated for shock must be carefully monitored to ensure that treatment is being effective and to avoid complications such as over-hydration. Animals that receive excessive quantities of fluid, or that have oliguria, heart failure, or vasculitis, are at high risk of developing signs of over-perfusion. The signs of over-perfusion include peripheral oedema, effusions, and pulmonary oedema, and these can become life threatening. Fluid therapy must be titrated to meet the requirements of the individual without inducing complications.

Clinical parameters are carefully and regularly assessed to monitor progress during fluid resuscitation. Heart rate, respiratory rate, mucous membrane colour, capillary refill time, and pulse quality are easily measured. Appropriate end points for resuscitation are when these key physiological parameters have returned to normal. Additional end points for resuscitation include mean arterial pressure of 80–100 mmHg or systolic blood pressure of 100–120 mmHg.

Hypotensive resuscitation for haemorrhagic shock

Aggressive fluid therapy in patients with haemorrhagic shock can be counterproductive, as the rapid increase in blood pressure may accelerate blood loss or disrupt blood clots, causing further bleeding. In these patients, *hypotensive resuscitation* may be more appropriate. During hypotensive resuscitation, the aim of initial resuscitation is to improve clinical parameters but not to the point where the patient becomes normotensive. Appropriate end points for this form of fluid therapy are mean arterial pressure of 60 mmHg or systolic blood pressure of 80 mmHg. This form of fluid therapy is sufficient to prevent severe hypoxia but minimizes the risk of accelerating blood loss. Once the cause of bleeding has been treated, fluid resuscitation using standard end points can be completed.

Blood products and oxygen-carrying colloids

Blood products (e.g. whole blood; packed red blood cells; plasma) are increasingly being used in small animal practice in the management of anaemia and hypoalbuminaemia. The decision to proceed with transfusion must be based on the assessment of the relative benefits and risks to the individual patient. However, transfusion could reasonably be considered when anaemia leads to weakness, dullness, or signs of hypovolaemic shock, or when acute blood loss leads to a haematocrit of 20% or less.

In most small animal practices, whole blood can be collected from donor dogs and delivered to recipients with comparative ease. In the UK, a nationwide canine blood donation service enables blood and blood products to be sourced externally within 24 or 48 h (www.petbloodbankuk.org), and similar facilities are available in other countries. Dogs rarely develop transfusion reactions when receiving a blood transfusion for the first time, but the risk increases with subsequent transfusions and in bitches that have previously been pregnant. Canine blood-antigen testing and cross-matching kits are available for in-practice use to reduce the risk of transfusion reaction.

Blood transfusion in cats is more dangerous as cats develop serious transfusion reactions if transfused with incompatible blood, even if they have not received blood products previously. The International Society of Feline Medicine (part of the Feline Advisory Bureau) provides information detailing the increased risks, and the methods of collection and administration of blood in cats (www.isfm.net). Consult experienced colleagues and specialist texts for advice before considering blood transfusion for the first time.

Haemoglobin-based oxygen-carrying colloids are synthetic products licensed for use in anaemic dogs. They deliver oxygen to tissues and have potent colloid properties. They can be stored and are compatible with all blood groups, removing the need to source a blood donor in an emergency. The main risk of using these products is inducing circulatory overload due to the rapid re-expansion of the vascular space that they achieve through their potent colloid properties. Follow the manufacturer's recommendations for total dose and rate of administration carefully and monitor for signs of circulatory overload. These products are contra-indicated in animals with pre-existing severe heart disease (e.g. congestive heart failure) or anuric renal failure. Cats are considered to be at greater risk of these adverse effects and, at the time of writing, the products are not licensed for use in this species.

Glucocorticoids

Previously, glucocorticoids have been recommended in the management of shock because their potent anti-inflammatory effects were thought to be beneficial in preventing cellular injury associated with shock. However, there is little evidence to suggest

that the use of glucocorticoids improves outcome in patients with shock, and their deleterious side effects are considered to be counterproductive. Glucocorticoids are no longer recommended for the treatment of shock unless patients are suffering from anaphylactic shock or Addisonian crisis.

Antibiotic therapy for shock and sepsis

During hypovolaemic shock, poor perfusion of the intestinal tract and liver enables bacteria to enter the bloodstream. Prophylactic antimicrobial therapy is often given to shocked patients. Conditions causing sepsis (e.g. peritonitis) also lead to septic shock. Gram-negative enteric organisms are often cultured from patients with septic shock but *Staphylococcus* spp., *Streptococcus* spp. and, in cats, *Pasteurella* spp. are also common. The early use of broad-spectrum antibiotics is indicated in the management of sepsis and is typically initiated intravenously. Selection of antimicrobials has similar limitations and restrictions to those found when selecting perioperative prophylactic antibiosis (see Chapter 2). Combinations of two or more bactericidal antimicrobials are generally recommended in veterinary texts but, in human medicine, there is a move away from this to targeted, single-agent therapy. Common protocols include:

- aminopenicillin (amoxycillin/ampicillin) plus aminoglycoside (gentamicin/amikacin): to capitalize on the synergistic effect of these groups of antibiotics;
- fluoroquinolone (marbofloxacin/enrofloxacin) plus clindamycin/metronidazole: to extend the spectrum of activity of the fluoroquinolone to include anaerobic organisms; and
- fluoroquinolone (marbofloxacin/enrofloxacin) plus aminopenicillin (amoxycillin/ampicillin): to extend the spectrum of activity of the fluoroquinolone (including anaerobic organisms).

The aminopenicillins used in these protocols are often augmented with clavulanic acid to counter the effects of bacterial beta-lactamases.

Pain relief

Patients in shock are often suffering from painful conditions and require pain relief. They are also at increased risk of drug side effects because their organs are poorly perfused. Non-steroidal anti-inflammatory drugs should be avoided in critically ill patients because of their potentially nephrotoxic and ulcerogenic properties. Most manufacturers recommend that they are not used in animals that are hypovolaemic.

Opioids provide good pain relief comparatively safely although they may cause dose-dependent cardiovascular and respiratory depression. Pethidine is a popular choice in critically ill patients as it: (i) has a short duration of action (so adverse effects will not be protracted); (ii) can be antagonized with naloxone; (iii) is licensed for use in dogs and cats in the UK; (iv) can be supplemented with additional boluses; and (v) provides good pain relief. One disadvantage is that pethidine must be administered intramuscularly and this may cause discomfort.

Investigating the Acute Abdomen Syndrome

The 'acute abdomen' is a clinical syndrome characterized by acute-onset abdominal pain usually accompanied by abdominal distension, shock, and collapse. The initial assessment of a patient with acute abdominal pain must include a rapid assessment of the risk of life-threatening acute deterioration, a process referred to as 'triage'. The initial assessment should include evaluation of the cardiovascular system, peripheral perfusion, respiratory system, and level of consciousness. If the patient has life-threatening signs, such as decompensatory shock, respiratory distress, or sepsis, immediate supportive care and shock treatment may be required before a detailed clinical history and physical examination can be carried out. However, it is important to ensure that a complete historical record is collected and a thorough physical examination is performed as soon as therapy has been started.

Historical findings

A thorough historical record will include details of:

- age, breed, sex;
- timing of last oestrus, pregnancy, or mating;
- vaccination and travel history;
- previous medical history; and
- current medications, allergies, access to toxins.

General signs:

- polydipsia;
- anorexia;
- pica (e.g. foreign body ingestion).

Gastrointestinal signs:

- retching/vomiting/regurgitation (e.g. blood; bile; food; frequency; volume);
- defecatory pattern (e.g. consistency; volume; frequency; blood; mucus).

Cardio-respiratory signs:

- exercise intolerance;
- respiratory distress;
- collapse.

Abdominal signs:

- abdominal distension;
- abdominal pain.

Urogenital signs:

- urination pattern and appearance (e.g. pyuria; haematuria; dysuria);
- vaginal discharge: (e.g. purulent or bloody vaginal discharge).

Physical findings

A thorough physical examination is performed, initially evaluating the cardiovascular and respiratory systems and abdomen, and includes assessment of the features shown below.

Body temperature

- Hyperthermia is associated with inflammation and sepsis.
- Hypothermia is associated with decompensatory shock.

Cardiovascular system

- Including evaluation of peripheral perfusion and hydration.

Respiratory system

- Including evaluation of adventitious lung sounds, altered resonance on thoracic percussion; displacement/muffling of cardiac apex beat.

Abdominal palpation

1. Abdominal pain.
2. Organomegaly:
   - hepatomegaly;
   - gastric distension;

- distended loops of intestine;
- splenomegaly;
- enlarged bladder;
- prostatomegaly;
- uterine distension.
3. Fluid thrill:
    - ballot the abdomen; a palpable thrill is highly suggestive of an abdominal effusion.
4. Tympany (gaseous distension of organs):
    - common in GDV and mesenteric volvulus.

Rectal examination

- Faecal sample: assess for blood or mucus;
- Prostate: size, position, symmetry, pain;
- Urethra: size, shape, pain, mass;
- Vagina: size, shape, pain, mass.

Vulval examination

- Discharge;
- Presence of fetus;
- Cranial vaginal cytology (assessment of stage of oestrus cycle).

Blood and urine analysis

The initial evaluation should include assessment of haematology, serum biochemistry, and urinalysis. These data help to assess hydration status, blood loss, and response to fluid therapy (see above). They may also identify an underlying systemic disease or inflammatory process that accounts for the acute presentation, and they provide baseline data for monitoring.

Diagnostic imaging

Abdominal imaging is an important step in investigating the 'acute abdomen' and helps to assess the severity of the problem and the need for surgery.

Abdominal radiography

Key radiographic features to assess include:

- *loss of serosal detail*: abdominal organs are normally delineated radiographically because of contrast between the serosal surface and the organ. However, even small volumes of abdominal fluid reduce this contrast and lead to loss of serosal detail;
- *free gas*: spontaneous accumulation of free gas in the peritoneal cavity usually indicates rupture

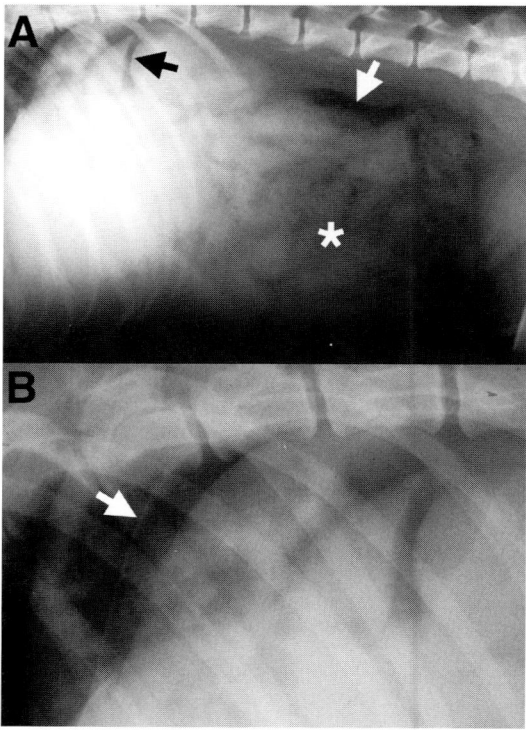

Fig. 13.2. Free gas in a case of peritonitis caused by a ruptured gastric ulcer: (A) free gas is seen dorsal to the colon (white arrow) and between the diaphragm and liver lobes (black arrow). There is also loss of serosal detail indicting a small peritoneal effusion (asterisk); (B) free gas in the abdomen can be difficult to distinguish from gas in the intestinal lumen. The best place to identify free gas is between the liver and diaphragm as this area should have no intestinal loops (arrow – diaphragm delineated by pocket of abdominal gas).

of a hollow organ (e.g. intestine) and is a clear indicator that exploratory surgery is warranted (Fig. 13.2);
- *dilatation and volvulus*: gaseous distension and compartmentalization lines are key features of organ torsion (e.g. GDV; mesenteric volvulus) (Fig. 13.3);
- *displaced organs*: e.g. abdominal hernia;
- *contrast leakage from hollow organs*: indicate rupture of the gastrointestinal or urinary tracts.

Abdominal ultrasound

Ultrasound is very sensitive for identifying abdominal fluid and assessing its character (e.g. flocculent

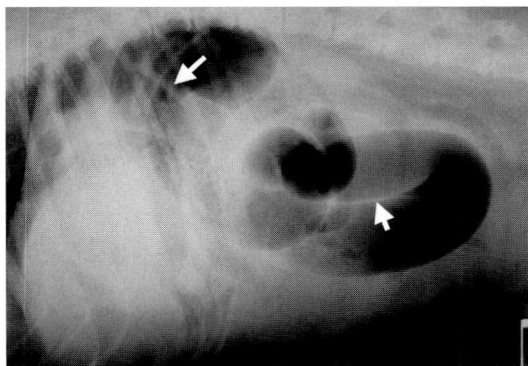

Fig. 13.3. Compartmentalization lines are characteristic of volvulus of a hollow organ and indicate that the patient has a life-threatening abdominal disease. This dog had mesenteric volvulus (volvulus of the intestinal tract around the root of the mesentery). Compartmentalization lines (soft tissue binds dividing hollow organs) are marked with arrows and are characteristic of volvulus.

fluid is suggestive of an exudate). It also enables detailed evaluation of the abdominal organs and facilitates abdominocentesis (see below).

Imaging the abdomen post-operatively

Evaluating patients for complications following abdominal surgery is hampered, as peritoneal fluid and gas, which inevitably collect in the abdomen during surgery, may remain for some time. Gas can take over 2 weeks to resorb fully and residual fluid may lead to loss of serosal detail and contain inflammatory cells. Neither gas nor fluid should continue to accumulate post-operatively, so sequential imaging helps to establish the significance of these findings.

Abdominal Fluid Analysis

A sample of ascitic fluid should always be collected and analysed as this is critical in order to establish the nature (and likely cause) of the effusion. Abdominocentesis can be performed by four-quadrant tap ('blind') or by ultrasound-guided collection. Ultrasound-guided abdominocentesis has the advantages of increasing the success of the procedure and ensuring that the bladder, spleen, and other organs are not punctured inadvertently.

Blind abdominocentesis

The abdomen is divided into four quadrants and each quadrant is sampled in turn until a positive sample is collected. The procedure can be performed with minimal sedation in compliant patients. Empty the bladder of urine (to avoid inadvertent cystocentesis). Position the patient in lateral recumbency. Clip and aseptically prepare the abdomen around the umbilicus. Use a 23-gauge needle attached to a 5 or 10 ml syringe. Introduce the needle 1–2 cm to the right of midline (to avoid the falciform fat), behind the umbilicus (to avoid the spleen), and aspirate. If no fluid is collected, repeat to the left of midline behind the umbilicus. If this is unsuccessful, repeat the tap in front of the umbilicus first to the right of midline and finally to the left of midline (the cranial left quadrant is tapped last as the spleen lies here).

Fluid analysis

Place samples of the ascitic fluid in EDTA tubes for cytology and plain tubes for biochemical analysis and culture. Samples can be submitted to commercial laboratories for detailed analysis but a great deal of information can be gathered from simple, in-house analysis and this facilitates reaching a diagnosis quickly.

Ascitic fluid is classified into four main groups:

- **exudate:** inflammatory fluid with high nucleated cell count and protein level. Exudates are caused by peritoneal inflammation due to infection or irritants (e.g. bile leakage; pancreatitis; septic peritonitis). Cell count >7000 cells/µl; protein >5.0 g/dl;
- **transudate:** serous effusion with low cell count and protein level caused by reduced oncotic pressure (e.g. hypoproteinaemia). Cell count <1500 cells/µl; protein <2.5 g/dl;
- **modified transudate:** low to moderate cell counts and increased protein levels (these values lie somewhere between those of pure transudates and those of exudates). Modified transudates form when fluid extravasates due to increased hydrostatic pressure (e.g. organ torsion; congestive heart failure) or increased vascular permeability (e.g. vasculitis). Cell count 1000–7000 cells/µl; protein 2.5–5.0 g/dl; and
- **haemorrhagic effusion:** resembles whole blood on fluid analysis but does not clot (see below).

Gross appearance

Assessment of opacity, colour, turbidity, and viscosity gives an initial impression of whether the fluid is a transudate or an exudate. Transudates are non-turbid, colourless, or serum-tinged, and not viscous. Exudates are turbid, opaque, and viscous. The colour of exudates ranges from creamy yellow to red depending on the cellular and biochemical constituents. Although the colour of abdominal fluid can indicate the likely aetiology of the effusion, other criteria should be used to confirm the diagnosis.

Cytological evaluation

Prepare a direct smear of the fluid, air dry it and stain it using in-house cytology and Gram-staining kits (Fig. 13.4). To increase the sensitivity of identifying features such as intracellular bacteria, the sample can be centrifuged to concentrate the cells into a pellet which is then resuspended before the smear is prepared (the 'sediment exam') (Fig. 13.5).

Initial microscopic evaluation of a direct smear using a low-powered objective (×10 or ×40) gives an indication of the cellularity of the sample: (i) low cell numbers are associated with transudates; (ii) high numbers of inflammatory cells (neutrophils and macrophages) are consistent with exudates; and (iii) large numbers of red blood cells with few white blood cells are consistent with haemorrhagic effusions. Evaluation using a high-powered objective (×100 with oil immersion) allows assessment of cellular morphology and the presence of bacteria (Fig. 13.6).

Cytological features to evaluate include:

- percentage of neutrophils, macrophages, and lymphocytes and their cellular morphology;
- red blood cells;
- extracellular bacteria: these usually indicate septic peritonitis but can be artefacts from sampling;
- intracellular bacteria (within macrophages and neutrophils): these indicate active infection and are always significant when present; and
- presence of bile salts or food material (indicate leakage of bile or intestinal contents).

Biochemical evaluation

Following centrifugation, the supernatant from abdominal fluid can be used for biochemical analysis (Fig. 13.5). To identify significant changes in ascitic fluid, there must be at least a twofold increase in the concentration of the solute in the

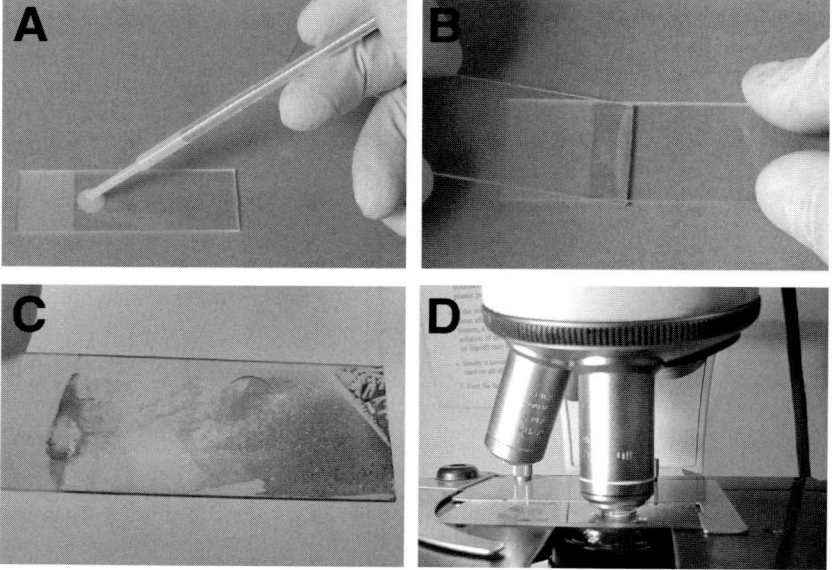

Fig. 13.4. Smear evaluation: (A) place a small aliquot of fluid on a glass slide; (B) create a smear and allow it to air-dry; (C) stain the slide using in-house cytology stains; (D) examine the smear under oil immersion.

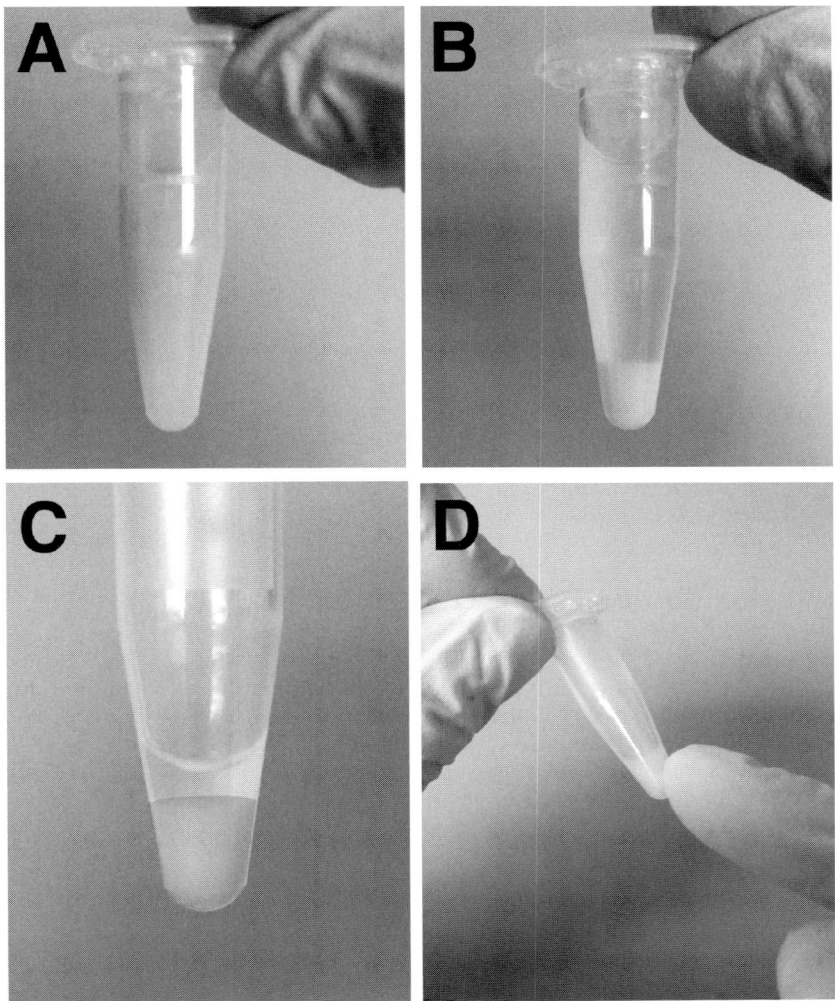

Fig. 13.5. Sediment preparation: (A) take a small aliquot of sample fluid and centrifuge it for 5 min at 2000 rpm; (B) cells and particulate material settle to the bottom of the tube leaving a clear supernatant. The sediment is used to create a smear for cytological analysis. The supernatant can be used for biochemical analysis; (C) use a pipette to remove most of the supernatant leaving only a small volume of supernatant in the tube; (D) resuspend the pellet of cells in this fluid by flicking the tube. The sediment sample can now be used to create a concentrated smear for analysis.

ascitic fluid compared with serum. Bile peritonitis causes increased bilirubin in ascitic fluid compared with serum. Uroabdomen causes increased creatinine, urea, and potassium in ascitic fluid compared with serum.

Peritonitis

Peritonitis is inflammation of the peritoneum and can become a life-threatening problem. In severe cases, peritonitis causes large inflammatory effusions and shock.

Classification

Peritonitis is classified on the speed of onset of signs, the extent of the lesions, and the aetiology.

Acute peritonitis is often associated with bacterial contamination of the abdomen (e.g. ruptured intestine). *Subacute* peritonitis may be caused by

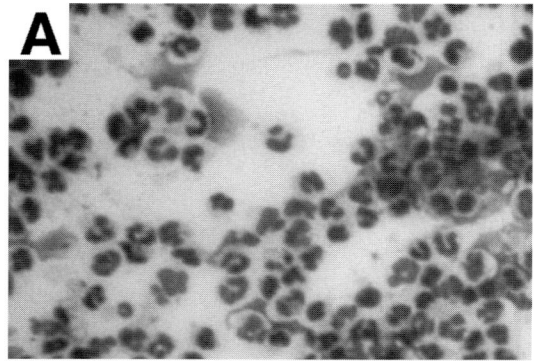

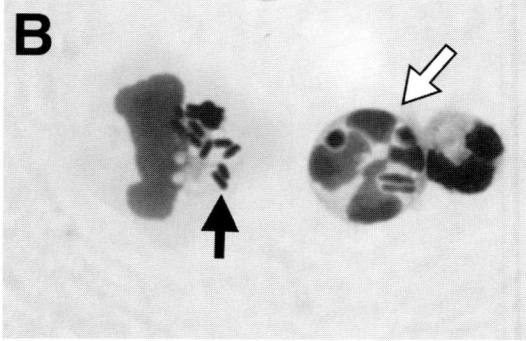

Fig. 13.6. Cytology from septic peritonitis abdominal tap: (A) sediment preparation with high numbers of degenerating neutrophils indicating inflammatory exudate; (B) neutrophil with intracytoplasmic bacteria (open arrow) and bacteria in the vicinity of a degenerating cell (closed arrow) indicating septic exudate. (Images courtesy of N. Reed.)

chemicals that cause peritoneal irritation (e.g. bile salts; urine). *Chronic* peritonitis may be associated with non-infected, focal disease (e.g. retained swab).

Focal peritonitis is confined to one area of the abdomen and surrounds a focal lesion (e.g. pancreatitis; retained swab; tumour). *Generalized peritonitis* affects the entire abdomen and is usually caused by infectious agents (e.g. bacteria; virus) or by ruptured abdominal organs (e.g. bile peritonitis). Generalized peritonitis is usually life-threatening.

Using the aetiological classification, peritonitis is described as being either *primary* or *secondary*, and as being either *septic* or *aseptic*. Primary peritonitis is caused by primary infection of the abdomen; secondary peritonitis is caused by other abdominal diseases (e.g. ruptured intestinal tract). Septic peritonitis is caused by infectious agents (e.g. bacterial; viral; fungal); aseptic peritonitis is caused by sterile irritants (e.g. urine; bile; foreign body).

Primary peritonitis

Primary peritonitis is caused by infection of the peritoneal cavity in the absence of predisposing abdominal disease. Feline coronavirus infection is the best described and commonest agent causing primary peritonitis in small animal patients. It leads to the syndrome of feline infectious peritonitis and is considered separately below. Other forms of primary peritonitis are extremely rare in dogs and cats but primary bacterial peritonitis is occasionally identified. The source of bacteria contaminating the abdomen is rarely found but may be from the bloodstream, from spread across the gastrointestinal wall, or from the uterus via the uterine tube.

FELINE INFECTIOUS PERITONITIS (FIP) Feline coronavirus infection is common in cats and can lead to a wide range of clinical signs including peritonitis. It is critical to distinguish primary viral peritonitis from secondary septic peritonitis when investigating cats with abdominal effusions. Key features to separate FIP from secondary septic peritonitis include: (i) failure to identify bacteria or other infectious agents microscopically; (ii) a very high protein count (>3.5 g/dl); (iii) a cellular population of predominantly monocytes and macrophages rather than neutrophils; and (iv) a low cell count (<5000 cells/μl). The effusions are often classified as modified transudates rather than as exudates and typically are clear, yellow, and viscous. Other clinical features that should raise suspicion of primary viral peritonitis in cats include involvement of multiple body systems, involvement of both thoracic and abdominal cavities, presence of neurological signs, and presence of ocular lesions such as uveitis. Patients with FIP have poor prognoses and generally will not benefit from surgery.

Secondary peritonitis

Secondary peritonitis is very common. It may be septic or aseptic but occurs secondary to other abdominal disease that causes peritoneal inflammation.

SECONDARY SEPTIC PERITONITIS Secondary septic peritonitis is the commonest form of peritonitis in dogs. It is caused by leakage of bacteria from a hollow organ or abscess, or contamination of the abdominal cavity following surgery or penetrating injury. The gastrointestinal tract is the commonest source of bacteria because of leakage following surgery, or from spontaneous rupture often associated with ulceration or neoplasia.

Less common causes of secondary septic peritonitis include ruptured pyometra, leakage of infected urine or bile into the abdomen, and rupture of an abscess within the abdomen (e.g. prostatic abscess).

SECONDARY ASEPTIC PERITONITIS Secondary aseptic peritonitis is caused by abdominal diseases that initiate peritoneal inflammation in the absence of bacterial infection. Bile salts and urine produce chemical peritonitis following leakage from the biliary and urinary tracts. Bile is an extreme irritant and will ultimately lead to severe peritonitis. Urine is less irritating and patients are likely to show signs of uraemia before peritonitis becomes obvious (see Chapter 16). Acute pancreatitis can also induce a severe chemical peritonitis. Foreign bodies (e.g. retained surgical swab or instrument) induce focal peritonitis (often termed mechanical peritonitis).

Diagnosis

Generalized septic peritonitis causes the acute abdomen syndrome leading rapidly to septic shock. Patients demonstrate signs consistent with shock, abdominal pain, and peritoneal inflammation as well as signs that relate directly to the underlying cause of peritonitis. There is often a history of gastrointestinal obstruction or surgery. The use of non-steroidal anti-inflammatory drugs for pain management has also been implicated in some cases of spontaneous gastrointestinal perforation in both dogs and cats.

Key findings to confirm the diagnosis are presence of free gas and fluid in the abdominal cavity, and the presence of large numbers of inflammatory cells, high protein levels, and extracellular and intracellular bacteria in ascitic fluid. Identifying bacteria on cytological evaluation of ascitic fluid is not always possible and, if the other features are present, septic peritonitis should still be considered as the most likely diagnosis.

Management of septic peritonitis

Successful management of septic peritonitis is difficult and surgery can be challenging. Costs of treatment are high. Management of peritonitis should not be undertaken by an inexperienced clinician without the support of an experienced colleague. Alternatively, refer cases to a specialist centre.

Figures 13.7–13.10 demonstrate a case-based example of surgical management of a case of generalized septic peritonitis in a cat. The key steps in management of septic peritonitis are:

1. treat shock and sepsis;
2. confirm diagnosis using imaging and abdominal fluid analysis;
3. perform exploratory surgery to identify the cause of abdominal contamination and to address it;
4. lavage the abdomen copiously;
5. place an abdominal drain;
6. provide supportive care.

Bacterial isolates from cases of septic peritonitis reflect the source of bacterial contamination of the abdomen. *Escherichia coli* is the most common bacterium isolated but other Gram-negative enteric organisms, Gram-positive organisms, and mixed bacterial populations are also common. Broad-spectrum antimicrobial therapy, modified following culture and sensitivity testing, is recommended (see 'Antibiotic therapy for shock and sepsis', p. 209).

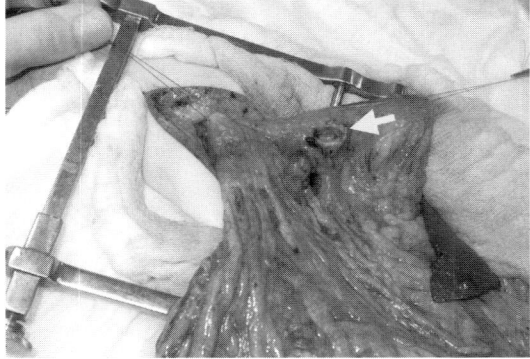

Fig. 13.7. Case example of peritonitis management – identifying the source of leakage. This cat had spontaneous perforation of a gastric ulcer (arrow) on the greater curvature of the stomach.

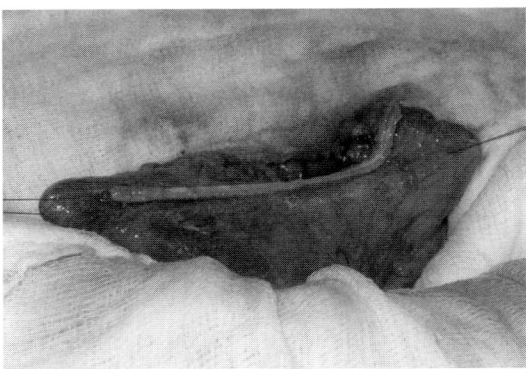

Fig. 13.8. Case example – treating the underlying cause of peritonitis. The gastric ulcer was resected along with the greater curvature of the stomach. A stapling device was used, producing this unusual appearance.

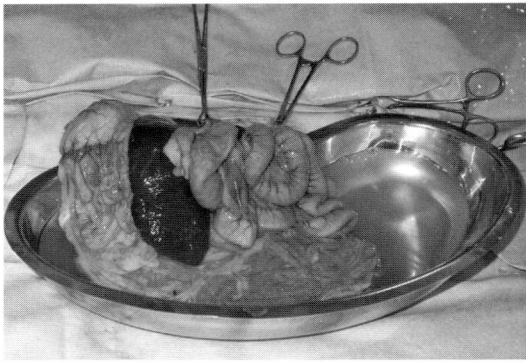

Fig. 13.9. Case example – lavaging to remove contaminants.

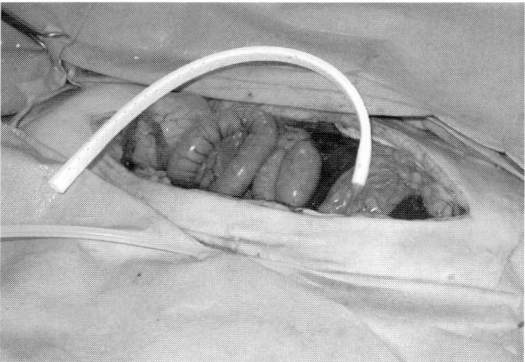

Fig. 13.10. Case example – placing an abdominal drain. This animal has an active, channel drain designed for use in the abdomen (Jackson-Pratt drain).

Prognosis

The prognosis for animals with peritonitis is guarded. Factors including the cause of peritonitis, the extent of damage by the time of diagnosis, and the presence of concurrent problems will influence the outcome. Mortality rates are reported to be around 30%.

Haemoabdomen

Haemoabdomen is a common syndrome diagnosed in general practice that leads to acute haemorrhagic shock. Haemoabdomen may occur spontaneously or follow trauma or abdominal surgery. Spontaneous haemoabdomen is most commonly caused by rupture of neoplastic abdominal organs (e.g. splenic haemangiosarcoma) but other diseases, such as splenic haematoma, hepatic necrosis, and coagulopathies, may also be responsible. Iatrogenic haemoabdomen occurs usually as a result of poor surgical technique (e.g. poor ligature placement). Traumatic haemoabdomen generally results from rupture of parenchymatous organs (e.g. spleen; liver; kidney).

Presentation and investigation

The severity of signs depends on the degree and speed of blood loss. Patients often present with severe haemorrhagic shock and obvious ascites. The key investigative steps are: (i) to confirm the diagnosis by performing abdominocentesis; (ii) to evaluate the degree of anaemia; (iii) to image the abdomen; and (iv) to screen for coagulation disorders. Initial assessment of the degree of blood loss can be misleading as the haematocrit of peripheral blood will remain high for several hours following major blood loss. This is because it takes several hours for fluid to redistribute into the vascular space, diluting the remaining blood, to compensate for the acute hypovolaemia. The haematocrit should be monitored regularly over the first few hours following acute blood loss.

It is possible to misdiagnose haemoabdomen by inadvertently aspirating blood from the spleen during abdominocentesis. To confirm that the sample is of free abdominal blood, place it in a metal dish or activated clotting tube. Free abdominal fluid will not form a clot whereas blood aspirated from the spleen will. This is because the clotting factors and platelets are sequestered into the intra-abdominal clot that forms initially following intra-abdominal bleeding, and the clot is subsequently disrupted by mechanical defibrination.

Treatment

Cases with haemoabdomen may benefit from hypotensive resuscitation (see p. 208) until the source of bleeding is addressed. They often require blood transfusion. Surgery is generally indicated except when haemoabdomen is the result of a bleeding disorder. The goals of surgery are to identify the source of bleeding, to prevent further blood loss, and to assess the extent of abdominal disease.

If the source of bleeding cannot be identified immediately, pack the abdomen with large laparotomy pads to get temporary control of bleeding and remove these one at a time until the source of haemorrhage is found. Procedures such as splenectomy may be required. When haemoabdomen is the result of trauma to the liver, it is often not possible to remove the affected portions of liver, but bleeding may be controlled by applying topical haemostatic agents and direct pressure. Further information about the management of conditions leading to haemoabdomen can be found in relevant chapters of this text.

Bibliography

Addie, D., Belák, S., Boucraut-Baralon, C., Egberink, H., Frymus, T., Gruffydd-Jones, T., Hartmann, K., *et al.* (2009) Feline infectious peritonitis: ABCD guidelines on prevention and management. *Journal of Feline Medicine and Surgery* 11, 594–604.

Jutkowitz, L.A. (2004) Blood transfusion in the perioperative period. *Clinical Techniques in Small Animal Practice* 19, 75–82.

Beal, M.W. (2005) Approach to the acute abdomen. *Veterinary Clinics of North America Small Animal Practice* 35, 375–396.

Brady, C.A. and Otto, C.M. (2001) Systemic inflammatory response syndrome, sepsis, and multiple organ dysfunction. *Veterinary Clinics in North America Small Animal Practice* 31, 1147–1162, v–vi.

Callan, M.B. and Rentko, V.T. (2003) Clinical application of a hemoglobin-based oxygen-carrying solution. *Veterinary Clinics of North America Small Animal Practice* 33, 1277–1293, vi.

Cariou, M., Lipscomb, V.J., Brockman, D.J., Gregory, S.P. and Baines, S.J. (2009) Spontaneous gastroduodenal perforations in dogs: a retrospective study of 15 cases. *Veterinary Record* 165, 436–441.

Cariou, M.P., Halfacree, Z.J., Lee, K.C. and Baines, S.J. (2010) Successful surgical management of spontaneous gastric perforations in three cats. *Journal of Feline Medicine and Surgery* 12, 36–41.

Chan, D.L. (2008) Colloids: current recommendations. *Veterinary Clinics of North America Small Animal Practice* 38, 587–593, xi.

Cruz-Arambulo, R. and Wrigley, R. (2003) Ultrasonography of the acute abdomen. *Clinical Techniques in Small Animal Practice* 18, 20–31.

Culp, W.T., Zeldis, T.E., Reese, M.S. and Drobatz, K.J. (2009) Primary bacterial peritonitis in dogs and cats: 24 cases (1990–2006). *Journal of the American Veterinary Medical Association* 234, 906–913.

Culp, W.T., Weisse, C., Kellogg, M.E., Gordon, I.K., Clarke, D.L., May, L.R. and Drobatz, K.J. (2010) Spontaneous hemoperitoneum in cats: 65 cases (1994–2006). *Journal of the American Veterinary Medical Association* 236, 978–982.

Day, T.K. (2006) Shock syndromes. In: Dibartola, S.P. (ed.) *Fluid Electrolyte and Acid–Base Disorders in Small Animal Practice*, 3rd edn. Saunders Elsevier, London, pp. 540–564.

Driessen, B. and Brainard, B. (2006) Fluid therapy for the traumatized patient. *Journal of Veterinary Emergency and Critical Care* 16, 276–299.

Dye, T. (2003) The acute abdomen: a surgeon's approach to diagnosis and treatment. *Clinical Techniques in Small Animal Practice* 18, 53–65.

Feldman, B.F. (1999) In-house canine and feline blood typing. *Journal of the American Animal Hospital Association* 35, 455–456.

Hansen, B.D. (2006) Technical aspects of fluid therapy. In: Dibartola, S.P. (ed.) *Fluid Electrolyte and Acid–Base Disorders in Small Animal Practice*, 3rd edn. Saunders Elsevier, London, pp. 344–376.

Hereen, V., Edwards, L. and Mazzaferro, E.M. (2004) Acute abdomen: diagnosis. *Compendium of Continuing Education for the Practicing Veterinarian* 26, 350–363.

International Society of Feline Medicine (2010a) Feline blood transfusions – practical guidelines for nurses. www.isfm. net/toolbox/info_sheets/transfusions_nurse.pdf, accessed 17 May 2011.

International Society of Feline Medicine (2010b) Feline blood transfusions – practical guidelines for vets. www.isfm.net/ toolbox/info_sheets/transfusions_vet.pdf, accessed 17 May 2011.

Kirby, B.M. (2003) Peritoneum and peritoneal cavity. In: Slatter, D.H. (ed.) *Textbook of Small Animal Surgery*, 3rd edn. Saunders, Philadelphia, Pennsylvania, pp. 414–445.

Lucas, R.L., Lentz, K.D. and Hale, A.S. (2004) Collection and preparation of blood products. *Clinical Techniques in Small Animal Practice* 19, 55–62.

Macintire, D.K. (2008) Pediatric fluid therapy. *Veterinary Clinics of North America Small Animal Practice* 38, 621–627, xii.

Manning, A.M. (2002) Oxygen therapy and toxicity. *Veterinary Clinics of North America Small Animal Practice* 32, 1005–1020, v.

Mathews, K.A. (2006) Monitoring fluid therapy and complications of fluid therapy. In: Dibartola, S.P. (ed.) *Fluid Electrolyte and Acid–Base Disorders in Small Animal Practice*, 3rd edn. Saunders Elsevier, London, pp. 377–391.

Mazzaferro, E.M. (2008) Complications of fluid therapy. *Veterinary Clinics of North America Small Animal Practice* 38, 607–619, xii.

Mensack, S. (2008) Fluid therapy: options and rational administration. *Veterinary Clinics of North America Small Animal Practice* 38, 575–586, xi.

Mongil, C.M., Drobatz, K.J. and Hendricks, J.C. (1995) Traumatic hemoperitoneum in 28 cases: a retrospective review. *Journal of the American Animal Hospital Association* 31, 217–222.

Moore, K.E. and Murtaugh, R.J. (2001) Pathophysiologic characteristics of hypovolemic shock. *Veterinary Clinics of North America Small Animal Practice* 31, 1115–1128, v.

Mueller, M.G., Ludwig, L.L. and Barton, L.J. (2001) Use of closed-suction drains to treat generalized peritonitis in dogs and cats: 40 cases (1997–1999). *Journal of the American Veterinary Medical Association* 219, 789–794.

Parsons, K.J., Owen, L.J., Lee, K., Tivers, M.S. and Gregory, S.P. (2009) A retrospective study of surgically treated cases of septic peritonitis in the cat (2000–2007). *Journal of Small Animal Practice* 50, 518–524.

Pintar, J., Breitschwerdt, E.B., Hardie, E.M. and Spaulding, K.A. (2003) Acute nontraumatic hemoabdomen in the dog: a retrospective analysis of 39 cases (1987–2001). *Journal of the American Animal Hospital Association* 39, 518–522.

Prittie, J.E. (2003) Triggers for use, optimal dosing, and problems associated with red cell transfusions. *Veterinary Clinics of North America Small Animal Practice* 33, 1261–1275.

Probst, C.W., Stickle, R.L. and Bartlett, P.C. (1986) Duration of pneumoperitoneum in the dog. *American Journal of Veterinary Research* 47, 176–178.

Quandt, J.E., Lee, J.A. and Powell, L.L. (2005) Analgesia in critically ill patients. *Compendium of Continuing Education for the Practicing Veterinarian* 27, 433–446.

Rakich, P.M. and Latimer, K.S. (2003) Cytology. In: Latimer, K.S., Mahaffey, E.A. and Prasse, K.W. (eds) *Duncan and Prasse's Veterinary Laboratory Medicine: Clinical Pathology*, 4 edn. Iowa State Press, Ames, Iowa, pp. 304–330.

Robertson, S.A. and Taylor, P.M. (2004) Pain management in cats – past, present and future. Part 2. Treatment of pain-clinical pharmacology. *Journal of Feline Medicine and Surgery* 6, 321–333.

Rozanski, E. and De Laforcade, A.M. (2004) Transfusion medicine in veterinary emergency and critical care medicine. *Clinical Techniques in Small Animal Practice* 19, 83–87.

Rudloff, E. and Kirby, R. (2001) Colloid and crystalloid resuscitation. *Veterinary Clinics of North America Small Animal Practice* 31, 1207–1229.

Rudloff, E. and Kirby, R. (2008) Fluid resuscitation and the trauma patient. *Veterinary Clinics of North America Small Animal Practice* 38, 645–652, xiii.

Swann, H. and Hughes, D. (2000) Diagnosis and management of peritonitis. *Veterinary Clinics of North America Small Animal Practice* 30, 603–615, vii.

Tocci, L.J. and Ewing, P.J. (2009) Increasing patient safety in veterinary transfusion medicine: an overview of pretrans-fusion testing. *Journal of Veterinary Emergency and Critical Care* 19, 66–73.

Vinayak, A. and Krahwinkel, D.J. (2004) Managing blunt trauma-induced hemoperitoneum in dogs and cats. *Compendium of Continuing Education for the Practicing Veterinarian* 26, 276–291.

Walters, J.M. (2003) Abdominal paracentesis and diagnostic peritoneal lavage. *Clinical Techniques in Small Animal Practice* 18, 32–38.

Walters, P.C. (2000) Approach to the acute abdomen. *Clinical Techniques in Small Animal Practice* 15, 63–69.

14 Ovarian and Uterine Surgery

caesarean section: surgical delivery of fetuses
dystocia: difficulty giving birth
ovariectomy: removal of the ovaries (uterus is left in place)
ovariohysterectomy: removal of the ovaries and uterus
pyometra: uterine infection
spay: colloquial term for ovariohysterectomy

The reader should be able to:

- list the indications for ovariohysterectomy in the dog and cat
- explain the advantages and disadvantages of ovariohysterectomy performed at 6 weeks, 6 months, and 6 years of age in a dog
- describe the legislation controlling who performs ovariohysterectomy on the dog in the UK
- explain the rationale for using triple clamp technique to ligate the ovarian pedicles in a bitch
- complete, with the assistance of a qualified veterinary surgeon, ovariohysterectomy in the bitch by midline approach including mobilization of the ovarian pedicle and application of triple clamp technique
- complete, with the assistance of a qualified veterinary surgeon, ovariohysterectomy in the queen by left flank approach
- list the complications of ovariohysterectomy in the dog
- recognize indications for emergency caesarean section in the bitch and queen
- calculate a safe date for elective caesarean section in the bitch from a known, single mating date using the information provided in the relevant sections of this text
- describe how to perform caesarean section in the dog or cat and how to manage the dam and the litter post-operatively

Ovariohysterectomy and Ovariectomy

The standard method for neutering dogs and cats is ovariohysterectomy (removal of the ovaries and uterus). Ovariectomy (removal of the ovaries in isolation) is also becoming popular. The beneficial effects of elective neutering are generally thought to outweigh the negative aspects of surgery, which include the risks of surgery and of post-neutering incontinence. The common prophylactic and therapeutic indications for ovariohysterectomy are listed.

Indications for prophylactic neutering

- Prevent pregnancy.
- Protect against mammary tumour.

- Prevent pyometra.
- Prevent oestrus-associated behaviour.
- Prevent recurrence of pseudopregnancy.
- Prevent recurrence of vaginal leiomyoma.

Indications for therapeutic neutering

- Pyometra.
- Dystocia with fetal death.
- Control vaginal hypertrophy and prolapse.
- Ovarian or uterine neoplasia.
- Improve management of diabetes mellitus.

Legislation

Prophylactic ovariohysterectomy is generally considered to be ethical because it prevents unwanted pregnancy, it protects against a range of diseases, and the benefits are perceived to outweigh the risks. However, this is not universally accepted and, in some countries, prophylactic neutering is considered to be an unjustifiable mutilation that prevents the expression of normal behaviour. For example, in Norway prophylactic neutering is considered to be unethical, and legislation limits neutering to surgery performed for therapeutic reasons only. Legislation also dictates a minimum standard of care. In the UK, ovariohysterectomy can only be performed by a qualified veterinary surgeon or by a veterinary student during the clinical part of their course, and while under the direct and continuous supervision of a qualified veterinary surgeon. Veterinary nurses cannot perform ovariohysterectomy. Veterinary surgeons must be familiar with the legislation governing veterinary practice where they are working.

Age at elective neutering

Elective neutering has traditionally been performed from *5 to 6 months* of age but the exact timing of neutering is controversial and may influence the complications and the prophylactic benefits of the procedure.

Neutering dogs is highly protective against the development of mammary tumours, but the protective effect diminishes as the age at neutering increases. Neutering before the first oestrus is associated with a 0.05% incidence of mammary tumour but the incidence rises to 8% if neutering is performed after the first oestrus. By 2.5 years of age, any protective effect of neutering is lost and the incidence of mammary tumour is 25%.

The timing of neutering dogs may also influence the incidence of acquired urinary incontinence, one of the main long-term complications of neutering. Some authors recommend neutering before the first oestrus to reduce the risk; others recommend neutering after the first oestrus for the same reason. There is conflicting evidence over which has the lower risk of incontinence later in life. However, what is clear is that, regardless of the timing of neutering, a proportion of dogs will develop incontinence.

Until a consensus can be reached on the influence of timing of neutering on incontinence, the author recommends neutering before the first oestrus to reduce the incidence of mammary tumours as much as possible, but also ensures that owners are aware that late-onset incontinence is a common complication of ovariohysterectomy.

In contrast, acquired urinary incontinence is not a significant complication of feline ovariohysterectomy and cats are neutered from 5 to 6 months of age, preferably before the onset of oestrus, to avoid unwanted pregnancy. Neutering at an early age in cats also appears to be highly protective against the development of mammary tumours later in life.

Early neutering from as early as 6 *weeks* of age is gaining in popularity, as this enables animals to be neutered before leaving the breeder, removing the risk of unwanted pregnancy, and taking the decision regarding breeding away from the new owner. There appear to be few additional adverse effects from early neutering and patients recover quickly from surgery.

Timing of neutering within the reproductive cycle

Ovariohysterectomy can take place at any stage of the reproductive cycle but ideally it should be performed on non-pregnant animals during anoestrus. Neutering is not performed routinely during oestrus because oestrogen induces a temporary coagulopathy and increases the vascularity of the ovaries and uterus. Neutering is not performed routinely in dioestrus as the sudden drop in progesterone following neutering may induce pseudopregnancy in dogs.

Canine elective ovariohysterectomy is performed either before the first oestrus or 3–4 months following a period of oestrus (by which time dioestrus should have ended). As cats have a seasonal breeding period and are induced ovulators, they do not have long periods of anoestrus, and ovariohysterectomy is often performed during oestrus or dioestrus through necessity. However, the smaller reproductive tract and low incidence of pseudopregnancy in this species reduces the complications associated with neutering during oestrus.

Canine Pyometra

Pyometra (uterine infection) is part of the spectrum of disease that includes cystic endometrial hyperplasia and is characterized by filling of the uterus with pus (Fig. 14.1). If the cervix is open, purulent fluid will leak from the vulva ('open pyometra') (Fig. 14.2). Pyometra develops in dioestrus and is dependent on the hormone progesterone. Bacteria colonize the uterus from the cranial vagina. *Escherichia coli*, *Staphylococcus* spp., *Streptococcus* spp., *Pseudomonas* sp., and *Proteus* sp. are common. Pyometra often leads to toxaemia, septicaemia, and hypovolaemic shock. Some dogs develop a secondary renal glomerulonephropathy and become azotaemic. Concurrent urinary tract infection is also very common. Occasionally, the uterus ruptures leading to peritonitis.

Historical and clinical findings

Pyometra is very common and affects 25% of entire bitches before the age of 10 years. It is generally considered to be a disease of older dogs but may occur as early as after the first oestrus in dogs less than a year of age. Clinical signs start 2–6 weeks after oestrus. Bitches may appear systemically well in the early stages but, as the condition progresses, they develop signs of infection and toxaemia including pyrexia, dullness, tachycardia, hypovolaemia, vomiting, and polydipsia. In severe cases, signs of life-threatening septic shock and peritonitis may be identified. Purulent vaginal discharge may be present. The abdomen is often distended and 'doughy' on palpation due to the enlarged uterus. Palpation must be performed carefully to avoid rupturing the uterus.

Investigation

Pyometra should be considered as a possible differential diagnosis of malaise, vomiting, or polydipsia in any intact bitch. The goals of investigation are to confirm the diagnosis, establish the extent of secondary problems, and to distinguish the condition from other causes of polydipsia, vomiting, or malaise.

Serum biochemistry and urinalysis are performed to document the degree of renal damage and the presence of urinary tract infection, and to screen for metabolic conditions that may mimic the syndrome (e.g. diabetes mellitus; liver disease; renal disease). A neutrophilia with left shift is consistent with an inflammatory process. The diagnosis can be confirmed by identifying the enlarged uterus by

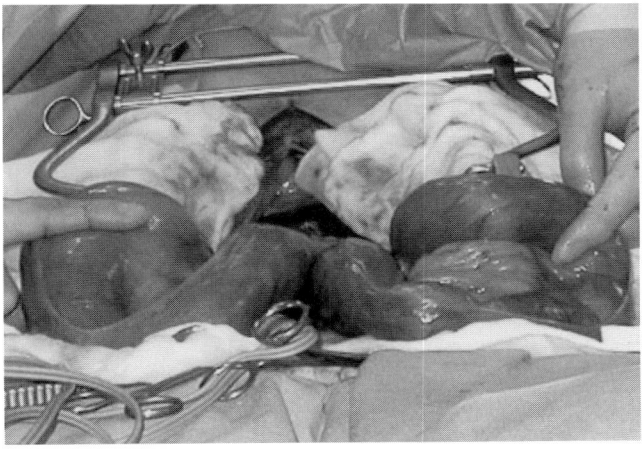

Fig. 14.1. Pyometra: uterus distended with pus.

ultrasound, the preferred imaging modality, or by radiography (Fig. 14.3).

Treatment

Most cases of pyometra are managed surgically as emergency ovariohysterectomy is a simple and effective treatment. All patients should receive fluid therapy and be rehydrated before being anaesthetized. Surgery should be performed as soon as the patient is stabilized, as delaying surgery increases the risk of peritonitis. Perform ovariohysterectomy modifying the technique as described below as required.

Medical management can be attempted as an alternative to surgery. The aims of medical therapy are to induce luteolysis to remove the influence of progesterone, and to cause cervical dilation and uterine contraction to expel pus from the uterus. Protocols using prostaglandins, dopamine agonists (e.g. prolactin), or progesterone receptor antagonists (e.g. aglepristone) have been described. A course of broad-spectrum antibiotics is also prescribed. Medical management might be selected for a patient that has a concurrent disease that makes it unsuitable for anaesthesia (e.g. congestive heart failure) or in a patient that is intended for breeding. Bitches have been successfully bred following medical management of pyometra. The disadvantages of medical management are that pyometra may recur after the next oestrus and some patients do not respond well to treatment.

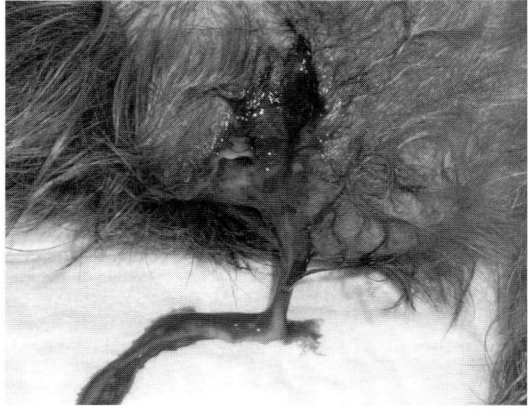

Fig. 14.2. Open pyometra: purulent fluid dripping from the vulva.

Feline Pyometra

Pyometra in cats is very uncommon. This may be due to the high incidence of elective neutering in this species or be because queens are induced ovulators so will only enter dioestrus if they are mated. Feline pyometra also can be managed either surgically or medically.

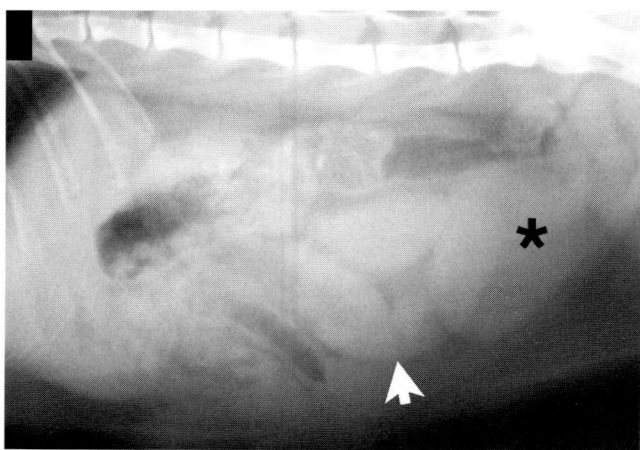

Fig. 14.3. Radiographic appearance of pyometra: the distended uterus is identified as a soft-tissue viscus in the caudal abdomen (arrow), originating between the bladder (asterisk) and the colon, and displacing the small intestinal tract cranially.

Chapter 14

Surgical Techniques

Surgical anatomy

The ovaries are located at the caudal pole of each kidney within the ovarian bursa. The cranial pole of the ovary is tethered in the dorsal abdomen by the *suspensory ligament*. This originates from the lumbar fascia near the last rib and runs caudoventrally, lateral to the kidney, to the ovary. The caudal pole of the ovary is attached to the uterine horn by the *proper ligament*. The ovary is attached to the dorsolateral body wall by the mesovarium. This contains a single ovarian artery arising directly from the aorta, and a plexus of ovarian veins draining into the caudal vena cava or renal vein. Together these form the *ovarian vascular pedicle* (Fig. 14.4).

The uterine horn runs from the ovary caudally in the paralumbar fossa lateral to the other abdominal organs. It converges with the contralateral uterine horn to form the uterine body. The uterine body lies between the bladder and colon. The mesometrium attaches the uterine body and horn to the dorsolateral body wall. A triangular fold runs from the mesometrium, through the inguinal canal, into the vaginal process and is called the *round ligament*. The uterine horn and body are supplied by the uterine artery and vein that run longitudinally within the mesometrium, having originated from the vaginal artery. Together, the mesovarium, mesosalpinx, and mesometrium form the *broad ligament*.

During ovariohysterectomy, it is important to appreciate that the ureter runs close to the base of the ovarian pedicle as it emerges from the renal hilus, and close to the cervix as it enters the bladder.

Midline ovariohysterectomy in the dog

There are many variations of ovariohysterectomy but the technique described here is simple and safe. It emphasizes the importance of adequate exposure of the ovarian pedicle for easier ligature placement, of good haemostasis, and of avoidance of damaging the ureters. Elective ovariohysterectomy is classified as a clean procedure and perioperative antimicrobials are not indicated (see Chapter 2).

Approach

Perform a midline coeliotomy from the umbilicus to halfway between the umbilicus and the pubis. Extending 1 or 2 cm cranial to the umbilicus facilitates ligation of the ovarian pedicles in deepchested dogs. Push the omentum that covers the abdominal viscera cranially.

Locate the uterus

Use a cupped hand to pull the intestinal tract cranially away from the bladder. The uterus is located in midline between the bladder and the colon (Fig. 14.5).

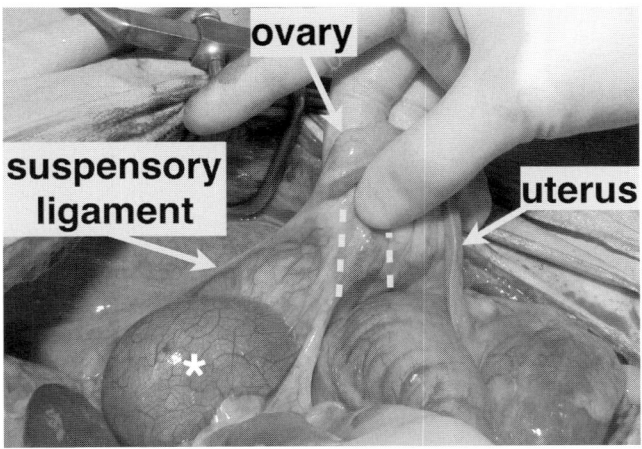

Fig. 14.4. Ovarian anatomy (left ovary viewed from medial side): the suspensory ligament, ovary and uterus are labelled. The kidney (asterisk) sits in front of the suspensory ligament. The dotted lines represent the width of the plexus of ovarian vessels that supply the ovary and run through the ovarian pedicle.

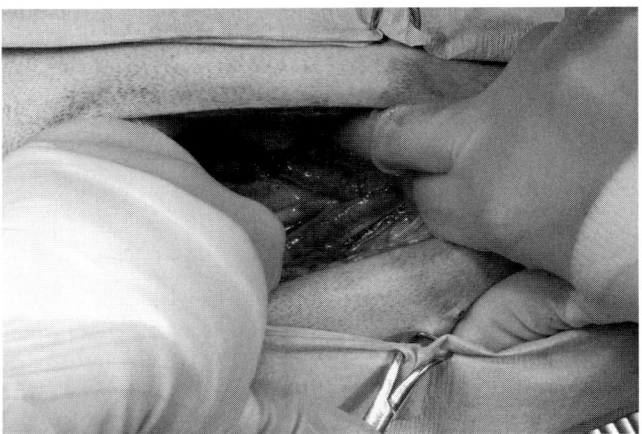

Fig. 14.5. Expose the uterus by pushing intestines cranially (left hand) and bladder caudally (right hand) – the 'Y' shaped uterine body is revealed (head towards left)

It is identified by its bifurcate structure, muscular wall, and longitudinal blood supply. Trace along the uterine horn to the ovary.

Break down the suspensory ligament

Disrupting the suspensory ligament enables the ovarian pedicle to be retracted from the abdomen and makes ligature placement much easier. Hold the ovary between the thumb and middle finger of your dominant hand. Apply caudal traction to the ovary (this stretches the suspensory ligament taut without stretching the ovarian vessels that run dorsoventrally in the pedicle). Push down and back on the suspensory ligament with the index finger of the same hand to further stretch the ligament (Fig. 14.6). Apply firm, continuous pressure. The ligament will begin to stretch and will then break with a mild popping sensation. This step takes time to master but is invaluable in improving access to the ovarian pedicle (Fig. 14.7). Ensure that all traction is applied to the ovary itself rather than to the uterine horn as the uterus can be avulsed from the ovary.

Ligate and transect the ovarian pedicle using 'triple clamp technique'

Retract the ovary and pedicle out of the abdomen and identify the ovarian vessels running in the mesovarium. Bluntly create a hole in the broad ligament caudal to the ovarian vessels to isolate the ovarian pedicle from the rest of the broad ligament. Place three bitch spay forceps ('clamps') onto the ovarian pedicle through this hole (Fig. 14.8).

The *proximal clamp* is placed closest to the aorta and vena cava. The *middle clamp* is placed at least 1 cm distal to the proximal clamp so that a transfixing ligature can be placed in the exposed ovarian pedicle. The *distal clamp* is placed between the middle clamp and ovary, ensuring that no ovarian tissue is caught in the clamp. When placing the clamps, take care not to catch the body wall, intestines, or omentum in the tips of the clamps. Lift the pedicle away from the abdominal viscera as the proximal clamp is placed, to ensure that the ureter is not inadvertently crushed by the clamp.

The proximal clamp creates a crush line in the tissue into which a circumferential ligature is placed. Pass suture material through the hole in the broad ligament and tie a surgeon's throw loosely around the proximal clamp. Release the proximal clamp as the surgeon's throw is tightened into the crush line (Fig. 14.9A). Place three additional single throws to secure the knot. Place a transfixing ligature through the pedicle between the first ligature and the middle clamp (Fig. 14.9B). This acts as the second point of haemostasis and resists slippage.

The middle clamp provides an additional crush line for added haemostasis. Transect the pedicle

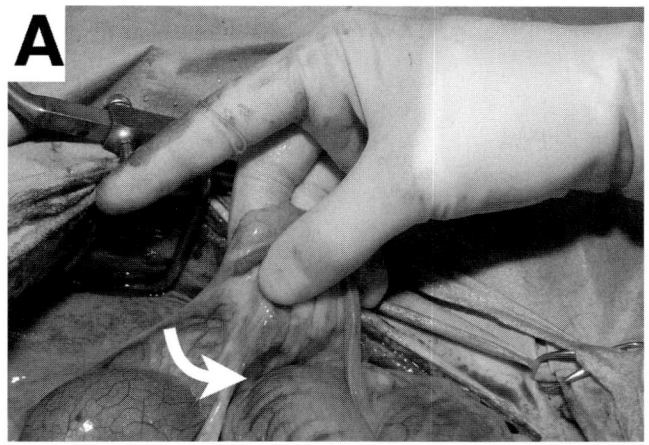

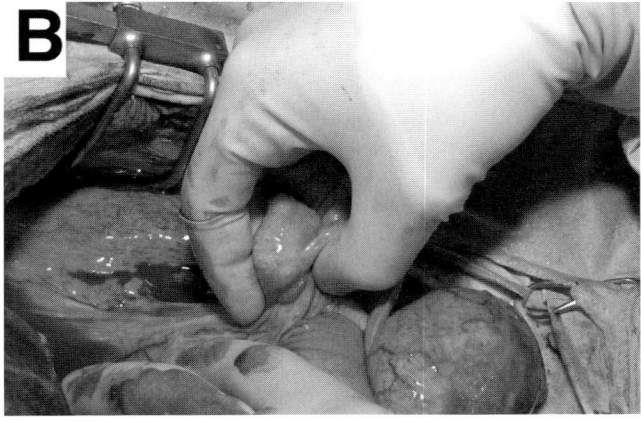

Fig. 14.6. Break down the suspensory ligament: (A) hold the ovary between the thumb and middle finger (see Fig. 14.4 for labels) and apply pressure on the suspensory ligament stretching it caudally (arrow shows direction); (B) pressure being applied to the suspensory ligament. These images were collected during exploratory coeliotomy performed for other reasons in an intact bitch. There is excellent exposure of these structures because a full abdominal incision has been made and abdominal retractors are being used. It is often difficult to visualize the suspensory ligament during ovariohysterectomy through a standard incision, but once a little traction is applied to the ovary, the suspensory ligament can be felt as a taut band running cranially, enabling this procedure to be completed.

between the middle and distal clamps using scissors or a scalpel blade (Fig. 14.10). The distal clamp separates the ovary from the transection site reducing the risk of leaving portions of the ovary and preventing back-bleeding.

A *modified triple clamp technique* can be used if there is insufficient room to place three clamps on the ovarian pedicle. This is identical to the technique described above except that the distal clamp is placed between the ovary and the uterine body to prevent back-bleeding (Fig. 14.11). If using this technique, greater care is required to ensure that

remnants of ovary are not left in the stump of the ovarian pedicle.

Check the pedicle for haemorrhage and release it

Hold the pedicle using non-traumatic dissecting forceps (do not hold the ligatures themselves) (Fig. 14.10B). Release the clamp and check for haemorrhage (Fig. 14.12). If there is no haemorrhage, replace the stump back into the abdomen so that it is not stretched, before releasing it. If there

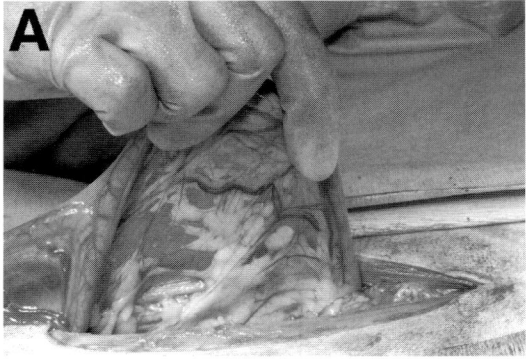

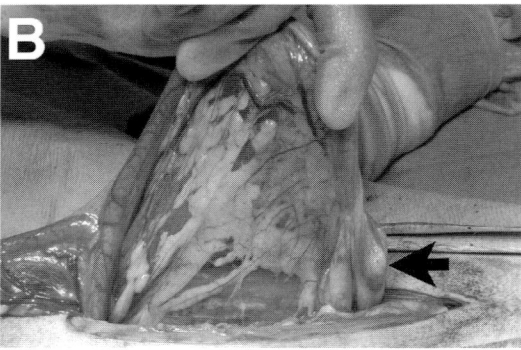

Fig. 14.7. Effect of disrupting the suspensory ligament (head towards right): (A) before disrupting the ligament, the ovary is below the level of the skin incision; (B) after disrupting the ligament, the ovary can be elevated out of the incision (arrow) exposing the ovarian pedicle.

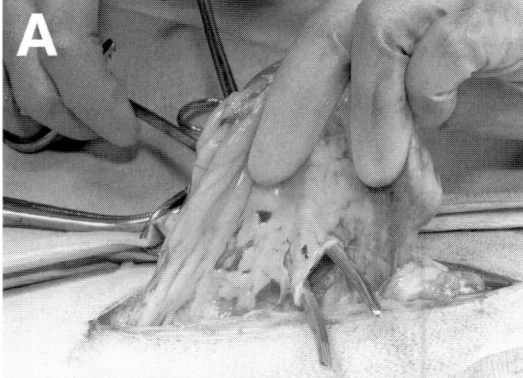

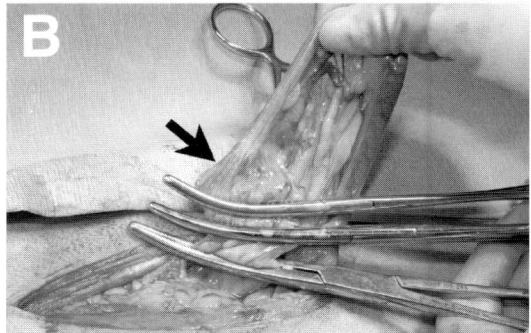

Fig. 14.8. Triple clamp technique part 1: (A) create window in broad ligament next to the ovarian pedicle (head to right); (B) apply three clamps to the ovarian pedicle proximal to the ovary (head to left; arrow marks ovary).

is haemorrhage, reapply the clamp and place an additional ligature.

Break down the broad ligament to free the uterine horn

Tear or cut the broad ligament to separate the uterine horn from its abdominal attachments (Fig. 14.13). Ensure that the uterine artery separates with the uterus. Continue until the uterine body is reached, avoiding the ureters that run close to the base of the broad ligament in this region.

Repeat these steps on the other ovary and uterine horn

Ligate and transect the uterine body

Palpate the uterine body and cervix. Place two transfixing ligatures around the distal uterine body.

Place two bitch spay forceps proximal to the ligatures and transect the uterus between the forceps (Fig. 14.14). Check the uterine stump for haemorrhage before releasing it.

Ovariohysterectomy for pyometra

This surgery is classified as a dirty procedure and perioperative antimicrobials are indicated. Continue these as a therapeutic course postoperatively and collect uterine fluid for culture and sensitivity testing.

Some modifications of the basic ovariohysterectomy technique may be required. Extend the abdominal incision as required to accommodate the enlarged uterus. The blood supply to the ovaries and uterus becomes engorged, and the broad ligament and ovarian pedicles become stretched and friable. Handle the ovarian pedicles carefully.

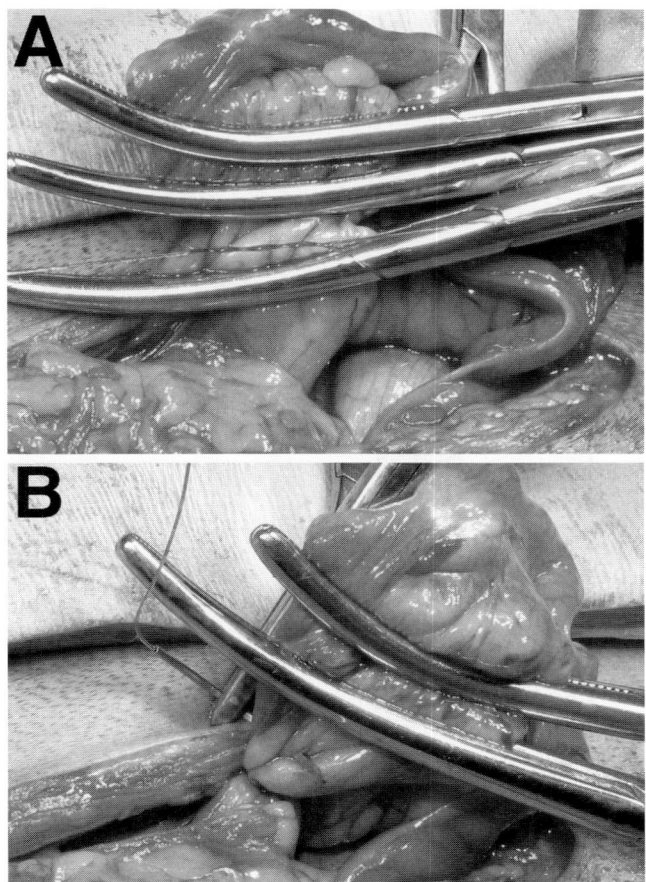

Fig. 14.9. Triple clamp technique part 2: (A) lay a circumferential ligature around the proximal clamp (shown), release the clamp and tie the ligature into the crush line; (B) place a transfixing ligature between the proximal ligature and the middle clamp.

If the pedicles are very friable, place ligatures before applying bitch spay forceps to reduce the risk of tearing the pedicles. Ligate the base of the broad ligament *en bloc* before tearing it to stop capillary haemorrhage. Transect the reproductive tract distal to the cervix if there is adequate exposure so that no infected endometrium is left. Do not transect through the cervix as this tissue is not compressible, making effective ligation impossible. This modification is not recommended for routine ovariohysterectomy, and is not always possible in cases with pyometra. This is because the ureters run in close proximity to the cranial vagina, just distal to the cervix, so this modification increases the potential for ureteral injury.

Flank ovariohysterectomy

Flank ovariohysterectomy is not recommended in the dog but remains popular for neutering cats. There are many variations and the method described here aims to provide a safe and simple technique for inexperienced surgeons.

Approach

Clip an area of the left flank, centring the clip caudodorsally, and prepare the animal for surgery. Position the patient in right lateral recumbency with the hind legs stretched back to ensure the cranial thigh muscles do not impinge

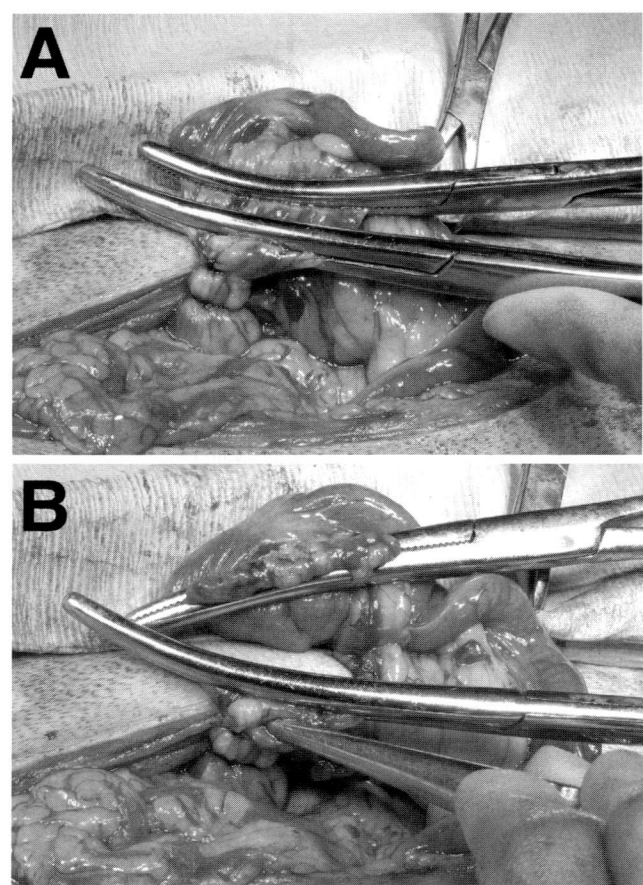

Fig. 14.10. Triple clamp technique part 3: (A) circumferential and transfixing ligatures in place; (B) transect between the middle and distal clamps. Thumb forceps are being used to hold the pedicle in preparation for releasing the middle clamp.

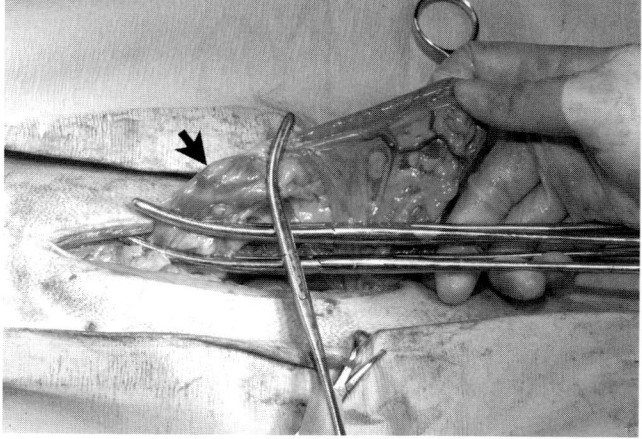

Fig. 14.11. Modified triple clamp technique (arrow indicates ovary)

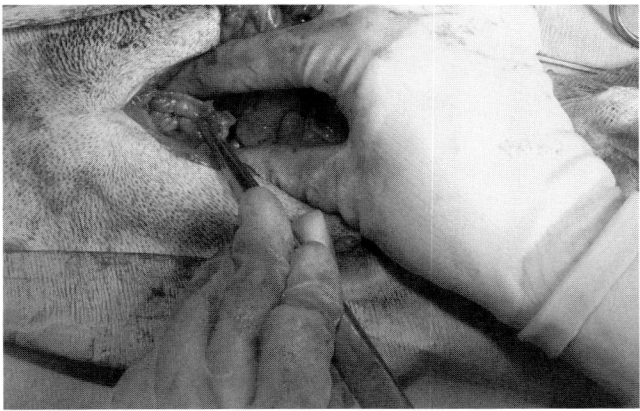

Fig. 14.12. Check for haemorrhage: hold the ovarian pedicle stump with non-traumatic forceps and release the remaining clamp. Place the pedicle back in the abdomen and check for further haemorrhage.

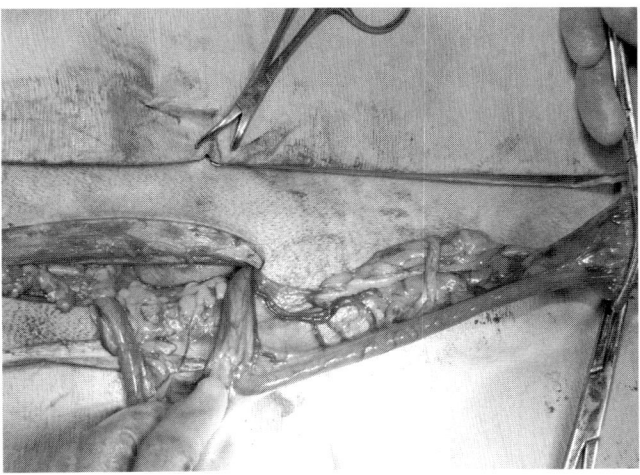

Fig. 14.13. The broad ligament has been broken to mobilize the entire uterine horn.

on the surgical approach (Fig. 14.15). Drape the surgical site.

Identify the flank incision site. Create an equilateral triangle using the greater trochanter of the hip and the wing of the ilium as two points. The third point marks the incision site (Fig. 14.15). Make a 1–2 cm, dorsoventral skin incision centred over this point, and extend the incision through the subcutaneous fat to expose the external rectus fascia. Tent the fascia using rat-toothed thumb forceps. Penetrate the abdomen by cutting with dissecting scissors. Extend the incision to the limits of the skin incision (Fig. 14.16).

Identify the reproductive tract

The left uterine horn runs across the surgical field and is the most lateral organ encountered during this approach. If it is visible, grasp it with non-traumatic forceps and pull it out of the abdominal incision. If it cannot be seen, use a finger or spay hook placed into the incision and drawn along the body wall in the immediate vicinity to locate and exteriorize it. It is often obscured by the lumbar fat pad at the dorsal extent of the incision. Ensure that the uterus rather than intestine has been retrieved by checking that it has linear blood supply (Fig. 14.17).

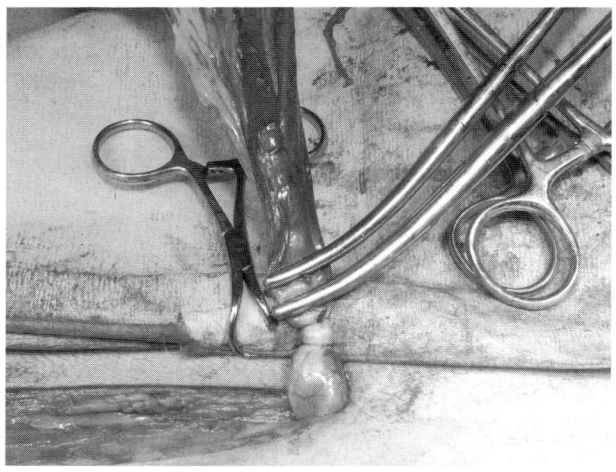

Fig. 14.14. Double ligate the uterine body, clamp and transect it.

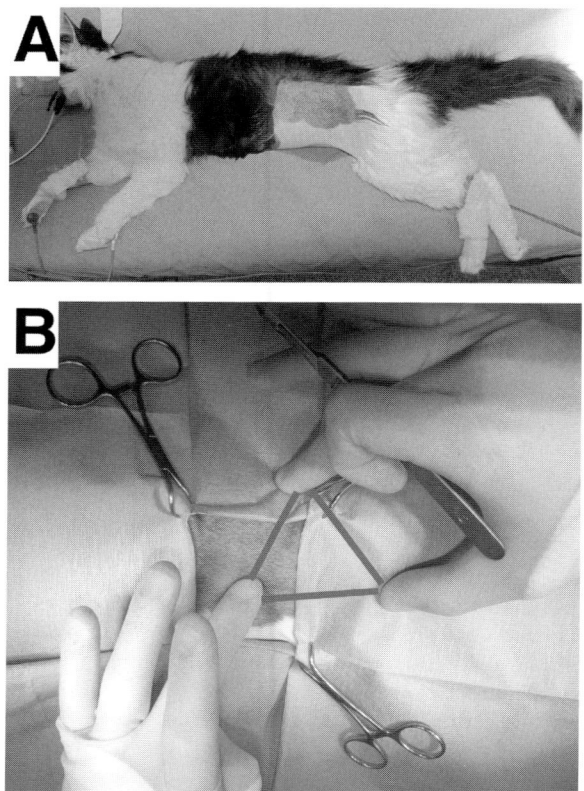

Fig. 14.15. Flank spay 1: (A) position the patient in right lateral recumbency with the hind legs tied back; (B) make the skin incision centred over the third point of an equilateral triangle with the wing of the ilium and the greater trochanter as the other two points.

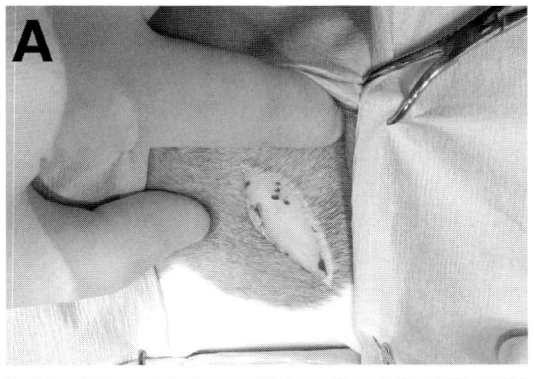

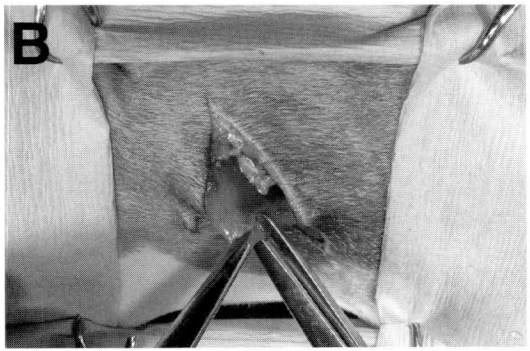

Fig. 14.16. Flank spay 2: (A) make a 2 cm skin incision running vertically or obliquely (craniodorsal to caudoventral) – the direction of incision is one of personal choice; (B) lift up the abdominal wall muscle and incise it with scissors.

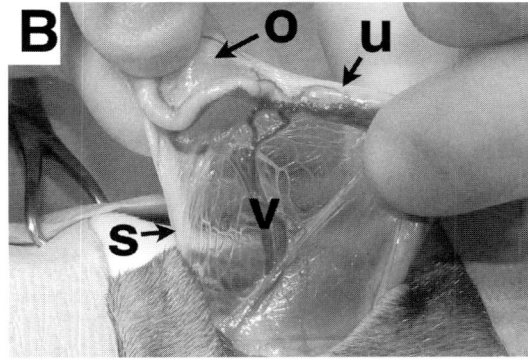

Fig. 14.17. Flank spay 3: (A) use a finger or a spay hook to lift the uterine horn out of the abdomen; (B) Trace the uterine horn to the ovary (ovary – 'o'; ovarian vessels – 'v'; suspensory ligament – 's'; uterine horn – 'u').

Ligate and transect the ovarian pedicles

Trace the uterine horn to the ovary (Fig. 14.17). There is limited space for forceps placement, the ovarian vessels are quite small, and the suspensory ligament is lax, so a modified ligation technique is used. Exteriorize the ovary. Create a hole in the broad ligament to isolate the ovarian pedicle. Place two haemostats proximal to the ovary. Double ligate the ovarian vessels below the haemostats using circumferential ligatures or a combination of circumferential and transfixing ligatures. Transect the pedicle between the haemostats. Hold the transected pedicle with non-traumatic thumb forceps before releasing the haemostat. Check for haemorrhage and replace the pedicle in the abdomen before releasing it (Fig. 14.18). It may be difficult to place two haemostats proximal to the ovary, so the second

haemostat may be placed between the ovary and the uterus instead.

Repeat to mobilize the right uterine horn and ovary

Trace the left uterine horn back, tearing the broad ligament to exteriorize the uterus. When the bifurcation of the uterine body is reached, retrieve the right uterine horn and repeat the steps to ligate and transect the ovarian pedicle and isolate the uterine horn (Fig. 14.19).

Ligate and transect the uterus

Exteriorize both uterine horns and ovaries and apply gentle traction. Place two haemostats across the uterus as far distally as possible. Due to the

Ovarian and Uterine Surgery

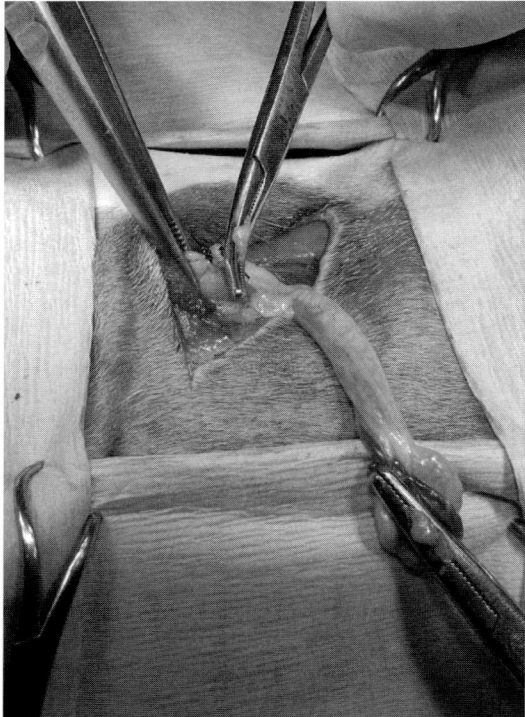

Fig. 14.18. Flank spay 4: clamp, ligate, and transect the ovarian pedicle.

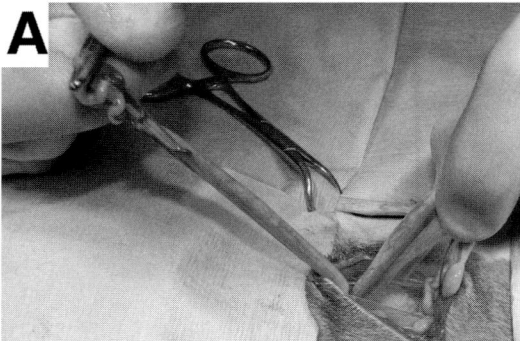

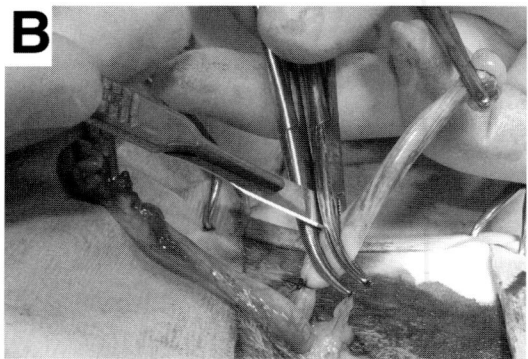

Fig. 14.19. Flank spay 5: (A) trace the uterus back to the uterine body, tearing the broad ligament to free the structures. Retrieve the second horn and ovary and ligate and transect the pedicle; (B) place ligatures around the uterine body, or each uterine horn, and amputate the ovaries and uterus.

limited access with this approach, a substantial portion of the uterine body is generally left *in situ*. Ligate the uterine body distal to the haemostats using one or two transfixing ligatures (Fig. 14.19). Transect the uterine body between the haemostats, check the stump for haemorrhage, and release it into the abdomen.

Close the laparotomy incision

Check for abdominal haemorrhage before closing the incision. Close all muscle layers in a single suture line using a simple continuous pattern of 3-0, monofilament, absorbable suture material (e.g. Glycomer™ 631; polydioxanone II). Close the subcutaneous fat and skin routinely.

Feline midline ovariohysterectomy

Feline midline ovariohysterectomy may be performed for elective neutering and is preferred over flank ovariohysterectomy for neutering cats that are heavily pregnant or in which the neutering status is unknown (e.g. from the stray cat population). It is the technique of choice for treating feline pyometra. It is also preferred for Siamese cats that get temperature-induced coat darkening in clipped areas of skin. The technique is very similar to midline ovariohysterectomy in the bitch but the coeliotomy incision is centred more caudally.

Ovariectomy

Ovariectomy (without hysterectomy) is becoming increasingly popular as an alternative to ovariohysterectomy because this is simpler to perform laparoscopically (i.e. by 'keyhole' surgery) than ovariohysterectomy. The outcomes and complications of ovariectomy appear to be very similar to those of ovariohysterectomy. The incidence of stump pyometra is not higher following ovariectomy because, although the uterus is left in place, there is no progesterone to promote the development of pyometra.

Complications

Ovariohysterectomy is generally well tolerated but a host of complications has been reported.

Haemorrhage

Haemorrhage is considered to be the commonest major perioperative complication of ovariohysterectomy. Bleeding may occur from the ovarian or uterine pedicles and is usually the result of poor ligature placement. If the bleeding pedicle cannot be located immediately, call for assistance, extend the incision cranially, place abdominal retractors, and use suction to remove blood. Perform the duodenal or colonic slings (see p. 138) to expose the paralumbar fossa and locate the ovarian pedicle caudal to the kidney. If haemorrhage obscures the area, pack the paralumbar fossa with swabs to get temporary control of haemorrhage and gradually remove these one at a time until the point of haemorrhage is located. The uterine pedicle is easily located by reflecting the bladder and pulling the descending colon forward.

If haemorrhage occurs post-operatively, there may be few external signs of bleeding. Signs that should prompt evaluation include prolonged recovery from anaesthesia, dripping of blood from the abdominal wound, abdominal distension, pallor, and other signs of hypovolaemic shock. Call for assistance from an experienced colleague and perform exploratory abdominal surgery.

Ureteral ligation

The ureters are occasionally trapped by the ovarian or cervical ligatures. This causes ureteral obstruction and hydronephrosis. These injuries are very difficult to manage and ureteral resection and anastomosis or nephrectomy may be required. Patients should be referred to specialist centres for management.

Weight gain

Weight gain is common. Food intake should be controlled to avoid obesity.

Behavioural changes

Behavioural problems, such as dominance aggression, may be exacerbated by ovariohysterectomy although these are likely to have been pre-existing conditions.

Coat changes

Coat colour may alter and hair coarseness may increase.

Urinary incontinence

Acquired sphincter mechanism incontinence (also referred to as post-spay incontinence or hormone-responsive incontinence) is common in dogs, affecting up to 20% of neutered bitches. This is a major complication of neutering in dogs which owners must be aware of before consenting to surgery (see p. 265). The syndrome is not recognized in cats.

Infantile vulva

Infantile vulva (juvenile vulva; recessed vulva) occurs in dogs that are neutered at a young age. The external genitalia do not develop to adult size. This is usually asymptomatic but may lead to the vulva becoming recessed and the development of perivulvar dermatitis (see p. 271).

Failure to remove all ovarian tissue

Portions of ovary are sometimes retained in the ovarian pedicle due to failure to isolate the ovary properly during ovariohysterectomy. Signs associated with remaining ovarian tissue may present months or years following neutering, in two ways:

1. **Ovarian remnant syndrome:** affected patients still have periods of oestrus because oestrogen is released from the ovarian remnant. Any animal showing signs of oestrus after neutering should be evaluated for an ovarian remnant.

2. **Stump pyometra:** endometrial infection in the stump of uterine body can develop under the influence of progesterone produced from corpora lutea in the ovarian remnant. Patients with stump pyometra may have open or closed pyometra and present identically to other cases with pyometra although, as they have been neutered, the condition is easily overlooked.

Confirming the presence of retained ovarian tissue is difficult. Abdominal ultrasound when the animal is showing signs of oestrus may identify the ovarian tissue. Various endocrine tests, including progesterone or luteinizing hormone assays, can be used. Exploratory surgery can combine confirmation of the diagnosis and definitive treatment in one procedure (Fig. 14.20). The goals of surgery are to remove the ovarian remnant and, if stump pyometra is present, to resect the uterine stump. Locating the retained ovarian tissue can be challenging and cases should be referred to an experienced colleague or specialist centre.

Caesarean Section

Caesarean section is commonly performed in small animal practice to manage dystocia. The British Veterinary Association and UK Kennel Club have introduced a reporting system in registered bitches to try to reduce the incidence.

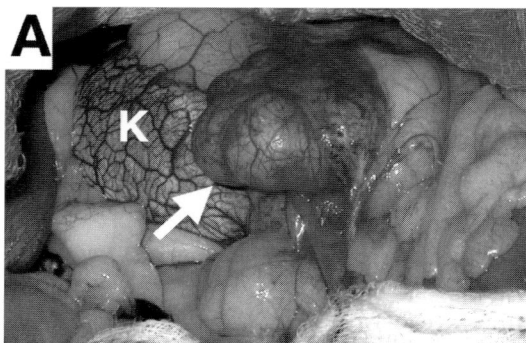

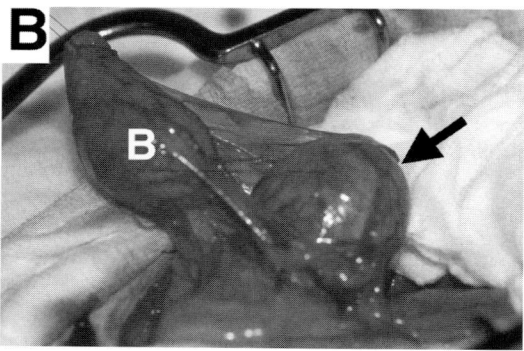

Fig. 14.20. (A) Retained ovary (arrow) at caudal pole of kidney ('K'); (B) Stump pyometra (arrow) sitting between the bladder ('B') and colon (images courtesy of E. Welsh).

Normal parturition

Normal parturition is divided into three phases. *First stage labour* is the start of uterine contraction and cervical dilation. It is recognized by nesting behaviour, restlessness, and mild straining, and lasts for 12–24 h.

Second stage labour is characterized by expulsion of the fetuses and follows immediately from the end of first stage labour. The start of second stage labour is identified by the onset of obvious abdominal contractions and straining, indicating that the first fetus is entering the birth canal for delivery. In the queen, the first fetus should be delivered within 60 min of the onset of abdominal contraction but, in the bitch, the first fetus may take considerably longer to be delivered. Lochia (green vulval discharge in the dog: dark brown discharge in the cat) may precede the delivery of each fetus and indicates the start of placental separation. Each fetus should be delivered within 20 min of lochia being seen. There may be pauses between the deliveries of each fetus in which the bitch or queen is relatively inactive. Although these gaps between fetuses are generally less than 60 min, they may be as long as 4 h.

Third stage labour is expulsion of the placentas. Second and third stage labour overlap and placentas are generally expelled between fetuses. Third stage labour should be complete within 2 h of delivery of the last fetus.

Mammary development may occur early in canine pregnancy and onset of lactation is an unreliable indicator of the end of gestation. Mammary development and lactation tend to occur towards the end of feline gestation. Failure of parturition to progress normally indicates dystocia.

Dystocia in dogs and cats

Dystocia is common in some breeds of dogs and cats (e.g. brachycephalic breeds, Scottish Terrier, French Bulldog, Devon Rex cat). Other risk factors include a previous history of dystocia or a familial history of dystocia.

Dystocia may be caused by fetal factors, maternal factors, or a combination of both. Fetal factors include malpresentation of fetuses, twin presentation of fetuses, and conformational abnormalities. Fetal conformational abnormalities may be associated with brachycephalic conformation, hydrocephalus, or the development of fetal monsters. Fetal oversize can lead to dystocia in a single-fetus pregnancy. Small litters may also produce insufficient cortisol to initiate first stage labour at the end of gestation.

Maternal causes of dystocia include physical obstruction to birthing, primary uterine inertia, and secondary uterine inertia. Obstruction of the birth canal may be caused by old pelvic injuries, vaginal masses, and vaginal strictures. Primary uterine inertia (failure of uterine contraction early during second stage labour) may have a familial basis although other factors such as small litter size may also contribute. Secondary uterine inertia may occur through uterine exhaustion, and is associated with prolonged parturition or with other factors that contribute to dystocia. Depletion of calcium is also often implicated in the pathogenesis of uterine inertia. Uterine inertia is recognized by cessation of delivery of fetuses or an extended period between the passage of fetuses in an animal that has started second stage labour. Failure of the Fergusson reflex (strong vaginal and uterine contraction in response to digital stimulation of the vagina) is an indication of uterine inertia and is a good marker that dystocia has occurred.

Emergency caesarean section for dystocia

Emergency caesarean section is performed when second stage labour has started but failed to progress. The procedure is performed as an emergency as the placentas may have started to detach which causes fetal distress and death. Criteria that are used to establish that dystocia has occurred include:

- Unproductive weak straining for more than 1–2 h.
- Unproductive vigorous straining for more than 20 min.
- Failure to deliver fetuses within 30 min of lochia (green or black vaginal discharge).
- Greater than 3 h between fetuses.
- Delivery of stillborn fetuses.
- Maternal distress or illness.
- Evidence of physical obstruction.

If uterine inertia is suspected without obstruction, oxytocin and calcium gluconate can be administered but caesarean section should be performed if no progress is made within a short period.

Caesarean section for prolonged gestation

Some animals fail to initiate parturition at the end of gestation. This may be because the litter size is small. These cases are challenging because it is difficult to confirm the exact stage of gestation. If an accurate mating date is known, caesarean section can be performed after 63 days of gestation in the cat. However, in dogs predicting the end of gestation is more difficult because of the possible delay between mating and conception caused by the protracted survival of spermatozoa and the variable timing of ovulation within the oestrus cycle. Canine pregnancy may extend naturally as late as 71 days following mating although the period from ovulation to parturition is predictably 63±1 day.

In dogs, the timing of surgery can be calculated from a documented luteinizing hormone (LH) surge during proestrus (parturition date 65±1 day) or from the postovulatory progesterone surge (parturition date 63±1 day). LH and progesterone can be assayed using ELISA kits or commercial laboratories, and are used to predict the optimal time of mating. The LH surge is short lived and LH assays must be repeated every 24 h during proestrus.

Luteolysis and a fall in progesterone levels occur 12–40 h before parturition and can also be used to predict the end of gestation. They are also associated with a drop in body temperature that can be identified effectively by the owner through regular (3–4 times daily) rectal temperature assessments.

Elective caesarean delivery

Elective caesarean delivery is performed before the start of parturition to prevent dystocia occurring. It can be performed from 63 days after ovulation although this time point can be difficult to predict (see above). Indications for elective caesarean delivery include a previous history of dystocia, concurrent problems that may cause dystocia (such as pelvic fracture), a familial history of dystocia, or a small litter size (and relative fetal oversize). As it is difficult to predict the timing from mating to conception in the dog, it may be prudent to wait until first stage labour has started before performing caesarean section in these patients to ensure that under-developed litters are not delivered.

Technique

During caesarean section, fetuses should be delivered as rapidly as possible and the duration of surgery and anaesthesia should be minimized to encourage rapid recovery of the dam. Pre-clip the abdomen before inducing anaesthesia. Tilt the table to elevate the thorax and reduce pressure on the diaphragm. Special consideration should be given to anaesthesia for caesarean section, taking into account the requirements for rapid recovery of the mother following surgery, provision of adequate pain relief postoperatively, the cardio-respiratory compromise of the dam, and the requirement to minimize the effects of anaesthetic drugs on the neonates. Refer to appropriate reference sources for further information.

Approach

Make a caudal, midline coeliotomy incision from cranial to the umbilicus running back towards the pubis. Avoid incising through hypertrophied mammary tissue. Take additional care to avoid penetrating the distended uterus during entry through the linea alba. Exteriorize the uterus, which is mobile due to stretching of the suspensory and broad ligaments, and isolate it from the abdomen using swabs to prevent peritoneal contamination (Fig. 14.21).

Delivering neonates

Make a longitudinal incision in the ventral surface of the uterine body. Palpate and select an area that is not directly over a fetus. Grasp the uterine wall with forceps and cut into the lumen with Metzenbaum scissors. Extend the incision longitudinally with Metzenbaum scissors (Fig. 14.21). Gently milk the fetus in the uterine body out of the incision. Immediately clear the fetal membranes from the head of the fetus (Fig. 14.22). Clamp the umbilical cord with haemostats, transect it, and pass the fetus to a non-sterile assistant for resuscitation. Extend the incision in the uterine wall to prevent tearing if necessary. Working quickly, repeat this process until all the fetuses are delivered. Separate incisions in the uterine horns may be required if the fetuses cannot easily be milked into the uterine body. Check the pelvic cavity for fetuses.

Delivery of placentas

If the placentas have started to detach, they can be removed as each fetus is delivered but, if they are firmly attached, they can be left to pass naturally. When elective caesarean section is performed before the start of labour, the cervix will not be dilated and the placentas may become retained. It is possible to strip the placentas carefully from the

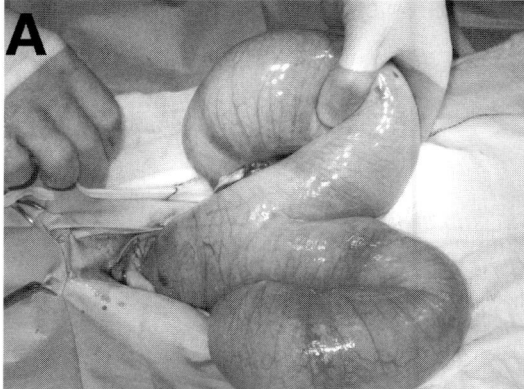

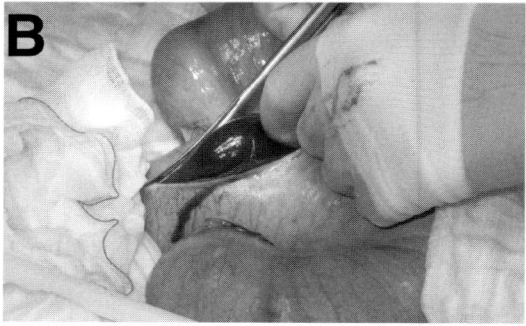

Fig. 14.21. Caesarean section: (A) exteriorize the uterus and isolate it from the abdomen with moistened swabs; (B) make a longitudinal incision into the uterine body, being careful to avoid damaging the fetuses, and extend the incision with Metzenbaum scissors.

endometrium but this may cause endometrial haemorrhage that sometimes necessitates emergency ovariohysterectomy.

Close the uterine incision

Close the uterine incision with a full-thickness, simple appositional, continuous pattern using 2-0–4-0, monofilament, absorbable suture material. This may be oversewn with a Cushing pattern to create an early serosal seal or an omental wrap can be placed (Fig. 14.23). Administer oxytocin once the uterine incision is closed, to stimulate uterine contraction (which reduces endometrial haemorrhage) and expulsion of placentas.

Close the abdomen

Lavage the abdomen and perform routine abdominal closure. Place intradermal sutures rather than

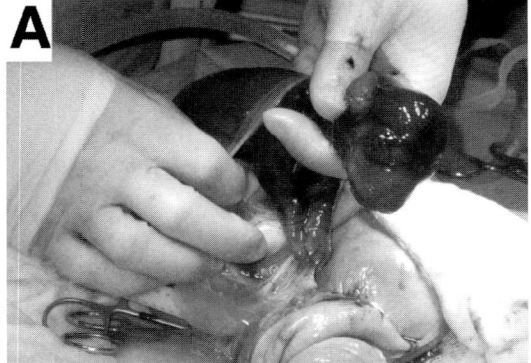

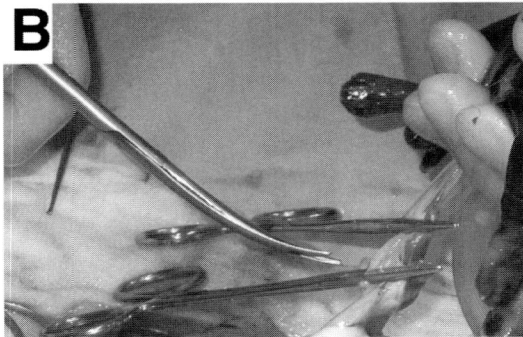

Fig. 14.22. Caesarean section: (A) remove the fetus and immediately clear the fetal membranes from its face; (B) clamp the umbilical cord with haemostats before transecting it.

skin sutures as suckling neonates may interfere with skin sutures.

Ovariohysterectomy combined with caesarean section

Ovariohysterectomy can be performed at the same time as caesarean section if desired (e.g. to prevent further pregnancy; to address uterine haemorrhage). Perform caesarean section as described above and, once all fetuses have been delivered, perform ovariohysterectomy.

Neonatal resuscitation

Neonates born by caesarean section generally require active resuscitation to stimulate spontaneous breathing. Prior to delivery of the neonates, prepare a warm, padded box for them. Prepare an oxygen delivery system (such as an Ayre's T Piece and small face mask), catheters and syringes for airway suction, clean towels for drying, and resuscitation drugs (doxapram to stimulate respiration; naloxone to reverse opioid drugs).

On delivery, the resuscitator should ensure that the nares and mouth are clear of membranes and fluids, and begin to revive the neonates. Vigorous rubbing along the body provides strong stimulation for spontaneous respiration. Oxygen

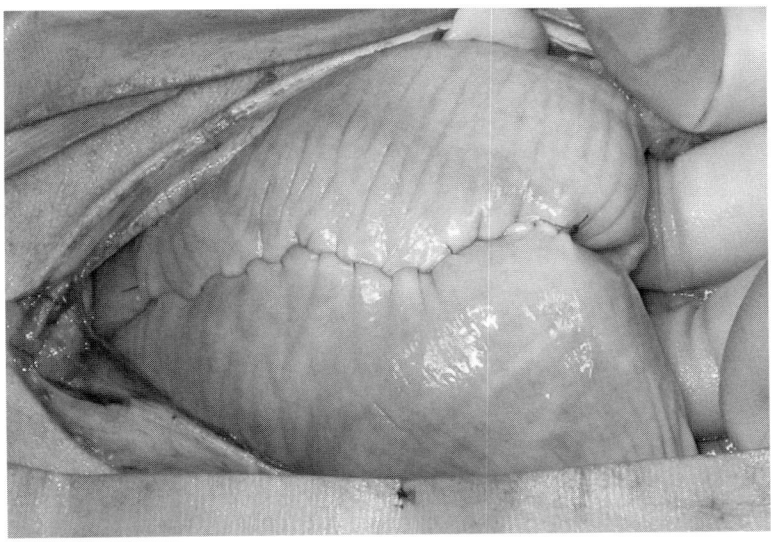

Fig. 14.23. Caesarean section – close the uterus in one or two layers.

supplementation by mask should be given during this period. An intravenous catheter and syringe can be used to clear the nares of fluid. Swinging of neonates to clear airways is not recommended because of the potential to induce serious injury.

Doxapram is given sublingually or by injection into the umbilical vein to stimulate respiration. Naloxone is given to reverse opioid drugs if required. The neonates can take several minutes to start to breathe well spontaneously, and the resuscitator should persevere during this period. Clean and ligate the umbilicus with short-acting, absorbable suture material.

Post-operative management

As soon as the dam has recovered sufficiently from anaesthesia, the neonates should be encouraged to feed. Check the dam for milk production and supplement the litter if required. Discharge the dam and litter as soon as possible (preferably the same day) to reduce stress and to limit contact between the litter and pathogens within the hospital environment. It is important to ensure that the dam has adequate pain relief and that drugs that have been prescribed are not contraindicated in lactating animals.

Complications

The prognosis for the dam following caesarean section is good but she may be predisposed to future episodes of dystocia, and it is generally recommended that she not be bred from again. Neonatal mortality may be as high as 20% in the first 7 days following caesarean section and is higher than the rate reported following unassisted delivery.

A range of complications, including eclampsia, retained placentas, and metritis, may occur following caesarean section. Eclampsia is a life-threatening condition that leads to hypocalcaemia in lactating bitches and queens due to the increased turnover of calcium within the body. Small breed dogs with large litters are at greatest risk. Eclampsia may develop around the time of parturition but most animals develop the condition between 2 and 4 weeks following parturition. Initially, animals may show signs including altered behaviour, weakness, vomiting, polydipsia, facial pruritis, and muscle tremors. Signs may progress to seizures and severe bradycardia. The diagnosis is made by combination of documenting hypocalcaemia (preferably by assessment of ionized calcium), clinical signs, and historical findings. It is treated by intravenous administration of calcium gluconate followed by oral calcium supplementation once signs have stabilized. Anticonvulsant therapy may be required in animals that are seizuring. The neonates should be removed from the dam for at least 12 h and fed a milk substitute. Consider early weaning of the litter.

Bibliography

Agudelo, C.F. (2005) Cystic endometrial hyperplasia-pyometra complex in cats. A review. *Veterinary Quarterly* 27, 173–182.

Anon (2010a) New Animal Welfare Act. www.regjeringen.no/en/doc/Laws/Acts/animal-welfare-act.html, accessed 21 May 2010.

Anon (2010b) Specific guidelines regarding the Animal Welfare Act. www.regjeringen.no/en/dep/lmd/whats-new/news/2009/mai-09/new-animal-welfare-act-/specific-guidelines-regarding-the-animal.html, accessed 21 May 2010.

Ball, R.L., Birchard, S.J., May, L.R., Threlfall, W.R. and Young, G.S. (2010) Ovarian remnant syndrome in dogs and cats: 21 cases (2000–2007). *Journal of the American Veterinary Medical Association* 236, 548–553.

BVA (2011) Veterinary reporting of caesarean sections. www.bva.co.uk/publications_and_resources/Forms.aspx, accessed 28 February 2011.

Coe, R.J., Grint, N.J., Tivers, M.S., Hotston Moore, A. and Holt, P.E. (2006) Comparison of flank and midline approaches to the ovariohysterectomy of cats. *Veterinary Record* 159, 309–313.

De Bleser, B., Brodbelt, D.C., Gregory, N.G. and Martinez, T.A. (2011) The association between acquired urinary sphincter mechanism incompetence in bitches and early spaying: a case-control study. *Veterinary Journal* 187, 42–47.

De Schepper, J., De Cock, I. and Capiau, E. (1989) Urinary gamma-glutamyl transferase and the degree of renal dysfunction in 75 bitches with pyometra. *Research in Veterinary Science* 46, 396–400.

Evans, H.E. and Christensen, G.C. (1993) The female genital organs. In: Evans, H.E. (ed.) *Miller's Anatomy of the Dog*, 3rd edn. W.B. Saunders, Philadelphia, Pennsylvania, pp. 531–558.

Evans, K.M. and Adams, V.J. (2010) Proportion of litters of purebred dogs born by caesarean section. *Journal of Small Animal Practice* 51, 113–118.

Fingland, R.B. (1998) Uterus. In: Bojrab, M.J. (ed.) *Current Techniques in Small Animal Surgery*, 4th edn. Williams and Wilkins, London, pp. 489–502.

Fransson, B.A. and Ragle, C.A. (2003) Canine pyometra: an update on pathogenesis and treatment. *Compendium of Continuing Education for the Practicing Veterinarian* 25, 602–612.

Gunn-Moore, D.A. and Thrusfield, M.V. (1995) Feline dystocia: prevalence, and association with cranial conformation and breed. *Veterinary Record* 136, 350–353.

Howe, L.M. (2006) Surgical methods of contraception and sterilization. *Theriogenology* 66, 500–509.

Jackson, P.G.G. (2004a) Cesarean section. *Handbook of Veterinary Obstetrics*, 2nd edn. Elsevier, Edinburgh, pp. 173–198.

Jackson, P.G.G. (2004b) Dystocia in the dog and cat. *Handbook of Veterinary Obstetrics*, 2nd edn. Elsevier, Edinburgh, pp. 141–166.

Jackson, P.G.G. (2004c) Normal birth. *Handbook of Veterinary Obstetrics*, 2nd edn. Elsevier, Edinburgh, pp. 1–12.

Kim, Y., Travis, A.J. and Meyers-Wallen, V.N. (2007) Parturition prediction and timing of canine pregnancy. *Theriogenology* 68, 1177–1182.

Kustritz, M.V. (2002) Early spay-neuter: clinical considerations. *Clinical Techniques in Small Animal Practice* 17, 124–128.

Lee, W.M., Kooistra, H.S., Mol, J.A., Dieleman, S.J. and Schaefers-Okkens, A.C. (2006) Ovariectomy during the luteal phase influences secretion of prolactin, growth hormone, and insulin-like growth factor-I in the bitch. *Theriogenology* 66, 484–490.

Luvoni, G.C. and Beccaglia, M. (2006) The prediction of parturition date in canine pregnancy. *Reproduction in Domestic Animals* 41, 27–32.

Moon-Massat, P.F. and Erb, H.N. (2002) Perioperative factors associated with puppy vigor after delivery by cesarean section. *Journal of the American Animal Hospital Association* 38, 90–96.

Nak, D., Nak, Y. and Tuna, B. (2009) Follow-up examinations after medical treatment of pyometra in cats with the progesterone-antagonist aglepristone. *Journal of Feline Medicine and Surgery* 11, 499–502.

O'Farrell, V. and Peachey, E. (1990) Behavioural effects of ovariohysterectomy on bitches. *Journal of Small Animal Practice* 31, 595–598.

Pretzer, S.D. (2008) Clinical presentation of canine pyometra and mucometra: a review. *Theriogenology* 70, 359–363.

RCVS (2008) Advice note 19 – Anaesthesia. www.rcvs.org.uk/advice-and-guidance/advice-notes, accessed 11 May 2010.

RCVS (2010) Guide to Professional Conduct. www.rcvs.org.uk/advice-and-guidance/guide-to-professional-conducts-for-veterinary-surgeons, accessed 17 May 2011.

Reichler, I.M. (2009) Gonadectomy in cats and dogs: a review of risks and benefits. *Reproduction in Domestic Animals* 44, 29–35.

Reichler, I.M., Welle, M., Eckrich, C., Sattler, U., Barth, A., Hubler, M., Nett-Mettler, C.S., *et al.* (2008) Spaying-induced coat changes: the role of gonadotropins, GnRH and GnRH treatment on the hair cycle of female dogs. *Veterinary Dermatology* 19, 77–87.

Robbins, M.A. and Mullen, H.S. (1994) En bloc ovariohysterectomy as a treatment for dystocia in dogs and cats. *Veterinary Surgery* 23, 48–52.

Ryan, S.D. and Wagner, A.E. (2006) Cesarean section in dogs: physiological and perioperative considerations. *Compendium of Continuing Education for the Practicing Veterinarian* 28, 34–43.

Smith, F.O. (2006) Canine pyometra. *Theriogenology* 66, 610–612.

Smith, F.O. (2007) Challenges in small animal parturition – timing elective and emergency cesarean sections. *Theriogenology* 68, 348–353.

Traas, A.M. (2008a) Resuscitation of canine and feline neonates. *Theriogenology* 70, 343–348.

Traas, A.M. (2008b) Surgical management of canine and feline dystocia. *Theriogenology* 70, 337–342.

Van Goethem, B., Schaefers-Okkens, A. and Kirpensteijn, J. (2006) Making a rational choice between ovariectomy and ovariohysterectomy in the dog: a discussion of the benefits of either technique. *Veterinary Surgery* 35, 136–143.

Verstegen, J., Dhaliwal, G. and Verstegen-Onclin, K. (2008) Mucometra, cystic endometrial hyperplasia, and pyometra in the bitch: advances in treatment and assessment of future reproductive success. *Theriogenology* 70, 364–374.

Wiebe, V.J. and Howard, J.P. (2009) Pharmacologic advances in canine and feline reproduction. *Topics in Companion Animal Medicine* 24, 71–99.

15 Testicular Surgery

closed castration: castration keeping the parietal tunic intact
cryptorchidism: failure of one or both testicles to descend into the scrotum
open castration: castration opening the parietal tunic

The reader should be able to:

- list the indications for castration in the dog and cat
- describe the anatomy of the spermatic cord
- define the difference between open and closed castration and explain the merits of each
- complete, with the assistance of a qualified veterinary surgeon, prescrotal castration in a dog (both open and closed techniques)
- complete, under the direct supervision a qualified veterinary surgeon, open scrotal castration in a cat
- describe the investigation and management of an adult cat that has no scrotal testicles but is suspected of being cryptorchid

Testicular surgery in the dog and cat is largely confined to elective castration to control breeding and modify behaviour. The health and management benefits of castration are generally thought to outweigh the disadvantages but, as for ovariohysterectomy, local practices may vary. Castration may be performed for prophylactic or therapeutic reasons.

Indications for prophylactic castration

- Prevent breeding.
- Behaviour modification: castration may reduce aggression, roaming, and inappropriate sexual behaviour if performed before these become learned traits; castration reduces urine spraying and the pungency of urine in tomcats.
- Prevent prostatic disease.
- Prevent testicular neoplasia.
- Prevent perineal hernia.

Indications for therapeutic castration

- Testicular neoplasia.
- Testicular torsion.
- Prostatic disease.
- Perianal adenoma.
- Prevent recurrence of perineal hernia following repair.
- Prevent recurrence of urethral prolapse.

Timing of Elective Castration

Prophylactic castration has traditionally been performed in dogs and cats from 5–6 months of age. Early castration, like early ovariohysterectomy, is also being promoted from 8 weeks of age to help population control and for other health benefits (e.g. the incidence of infectious disease is lower in castrated, compared to entire, cats). Early castration does not appear to increase the rate of complications, and patients recover very quickly, but it can only be performed in patients that have both testicles descended into the scrotum. In male cats, concerns have been raised that early castration may increase the incidence of lower urinary tract disease but there is little evidence to support this.

Legislation

The legislation controlling castration is similar to that controlling ovariohysterectomy and legislation differs between countries (see Chapter 14).

Testicular Neoplasia

Testicular tumours are common in dogs. The commonest forms are seminoma, interstitial cell tumour, and Sertoli cell tumour. Cryptorchidism is a major risk factor for the development of Sertoli cell tumour and seminoma. Testicular tumours have a low metastatic rate and castration is usually curative. The main clinical finding is testicular enlargement, but Sertoli cell tumours may cause *feminization syndrome* through production of oestrogen. Signs include attractiveness to male dogs, pendulous prepuce, gynaecomastia, atrophy of the contralateral testicle, symmetrical alopecia, melanosis (heavily pigmented skin) and, in severely affected cases, myelosuppression. In contrast, male cats rarely get testicular neoplasia probably because of the high rate of prepubertal castration.

The treatment of choice for testicular tumours is castration. Animals with severe myelosuppression due to hyperoestrogenism are at increased risk of bleeding during surgery and may require preoperative blood transfusion.

Cryptorchidism

Cryptorchidism (retained testicle) can affect one or both testicles. The undescended testicle may be located in the abdomen, the inguinal canal, or subcutaneously under the inguinal skin. Normally, the testicles descend into the scrotum by 2 months of age. If they have not descended by 6 months of age, it is unlikely that they will descend. Cryptorchidism can be diagnosed by scrotal palpation but it can be difficult to locate the retained testicle. Inguinal testicles are usually palpable but can be difficult to find if the testicles are small or obscured by fat. Abdominal testicles are rarely palpable and can be missed easily during abdominal ultrasound. The general recommendation is to castrate cryptorchid animals because of the association with testicular neoplasia, and because the condition is heritable.

Many dogs and cats are rehomed as adults and, having no palpable scrotal or inguinal testicles, are assumed to be castrated. It is possible, however, that they have cryptorchidism. To investigate cryptorchidism, abdominal ultrasound or hormone assays (gonadotrophin-releasing hormone (GnRH) or human chlorionic gonadotrophin (hCG) stimulation tests that check for induced testosterone surges) can be performed. Uncastrated male cats develop seasonal penile spurs during the spring and summer months that can be helpful in distinguishing between castrated and cryptorchid cats (Fig. 15.1).

Techniques

There are numerous castration methods and a selection of simple ones to meet most clinical scenarios is presented here. Castration is classified as a clean procedure and perioperative prophylactic antimicrobials are not indicated.

Anatomy

The regional anatomy of the male genitalia differs between the dog and cat and this influences the approach to routine castration in the two species. In cats, the penis and scrotum are positioned caudally in the perineal region, preventing prescrotal castration.

The testicles and spermatic structures (testicular artery, pampiniform plexus of testicular veins, ductus deferens, testicular nerve, and lymphatic vessels) are enclosed within a double sheath of

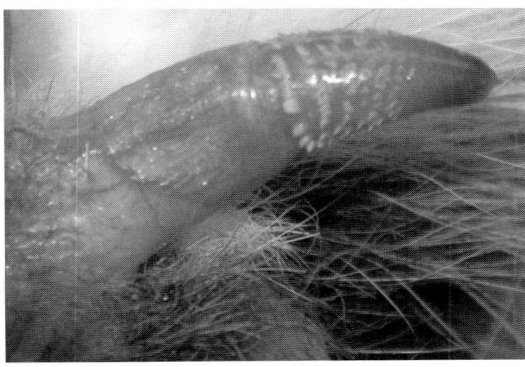

Fig. 15.1. Penile spines indicate that the cat is intact.

mesothelium. This is an extension of the peritoneal lining. The visceral tunic (inner sheath) is intimately apposed to the surface of the testicle and the structures running to and from it. The parietal tunic (outer sheath) is separated from the visceral tunic by a potential space that is contiguous with the peritoneal cavity. The ligament of the tail of the epididymis is the remnant of the gubernaculum. It runs between the visceral and parietal tunics at the caudal pole of the testicle, anchoring the testicle in the scrotum. The internal and external spermatic fasciae arise from the abdominal fascia. The internal spermatic fascia is intimately apposed to the parietal tunic and together these form a thick sheath over the testicle. The external spermatic fascia lies subcutaneously and is separated from the internal spermatic fascia by loose connective tissue. The cremaster muscle, which retracts the testicle, is an extension of the internal abdominal oblique muscle and runs with the internal spermatic fascia in close association with the parietal tunic.

The testicular artery originates from the aorta. The testicular veins drain into the caudal vena cava or renal vein. The ductus deferens has a smaller, distinct blood supply originating from the prostatic vessels.

Closed versus open castration

Closed castration is castration without incising into the parietal tunic. This means that the potential space that extends into the peritoneal cavity between the parietal and visceral tunics is not penetrated. The advantages of closed castration are that there is little risk of ascending infection into the abdomen or of evisceration if the patient has an undiagnosed scrotal hernia. The disadvantage is that ligatures are applied around the parietal tunic rather than directly on to the testicular vessels, and may be less effective.

Open castration is castration with incision into the parietal tunic to expose the visceral tunic and spermatic structures. Haemostasis is better than in closed castration because the vessels are ligated directly, but evisceration of herniated organs and peritonitis may be more likely.

There are no comparative studies of these techniques in the dog or cat and, as evisceration, peritonitis, and life-threatening haemorrhage are all rare complications of castration in these species, the decision of which to perform remains one of personal choice. Some authors recommend that

open castration is performed in larger dogs (e.g. >20 kg).

Prescrotal castration – closed (dog)

Prescrotal castration is the standard technique performed in dogs. Both testicles are removed through a single skin incision immediately in front of the scrotum. This technique avoids making incisions into the scrotal skin as it is thin, sensitive, and difficult to prepare aseptically.

Approach

Position the dog in dorsal recumbency. Clip hair from the cranial scrotum to halfway along the penis. Drape the scrotum just out of the surgical field but ensure that the testicles can be manipulated through the drapes and pushed into the prescrotal position (Fig. 15.2). Push the first testicle forward through the drapes until it sits subcutaneously in front of the scrotum within the surgical field. Stabilize it and

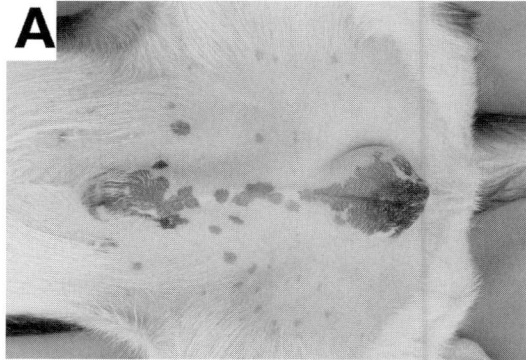

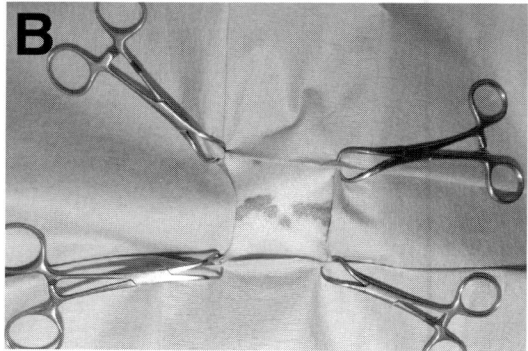

Fig. 15.2. Prescrotal castration: (A) positioning and clip; (B) drape just in front of the scrotum.

make a ventral midline skin incision along the length of the testicle. Continue the incision through the subcutaneous fat and the external spermatic fascia until the parietal tunic is exposed (do not incise the parietal tunic) (Fig. 15.3).

Exteriorize the testicle

Squeeze the testicle (within the parietal tunic) out of the skin incision by applying firm pressure on either side (Fig. 15.4). Extend the incision in the spermatic fascia if necessary. Hold the testicle up and break down the firm, caudal attachments of the parietal tunic to the scrotum using a combination of blunt and sharp dissection (Fig. 15.5).

Ligate the spermatic cord and amputate the testicle

Clear fat away from the spermatic cord with a swab. Identify the cremaster muscle running along

the caudal edge of the parietal tunic. Use triple clamp technique as described for ovariohysterectomy (see p. 225). Apply three haemostats to the parietal tunic and spermatic cord, starting close to

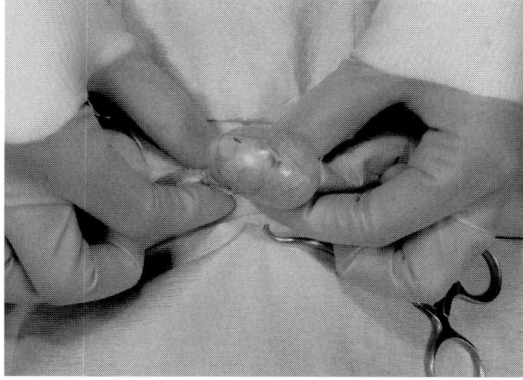

Fig. 15.4. Prescrotal castration: squeeze to prolapse the testicle out of the incision.

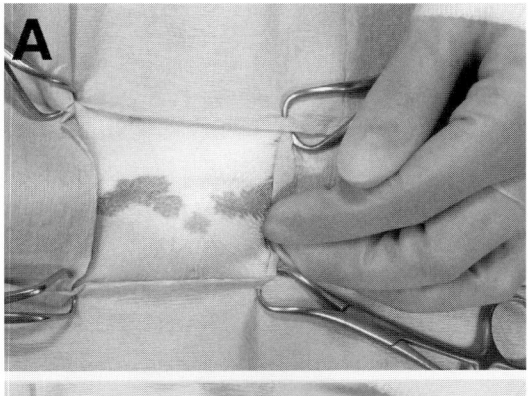

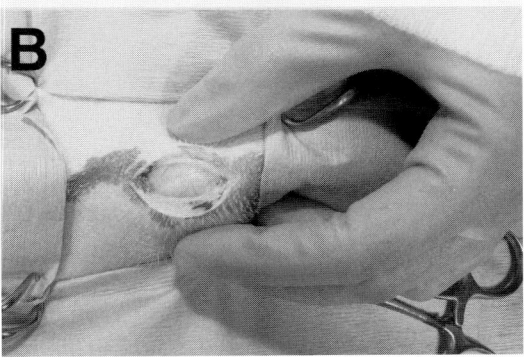

Fig. 15.3. Prescrotal castration: (A) push first testicle up into position; (B) incise over testicle without penetrating the parietal tunic.

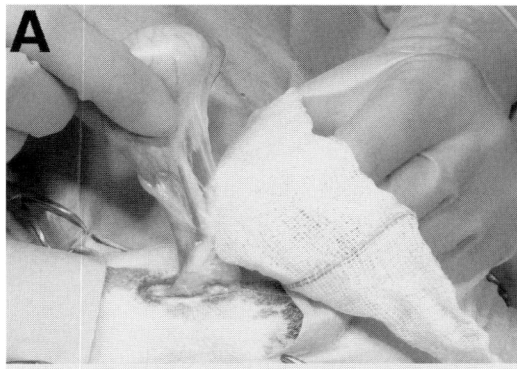

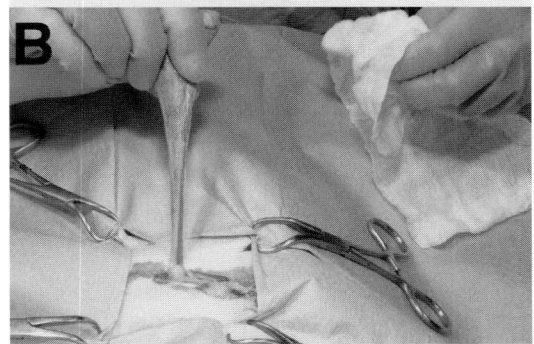

Fig. 15.5. Prescrotal castration: break down the fascial attachments to the caudal aspect of the testicle (A) to fully exteriorize the testicle (B).

the skin incision, and avoiding the pampiniform plexus near the testicle. Leave a gap between the proximal and middle haemostats to enable the placement of a transfixing ligature. Tie a circumferential ligature into the crush line created by the proximal haemostat. Place a transfixing ligature into the spermatic cord between the proximal and middle clamps, anchoring this into the cremaster muscle to prevent slippage of the suture if the muscle contracts (Fig. 15.6). Amputate the testicle by incising between the middle and distal clamps. Hold the stump with non-traumatic forceps and release the clamp. Check the pedicle for bleeding before returning it into the skin incision and releasing it (Fig. 15.7B).

Remove second testicle

Push the second testicle cranially into the surgical field (Fig. 15.7B). Incise through the spermatic

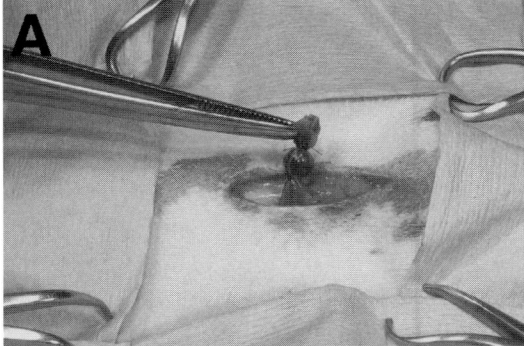

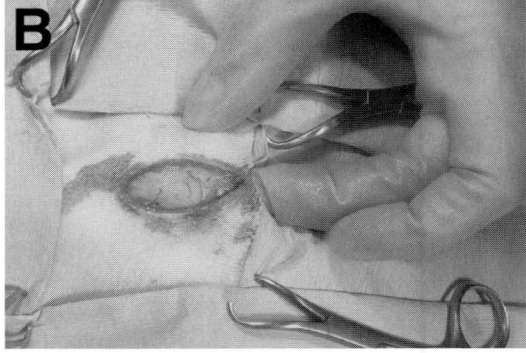

Fig. 15.7. Prescrotal castration: (A) having amputated the testicle between the middle and distal haemostat, check for haemorrhage of the stump before releasing it; (B) push the second testicle into position and proceed as before.

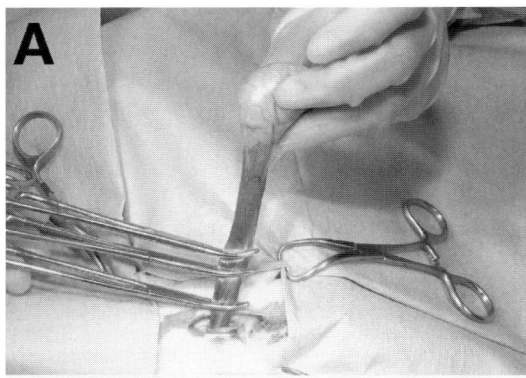

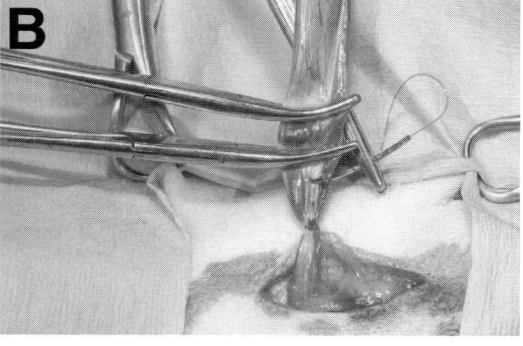

Fig. 15.6. Prescrotal castration: (A) apply three haemostats to the testicle; (B) place a circumferential ligature in the crush line of the proximal clamp and a transfixing ligature between the first ligature and the middle clamp.

fascia overlying this testicle (via the original skin incision) and proceed as above to exteriorize and resect the testicle.

Closure

Suture the outer edges of both spermatic fascia incisions to each other with a simple continuous pattern of absorbable, short-lasting, monofilament suture material (Fig. 15.8). Close the subcutaneous tissue. Place an intradermal suture pattern to appose the skin edges (skin sutures cause irritation through rubbing on the inner thigh).

Prescrotal castration – open (dog)

To perform open castration, proceed as described above. Push the testicle into the prescrotal position. Incise the skin and the external spermatic fascia over it.

Continue the incision through the parietal tunic to expose the testicle and visceral tunic. Squeeze firmly to prolapse the testicle out of the parietal tunic (Fig. 15.9). The testicle remains tethered by the

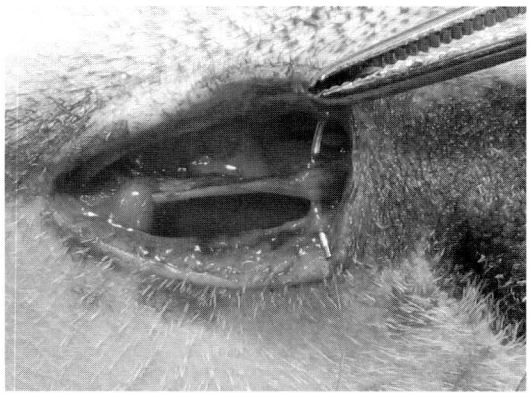

Fig. 15.8. Prescrotal castration: suture the edges of the incisions in the external spermatic fascia together before closing the subcutaneous tissues and skin separately. Take care not to include the urethra.

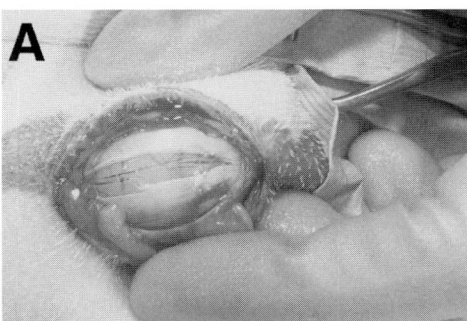

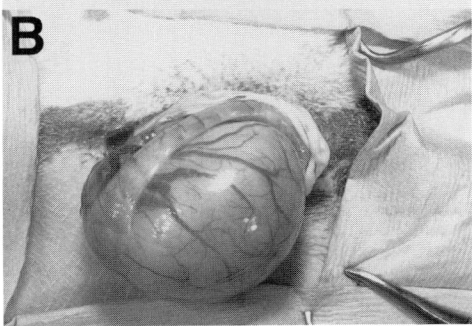

Fig. 15.9. Open castration: (A) incise directly over the testicle and into the parietal tunic; (B) prolapse the testicle from within the parietal tunic.

proper ligament between the caudal pole of the testicle and the parietal tunic. Disrupt the proper ligament by tearing it off the testicle to mobilize the testicle completely (Fig. 15.10). Apply three haemostats to the spermatic structures below the pampiniform plexus (Fig. 15.11). Release the proximal clamp and tie a circumferential ligature into the crush line. Place a transfixing ligature between the proximal ligature and middle haemostat. Amputate the testicle between the middle and distal haemostats. Hold the pedicle with plain forceps, release the haemostat, and check for bleeding before releasing the pedicle into the incision. Repeat the process for the second testicle. Close the external spermatic fascia, subcutaneous tissues, and skin as described above.

Castration with scrotal ablation

Castration can be combined with removal of the scrotum (*en bloc* resection of the testicles). This is

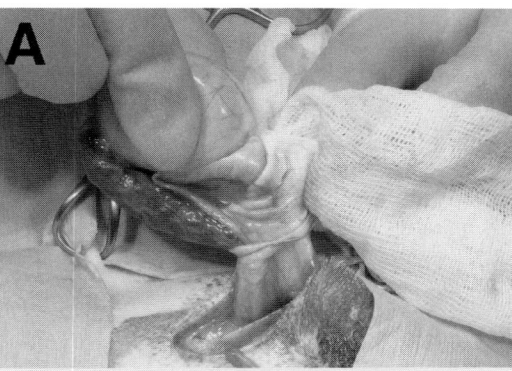

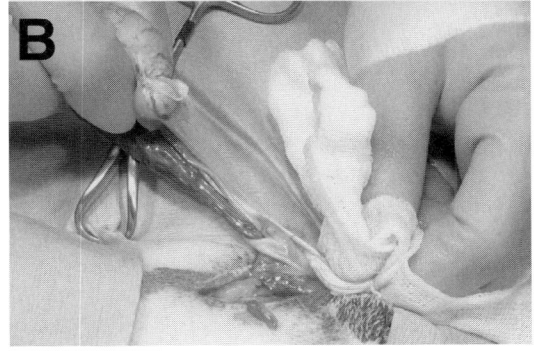

Fig. 15.10. Open castration: break down the proper ligament between the caudal pole of the testicle and the parietal tunic by avulsing the tunic from the testicle: (A) before; (B) after.

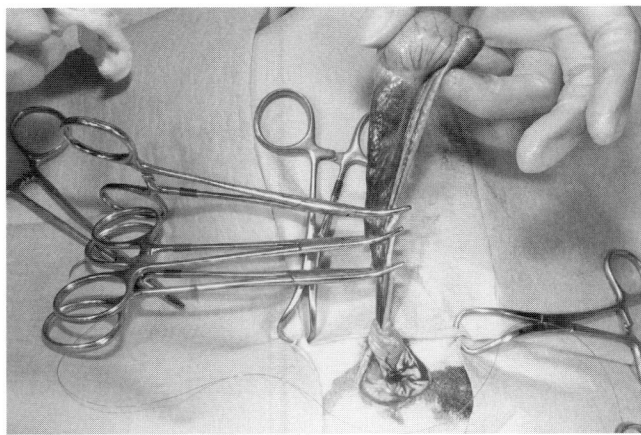

Fig. 15.11. Open castration: apply haemostats, ligate the spermatic structures and amputate the testicle.

indicated for castration when the scrotum is also diseased (e.g. scrotal mast cell tumour; adherent testicular tumour).

Clip and prepare the scrotum and surrounding skin. Make an incision that encircles the base of the scrotum. The incision should be made just outside the border between the scrotal and inguinal skin, ensuring that inguinal rather than scrotal skin is incised (Fig. 15.12A). Dissect the fascia and fat using a combination of blunt and sharp dissection to expose the spermatic cords within the parietal tunics (Fig. 15.12B). Proceed as described above for closed castration. Close the wound using the same principles as described for prescrotal castration.

Scrotal castration (cat)

Open scrotal castration is the standard method of castration in the cat. The testicles are removed through two separate skin incisions in the scrotum as there is no space to perform prescrotal castration.

Technique

The scrotum is clipped or plucked and prepared for surgery. Squeeze the testicles into the base of the scrotum so that the scrotal skin is taut against them. Make a vertical incision in the scrotum directly over the first testicle and to one side of midline to avoid damaging the prepuce (Fig. 15.13A). Extend the skin incision through the parietal tunic to expose the testicle. Squeeze gently to prolapse the testicle out of the parietal tunic.

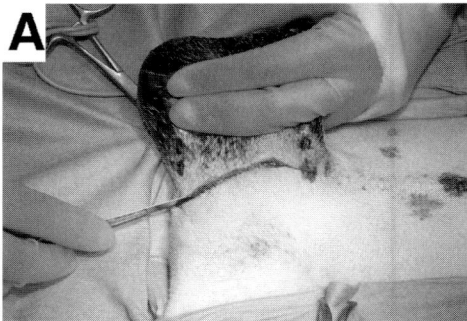

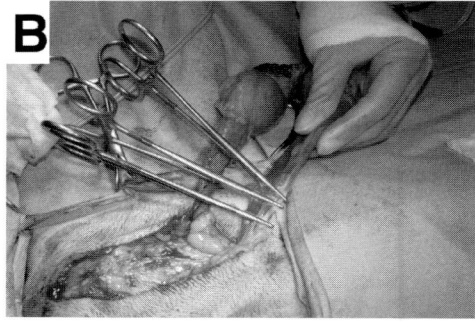

Fig. 15.12. Scrotal ablation: (A) incise round base of scrotum; (B) dissect to locate spermatic cord then proceed as described above.

Take care when prolapsing the testicle not to apply excessive pressure as this can cause the testicle to rupture. Tear the proper ligament between testicle and parietal tunic and draw the testicle away from the body (Fig. 15.13B). Separate the ductus deferens

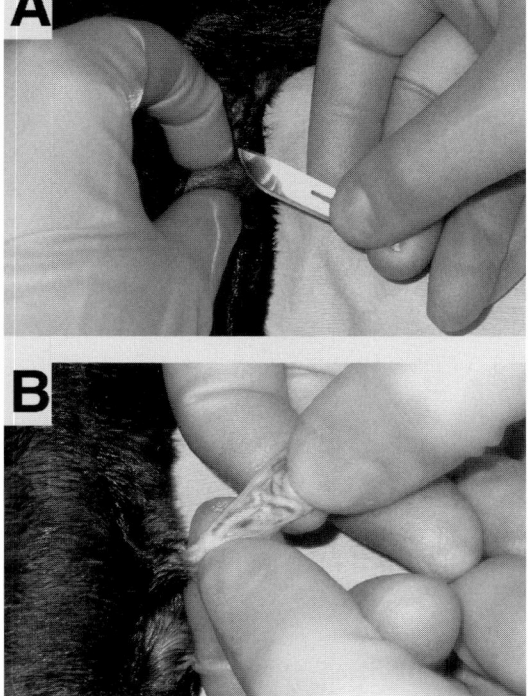

Fig. 15.13. Open scrotal castration: (A) squeeze testicles into scrotum and make vertical incision into the parietal tunic; (B) disrupt proper ligament to withdraw testicle.

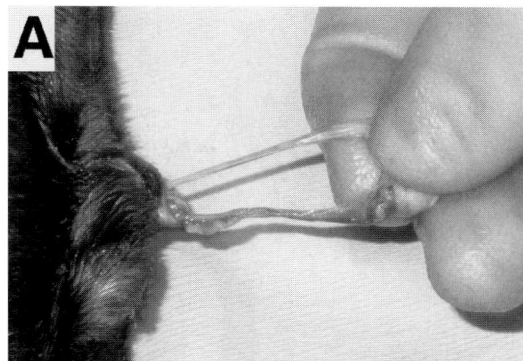

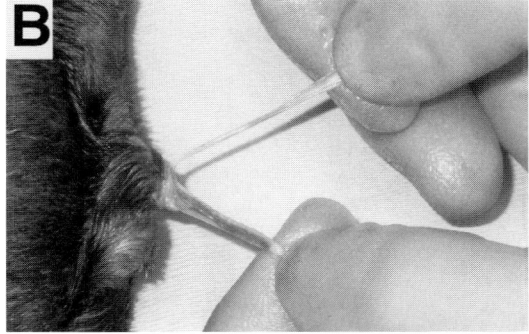

Fig. 15.14. Open scrotal castration: (A) separate ductus deferens from vessels; (B) tear ductus deferens off testicle.

from the testicular vessels and tear it from the testicle (Fig. 15.14). Tie a four-throw, square knot between the ductus deferens and vessels to achieve haemostasis. Amputate the testicle distal to the knot (Fig. 15.15). Check for haemorrhage and return the spermatic structures to the scrotum. Make a second skin incision in the scrotum over the second testicle and repeat this process.

Cryptorchid castration

If the undescended testicle cannot be located pre-operatively, be prepared to explore both the inguinal region and the abdomen.

Inguinal testicles

Make a longitudinal incision directly over the testicle in the inguinal canal. Extend through the subcutaneous fat, fascia, and parietal tunic to expose the testicle. Proceed as described for open castration above.

Abdominal testicles

Clip and prepare the abdomen for exploratory surgery. Perform a caudal midline coeliotomy (through a parapreputial skin incision in male dogs, see p. 132) and locate the testicle. The testicle is usually identified as the most lateral structure in the abdomen, lying in the paralumbar fossa between the caudal pole of the kidney and the inguinal canal (Fig. 15.16). If it cannot be located easily, trace the ductus deferens from the bladder neck back to the testicle. Enlarged abdominal testicles may migrate away from this position and the abdominal incision may need to be extended to locate and remove the testicle. Once the testicle is located, double ligate and divide the testicular vessels and the ductus deferens separately to amputate the testicle.

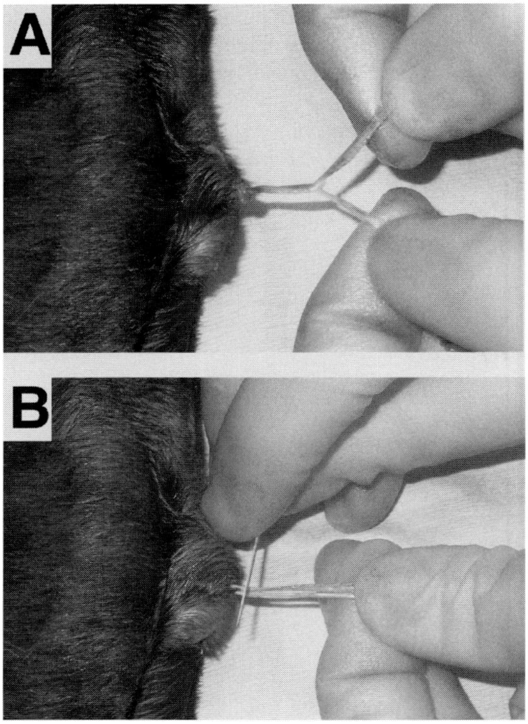

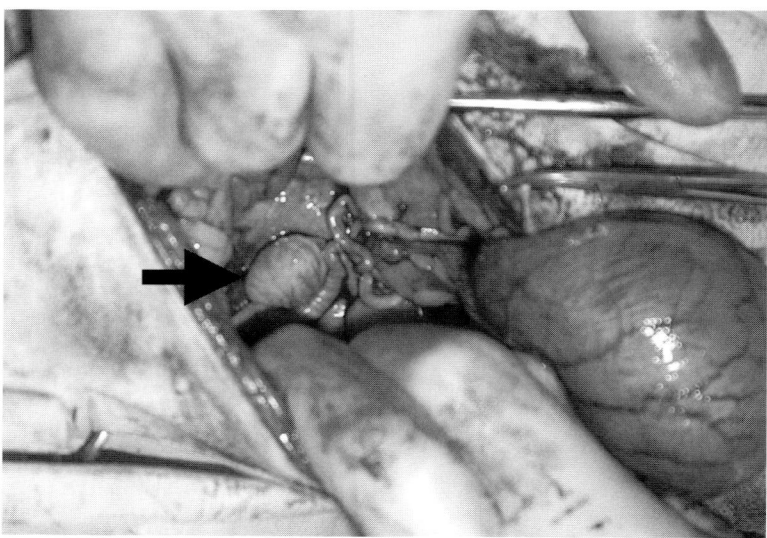

Fig. 15.15. Open scrotal castration: (A) tie square knot between ductus deferens and testicular vessels; (B) amputate testicle distal to the knot.

Testicle in inguinal canal

Occasionally a retained testicle gets lodged in the inguinal canal, complicating retrieval. Although the testicle is not palpable in the inguinal region, it cannot be identified by an abdominal approach (the ductus deferens and vessels enter the inguinal canal normally). Either the testicle can be pulled into the abdomen by gentle traction on the ductus deferens (taking care not to avulse it) or a direct approach through the skin to the inguinal canal can be made.

Complications

Scrotal haematomas may develop post-operatively because of capillary haemorrhage within the scrotum and parietal tunic. Most cases can be managed conservatively but, if the haematoma is associated with dysuria, extreme discomfort, or ongoing haemorrhage, revisional surgery is required. Either evacuate the haematoma through the original incision and ligate any bleeding vessels, or perform scrotal ablation.

Significant haemorrhage from the testicular artery or vein is rare but can lead to life-threatening blood loss. There may be few external signs of bleeding. The testicular vessels may retract back into the abdomen leading to abdominal, rather

Fig. 15.16. Abdominal testicle located between the bladder and the body wall (bladder has been reflected caudally).

than scrotal, bleeding. Signs that should prompt evaluation include prolonged recovery from anaesthesia, dripping of blood from the castration incision, abdominal distension, pallor, and other signs of hypovolaemic shock. Emergency surgery to isolate and ligate the vessels is required. This may necessitate extending the prescrotal incision towards the inguinal canal to locate the bleeding stump, or performing exploratory coeliotomy and following principles similar to those described for addressing ovarian pedicle haemorrhage (see Chapter 14). Call for assistance from an experienced colleague.

Acquired urinary incontinence in male dogs associated with neutering is rare, but leads to a similar syndrome to acquired sphincter mechanism incompetence in female dogs (see Chapter 14). This complication does not occur in cats.

Bibliography

Birchard, S.J. and Nappier, M. (2008) Cryptorchidism. *Compendium of Continuing Education for the Practicing Veterinarian* 30, 325–336; quiz 336–327.

Evans, H.E. and Christensen, G.C. (1993) The male genital organs. In: Evans, H.E. (ed.) *Miller's Anatomy of the Dog*, 3rd edn. W.B. Saunders, Philadelphia, Pennsylvania, pp. 504–531.

Grieco, V., Riccardi, E., Greppi, G.F., Teruzzi, F., Iermano, V. and Finazzi, M. (2008) Canine testicular tumours: a study on 232 dogs. *Journal of Comparative Pathology* 138, 86–89.

Hardie, E.M. (1984) Selected surgeries of the male and female reproductive tracts. *Veterinary Clinics of North America Small Animal Practice* 14, 109–122.

Howe, L.M. (2006) Surgical methods of contraception and sterilization. *Theriogenology* 66, 500–509.

Howe, L.M., Slater, M.R., Boothe, H.W., Hobson, H.P., Fossum, T.W., Spann, A.C. and Wilkie, W.S. (2000) Long-term outcome of gonadectomy performed at an early age or traditional age in cats. *Journal of the American Veterinary Medical Association* 217, 1661–1665.

Kustritz, M.V. (2002) Early spay-neuter: clinical considerations. *Clinical Techniques in Small Animal Practice* 17, 124–128.

Liao, A.T., Chu, P.Y., Yeh, L.S., Lin, C.T. and Liu, C.H. (2009) A 12-year retrospective study of canine testicular tumors. *Journal of Veterinary Medical Science* 71, 919–923.

McEntee, M.C. (2002) Reproductive oncology. *Clinical Techniques in Small Animal Practice* 17, 133–149.

Memon, M.A. (2007) Common causes of male dog infertility. *Theriogenology* 68, 322–328.

Reichler, I.M. (2009) Gonadectomy in cats and dogs: a review of risks and benefits. *Reproduction in Domestic Animals* 44, 29–35.

Romagnoli, S.E. (1991) Canine cryptorchidism. *Veterinary Clinics of North America Small Animal Practice* 21, 533–544.

Stubbs, W.P. (1998) Testicles. In: Bojrab, M.J. (ed.) *Current Techniques in Small Animal Surgery*, 4th edn. Williams and Wilkins, London, pp. 511–526.

Turek, M.M. (2003) Cutaneous paraneoplastic syndromes in dogs and cats: a review of the literature. *Veterinary Dermatology* 14, 279–296.

16 Urinary Tract Surgery

crystalluria: microscopic crystals in urine
cystotomy: incision into the bladder
dysuria: difficulty passing urine
haematuria: bloody urine
pollakiuria: increased frequency of urination
prostatomegaly: prostatic enlargement
stranguria: straining to urinate
urethrostomy: creation of a permanent stoma into the urethra
urethrotomy: incision into the urethra
urine scald: contact dermatitis caused by urine
uroabdomen: urine leakage into the abdomen
urolith: a stone from the urinary tract (also nephrolith, ureterolith, cystolith)

The reader should be able to:

- formulate an investigation and treatment plan for a male dog with urolithiasis that presents with dysuria
- formulate an investigation and treatment plan for a male cat that presents with stranguria and a previous history of feline lower urinary tract disease (FLUTD)
- catheterize a male dog and female cat
- catheterize a female dog and male cat with the assistance of an experienced veterinary surgeon
- describe how to perform retrograde hydropulsion of urethral uroliths in a male dog
- describe how to perform cystotomy, urethrotomy, and urethrostomy in a male dog with urolithiasis
- list the common causes of prostatomegaly in the male dog and how to differentiate between them using historical and physical findings and abdominal ultrasound
- recognize urethral prolapse in the dog
- describe how to investigate a dog for possible urinary tract trauma following extensive abdominal and pelvic injuries

The main indication for urinary tract surgery is management of urolithiasis, and the key techniques of urethral catheterization, cystotomy, urethrotomy and urethrostomy are described within this context.

Canine Urolithiasis

Minerals salts excreted in urine precipitate to form microscopic crystals (crystalluria) that cause inflammation and predispose to urinary tract infection. The minerals precipitate because of factors like supersaturation of urine with mineral and the presence of urease-producing bacteria. Systemic disorders may also predispose to urolith formation (e.g. liver disease; hypercalcaemia). Ultimately, the crystals enlarge to form visible uroliths that can cause urinary tract obstruction. There are various forms of urolith and their chemical composition influences their management (summarized in Table 16.1). *Calcium oxalate* and *struvite* (magnesium ammonium phosphate) uroliths are the most common.

Historical and clinical findings

Patients with urolithiasis have signs of cystitis including haematuria, dysuria, and pollakiuria. Male dogs may also develop signs of urinary tract obstruction because their long, narrow urethras are easily blocked by small uroliths. Obstruction leads to unproductive straining to urinate and the bladder becomes large and distended with urine. As pressure builds up in the bladder, overflow incontinence (dripping of urine from the penis) may also be seen. In contrast, female dogs rarely develop urethral obstruction because they have short, wide urethras that allow uroliths to pass easily. Occasionally, large uroliths can be palpated in the bladder or in the urethra by abdominal, rectal, or perineal examination.

Investigation

The major differential diagnoses for urolithiasis are urinary tract infection (UTI) and neoplasia, which are also common and produce similar signs. UTI and urolithiasis also frequently occur together. The aims of investigation are to:

- confirm the diagnosis;
- establish the composition of uroliths;
- identify predisposing factors; and
- assess location and size of uroliths to plan treatment.

Urinalysis

Urinalysis involves microscopic examination of urine, biochemical testing with urine test strips, and urine culture. Urine can be collected from the middle of a stream of urine as it is being passed ('free-catch'), by urethral catheterization, or by cystocentesis. Of these methods, cystocentesis is

Table 16.1. Types of urolith, their predisposing causes, and management options.

Composition	Aetiology and risk factors	Prevention protocols
Struvite (also amenable to dissolution)	Urease-producing bacterial urinary tract infection (UTI) (most common) Idiopathic	Increase water intake[1] Feed magnesium and phosphate-restricted, urine-acidifying diets[2] Treat UTI
Calcium oxalate	Hypocalcaemia Dietary calcium supplementation Acidic urine	Treat hyperkalaemia Increase water intake Feed diets with adequate oxalate and phosphorus that alkalinize urine Potassium citrate supplementation[3] if urine pH<6.5 Consider thiazide diuretics
Urate	Portosystemic shunt Breed-association in Dalmatians and bulldogs (breeds excreting uric acid)	Treat liver disease if present Increase water intake Feed purine-restricted urine-alkalinizing diets Consider allopurinol Consider potassium citrate
Silica	Dietary intake of plant proteins such as corn gluten and soybean hulls	Increase water intake Avoid diets with high plant protein content Avoid urine acidification
Cystine (also amenable to dissolution)	Primary defect in cystine metabolism	Increase water intake Feed protein-restricted, alkalinizing diets Consider long-term 2-MPG therapy[4]: aim for urine cystine <200 mg/l

[1]Increased water intake: change from dry to tinned food; add additional water to food.
[2]Vitamin C: urine acidifier.
[3]Potassium citrate: urine alkalinizer.
[4]2-MPG: n-(2-mercaptoropionyl)-glycine.

preferred as the sample is least likely to become contaminated with bacteria during sampling. The mineral composition of urinary crystals can be determined by examining their morphology microscopically. However, the sample should be evaluated within 1 h of collection, as salts in urine can precipitate if the sample is left standing, leading to a false positive diagnosis of crystalluria. Urine collected by cystocentesis can be cultured to confirm the presence of bacterial infection.

Urolith analysis

To manage urolithiasis successfully, it is important to identify the composition of uroliths accurately. Occasionally, small uroliths are passed freely in urine and can be collected for analysis, but the main source of uroliths for analysis is from surgical removal. A variety of different methods are used to analyse the mineral content of uroliths. Many laboratories provide this service, but (at the time of writing) the Minnesota Urolith Center provides a free international service as part of an ongoing research programme to pool data on feline and canine uroliths from around the world. Details of the submission process can be obtained from www.cvm.umn.edu/depts/minnesotaurolithcenter/home.html.

Serum biochemistry

A range of systemic disorders may predispose to urolithiasis (Table 16.1). Serum biochemistry is used to screen for predisposing causes of urolithiasis and to monitor renal function in cases with urinary tract obstruction.

Imaging studies

Radiography and ultrasound are invaluable in confirming the diagnosis of uroliths, identifying their location, and planning treatment. Abdominal ultrasound is very sensitive in screening the bladder for uroliths and for differentiating between bladder neoplasia and other causes of dysuria. However, ultrasound provides little information about the urethra as it passes through the pelvic cavity and os penis, and is often inadequate for screening for urethral obstruction with uroliths.

Radiographic studies provide additional information, particularly about the urethral lumen. Radiodense uroliths may be visible on plain radiographs, but radiolucent or small uroliths are not (Fig. 16.1). Contrast radiographic studies increase the sensitivity of radiography. Positive-contrast studies use radio-opaque dyes to fill the urinary tract and outline radiolucent uroliths and points of obstruction. The *positive-contrast urethrogram* (contrast filling the urethra) is most useful for screening for urethral obstruction and should be performed in patients with suspected urethral uroliths (Figs 16.2 and 16.3). Double-contrast studies combine a positive-contrast agent and gas (CO_2 or NO_2) to delineate surface detail. The *double-contrast cystogram* is useful for identifying radiolucent uroliths and other bladder lesions such as neoplasia (Fig. 16.4). Use positive-contrast agents specifically indicated for use in the urinary tract (e.g. iothalamate meglumine).

Management of bladder uroliths without obstruction

Uroliths that are not causing obstruction can be managed either medically or surgically depending on the type of urolith and the severity of signs.

Medical dissolution

Medical dissolution of uroliths is possible for struvite uroliths that are not causing obstruction. Medical dissolution is achieved by dietary modification to reduce the saturation of mineral salts and increase acidity of urine. Drugs such as ascorbic acid may also be prescribed to acidify urine. If there is concurrent urinary tract infection, this must be treated, as urease-producing bacteria act as precipitating factors for struvite urolith formation. Medical dissolution avoids the need for surgery but it does not provide immediate relief from clinical signs. Diets used to dissolve struvite crystals may also exacerbate the formation of other forms of crystal. For example, therapy to dissolve struvite uroliths causes precipitation of calcium oxalate.

A variety of prescription diets are available for medical dissolution. Once the uroliths have been dissolved, the diet is changed to a maintenance diet to prevent uroliths forming again. Summaries of medical options for management of urolithiasis are available from a range of reference sources including the Minnesota Urolith Center (see above). Cystine uroliths are also amenable to medical dissolution but other forms, such as calcium oxalate, cannot be dissolved.

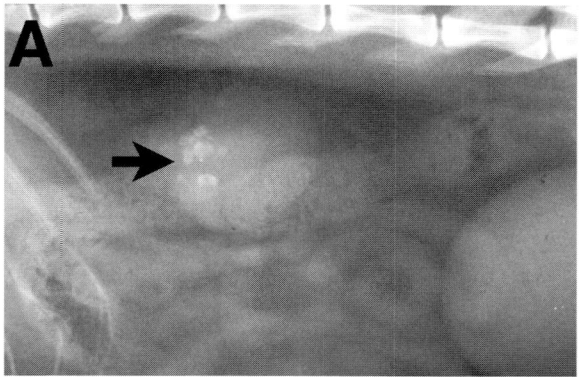

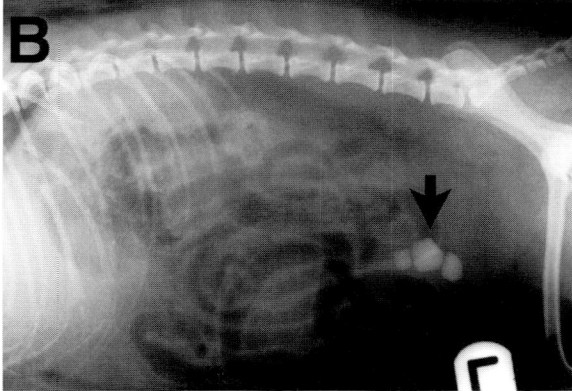

Fig. 16.1. Plain radiographs. Arrows indicate: (A) radiolucent nephroliths; (B) cystoliths.

Surgical removal

Surgical removal of uroliths that are not causing obstruction is indicated for patients with severe signs of cystitis or uroliths that are not dissolvable (e.g. calcium oxalate).

Management of uroliths causing urethral obstruction

A two-step approach is required to manage urethral obstruction: first the obstruction must be relieved, and then further urolith formation must be prevented. Uroliths should be collected and submitted for mineral analysis to enable long-term management to prevent recurrence.

Relieve urethral obstruction

Uroliths lodged in the male urethra can usually be dislodged and pushed back into the bladder by urethral catheterization and *retrograde hydropulsion* (see below). Once the obstruction has been relieved, if the uroliths are of a composition amenable to medical dissolution, this can attempted, but there is some risk that the patient will obstruct again before the uroliths have dissolved. Alternatively, *cystotomy* to remove the uroliths can be performed. This is well tolerated, removes the risk of early re-obstruction, enables uroliths to be collected for analysis, and is effective independent of the type of urolith present.

If the obstruction cannot be relieved, *urethrotomy* (direct incision over the urolith to remove it) is performed. However, as this is not as well tolerated as cystotomy, it should only be considered in cases that cannot be managed by retrograde hydropulsion and cystotomy. In some cases, uroliths cannot be removed even by urethrotomy (e.g. stones lodged within the os penis) and *urethrostomy* (creating a permanent stoma into the urethra)

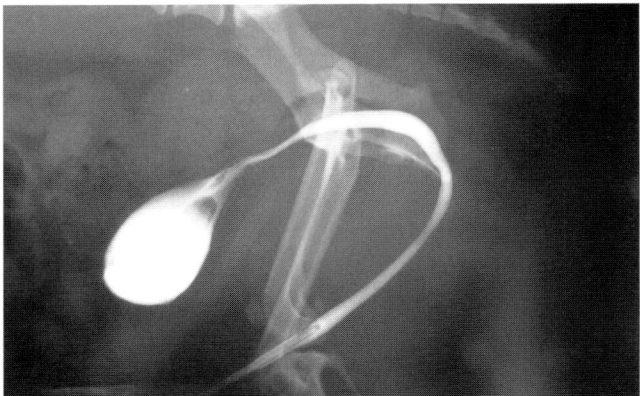

Fig. 16.2. Normal retrograde urethrogram: a wide column of contrast runs all the way to the bladder. The pelvic and prostatic urethra is wider than the perineal urethra. To perform this technique, preload a urinary catheter with an appropriate positive contrast agent (to prevent air bubbles); insert the catheter a short way into the urethra; inject 5–10 ml of contrast under pressure; take a radiograph immediately.

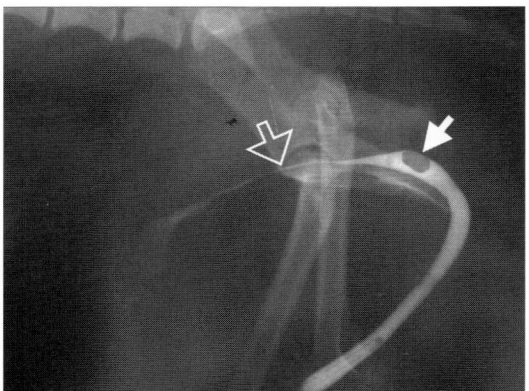

Fig. 16.3. Urethral obstruction: a urolith is partially obstructing the urethra. The wall of the urethra distorts around the urolith (solid arrow). Open arrow indicates point where urethral pressure was applied during retrograde hydropulsion to return these uroliths to the bladder (see p. 259).

proximal to the site of obstruction is necessary to provide an alternative route for urination.

Prevent recurrence

Once the obstruction has been relieved, steps to prevent recurrence by starting appropriate prescription

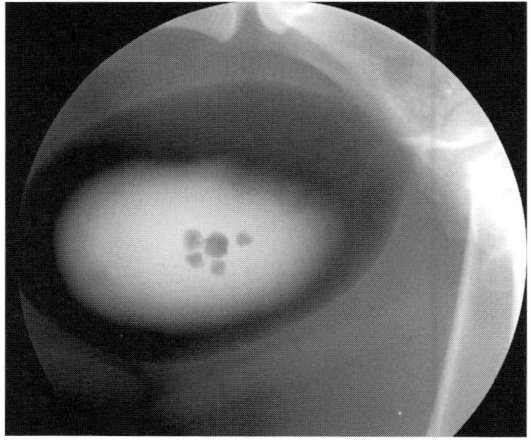

Fig. 16.4. Double-contrast cystogram demonstrating radiolucent uroliths. A retrograde urethrogram was performed (see Fig. 16.2 for details of technique) after 5–10 ml/kg of CO_2 had been introduced into the bladder (do not to inject under pressure). The positive contrast coats the mucosal lining and highlights mucosal damage (e.g. inflammation; neoplasia). The negative contrast provides better delineation of the surface detail. In this case, the mucosal lining of the bladder is normal. Positive contrast also pools in the dependent part of the bladder where uroliths collect. Five radiolucent uroliths are delineated by the voids that they create within the pool of contrast. (Image courtesy of T. Schwarz.)

diets and treating predisposing factors must be taken. The results of chemical analysis of uroliths help to plan appropriate therapy.

Some male dogs have recurrent episodes of urethral obstruction throughout their lives, and permanent urethrostomy may be considered as a palliative measure. Prescrotal urethrostomy produces a stoma that is wider than the narrowest portion of the urethra (the os penis) and uroliths usually pass out of the urethrostomy site without causing obstruction. Although this is a good solution in some dogs, it is associated with a range of complications and should not be performed without good justification.

Management of uroliths in the kidney or ureter

Uroliths can also form in the renal pelvis or move into the ureter. Ultimately these can cause irreversible renal damage or hydroureter. Managing nephroliths and ureteroliths is difficult. If nephroliths do not cause hydronephrosis or azotaemia, they may be managed conservatively or medical dissolution may be attempted. If they cause renal impairment, referral to a specialist centre for retrieval should be considered, but kidney damage may be irreversible. Ureteroliths may pass into the bladder over a few days but, if they do not, cases should be referred for management.

Feline Lower Urinary Tract Disease

Cats, like dogs, suffer from urolithiasis but this is part of a wider range of related conditions termed feline lower urinary tract disease (FLUTD). FLUTD may affect any sex or breed of cat but neutered, male, middle-aged cats are predisposed. Other predisposing factors include being overweight, getting little access outside, and being fed a dry diet. The Persian breed is also predisposed. Diet, lifestyle, and stress may be important in the pathogenesis of this syndrome.

Conditions associated with FLUTD include:

- Feline idiopathic cystitis (with or without urethral obstruction): this is the commonest cause of FLUTD but the pathogenesis is unclear.
- Urethral plugs: these are common and are composed of mucoproteins and urine crystals.
- Urolithiasis: these are less common than urethral plugs. Most are calcium oxalate or struvite.

- UTI: this is comparatively uncommon. It is identified in less than 12% of cases and plays less of a part in urinary tract disease in the cat than in the dog.
- Neoplasia.
- Behavioural disorders.
- Anatomic defects.

Historical and clinical findings

Affected cats have recurrent signs of dysuria, pollakiuria, haematuria, and urge incontinence that last for several days. The bladder is usually small unless the urethra is obstructed. Patients with urethral obstruction present with severe dysuria and have large, painful, distended bladders. They develop progressive postrenal azotaemia and hypovolaemic shock, and may be severely depressed. Hyperkalaemic patients may develop bradycardia and shock.

Investigation

The aims of investigation are to identify specific conditions that contribute to FLUTD, and to distinguish between obstructive and non-obstructive causes. Investigative tools include urinalysis, ultrasound, and radiographic contrast studies.

Management of FLUTD

Management of FLUTD aims to treat specific contributory causes, to prevent recurrence, and to manage acute urethral obstruction when it occurs. This is a complex and evolving field and readers should refer to specific reference sources detailing current recommendations for the treatment of this condition. An overview of medical management and indications for surgical management are presented here.

Management of cases without urethral obstruction

Feline idiopathic cystitis is usually self-limiting, with signs resolving within 5–10 days, but recurrence is very common. Management strategies include:

- *Stress-reducing measures*: reduce overcrowding; ensure adequate access to litter trays; site litter trays in 'safe environment'; use of feline facial pheromone.

- *Dietary modification*: promote formation of dilute urine (move from dry to wet diets; ensure free access to water).
- *Glycosaminoglycan supplementation*: may replenish depleted glycosaminoglycans that line the bladder and provide protection to the mucosa.
- *Antimicrobial therapy*: indicated only if UTI is confirmed.

Management of cases with urethral obstruction

Urethral obstruction is predominantly seen in male cats. Cases with urethral obstruction may present in a collapsed state with metabolic acidosis, hyperkalaemia, and hypovolaemic shock. Severely debilitated patients are best referred to an experienced colleague or a specialist centre for stabilization and treatment. Animals with urethral obstruction may have urethral spasm, physical blockage (urethral plugs or uroliths), or a combination of both. Strategies to relieve obstruction include:

1. Urethral catheterization: stabilize and anaesthetize the patient before attempting urethral catheterization. Catheterization can be difficult because of physical obstruction or urethral spasm (see below). Use a urethral catheter with an end port (rather than side ports), lubricate it well, and flush with saline as the catheter is advanced to dislodge urethral plugs and uroliths. Do not force the catheter, as urethral trauma, or even rupture, can occur. Once the catheter is in place, attach it to a closed urine collection system and instigate medical therapy. If uroliths are present, remove them by cystotomy.

2. Treatment of urethral spasm: smooth muscle relaxants are prescribed to relieve spasm. Acepromazine has a rapid onset of effect. For longer-term effect, a combination of smooth and skeletal muscle relaxants is given. Smooth muscle relaxants commonly used include prazosin (0.25–1.0 mg per cat PO q8–12 h) or phenoxybenzamine (0.5–1.0 mg/kg PO q12 h (has a delayed-onset effect)). The skeletal muscle relaxant, dantrolene (0.5–2.0 mg/kg PO q12 h), is often prescribed. These drugs are not licensed for treatment of urethral spasm in the cat and may cause side effects.

3. Cystotomy: if uroliths can be hydropulsed into the bladder, cystotomy can be performed to remove them. Calcium oxalate uroliths should always be removed surgically from the bladder. Struvite uroliths can be managed by medical dissolution or surgical removal. Surgery has the advantage that it enables uroliths to be collected for mineral analysis.

4. Feline perineal urethrostomy: male cats can have recurrent and debilitating episodes of urethral obstruction or develop severe urethral injury following repeated urethral catheterization. These cases are candidates for feline perineal urethrostomy. The procedure involves amputating the penis and creating a new urethral opening in the wide pelvic urethra just at the ischial arch (Fig. 16.5). This is an aggressive surgery that can lead to a host of post-operative problems, including urethral stricture, recurrent UTI, and incontinence. When performed competently, surgery is generally well tolerated and is effective in relieving urinary tract obstruction. However, 50% of patients will continue to show signs of FLUTD due to ongoing cystitis, although they should not develop urethral obstruction. Refer cases to an experienced colleague or a specialist centre for this procedure.

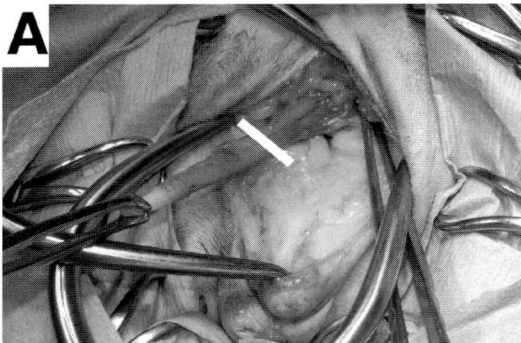

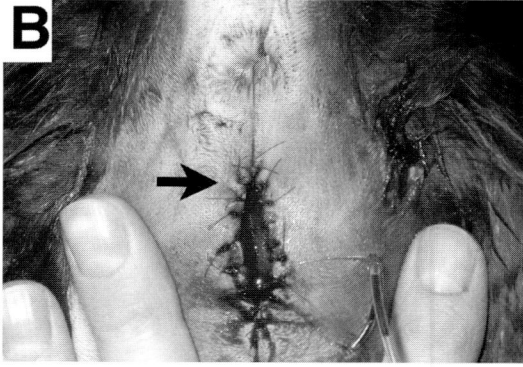

Fig. 16.5. Feline perineal urethrostomy: (A) the penis has been dissected and is about to be amputated (line marks amputation site); (B) the completed perineal urethrostomy with a ventral baffle plate of urethral mucosa (arrow marks entry into the urethra).

Prognosis

The prognosis for FLUTD is guarded as most cats have recurrent episodes despite treatment. The condition requires ongoing management to reduce predisposing factors, prevent urolith formation, and to manage acute episodes of dysuria.

Techniques

Anatomy

The bladder wall is composed of four layers: (i) the serosa; (ii) the detrusor muscle (smooth muscle); (iii) the submucosa; and (iv) the mucosa (transitional epithelium). The bladder narrows caudally to the bladder neck that leads into the urethra near the pubic brim. The ureters enter the bladder dorsally near the bladder neck at the trigone. In male dogs, the prostate envelops the urethra and caudal portion of the bladder neck, and the ductus deferentes penetrate the dorsal prostatic capsule and empty into the prostatic urethra. The prostate is small in castrated dogs and difficult to identify in castrated cats.

The urethra has an external layer of skeletal muscle and an internal layer of smooth muscle. Together these form a sphincter mechanism along the length of the urethra. In females, the urethra terminates in the vestibule, just distal to the vagino-vestibular junction, as it runs over the caudal border of the ischial arch. In male dogs and cats, the retractor peni muscle runs onto the outer surface of the urethra as the urethra passes over the ischium. The cat penis terminates in the prepuce just ventral to the scrotum in the perineal region and may have a small os penis. In the dog, the urethra continues between the hind legs into the penis on the ventral abdominal wall running through a ventral channel in the os penis.

Urethral catheterization

Male dogs do not require anaesthesia for urethral catheterization, but female dogs and both sexes of cat must be anaesthetized. The main risk of urethral catheterization is ascending infection so the procedure should be performed with clean or aseptic technique. Clip hair around the genital orifice. Wipe the penis or flush the vulva with dilute povidone-iodine. Use urinary catheters specifically designed for catheterization of male dogs (6–10 Fr) and cats (3–4 Fr). Female dogs can be catheterized with rigid male urinary catheters or rubber urinary catheters with inflatable bulbs (e.g. Foley catheters; 10 Fr and 12 Fr). Lubricate catheters well with sterile, water-soluble gels. During catheterization, do not advance the catheter if there is any resistance, to avoid damaging the urethra. Antibiotic therapy is contraindicated unless a UTI is confirmed, as indiscriminate use of antibiotics in catheterized patients is likely to lead the selection of organisms with antimicrobial resistance.

Male dog

Extrude the penis by holding it behind the bulb and pushing it forward as the prepuce is drawn back. Feed the catheter along the urethra into the bladder. Slight resistance may be encountered as the catheter passes through the os penis and as it rounds the ischial arch (Fig. 16.6).

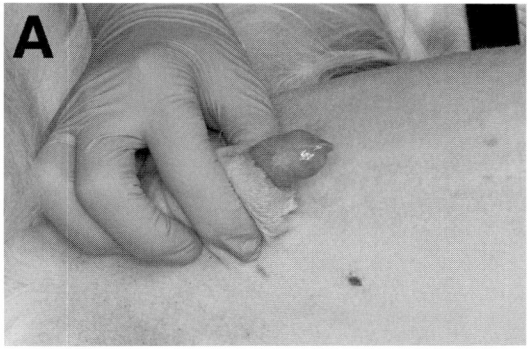

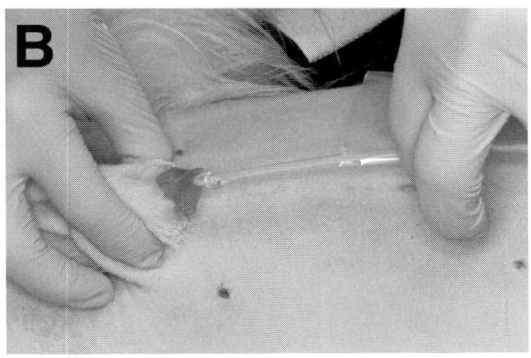

Fig. 16.6. Male dog urethral catheterization: (A) extrude the penis; (B) pass a lubricated urinary catheter into the urethral orifice. The catheter is kept within its protective sleeve to prevent contamination as it is advanced into the urethra.

Male cat

Extrude the penis by pushing the prepuce down the shaft of the penis. The penis has a sigmoid flexure that must be straightened before the catheter can be advanced. Engage the urethral catheter in the tip of the penis. Pull the penis (or prepuce) caudally and dorsally to stretch out the sigmoid flexure and advance the catheter into the bladder (Fig. 16.7).

Female dog

Use a vaginal speculum or vaginoscope to visualize the urethral orifice and papilla just caudal to the vagino-vestibular junction at the level of the ischial arch. Advance a rigid urinary catheter or soft catheter with a stylet into the urethral orifice. If using a Foley catheter, inflate the bulb to keep the catheter in position (Fig. 16.8). Alternatively, the urinary catheter can be passed under digital palpation, ensuring that the tip of the catheter is directed

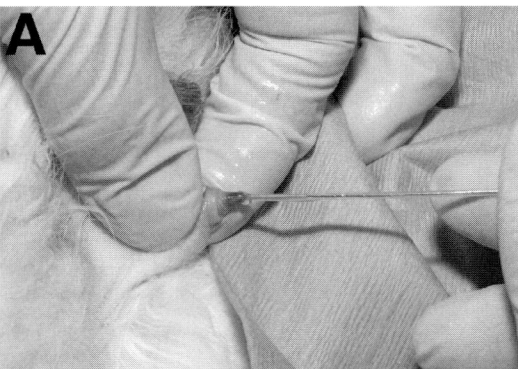

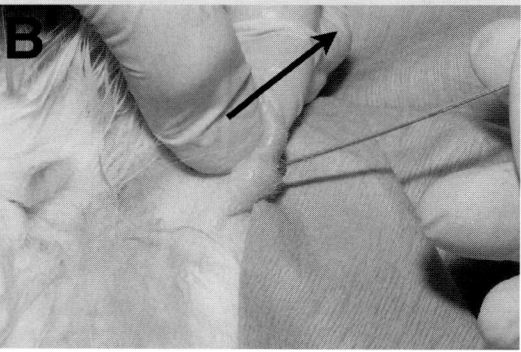

Fig. 16.7. Male cat urethral catheterization: (A) extrude the penis and insert the tip of the urinary catheter; (B) pull the penis (or prepuce) caudally and dorsally (direction of arrow) and advance the catheter.

along the ventral floor of the vestibule as it passes over the ischial arch.

Female cat

Position the cat in dorsal recumbency. Pass a catheter into the vulva on midline and advance it (Fig. 16.9). The natural path for the catheter to follow is directly into the urethra and bladder. If this is not successful, repeat, ensuring that the catheter is being advanced on midline.

Retrograde hydropulsion

Retrograde hydropulsion is used in male dogs and cats to force urethral stones into the bladder. Pass a urethral catheter until the point of obstruction is reached. Perform a rectal examination and apply downward pressure to the urethra in front of the obstruction by pushing down onto the pelvic floor to occlude the urethra (Fig. 16.3). Flush saline into the urethra until some resistance is met. Release the occlusion of the urethra while continuing to flush, and repeat until the obstruction is relieved. This technique enables back-pressure to build up distal to the urolith and the saline pushes the urethral mucosa away from the stone to dislodge it. When digital pressure is released from the urethra, the force of saline behind the urolith carries it forwards into the bladder.

Cystotomy

Cystotomy is performed regularly in dogs and cats in general practice, predominantly for the management of uroliths.

Patient preparation

Position the patient in ventral recumbency and prepare the abdomen for exploratory surgery. If surgery is being performed to remove uroliths, extend the clip caudally to include the vulva or prepuce and prepare these so that they can be included in the surgical field for catheterization during surgery (Fig. 16.10). Catheterize and empty the bladder to reduce urine leakage before surgery, if possible.

Approach

Perform a ventral midline coeliotomy incision from the umbilicus to the pubis to give adequate exposure

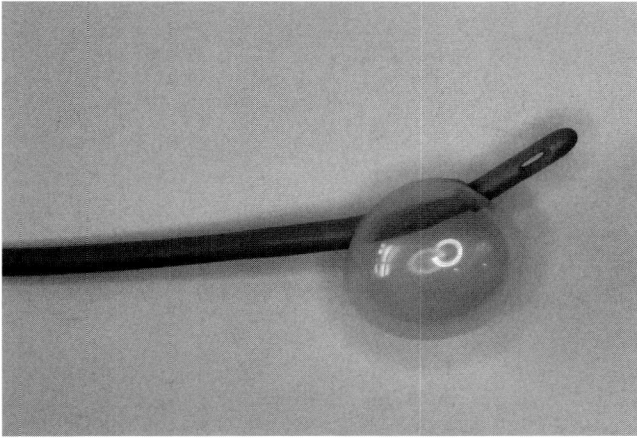

Fig. 16.8. Foley catheter: these catheters have an inflatable balloon at one end to help maintain them in position.

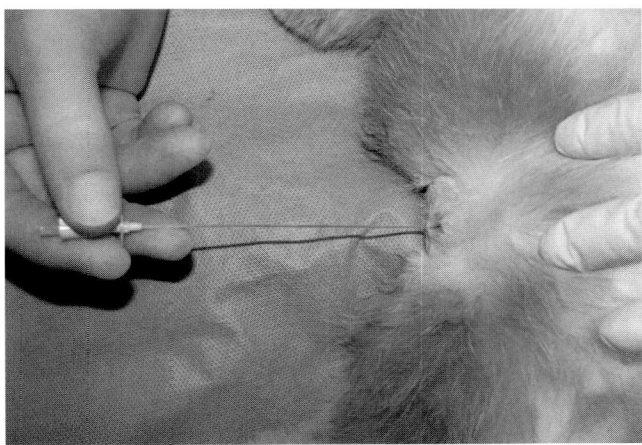

Fig. 16.9. Female cat catheterization.

to the bladder neck. Isolate the bladder with moistened laparotomy pads. Place a stay suture in the bladder apex. If the bladder is full, empty it by cystocentesis to reduce urine spillage during cystotomy (Fig. 16.11).

Incise the bladder

Make a stab incision into an avascular portion of the ventral surface of the bladder using a no. 11 scalpel blade. Extend the incision longitudinally using Metzenbaum scissors. The incision may extend as far as the bladder neck to enable retrieval of uroliths if required (Fig. 16.12). To improve exposure, two additional stay sutures may be placed midway along the incision on either side to provide lateral retraction of the incision.

Remove uroliths

Pick uroliths out of the bladder and bladder neck with forceps. Catheterize the urethra from the vulva or penis and flush uroliths from the urethra into the bladder. Perform vigorous flushing to

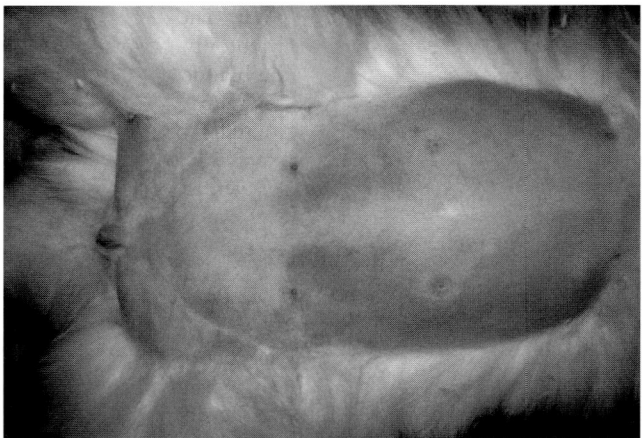

Fig. 16.10. Positioning and clip for urolith removal: the penis and prepuce have been included in the surgical clip to enable the urethra to be catheterized intra-operatively.

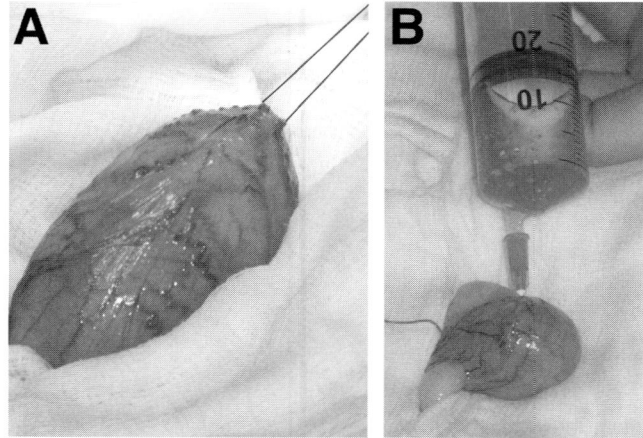

Fig. 16.11. Cystotomy: (A) place a stay suture in the bladder apex to facilitate manipulation (pass a loop of suture through the bladder apex using a needle; keep the suture ends long and clamp them with a haemostat); (B) perform cystocentesis before incising the bladder.

ensure all uroliths are removed. Finally, ensure that a large-bore urethral catheter can pass along the urethra without difficulty.

Close the incision

Close the incision using a single layer, full thickness, simple, continuous suture pattern. Use 3-0, monofilament, absorbable suture material suitable for urinary tract surgery (e.g. Glycomer™ 631). Ensure that the submucosa is included in the suture line.

If the bladder wall has become very thick, a double-layered closure may be easier to perform. Suture material that penetrates the bladder lumen can act as a nidus for urolith formation, so long-lasting and permanent suture materials should be avoided.

Complications

Most animals recover well from cystotomy without major complications. Self-limiting haematuria and dysuria are common for the first 48 h. Rarely, urine leaks from the cystotomy incision leading to uroabdomen and requires emergency reparative surgery. Uroliths are also occasionally left in the bladder. This complication can be reduced by counting uroliths on preoperative radiographs, flushing the urethra and bladder neck intra-operatively, and repeating radiographic studies at the end of surgery.

Urethrotomy (prescrotal)

Urethrotomy is performed regularly in male dogs in general practice.

Patient preparation

Urethrotomy is performed directly over the site of urethral obstruction which may be anywhere from the base of the os penis to the ischial arch in the dog. However, most obstructions occur just behind the os penis, as the urethra is narrowest at this

point. The procedure is generally combined with cystotomy to allow uroliths to be removed from the bladder. Position the dog in dorsal recumbency and clip and prepare the area. Extend the clip cranially to include the prepuce, which has been prepared for catheterization during surgery, and the ventral abdomen, to enable cystotomy to be performed.

Approach

Place a rigid urinary catheter up to the point of obstruction to act as a guide. Make a 2–4 cm long skin incision directly over the obstruction. Continue the incision through the subcutaneous fat and fascia to expose the urethra (Fig. 16.13). Reflect the retractor peni muscle from the ventral surface of the urethra laterally (the muscle is very small and loosely attached to the ventral surface of the

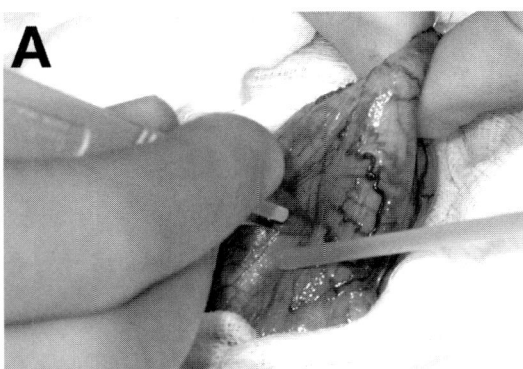

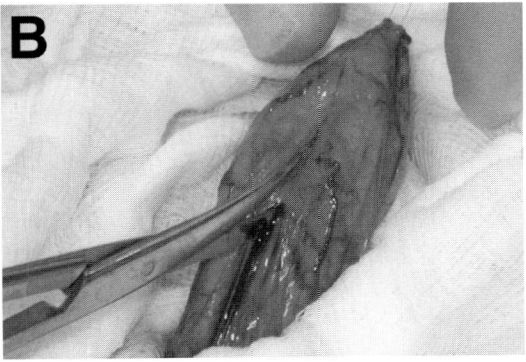

Fig. 16.12. Cystotomy: (A) make a stab incision in the ventral surface of the bladder; (B) extend the incision longitudinally using Metzenbaum scissors.

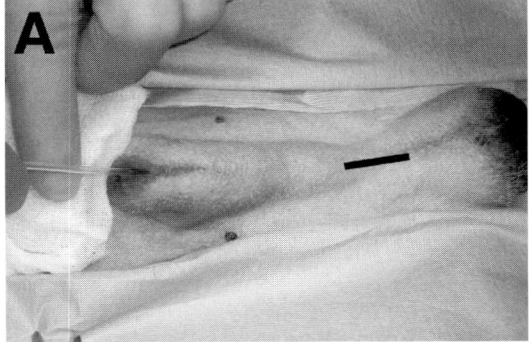

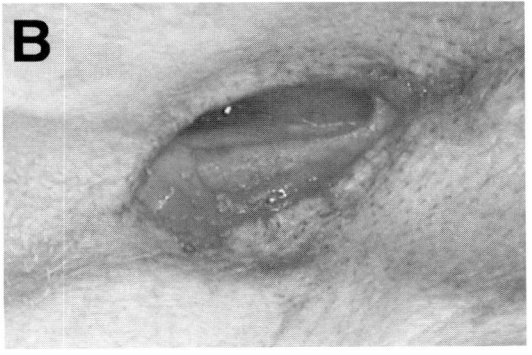

Fig. 16.13. Prescrotal urethrotomy: (A) place a rigid urinary catheter into the urethra to the point of obstruction (line marks site of urethrotomy incision); (B) make a skin incision between the base of the scrotum and the os penis to expose the urethra.

urethra). Incise directly into the urethral lumen on the ventral midline with the tip of a no. 11 scalpel blade using the urinary catheter as a guide. Remove the urolith (Fig. 16.14). Leave the urethrotomy incision open to heal by second intention.

Post-operative care

Place an Elizabethan collar for 2 weeks until the site has healed, to prevent self-inflicted trauma. Warn owners that haematuria will continue for several days following surgery. The patient may urinate through the urethrotomy site for several days until it closes. Apply barrier creams (e.g. Vaseline®) to prevent urine scald if urine dribbles onto the inner thigh.

Complications

The prognosis for dogs following urethrotomy is reasonable as most animals respond well to surgery.

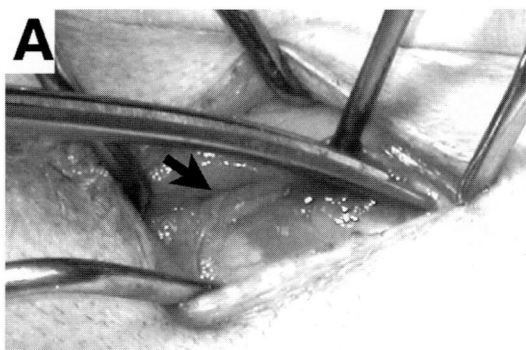

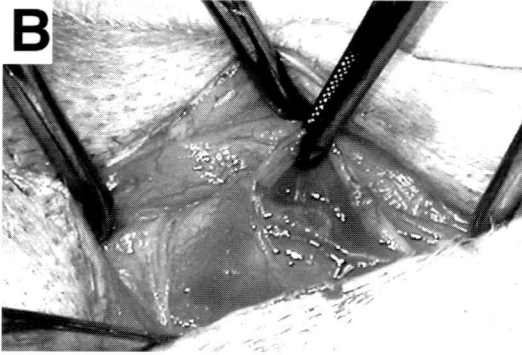

Fig. 16.14. Prescrotal urethrotomy: (A) dissect the retractor peni muscle off the ventral surface of the urethra and retract it laterally (arrow); (B) make a longitudinal incision in the urethra to retrieve the obstruction.

However, recurrence of signs may occur if the primary problem is not addressed, or if stenosis occurs at the surgery site. Haematuria is also inevitable following urethrotomy due to bleeding from the incised urethral mucosa. The bleeding can be profuse and may continue for up to 14 days following surgery, and owners must be warned of this preoperatively.

Urethrostomy (canine)

Urethrostomy is performed either directly over the site of obstruction (allowing retrieval of the obstruction) or proximal to the obstruction (if the obstruction cannot be retrieved). As most obstructions occur at the level of the os penis, prescrotal and scrotal urethrostomies are most common. Scrotal urethrostomy is the best technique, as there is plenty of room to create the stoma, but dogs must be castrated. Prescrotal urethrostomy can be performed in intact dogs but the scrotum limits the length of incision that can be made and may become scalded with urine.

Prescrotal and scrotal urethrostomies are regularly performed in general practice. Canine perineal urethrostomy is more difficult to perform as the perineal urethra does not sit in as prominent a subcutaneous position.

Prescrotal urethrostomy

Position and prepare the patient in the same manner as described for urethrotomy. The initial approach and incision into the urethra is identical to that described for prescrotal urethrotomy. Make a 3–6 cm incision in the urethra. The incision must be long as the stoma will contract by up to 50% postoperatively. Once the urethra is incised, suture the urethral mucosa to the skin to create the permanent stoma. Use either a simple, continuous pattern of 4-0 or 5-0, monofilament, short-lasting material (e.g. poliglecaprone) or a simple interrupted pattern of 3-0 or 4-0, monofilament, non-absorbable material (e.g. polypropylene). Continuous patterns of absorbable suture do not require removal. Remove other skin sutures after 7–10 days.

Scrotal urethrostomy

If the dog is entire, perform castration by scrotal ablation and proceed to complete the urethrostomy as described above through the scrotal ablation incision. If the dog has been castrated, resect the scrotum and proceed to complete the urethrostomy through the incision (Fig. 16.15).

Complications

Urethrostomy is associated with similar short-term complications to urethrotomy, of which haematuria is the most common. Post-operative haematuria may be reduced if the site is closed with the continuous suture pattern and if a bite of the deeper (submucosal) tissues is incorporated into each pass of the suture.

The prognosis following urethrostomy is reasonable but long-term complications may occur. Urine scald may develop if the dog urinates onto his inner thigh. Some dogs learn to squat or alter their urination stance, but others require barrier

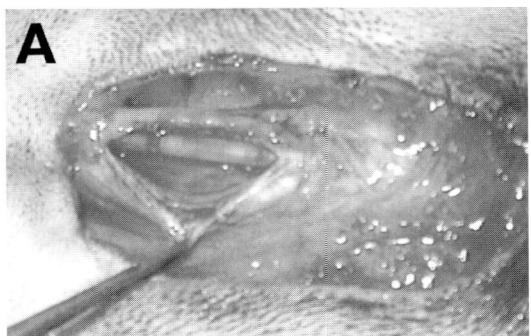

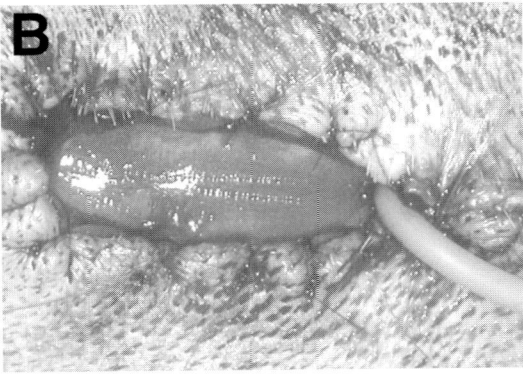

Fig. 16.15. Scrotal urethrostomy: (A) perform scrotal ablation; expose the ventral surface of the urethra and make a longitudinal incision using the rigid urinary catheter as a guide; (B) create a large stoma by suturing the incised urethra to the skin. The caudal aspect of the skin incision has been closed over the scrotal ablation site.

creams and frequent cleaning to prevent dermatitis. The urethrostomy incision will contract and may close completely. If this occurs, the procedure can be repeated proximally along the urethra. Permanent urethrostomy may predispose to ascending urinary tract infection and recurrent cystitis. Hair must be clipped from around the site regularly to reduce the incidence of stomal dermatitis and ascending infection.

Urinary Incontinence

Urinary incontinence is defined as involuntary voiding of urine. It can be either congenital or acquired. There are many possible causes but the majority of cases fall into one of these categories:

1. urge incontinence;
2. sphincter mechanism incompetence;
3. ectopic ureter;
4. neurogenic incontinence.

Investigating urinary incontinence

Most patients with inappropriate patterns of urination have urge incontinence due to UTI or urolithiasis. UTI is also extremely common as a secondary problem in animals with other forms of incontinence. All animals presenting with urinary incontinence should be investigated for UTI and urolithiasis before other causes of incontinence are investigated. The minimum investigation of a patient presenting for the first time with incontinence should include collection of a detailed history, performance of a full clinical evaluation, and in-house analysis of a free-catch urine sample.

History

Take a history that includes details of neutering status, urination pattern, and incontinence pattern. Key questions to answer include:

- What are the sex, breed, and age of the patient?
- Has it been neutered?
- When did incontinence start and how does this relate to neutering or oestrus?
- Is the patient aware of urinating involuntarily?
- What is the pattern of incontinence:
  - Are large pools of urine passed infrequently?
  - Is incontinence associated with particular postures or states (e.g. lying down, sleeping)?

- Is incontinence associated with dysuria, haematuria or pyuria?
- Is the patient polydipsic (normal water intake: 50–100 ml/kg/day in dogs)?
- Are there signs of systemic disease?
- Are there signs of neurological dysfunction (e.g. ataxia; seizures; abnormal behaviour)?

Clinical examination

Perform a through physical examination. Examine the external genitalia for gross abnormalities, discharges, urine leakage, and urine scald. Palpate the bladder and perform a rectal examination. Palpate the urethra running ventrally along the pelvic floor for irregularities, masses, and pain. In males, palpate the prostate (see below). Perform a neurological examination paying particular attention to tests of pelvic limb proprioception, spinal reflexes, and tests of sacral spinal segment function. Withdraw the prepuce and evaluate the penis. Perform a digital vaginal examination checking for evidence of vaginal masses and strictures. Perform vaginoscopy and evaluate the external urethral orifice. Some of these investigations will necessitate general anaesthesia.

Urinalysis

Urine is examined for evidence of UTI and crystalluria. Culture is performed on samples collected by cystocentesis if required. Urine is also used in combination with serum biochemistry to evaluate for the presence of systemic diseases that may contribute to polydipsia and urge incontinence.

Imaging of the urinary tract

Ultrasound and radiography are very useful for investigating causes of incontinence in many cases. In experienced hands, ultrasound provides more information than radiography for evaluation of kidney and bladder disorders but contrast radiography still provides additional information about the urethra and ureters. More advanced techniques, including contrast computed tomography and cystoscopy, are also used for the investigation of specific syndromes but are only available in specialist centres. The imaging findings of the individual causes of urinary incontinence are discussed below.

Urge incontinence

Urge incontinence usually occurs in animals with cystitis. It may also be caused by conditions that lead to rapid bladder filling (e.g. polyuria) or space-occupying bladder lesions (e.g. tumours; large uroliths). Patients are aware that they are voiding urine but are unable to override the micturition reflex to delay urinating until an appropriate time. They squat and urinate frequently, may appear dysuric, and demonstrate urgency when urinating, often passing urine in the house or missing the litter tray. Animals presenting for urinary incontinence will be investigated for the common causes of urge incontinence and, where appropriate, additional imaging may be performed. Treatment is aimed at treating the underlying causes.

Sphincter mechanism incompetence

Acquired sphincter mechanism incompetence (SMI) (also known as *hormone-responsive incontinence* or *post-spay incontinence*) is the commonest form of chronic acquired incontinence in the dog. SMI can be seen in any breed or age of dog but predominantly affects female, neutered dogs. It is usually diagnosed in middle-aged or older dogs, typically 2–3 years after neutering. Large-breed dogs are predisposed to the condition. Occasionally, acquired SMI is diagnosed in entire bitches and in castrated male dogs.

The aetiology of SMI is unknown but loss of oestrogen following neutering, obesity, and bladder neck position may all be linked to the development of the condition. Oestrogen deficiency is implicated as most cases are neutered, female dogs, and because oestrogen replacement resolves the problem in a percentage of cases. Similarly, many dogs are obese and weight loss alone can lead to improvement in signs. Bladder position seems to be important in the development of the condition, as many affected dogs have a caudally positioned bladder with an intrapelvic bladder neck, and because surgery to reposition the bladder neck can be effective in managing the condition.

Impaired urethral sphincter function allows urine to leak passively from the bladder, particularly when the patient is recumbent or relaxed. Typically, patients leave large pools of urine where they have been lying (e.g. bed-wetting overnight) but are continent most of the time. Usually the patient is unaware of leaking urine. However, the pattern of incontinence varies greatly between individual animals.

Juvenile SMI also occurs occasionally as a congenital form of incontinence in prepubertal female dogs. The influence of hormones also appears to be linked to the development of this problem as 50% of cases resolve following their first oestrus. Juvenile SMI and ectopic ureter occur concurrently in many cases (see below).

Investigation

SMI is diagnosed largely through exclusion of other causes of incontinence. Evaluate patients for UTI, urolithiasis, bladder masses, neurological disease, and undiagnosed congenital lesions such as ectopic ureter. Identification of an intrapelvic bladder is suggestive of, but not diagnostic for, the condition (Fig. 16.16).

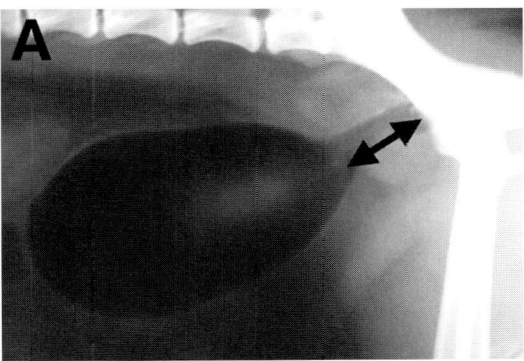

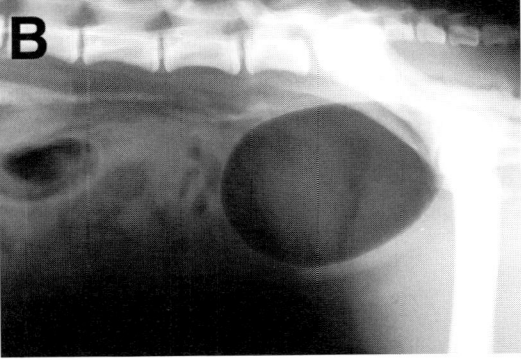

Fig. 16.16. Bladder neck position – double contrast cystogram: (A) normal position – double-headed arrow indicates space between bladder neck and entrance to pelvic cavity; (B) intrapelvic bladder – the bladder neck is positioned caudal to the wing of the ilium (the radiographic landmark for the start of the pelvic cavity).

Treatment

Affected animals commonly have concurrent UTIs that can exacerbate the signs of incontinence. UTI should be investigated and treated in every case. Obese patients should be placed on weight-control diets as reducing body weight can also lessen the severity of signs. Specific therapies include surgical and medical treatments. Unfortunately, no single treatment is completely effective in resolving incontinence and it may be more reasonable to aim to improve, rather than to stop, signs. Many patients ultimately end up receiving a combination of all treatments to control their problem:

1. Oestrogen therapy: oestrogen supplementation in neutered bitches may resolve the condition. Short-acting oestrogens (e.g. estriol) are used as they have less adverse effects than long-acting oestrogens (e.g. myelosuppression; attractiveness to male dogs). Oestrogen therapy should not be given to prepubertal dogs.

2. Alpha-adrenergic agonists: phenylpropanolamine increases internal urethral sphincter tone and can be very effective at managing sphincter mechanism incompetence. Treatment is generally well tolerated but behavioural changes (including aggression) and cardiovascular effects may occur.

3. Colposuspension: a range of surgical procedures to position the bladder more proximally and to increase urethral sphincter tone have been described, however none has proven to be completely successful. Colposuspension is popular as it is well tolerated and has reasonable results. It involves pulling the bladder neck forward by anchoring the cranial vagina to the prepubic tendon. Few dogs become completely continent but many show a marked improvement or a better response to medical therapy after colposuspension has been performed. Despite the limitations of surgery, owner satisfaction is high with this procedure. Consider referring patients for specialist evaluation for this surgery.

Ectopic ureter

Ectopic ureter is the commonest cause of congenital urinary incontinence. The ureter is malpositioned and empties into the urethra or vagina instead of the bladder (Fig. 16.17). Ectopic ureter may be unilateral or bilateral and is frequently

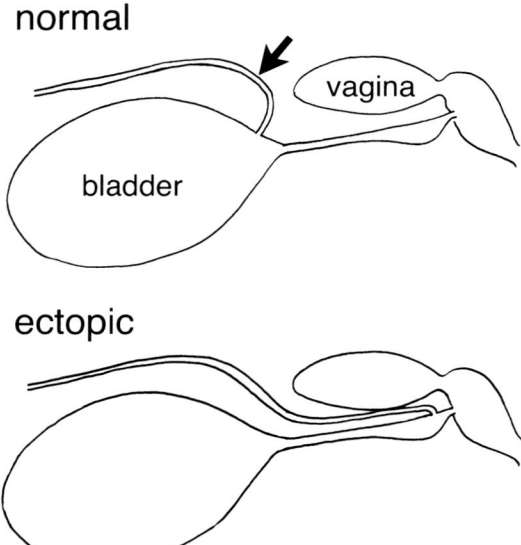

normal

vagina

bladder

ectopic

Fig. 16.17. Diagram of ectopic ureter: arrow shows entry of normal ureter into bladder neck; the ectopic ureter in this diagram empties into the distal urethra near the urethral orifice.

accompanied by hydroureter and hydronephrosis. These may be caused by partial obstruction of urine through the ectopic ureter.

In most cases, the condition is diagnosed in female dogs in the first few weeks of life. Labrador and golden retrievers are predisposed. Usually, urine dribbles continuously from the vulva but the pattern of incontinence is variable. Occasionally, ectopic ureters are diagnosed in male dogs in which the onset of signs is often delayed. This may be because the longer urethra in male dogs provides more resistance to urine leakage distal to the point where the ectopic ureter enters the urethra. Occasionally, bitches may present for the first time in adulthood and subsequently be found to have an ectopic ureter that was clinically silent for several months or years. It is prudent to screen for this condition in older animals with chronic incontinence problems, even if they do not fit the typical pattern of presentation.

Investigation

The diagnosis of ectopic ureter can be difficult to confirm using conventional imaging studies. The opening of the ureter into the vagina may be seen by vaginoscopy. Contrast radiography has been the mainstay of investigation but often fails to produce a definitive diagnosis. The most useful study is the *intravenous urogram* in which a contrast agent is given intravenously and highlights the ureters as it is excreted rapidly in urine. However, other specialist techniques including contrast CT and cystoscopy (endoscopic examination of the urethra and bladder) provide more consistent results. Many cases are referred for imaging studies to establish the diagnosis.

Treatment

Once the diagnosis is reached, ectopic ureters should be corrected without delay, as progressive kidney damage may occur due to hydronephrosis. A variety of specialist techniques are used to redirect urine into the bladder from the ectopic ureter but, if there is severe secondary renal damage, nephrectomy (removal of the kidney) may be performed as an alternative. Patients should be referred to a specialist practice for assessment and surgery.

Complications and prognosis

The most significant problem following surgery is continuing urinary incontinence that affects up to 50% of cases. Juvenile SMI is commonly diagnosed concurrently with ectopic ureter and is thought to account for ongoing incontinence in many cases post-operatively. Careful preoperative counselling of owners is required to ensure that they appreciate that incontinence may not resolve following surgery and that ongoing treatment may be required. Other complications include stenosis of the ureter and secondary hydronephrosis.

Neurogenic incontinence

Neurological disorders leading to incontinence usually affect bladder contraction or urethral tone. Neurogenic incontinence is a complex area but two examples demonstrate common presentations that may be seen:

1. Animals with spinal lesions between the brainstem and the caudal lumbar spinal segments (e.g. a thoracolumbar intervertebral disc extrusion) have disruption of pathways providing upper motor neuron control of the external urethral sphincter and providing conscious control of urination. This leads to increased urethral tone. The bladder

becomes distended and is difficult to express. *Overflow incontinence* may develop when the pressure in the overfilling bladder exceeds that of the urethra, leading to dribbling of urine. Patients may recover if the spinal cord injury can be addressed.

2. Patients with sacral spinal cord segment injuries (e.g. sacral and tail injuries) have damage to the lower motor neurons of the external urethral sphincter and the autonomic pathways to the bladder and urethra. The bladder loses the innervation to induce contraction and the urethra loses tone, leading to continuous dribbling of urine from a flaccid bladder. The bladder is easily expressed as there is low urethral tone but no active bladder contraction is seen. The prognosis for recovery from this injury is poor.

These examples demonstrate severe incontinence associated with common lesions but oversimplify this complex area. Consult specialist texts for more information.

Feline incontinence

Urge incontinence (usually as a result of FLUTD) and neurogenic incontinence (following sacral and tail injuries) are common in the cat. Other forms of incontinence are rare. Cats occasionally present with ectopic ureter (male and female cats are equally represented) but other congenital forms of incontinence are very uncommon and are usually associated with severe urogenital tract abnormalities conferring a poor prognosis. Sphincter mechanism incompetence is not recognized as a distinct syndrome associated with neutering in cats.

Prostatic Disease

Prostatic disease is common in older, entire, male dogs. Male cats develop prostatic disease but the incidence is very low.

Aetiopathogenesis

A range of diseases affects the prostate, and multiple diseases are commonly found in the same patient. Prostatic enlargement causes urethral obstruction and impinges on the rectum causing tenesmus. Secondary UTIs are common as bacteria are comparatively protected from the body's defence mechanisms within the prostatic parenchyma. Prostatic disease may also cause infertility.

Benign prostatic hyperplasia

Most older, intact dogs develop benign prostatic hyperplasia. The condition is caused by prostatic hyperplasia due to chronic androgen stimulation.

Prostatic cyst

Prostatic cysts are often associated with benign prostatic hyperplasia. As the gland enlarges, ducts become obstructed leading to cyst formation within the parenchyma.

Paraprostatic cyst

Paraprostatic cysts are congenital and develop from Müllerian duct remnants that form fluid-filled cysts around the bladder neck and prostate. They increase in size slowly, eventually becoming clinically apparent in mature dogs.

Prostatitis

Bacterial prostatitis ranges from a subclinical infection that leads to recurrent bouts of UTI, through chronic, low-grade infection to acute, severe prostatitis. Acute prostatitis is associated with severe inflammation of the gland, pyrexia, and malaise.

Prostatic abscess

Prostatic abscess is a life-threatening condition that develops rapidly and causes septic shock. The abscess erodes through adjacent prostatic tissue and may cause urethral erosion or leakage of pus into the abdomen. Uroabomen and septic peritonitis can develop.

Prostatic adenocarcinoma

In older dogs, prostatic adenocarcinoma is an aggressive tumour that rapidly metastasizes. The tumour may become partly mineralized. Unlike other prostatic diseases, androgens are not linked to the development of prostatic adenocarcinoma and castration does not prevent adenocarcinoma developing.

Historical and clinical findings

Patients often have dysuria, haematuria, and other signs of urinary tract disease. Dogs with severe urethral obstruction may be unable to urinate or demonstrate overflow incontinence. Dyschezia and formation of ribbon-shaped stools is often associated with prostatic enlargement.

On clinical evaluation, the enlarged prostate may be palpable as a caudal abdominal mass. A great deal of information can be obtained from rectal examination (see below). Marked pain is associated with prostatitis, abscess, and neoplasia. Animals with prostatic abscess may present in septic shock or with signs of serious infection such as pyrexia, malaise, or septic peritonitis.

Investigation of prostatic disease

Rectal examination and ultrasound are invaluable in the investigation of prostatic disease:

1. Normal prostate: in young dogs, the prostate is small and sits within the pelvic cavity. On rectal examination, it has a smooth, symmetrical, bilobed shape with an obvious dorsal median sulcus. It fills 50–70% of the height of the pelvic canal. Prostatic examination should not be resented. On ultrasound examination, the prostate has a bilobed appearance with even echotexture and the urethra sits centrally within the gland.

2. Benign prostate hyperplasia: in older intact dogs, as benign prostatic hyperplasia develops, the prostate enlarges and moves forward into the caudal abdomen but it retains its features on rectal and ultrasound examinations.

3. Prostatic cysts: on rectal examination, the cyst causes asymmetric prostatomegaly but the prostate is not painful. Ultrasound examination shows asymmetric prostatic enlargement and single or multiple fluid-filled cavities within the prostatic parenchyma.

4. Prostatitis: on rectal examination, the prostate enlarges symmetrically and loses definition of the dorsal median sulcus. It may move forward into the abdomen. In acute prostatitis, the prostate is extremely painful and rectal examination can be very difficult. Ultrasound evaluation shows symmetrical prostatomegaly with a centrally positioned urethra and increased echogenicity of the parenchyma.

5. Prostatic abscess: rectal examination is resented as the prostate is extremely painful. The prostate is asymmetrically enlarged and may have an appreciable fluid-filled swelling in one lobe. Ultrasound confirms asymmetric prostatic enlargement with the urethra displaced from midline. One or several cavitated lesions are seen filled with flocculent

fluid. The presence of free abdominal fluid may indicate that uroabdomen or peritonitis has developed due to erosion of the prostatic capsule.

6. Prostatic carcinoma: on rectal examination, the prostate is extremely painful and enlarged. Ultrasound examination identifies increased echogenicity of the prostatic parenchyma and may demonstrate erosion around the urethra. Prostatic neoplasia is difficult to distinguish from acute prostatitis without biopsy. Other features seen with prostatic neoplasia include periosteal reaction around the lumbar spine and ilium and mineralization of the prostatic parenchyma.

Treatment

Treatment for prostatic disease involves castration, antimicrobial therapy, and surgical drainage of cysts and abscesses.

Castration

Castration is generally beneficial as it stops androgen-dependent prostatic enlargement, leads to shrinkage of the prostate, and prevents recurrence of disease. It should be performed in all patients with prostatic disease. Anti-androgen therapy (e.g. delmadinone acetate injections) can be considered as an alternative.

Antimicrobial therapy

Antimicrobial therapy is indicated when bacterial prostatitis or prostatic abscess are diagnosed. Many antimicrobials do not penetrate into the prostatic parenchyma well. Fluoroquinolones, clindamycin and trimethoprim-sulfonamides penetrate better than the beta-lactam antibiotics.

Surgery

Surgical management of prostatic disease is technically demanding. Complications of prostatic surgery include neurological injury leading to incontinence, copious bleeding, and iatrogenic urethral injury. Cases should be referred to specialist centres or experienced colleagues for surgery. Omentum is often packed into prostatic cysts and abscesses to act as a physiological drain, a technique called *omentalization*. Animals with prostatic abscesses require aggressive therapy for septic shock and for peritonitis. Prostatic carcinoma is very difficult to treat as prostatectomy (removal of the prostate) is associated with high morbidity and mortality rates, and is rarely performed.

Prognosis

The prognosis for benign prostatic hyperplasia, prostatitis, prostatic cyst, or paraprostatic cysts is good following appropriate therapy. The prognosis for prostatic abscess is guarded due to the severity of signs and the destructive nature of the condition. The prognosis for prostatic adenocarcinoma is poor.

Penile Surgery

Urethral prolapse and penile laceration are quite common and are usually managed in general practice. Other conditions such as tumours of the prepuce or penis, fracture of the os penis, or severe balanitis (penile inflammation) are rare and cases should be referred to an experienced colleague or specialist centre for management. Management of these more uncommon problems may entail penile amputation.

Urethral prolapse

Urethral prolapse occurs when the mucosa at the external urethral orifice of a male dog prolapses. The prolapsed mucosa becomes oedematous, bleeds easily, and may become necrotic. Urethral prolapse is typically seen in young, male, entire brachycephalic dogs and is associated with sexual activity. Animals present with signs of haematuria, penile irritation, and dysuria. The prolapsed mucosa has a characteristic appearance (Fig. 16.18).

Treatment

Treatment consists of castration to reduce sexual activity, and excision of the prolapsed tissue. To excise the prolapsed mucosa, extrude the penis from prepuce and hold it in position by tying a Penrose drain around the base of the penis (Fig. 16.18). Prepare the penis with dilute povidone-iodine solution and place a rigid urinary catheter through the centre of the prolapse into the urethra to act as a marker of the urethral lumen. Excise one-quarter segment of the prolapsed tissue with a no. 15 blade ensuring that the mucosa is trimmed as short as possible. Suture the edges of the incised

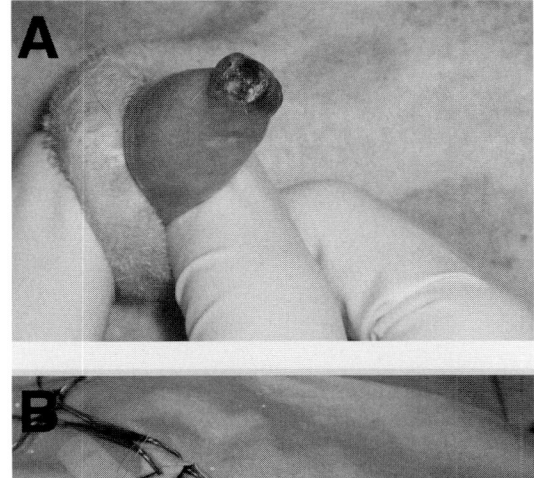

Fig. 16.18. Urethral prolapse: (A) prolapsed mucosa at the tip of the penis; (B) positioning for surgery using a Penrose drain tied around the base of the penis to keep the penis extruded and a rigid urinary catheter as a guide.

mucosa to the skin at the external urethral orifice using 4-0 or 5-0 monofilament, permanent suture material (e.g. polypropylene to reduce tissue reaction) in a simple interrupted pattern (Fig. 16.19). Resect the next segment of prolapsed tissue and repeat until all of the tissue is excised. The prolapse is excised in sections as, if it is amputated with a single incision, the urethral mucosa retracts into the penis and is difficult to suture.

Haemorrhage from the incision line can continue for several days after surgery, and self-inflicted injury must be prevented by use of an Elizabethan collar. Sedate or anaesthetize the patient for suture removal after 7–10 days.

Prognosis

The prognosis for urethral prolapse is reasonable. Complications such as stenosis at the surgery site are rare but the prolapse may recur. If urethral

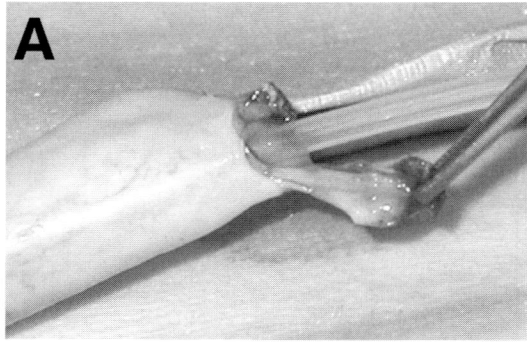

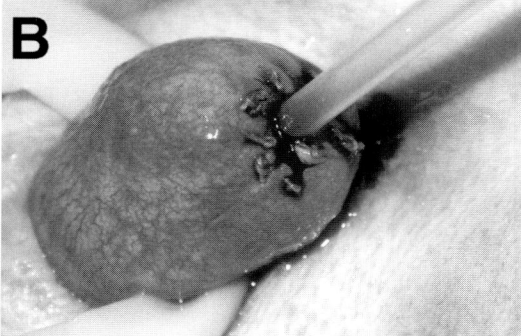

Fig. 16.19. Urethral prolapse: (A) resect the prolapsed tissue in sections and suture the mucosa to the penile skin; (B) completed resection.

prolapse becomes a recurrent problem, urethropexy or partial penile amputation can be performed.

Penile laceration

Penile laceration results from direct trauma and typically occurs when the penis is caught as a dog jumps over a wire fence. Profuse bleeding occurs but is unlikely to be life-threatening. Anaesthetize the patient and retract the prepuce to access the penis. Lavage the laceration, debride devitalized edges, and suture with short-acting, absorbable suture material. Small lacerations can be managed as open wounds. Haemorrhage usually continues for several days following the injury. Keep the patient quiet and avoid stimulating him. Consider using low-dose sedative agents such as acepromazine for the first few days. Sexual arousal in intact dogs may stimulate further haemorrhage. Consider castration or anti-androgen therapy.

Vulval Surgery

There are few indications for vulval surgery in general practice.

Episiotomy

Episiotomy is a procedure that involves incising into the dorsal aspect of the vulva to give access to the vestibule and vagina. The main indication is for removal of vaginal masses (e.g. leiomyoma). The incision is made on midline, running from the dorsal commissure of the vulva to a point level with the ischial arch (Fig. 16.20). The incision is closed in three layers (mucosa, fascia/fat, and skin).

Episioplasty

Episioplasty is a reconstructive surgery to reshape the vulva. The main indication is for removal of dorsal perivulvar skin folds, often associated with recessed juvenile vulvas, which cause perivulvar dermatitis or recurrent UTIs (Fig. 16.21). Judgement for resection of tissue is critical and these procedures should be performed by experienced clinicians.

Urinary Tract Trauma

Urinary tract trauma sustained during blunt abdominal trauma (e.g. RTA) may lead to uroabdomen. Trauma to the urethra may also occur following pelvic and sacral fractures. Urinary tract injuries include:

- ureteral rupture with separation of the ends;
- ureteral avulsion from trigone;
- bladder tear;
- urethral tear;
- urethral rupture with separation of the ends; and
- urethral avulsion from the bladder neck.

Uroabdomen may also result from leakage following urinary tract surgery.

Presentation

It may take 2–3 days for signs to become apparent. Uroabdomen is easily missed during the initial evaluation of a trauma patient and any patient deteriorating 2 or 3 days following trauma should be re-evaluated for urinary tract and other soft-tissue injuries that were not apparent at initial presentation.

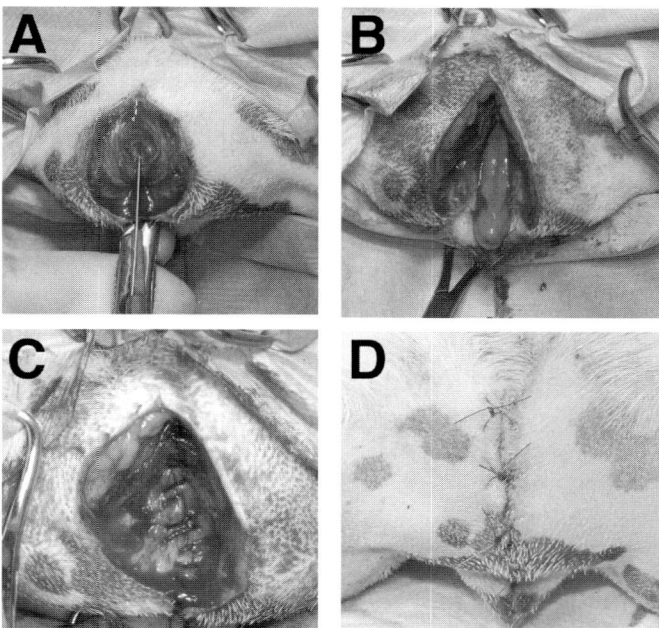

Fig. 16.20. Episiotomy: (A) make a midline incision in the vulva using probe (haemostat in this case) inserted into the vulva as a guide; (B) the vaginal floor exposed; (C) close the incision in three layers; (D) appearance post-operatively

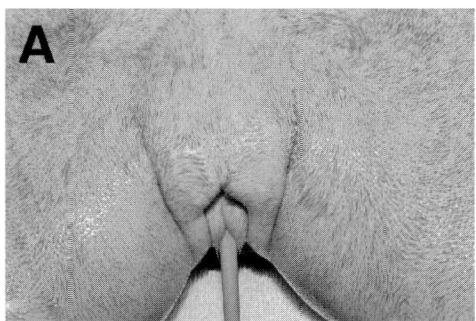

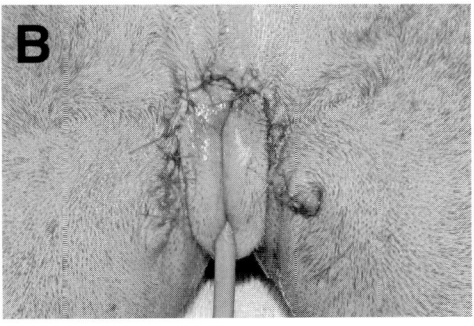

Fig. 16.21. Episioplasty: (A) large perivulvar skin fold; (B) appearance following episioplasty.

Initial signs may include haematuria and dysuria, but patients may pass a normal stream of urine despite having severely traumatized urinary tracts. As urine accumulates in the abdomen, signs of azotaemia, hyperkalaemia, hypovolaemic shock, and ascites develop over 48–72 h and lead to rapid deterioration of the patient.

Investigation

1. Serum biochemistry: immediately following trauma, serum biochemistry is usually normal but, as urine accumulates in the abdomen, azotaemia and hyperkalaemia will develop and comparison of biochemistry immediately following trauma and 48 h later is highly informative.

2. Abdominocentesis: a definitive diagnosis of uroabdomen can be confirmed by comparing creatinine concentrations of serum with abdominal fluid. If the level of creatinine in abdominal fluid exceeds that of serum by twofold or more, this is diagnostic for uroabdomen (see Chapter 13).

3. Radiography: plain abdominal radiography is of limited value. Initially, the abdomen may be radiographically normal. As urine accumulates,

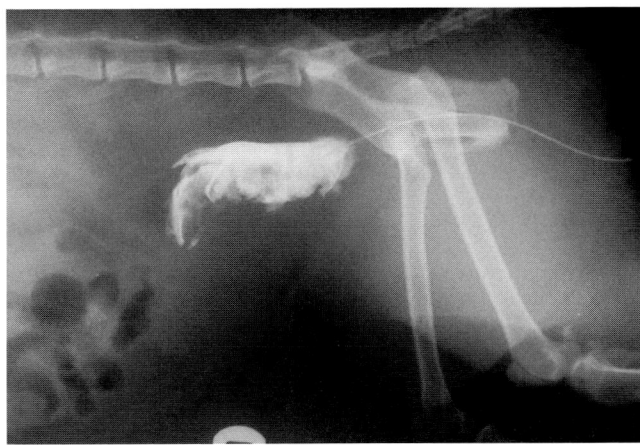

Fig. 16.22. Cat with urethral rupture: positive contrast retrograde urethrogram identified urethral leakage of contrast (there is no bladder filling).

loss of serosal detail indicates accumulation of free abdominal fluid but is a non-specific finding. However, *positive contrast radiography* is of great diagnostic value as it enables disruption of the urinary tract to be demonstrated directly. Retrograde urethrocystography and intravenous urography enable the entire urinary tract to be imaged (Fig. 16.22).

Treatment

Management of urinary tract trauma is complex and challenging. The prognosis is guarded and cases should be referred to an experienced colleague or specialist practice for management. Ureteral injuries are difficult to repair and nephrectomy may be considered as an alternative. Bladder ruptures are repaired by debridement and suturing following the principles of cystotomy closure. Partial urethral tear can be managed by placing an indwelling urethral catheter attached to a closed collection system and leaving it in place for 14 days while the urethra heals around the catheter. Complete urethral rupture with separation is challenging to manage and may require pelvic osteotomy to gain access to the urethra.

Bibliography

Abell, K. and Waldrop, J. (2009) Uroadbomen. *Compendium of Continuing Education for the Practicing Veterinarian* 11, 1–11.

Aumann, M., Worth, L.T. and Drobatz, K.J. (1998) Uroperitoneum in cats: 26 cases (1986–1995). *Journal of the American Animal Hospital Association* 34, 315–324.

Bass, M., Howard, J., Gerber, B. and Messmer, M. (2005) Retrospective study of indications for and outcome of perineal urethrostomy in cats. *Journal of Small Animal Practice* 46, 227–231.

Boothe, H.W. (2000) Managing traumatic urethral injuries. *Clinical Techniques in Small Animal Practice* 15, 35–39.

Bradbury, C.A., Westropp, J.L. and Pollard, R.E. (2009) Relationship between prostatomegaly, prostatic mineralization, and cytologic diagnosis. *Veterinary Radiology and Ultrasound* 50, 167–171.

Cornell, K.K. (2000) Cystotomy, partial cystectomy, and tube cystostomy. *Clinical Techniques in Small Animal Practice* 15, 11–16.

Davidson, A.P. and Baker, T.W. (2009) Reproductive ultrasound of the dog and tom. *Topics in Companion Animal Medicine* 24, 55–63.

Essman, S.C. (2005) Contrast cystography. *Clinical Techniques in Small Animal Practice* 20, 46–51.

Gerber, B., Eichenberger, S. and Reusch, C.E. (2008) Guarded long-term prognosis in male cats with urethral obstruction. *Journal of Feline Medicine and Surgery* 10, 16–23.

Grant, D.C. Harper, T.A. and Werre, S.R. (2010) Frequency of incomplete urolith removal, complications, and diagnostic imaging following cystotomy for removal of uroliths from the lower urinary tract in dogs: 128 cases (1994–2006). *Journal of the American Veterinary Medical Association* 236, 763–766.

Gregory, S.P. (1994) Developments in the understanding of the pathophysiology of urethral sphincter mechanism incompetence in the bitch. *British Veterinary Journal* 150, 135–150.

Gunn-Moore, D.A. (2003) Feline lower urinary tract disease. *Journal of Feline Medicine and Surgery* 5, 133–138.

Hardie, E.M. (1984) Selected surgeries of the male and female reproductive tracts. *Veterinary Clinics of North America Small Animal Practice* 14, 109–122.

Heuter, K.J. (2005) Excretory urography. *Clinical Techniques in Small Animal Practice* 20, 39–45.

Holt, P.E. (1985) Importance of urethral length, bladder neck position and vestibulovaginal stenosis in sphincter mechanism incompetence in the incontinent bitch. *Research in Veterinary Science* 39, 364–372.

Holt, P.E. (2000) Investigation and therapy of incontinent animals. *European Journal of Companion Animal Practice* 10, 111–116.

Holt, P.E. and Gibbs, C. (1992) Congenital urinary incontinence in cats: a review of 19 cases. *Veterinary Record* 130, 437–442.

Holt, P.E. and Moore, A.H. (1995) Canine ureteral ectopia: an analysis of 175 cases and comparison of surgical treatments. *Veterinary Record* 136, 345–349.

Johnston, G.R., Feeney, D.A., Rivers, B. and Walter, P.A. (1991) Diagnostic imaging of the male canine reproductive organs: methods and limitations. *Veterinary Clinics of North America: Small Animal Practice* 21, 553–589.

Krawiec, D.R. and Heflin, D. (1992) Study of prostatic disease in dogs: 177 cases (1981–1986). *Journal of the American Veterinary Medical Association* 200, 1119–1122.

Lane, I.F. (2000) Diagnosis and management of urinary retention. *Veterinary Clinics of North America: Small Animal Practice* 30, 25–57.

Langston, C., Gisselman, K., Palma, D. and McCue, J. (2008) Diagnosis of urolithiasis. *Compendium of Continuing Education for the Practicing Veterinarian* 30, 447–450, 452–444; quiz 455.

Lanz, O.I. and Waldron, D.R. (2000) Renal and ureteral surgery in dogs. *Clinical Techniques in Small Animal Practice* 15, 1–10.

Lightner, B.A., McLoughlin, M.A., Chew, D.J., Beardsley, S.M. and Matthews, H.K. (2001) Episioplasty for the treatment of perivulvar dermatitis or recurrent urinary tract infections in dogs with excessive perivulvar skin folds: 31 cases (1983–2000). *Journal of the American Veterinary Medical Association* 219, 1577–1581.

Mandigers, P.J.J. and Nell, T. (2001) Treatment of bitches with acquired urinary incontinence with oestriol. *Veterinary Record* 149, 764–767.

Mathews, K.G. (2001) Surgery of the canine vagina and vulva. *Veterinary Clinics of North America Small Animal Practice* 31, 271–290.

McLoughlin, M.A. and Chew, D.J. (2000) Diagnosis and surgical management of ectopic ureters. *Clinical Techniques in Small Animal Practice* 15, 17–24.

McLoughlin, M.A. and Chew, D.J. (2009) Surgical views: surgical treatment of urethral sphincter mechanism incompetence in dogs. *Compendium of Continuing Education for the Practicing Veterinarian* 31, 360–373.

Meige, F., Sarrau, S. and Autefage, A. (2008) Management of traumatic urethral rupture in 11 cats using primary alignment with a urethral catheter. *Veterinary and Comparative Orthopedics and Traumatology* 21, 76–84.

Olson, P.N., Wrigley, R.H., Thrall, M.A. and Husted, P.W. (1987) Disorders of the canine prostate gland: pathogenesis, diagnosis, and medical therapy. *Compendium of Continuing Education for the Practicing Veterinarian* 9, 613–623.

Osborne, C.A., Lulich, J.P. and Polzin, D.J. (1999) Canine retrograde urohydropropulsion. Lessons from 25 years of experience. *Veterinary Clinics of North America Small Animal Practice* 29, 267–281.

Osborne, C.A., Lulich, J.P., Forrester, D. and Albasan, H. (2009a) Paradigm changes in the role of nutrition for the management of canine and feline urolithiasis. *Veterinary Clinics of North America Small Animal Practice* 39, 127–141.

Osborne, C.A., Lulich, J.P., Kruger, J.M., Ulrich, L.K. and Koehler, L.A. (2009b) Analysis of 451,891 canine uroliths, feline uroliths, and feline urethral plugs from 1981 to 2007: perspectives from the Minnesota Urolith Center. *Veterinary Clinics of North America Small Animal Practice* 39, 183–197.

Papazoglou, L.G. and Kazakos, G.M. (2002) Surgical conditions of the canine penis and prepuce. *Compendium: Continuing Education for Veterinarians* 24, 204–217.

Radasch, R.M., Merkley, D.F., Wilson, J.W. and Barstad, R.D. (1990) Cystotomy closure. A comparison of the strength of appositional and inverting suture patterns. *Veterinary Surgery* 19, 283–288.

Rawlings, C., Barsanti, J.A., Mahaffey, M.B. and Bement, S. (2001) Evaluation of colposuspension for treatment of incontinence in spayed female dogs. *Journal of the American Veterinary Medical Association* 219, 770–775.

Reine, N.J. and Langston, C.E. (2005) Urinalysis interpretation: how to squeeze out the maximum information from a small sample. *Clinical Techniques in Small Animal Practice* 20, 2–10.

Saevik, B.K., Trangerud, C., Ottesen, N., Sorum, H. and Eggertsdottir, A.V. (2011) Causes of lower urinary tract disease in Norwegian cats. *Journal of Feline Medicine and Surgery* 13, 410–417.

Scott, L., Leddy, M., Bernay, F. and Davot, J.L. (2002) Evaluation of phenylpropanolamine in the treatment of urethral sphincter mechanism incompetence in the bitch. *Journal of Small Animal Practice* 43, 493–496.

Silverman, S. and Long, C.D. (2000) The diagnosis of urinary incontinence and abnormal urination in dogs and cats. *Veterinary Clinics of North America: Small Animal Practice* 30, 427–448.

Smeak, D.D. (2000) Urethrotomy and urethrostomy in the dog. *Clinical Techniques in Small Animal Practice* 15, 25–34.

Smith, C.W. (2002) Perineal urethrostomy. *Veterinary Clinics of North America: Small Animal Practice* 32, 917–925.

Smith, J. (2008) Canine prostatic disease: a review of anatomy, pathology, diagnosis, and treatment. *Theriogenology* 70, 375–383.

Teske, E., Naan, E.C., Van Dijk, E.M., Van Garderen, E. and Schalken, J.A. (2002) Canine prostate carcinoma: epidemiological evidence of an increased risk in castrated dogs. *Molecular and Cellular Endocrinology* 197, 251–255.

Thomas, P.C. and Yool, D.A. (2010) Delayed-onset urinary incontinence in five female dogs with ectopic ureters. *Journal of Small Animal Practice* 51, 224–226.

Threlfall, W.R. and Chew, D.J. (1999) Diagnosis and treatment of canine bacterial prostatitis. *Compendium of Continuing Education for the Practicing Veterinarian* 21, 73–86.

Tursi, M., Costa, T., Valenza, F. and Aresu, L. (2008) Adenocarcinoma of the disseminated prostate in a cat. *Journal of Feline Medicine and Surgery* 10, 600–602.

Weisse, C., Aronson, L.R. and Drobatz, K. (2002) Traumatic rupture of the ureter: 10 cases. *Journal of the American Animal Hospital Association* 38, 188–192.

White, R.A.S. (2000) Prostatic surgery in the dog. *Clinical Techniques in Small Animal Practice* 15, 46–51.

Williams, J. (2009) Surgical management of blocked cats. Which approach and when? *Journal of Feline Medicine and Surgery* 11, 14–22.

17 Splenic Surgery

partial splenectomy: removal of a portion of the spleen
splenomegaly: splenic enlargement (focal or generalized)
total splenectomy: removal of the whole spleen

The reader should be able to:

- list causes of focal and of generalized splenomegaly in the dog
- describe the vascular anatomy of the spleen relevant to performing total splenectomy in the cat
- describe how to perform total splenectomy in the dog

Anatomy

The spleen is a long, strap-like organ suspended in the greater omentum. The omentum attaches along the hilus that runs the length of the spleen. The head of spleen lies between the fundus of the stomach and the left lateral abdominal wall. It continues into the body and tail that follow the greater curvature of the stomach ventrally across midline. The splenic artery, a branch of the coeliac artery, runs in the deep leaf of the greater omentum close to the left limb of the pancreas, to which it supplies a branch. A few centimetres from the hilus, the splenic artery divides into two or three large branches and these further divide into 20 or 30 smaller vessels before penetrating the hilus of the spleen (Fig. 17.1). At the head of the spleen, vessels run from the splenic vessels to the fundus of the stomach (Fig. 17.2). These are called short gastric vessels and partly contribute to the blood supply of the fundus.

Splenic Disease

Splenic disease is often identified during the evaluation of haemoabdomen which is discussed in Chapter 13. Splenic pathology may also be identified as an incidental finding during abdominal palpation, surgery, or ultrasound.

Focal splenomegaly

Focal splenomegaly is usually caused by splenic tumours in the dog (Fig. 17.3). German Shepherd dogs and retrievers are predisposed to developing them. Splenic haemangiosarcoma is the commonest form and usually has metastasized by the time of diagnosis. Non-cancerous splenic masses may also be identified. Splenic haematoma is quite common. It is grossly indistinguishable from a splenic tumour and may also lead to haemoabdomen. Histopathology should always be performed to distinguish between different forms of splenic mass. Other causes of focal splenomegaly include splenic abscess, hyperplastic splenic nodules, and extramedullary haematopoiesis.

Generalized splenomegaly

A range of conditions cause generalized splenomegaly.

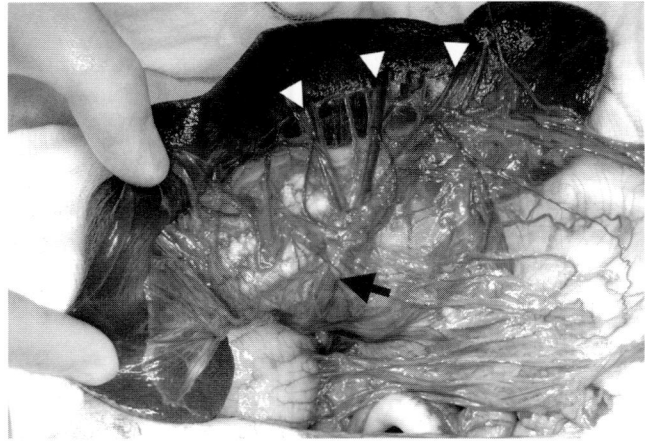

Fig. 17.1. The splenic artery (black arrow) runs through the deep leaf of the omentum and branches to supply many small vessels along the splenic hilus (white arrowheads).

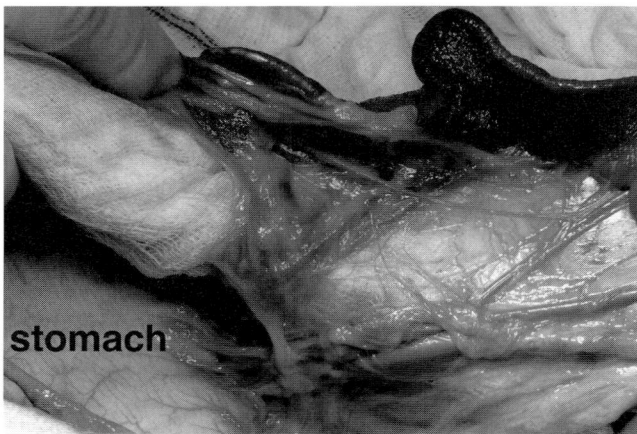

Fig. 17.2. Short gastric arteries arise from the terminal branches of the splenic artery near the hilus of the spleen and run from the head of the spleen to the fundus of the stomach.

Splenic congestion

Splenic congestion is usually induced by vasodilatory drugs (e.g. acepromazine; barbiturates) given during anaesthesia and is of no clinical significance. It may also occur secondary to splenic displacement if the vascular pedicle to the spleen becomes compromised. This occurs commonly in animals with gastric dilatation and volvulus (GDV), but the congestion will resolve within 10–15 min once the spleen is returned to its normal position. Splenectomy should only be considered if the spleen is necrotic, if congestion does not resolve 15 min after the spleen has been repositioned, or if the splenic vessels are damaged (e.g. avulsed from the hilus; thrombosed).

Splenic infarction

Splenic infarction is an uncommon cause of splenomegaly associated with hypercoagulable states or with conditions predisposing to thromboembolic disease. Splenectomy is usually indicated but the underlying cause of infarction should be investigated and may carry a poor prognosis.

Splenic torsion

Spontaneous splenic torsion is uncommon and can lead to hypovolaemic shock through sequestration of blood in the spleen (Fig. 17.4). Splenic torsion occurs spontaneously and affects large-breed dogs. Great Danes are predisposed. Body conformation and prior GDV have also been implicated in the aetiology. Dogs may present with rapid-onset signs of abdominal discomfort, abdominal enlargement, shock, and collapse, but chronic and less dramatic signs are also reported. Investigations identify massive splenomegaly and displacement of other organs, anaemia, and acid–base disorders. The prognosis following splenectomy is good but some dogs have subsequently developed GDV leading to the recommendation to perform gastropexy at the time of splenectomy for splenic torsion (see below).

Splenic infiltration

Neoplastic and other infiltrative conditions, such as lymphoma, mastocytosis, and systemic histiocytosis, may cause focal or generalized splenomegaly. Splenectomy may be of value depending on the primary condition.

Incidental splenic pathology

Insignificant splenic pathology is commonly identified during abdominal surgery. Accessory splenic tissue forms small nodules of dark red material in the omentum and can be mistaken for neoplastic nodules. Haemosiderin (a by-product of iron metabolism) collects on the surface of the spleen leading to golden-brown plaques of no clinical significance (Fig. 17.5). Extramedullary haematopoiesis and hyperplastic splenic nodules may also cause focal enlargement.

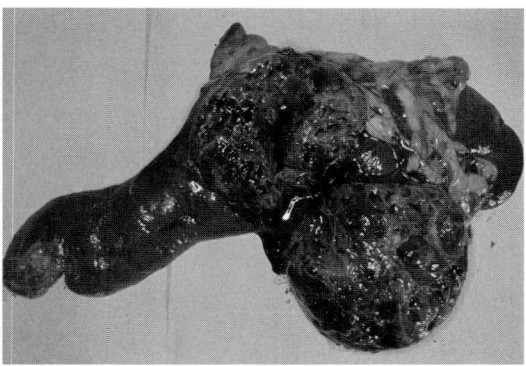

Fig. 17.3. Spleen removed from a German Shepherd dog that presented with acute haemoabdomen. This dog had a splenic haemangiosarcoma. The disorganized vascular channels through the tumour can be seen where it has been sectioned.

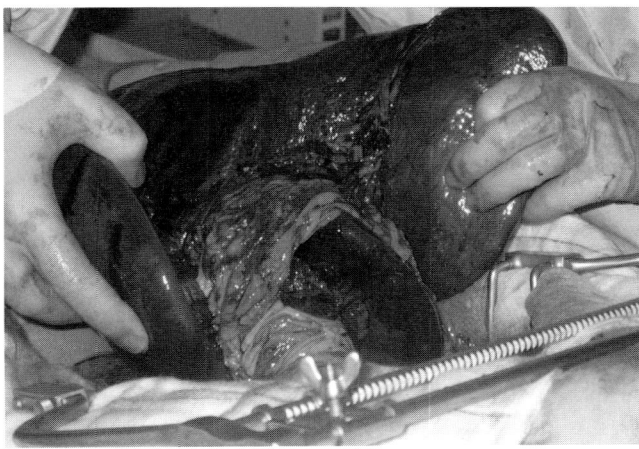

Fig. 17.4. Splenic torsion in a Great Dane. The spleen weighed 10% of the body weight of this dog and the patient had signs of acute hypovolaemic shock because of sequestration of blood within the engorged spleen. Splenectomy and gastropexy were performed and the dog made a complete recovery.

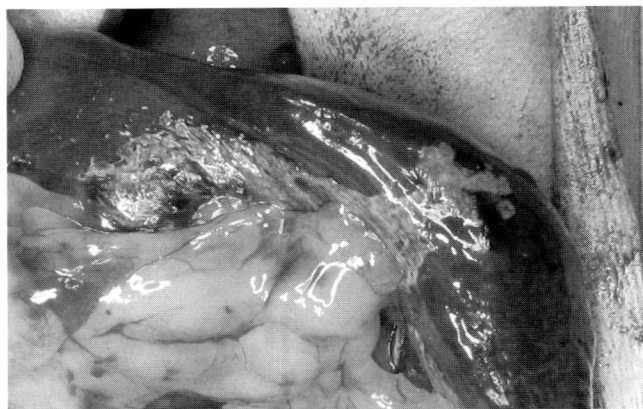

Fig. 17.5. Haemosiderin plaques on the surface of a spleen.

Association with ventricular arrhythmias

There is a strong association between splenic disease and the development of ventricular arrhythmias. Thirty per cent of dogs with splenomegaly develop arrhythmias perioperatively. The cause of the arrhythmias is not known but factors including myocardial hypoxia and release of toxins from hypoxic pancreas in shocked patients, and metastatic deposits within the myocardium from splenic tumours, have all been implicated. These arrhythmias are rarely fatal but may require treatment.

Feline splenic disease

Cats suffer from a similar range of splenic diseases to dogs. Infiltration of the spleen with mast cells associated with systemic mastocytosis is the commonest cause of splenomegaly (see Chapter 9). Haemangiosarcoma and lymphoma are also reported. Non-neoplastic conditions, including extramedullary haematopoiesis, may also lead to splenomegaly.

Investigation

The mainstays of investigation of splenic disease are preoperative imaging and histopathological analysis of splenic tissue.

Imaging

Ultrasound is the imaging modality of choice for splenic disease as it provides most information about splenic lesions, metastatic spread, and haemoabdomen. Radiography can also be used to assess splenic size, shape, and position. The spleen should be clearly identified on left lateral abdominal views as a strap-like organ lying caudal to the stomach and parallel to the gastric axis. The body should be identified on the left and the tail on the right of dorsoventral or ventrodorsal abdominal views. On the right lateral view, only the tail of the spleen sitting in the ventral abdomen just caudal to the pylorus should be seen. Splenic masses may cause displacement of the small intestines caudally (lateral view) or gastric fundus towards midline (ventrodorsal view) (Fig. 17.6).

Animals with splenic tumours often have metastatic lesions detected in the liver, omentum, and lungs. These may be detectable using abdominal ultrasound and thoracic radiography. Splenic haemangiosarcoma may also metastasize to the heart.

Splenic biopsy

Preoperative needle-core or incisional splenic biopsies may cause significant abdominal bleeding and are rarely performed. Splenic fine-needle aspirate is well tolerated and can be useful for investigating infiltrative disease, although the aspirate results often do not correlate with the final histopathological diagnosis. Often preoperative biopsy is not performed and the diagnosis is only reached following analysis of the whole spleen after splenectomy. As total splenectomy is comparatively safe and is the procedure of choice for managing most splenic disease, it is common to forego preoperative biopsy and to proceed straight to exploratory abdominal surgery after imaging studies.

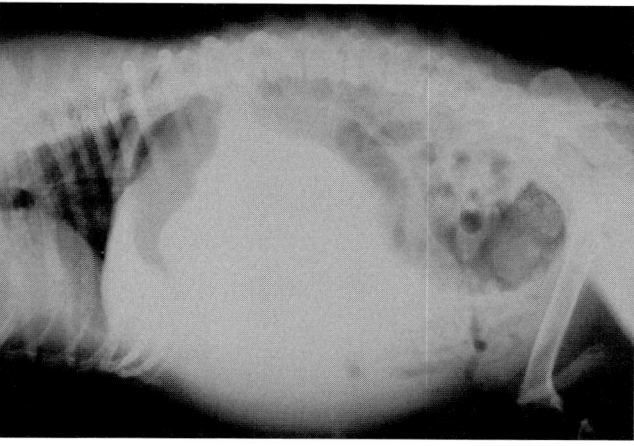

Fig. 17.6. Radiograph of a dog with splenomegaly. The grossly enlarged spleen fills the central abdomen and has displaced the stomach and small intestine.

Surgery

Splenic disease can be managed by total or partial splenectomy. Total splenectomy is technically easy to perform, quick, and associated with a low rate of post-operative haemorrhage. Total splenectomy also removes all splenic tissue, reducing the risk of local recurrence of splenic tumours. In contrast, partial splenectomy is technically more difficult and more likely to result in haemorrhage. For these reasons, total splenectomy is generally performed in preference to partial splenectomy.

Animals undergoing splenic surgery often have severe haemorrhagic shock and may require resuscitation prior to surgery (see Chapter 13). If haemoabdomen has resulted from trauma, they may also have concurrent injuries, including diaphragmatic rupture or pulmonary contusions, which require separate evaluation and treatment.

Total splenectomy

Make a ventral midline coeliotomy incision from the xiphisternum to near the pubis and explore the abdomen before performing splenectomy. Be prepared to remove large volumes of free abdominal blood using suction. Collect biopsies of possible metastatic lesions.

Gently exteriorize the spleen from the abdomen. If there is active haemorrhage, apply bitch spay forceps along the hilus of the spleen to achieve temporary haemostasis. Working from the tail towards the head of the spleen, isolate individual vessels entering the hilus by blunt dissection, double ligate them, and divide them between the ligatures. Incise the omental attachments to the hilus as you proceed. Use 2-0 or 3-0 absorbable, synthetic, monofilament suture material (Fig. 17.7). Once the last hilar vessels at the head of the spleen have been transected, cut any remaining omental attachments and remove the spleen (Fig. 17.8). Check carefully for bleeding before closing the abdominal incision.

Post-operative care

Monitor the patient for signs of haemoabdomen and shock in the immediate post-operative period. Submit excised tissues for histopathological analysis.

Complications

The physiological consequences of splenectomy are minor but some haematological abnormalities have been noted such as increased numbers of Howell–Jolly bodies, nucleated red blood cells, and target cells. Most complications relate to progression of the underlying disease, and specific complications of surgery are uncommon. Severe post-operative haemorrhage may occur if haemostasis is inadequate. Ventricular arrhythmias may develop

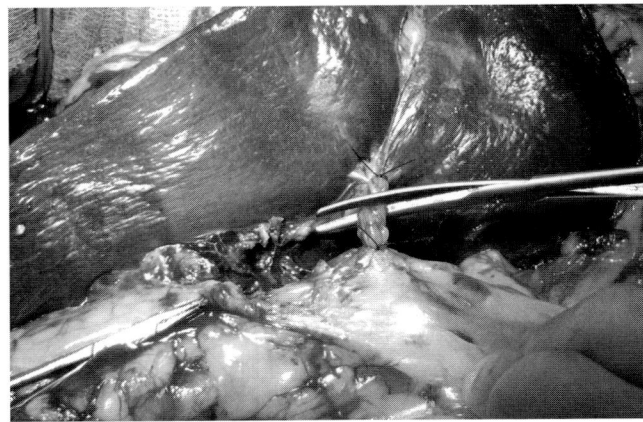

Fig. 17.7. Total splenectomy: the splenic vessels are double ligated and divided as they enter the hilus of the spleen.

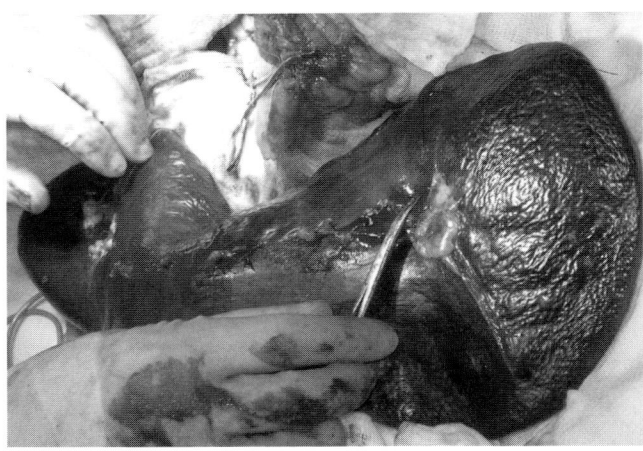

Fig. 17.8. Spleen following removal showing ligature line along the hilus.

post-operatively (see p. 279). Resurgence of blood-borne disease has also been reported following splenectomy in infected animals.

GDV has been reported in a small number of dogs following splenectomy and there has been some speculation that splenomegaly and subsequent splenectomy may predispose dogs to GDV. There is no evidence that performing prophylactic gastropexy at the time of splenectomy is warranted in most cases. However, splenic torsion and GDV share common epidemiological features and there seems to be a genuine association between these two conditions, prompting the recommendation to perform prophylactic gastropexy following splenectomy in dogs with splenic torsion.

Prognosis

The prognosis for patients with splenic rupture following trauma is good if they survive the immediate perioperative period. The prognosis for cats with splenic mastocytosis is reasonable as median survival times of over 1 year are reported following splenectomy (although most animals ultimately succumb to the disease). The prognosis for animals with splenic haemangiosarcoma is, in contrast, very poor as they are likely to succumb to metastatic disease quickly. For example, dogs with haemangiosarcoma are reported to have median survival times of only 86 days following splenectomy alone, and of only 114 days if this is combined with epirubicin therapy.

Bibliography

Allan, R., Halsey, T.R. and Thompson, K.G. (2000) Splenic mast cell tumour and mastocytaemia in a cat: case study and literature review. *New Zealand Veterinary Journal* 48, 117–121.

Aronsohn, M.G., Dubiel, B., Roberts, B. and Powers, B.E. (2009) Prognosis for acute nontraumatic hemoperitoneum in the dog: a retrospective analysis of 60 cases (2003–2006). *Journal of the American Animal Hospital Association* 45, 72–77.

Ballegeer, E.A., Forrest, L.J., Dickinson, R.M., Schutten, M.M., Delaney, F.A. and Young, K.M. (2007) Correlation of ultrasonographic appearance of lesions and cytologic and histologic diagnoses in splenic aspirates from dogs and cats: 32 cases (2002–2005). *Journal of the American Veterinary Medical Association* 230, 690–696.

Bezuidenhout, A.J. (1993) The lymphatic system. In: Evans, H.E. (ed.) *Miller's Anatomy of the Dog*, 3rd edn. W.B. Saunders, Philadelphia, Pennsylvania, pp. 716–757.

Bischoff, M.G. (2003) Radiographic techniques and interpretation of the acute abdomen. *Clinical Techniques in Small Animal Practice* 18, 7–19.

Culp, W.T., Drobatz, K.J., Glassman, M.M., Baez, J.L. and Aronson, L.R. (2008) Feline visceral hemangiosarcoma. *Journal of Veterinary Internal Medicine* 22, 148–152.

Culp, W.T., Weisse, C., Kellogg, M.E., Gordon, I.K., Clarke, D.L., May, L.R. and Drobatz, K.J. (2010) Spontaneous hemoperitoneum in cats: 65 cases (1994–2006). *Journal of the American Veterinary Medical Association* 236, 978–982.

Day, M.J., Lucke, V.M. and Pearson, H. (1995) A review of pathological diagnoses made from 87 canine splenic biopsies. *Journal of Small Animal Practice* 36, 426–433.

Dobson, J., Villiers, E., Roulois, A., Gould, S., Mellor, P., Hoather, T. and Watson, P. (2006) Histiocytic sarcoma of the spleen in flat-coated retrievers with regenerative anaemia and hypoproteinaemia. *Veterinary Record* 158, 825–829.

Evans, H.E. (1993) Unpaired visceral branches of abdominal aorta. In: Evans, H.E. (ed.) *Miller's Anatomy of the Dog*, 3rd edn. W.B. Saunders, Philadelphia, Pennsylvania, pp. 651–657.

Furneaux, R.W. (1975) Symposium on surgical techniques in small animal practice. Surgical techniques for the spleen and liver. *Veterinary Clinics of North America* 5, 363–381.

Goldhammer, M.A., Haining, H., Milne, E.M., Shaw, D.J. and Yool, D.A. (2010) Assessment of the incidence of GDV following splenectomy in dogs. *Journal of Small Animal Practice* 51, 23–28.

Gordon, S.S., McClaran, J.K., Bergman, P.J. and Liu, S.M. (2010) Outcome following splenectomy in cats. *Journal of Feline Medicine and Surgery* 12, 256–261.

Hammond, T.N. and Pesillo-Crosby, S.A. (2008) Prevalence of hemangiosarcoma in anemic dogs with a splenic mass and hemoperitoneum requiring a transfusion: 71 cases (2003–2005). *Journal of the American Veterinary Medical Association* 232, 553–558.

Hardie, E.M., Vaden, S.L., Spaulding, K. and Malarkey, D.E. (1995) Splenic infarction in 16 dogs: a retrospective study. *Journal of Veterinary Internal Medicine* 9, 141–148.

Hosgood, G., Bone, D.L., Vorhees III, W.D. and Reed, W.M. (1989) Splenectomy in the dog by ligation of the splenic and short gastric arteries. *Veterinary Surgery* 18, 110–113.

Kemming, G., Messick, J.B., Mueller, W., Enders, G., Meisner, F., Muenzing, S., Kisch-Wedel, H., *et al.* (2004) Can we continue research in splenectomized dogs? *Mycoplasma haemocanis*: old problem – new insight. *European Surgical Research* 36, 198–205.

Keyes, M.L., Rush, J.E., Autran De Morais, H.S. and Couto, C.G. (1993) Ventricular arrhythmias in dogs with splenic masses. *Journal of Veterinary Emergency and Critical Care* 3, 33–38.

Kim, S.E., Liptak, J.M., Gall, T.T., Monteith, G.J. and Woods, J.P. (2007) Epirubicin in the adjuvant treatment of splenic hemangiosarcoma in dogs: 59 cases (1997–2004). *Journal of the American Veterinary Medical Association* 231, 1550–1557.

Knapp, D.W., Aronsohn, M.G. and Harpster, N.K. (1993) Cardiac arrhythmias associated with mass lesions of the canine spleen. *Journal of the American Animal Hospital Association* 29, 122–128.

Lamb, C.R. (1990) Abdominal ultrasonography in small animals: examination of the liver, spleen and pancreas. *Journal of Small Animal Practice* 31, 5–14.

Marino, D.J., Matthiesen, D.T., Fox, P.R., Lesser, M.B. and Stamoulis, M.E. (1994) Ventricular arrhythmias in dogs undergoing splenectomy: a prospective study. *Veterinary Surgery* 23, 101–106.

Neath, P.J., Brockman, D.J. and Saunders, H.M. (1997) Retrospective analysis of 19 cases of isolated torsion of the splenic pedicle in dogs. *Journal of Small Animal Practice* 38, 387–392.

Spangler, W.L. and Culbertson, M.R. (1992a) Prevalence and type of splenic diseases in cats: 455 cases (1985–1991). *Journal of the American Veterinary Medical Association* 201, 773–776.

Spangler, W.L. and Culbertson, M.R. (1992b) Prevalence, type, and importance of splenic diseases in dogs: 1480 cases (1985–1989). *Journal of the American Veterinary Medical Association* 200, 829–834.

Stefanello, D., Valenti, P., Faverzani, S., Bronzo, V., Fiorbianco, V., Pinto Da Cunha, N., Romussi, S., *et al.* (2009) Ultrasound-guided cytology of spleen and liver: a prognostic tool in canine cutaneous mast cell tumor. *Journal of Veterinary Internal Medicine* 23, 1051–1057.

Tillson, D.M. (2003) Spleen. In: Slatter, D.H. (ed.) *Textbook of Small Animal Surgery*, 3rd edn. Saunders, Philadelphia, Pennsylvania, pp. 1046–1062.

Vinayak, A. and Krahwinkel, D.J. (2004) Managing blunt trauma-induced hemoperitoneum in dogs and cats. *Compendium of Continuing Education for the Practicing Veterinarian* 26, 276–291.

Wrigley, R.H. (1991) Ultrasonography of the spleen. Life-threatening splenic disorders. *Problems in Veterinary Medicine* 3, 574–581.

18 Hepatic Surgery

cholecystectomy: removal of the gall bladder
cholecystoduodenostomy: creation of a stoma between the gall bladder and duodenum
partial hepatectomy: removal of a portion of liver (e.g. a lobe)
portosystemic shunt: an abnormal vessel that allows portal blood to bypass the liver and enter the systemic circulation

The reader should be able to:

- perform liver biopsy
- discuss options for treatment of congenital portosystemic shunt with a pet owner
- recognize the signs of hepatic encephalopathy and implement medical management of the condition

Liver biopsy is simple and is often performed in general practice. However, other hepatobiliary procedures are technically demanding and require careful preoperative planning and post-operative management.

Anatomy

The liver is divided into the caudate (with caudate and papillary processes), right lateral, right medial, quadrate, left medial and left lateral lobes. The biliary tree drains bile from the liver into the proximal duodenum via the common bile duct. It consists of 2–5 hepatic ducts from the liver lobes that coalesce to form the common bile duct. The common bile duct runs through the lesser omentum before entering the mesenteric border of the proximal duodenum. It runs for a short distance through the wall of the duodenum before emptying into the lumen. The gall bladder stores bile between feeding and is joined to the common bile duct by the cystic duct. The gall bladder lies between the right medial and quadrate lobes.

The hepatic artery, a branch of the coeliac artery, supplies 20% of the blood supply to the liver. The portal vein drains blood from the gastrointestinal tract, pancreas and spleen and supplies 80% of the blood supply to the liver. These vessels run parallel to the common bile duct into the hilus of the liver. The hepatic veins drain blood from the liver into the caudal vena cava, which is embedded dorsally within the hepatic parenchyma on the right.

Liver Biopsy

Liver biopsy is indicated for the evaluation of diffuse liver disease or for investigation of discrete liver lesions. Animals with diffuse liver pathology cannot metabolize anaesthetic agents efficiently and anaesthetic protocols must be adjusted accordingly. These patients may also have coagulopathies. Preoperative assessment for clotting disorders and strategies for dealing with intra-operative bleeding must be considered.

Approach

To carry out liver biopsy for diffuse liver disease, a cranial midline coeliotomy from the umbilicus to the xiphisternum is adequate (Fig. 10.3B). However, for full evaluation of all liver lobes and biopsy of focal lesions, a full exploratory coeliotomy incision should be performed.

Technique 1 (guillotine technique)

To biopsy the tip of a liver lobe, place a ligature of 2-0 or 3-0 monofilament, absorbable suture material around the tip of the lobe (Fig. 18.1). Tighten the ligature to crush though the tissue before tying. The ligature ensnares larger vessels, preventing bleeding. Transect the tip of the liver lobe distal to the ligature. Alternatively, place a transfixing ligature in a similar manner.

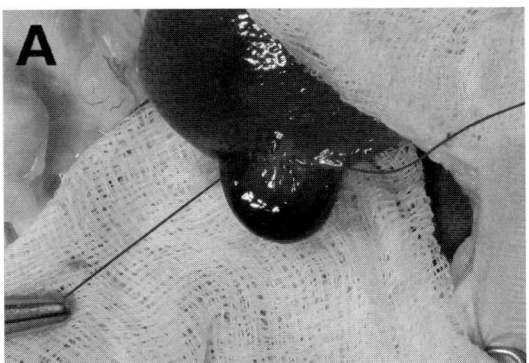

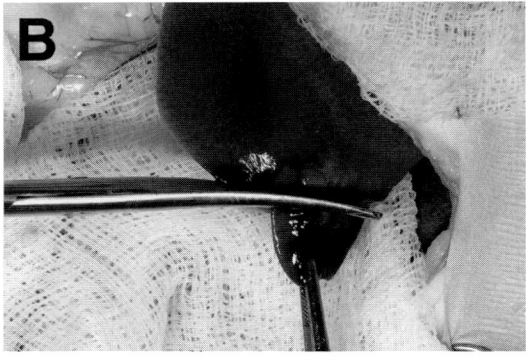

Fig. 18.1. Liver biopsy technique 1: (A) encircle the tip of a liver lobe with a ligature; (B) remove the tip.

Technique 2

To biopsy a lesion at the edge of a liver lobe, isolate the lesion with two or three overlapping ligatures (which create a semi-circle around the lesion). Then excise the tissue isolated within the suture line (Fig. 18.2).

Alternative techniques

Lesions on the surface of the liver that are not near the edge of the lobe can be biopsied using a skin punch biopsy knife to remove a core (Fig. 18.3). Close the defect with one or two mattress sutures. This technique causes more bleeding, and topical haemostatic agents (e.g. collagen swabs) may be required. It should not be performed near to the base of a liver lobe as the hepatic vessels are larger in this region. Do not push the biopsy punch deeply into the liver to avoid the larger, deeper vessels. Ultrasound-guided needle-core biopsy and laparoscopic biopsy are alternative techniques.

Congenital Portosystemic Shunt

Congenital portosystemic shunts (PSS) can be managed medically or surgically. Confirming the diagnosis and operating successfully require considerable experience. The aim of this section is to provide background information to enable the clinician to initiate medical management and discuss treatment options with an owner prior to referral.

Aetiology and morphology

Congenital PSS is a developmental vascular anomaly that allows portal blood from the intestines to bypass the liver and empty directly into the systemic circulation. The shunt is often a single vessel running between the portal vein and caudal vena cava (Fig. 18.4). It may run outside the liver (extrahepatic) or be buried within the liver (intrahepatic). Small-breed dogs tend to have extrahepatic PSS whereas large-breed dogs tend to have intrahepatic PSS. Cats can have either form. Other variations also occur in both species.

Pathophysiology

The portal circulation collects blood from the gastrointestinal tract and delivers it to the liver where nutrients and toxins from the intestinal tract are metabolized before being released into the systemic

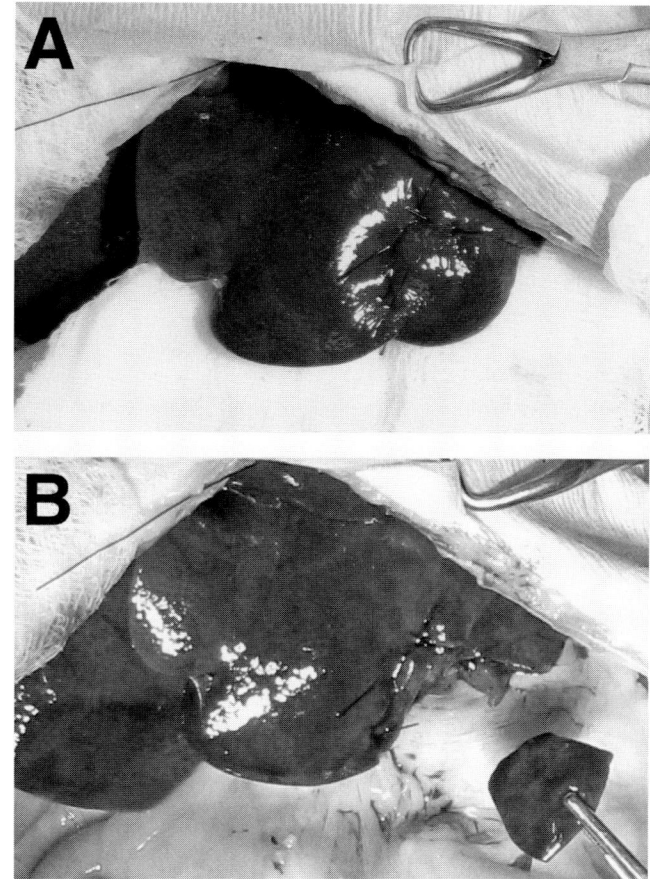

Fig. 18.2. Liver biopsy technique 2: (A) encircle the lesion with overlapping ligatures; (B) remove the isolated section.

circulation. PSS enables portal blood to bypass the liver and leads to a range of metabolic disorders.

Microhepatica and inadequate liver function

The portal vein provides trophic factors, nutrients, and 80% of the blood supply to the liver. Animals with PSS have microhepatica and poor liver function. They are often stunted and lean. Reduced protein production leads to hypoalbuminaemia and coagulation disorders. Animals are prone to hypoglycaemia due to poor hepatic gluconeogenesis. Inadequate liver function also leads to poor drug metabolism that manifests as prolonged recovery from general anaesthesia and profound sedation with opioids and other drugs.

Metabolic encephalopathy

Endogenous colonic bacteria and the intestinal mucosa generate toxins (e.g. ammonia) through metabolism of proteins in the diet. An important function of normal enterohepatic circulation is to remove these toxins before blood from the intestinal tract enters the general circulation. Release of these toxins directly into the bloodstream leads to hepatic encephalopathy in animals with PSS.

Urate urolithiasis

Disruption of urea and ammonia metabolism predisposes to urate urolithiasis that cause signs in 30% of cases.

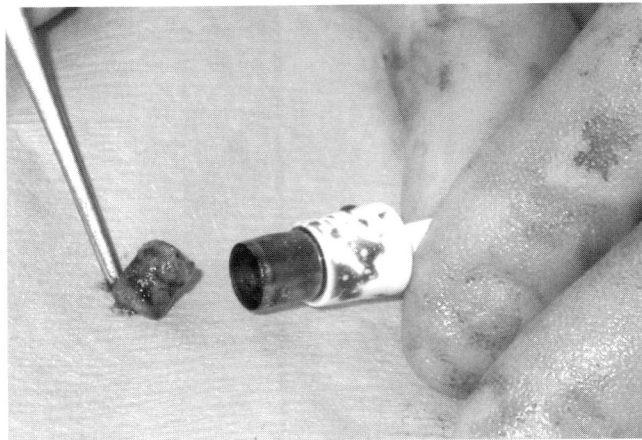

Fig. 18.3. Liver biopsy technique 3: circular skin punch.

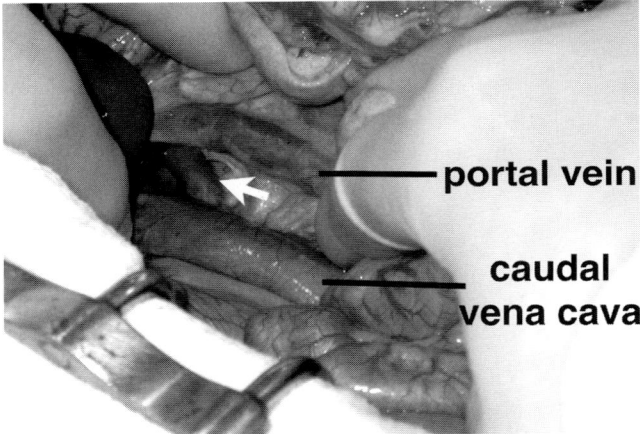

Fig. 18.4. Congenital, extrahepatic PSS (arrow) running between portal vein and caudal vena cava just distal to the hepatic hilus (viewed having performed the duodenal sling manoeuvre).

Presentation

Dogs and cats with PSS typically present within the first 6 months of life with a range of signs:

- stunting and poor body condition;
- quiet demeanour in comparison to littermates;
- urinary tract signs caused by urate urolithiasis;
- hepatic encephalopathy: typically occurs shortly after feeding; signs include ataxia, altered behaviour, central blindness, dullness, unresponsiveness, aimless wandering, head pressing, seizures, stupor, or coma;
- polydipsia.

Some animals present older, having shown few or no signs of PSS for the first few years of life. The reason why these cases are unaffected for so long is unknown.

Investigation

A high index of suspicion of PSS can be reached when juvenile patients present with signs of hepatic encephalopathy or with urate urolithiasis. Investigation aims to confirm the diagnosis and to assess the feasibility and value of surgery. Differential diagnoses to consider include acquired hepatopathies (e.g. viral hepatopathy), conditions related to PSS such as microvascular dysplasia, and breed-associated urate urolithiasis.

Serum biochemistry

Hypoalbuminaemia, low urea, and mild to moderate elevations in liver enzymes may be seen. Hyperbilirubinaemia is not a feature of PSS.

Elevated serum *ammonia* levels after eating are consistent with hepatic encephalopathy but will fall to normal quickly. Ammonia must be evaluated within a few minutes of sampling as ageing blood samples spontaneously produce ammonia from breakdown of nitrogenous chemicals.

Serum *bile acids* are elevated in patients with PSS. Bile acids are released into the duodenum by gall bladder contraction during feeding and are resorbed by the intestinal tract into the portal circulation. Most bile acids (~95%) are removed from the circulation by the liver during first-pass hepatic metabolism. Animals with PSS do not sequester bile acids in the liver following feeding, as the shunt delivers the bile acids directly into the general circulation. This causes serum bile acid levels to rise rapidly immediately after feeding and then gradually fall over several hours (normally, they would only rise marginally postprandially). The bile acid stimulation test is useful for screening for PSS. A sample is collected for a fasting serum bile acid assay. The patient is fed and the assay is repeated after 2 h. Animals with PSS may have normal or moderately elevated resting bile acid levels but show massive elevation of bile acids after feeding. This test is very useful but it is not specific for PSS, as high values are associated with other hepatopathies.

Haematology

Patients with PSS often have microcytic anaemia due to altered iron metabolism. Mild coagulation disorders may also be identified.

Imaging

Contrast radiography, abdominal ultrasound, and scintigraphy are all sensitive methods for detecting PSS but require experience to interpret accurately.

Treatment

Patients may be treated medically or with combined medical and surgical therapy. The long-term prognosis is best with combined medical and surgical therapy, but surgery carries a moderate risk of fatal complications. Medical management should be instigated as soon as a diagnosis is reached.

Medical management

Medical management is mainly aimed at managing hepatic encephalopathy with dietary modification, lactulose, and antibiotics. During severe episodes of hepatic encephalopathy, lactulose enemas, anticonvulsants, and supportive care may also be required.

DIETARY MODIFICATION Protein-restricted hepatic diets are fed as they have lower levels of aromatic amino acids that generate most neurotoxins. However, these diets are not designed to support growth in young animals and may precipitate hypoalbuminaemia. In young animals, protein-restricted diets can be supplemented with dairy proteins (cottage cheese 100 g per 450 g tin of hepatic diet) that help to maintain a positive nitrogen balance in the actively growing patient. The daily ration is divided into several small meals spaced through the day to reduce the level of neurotoxins being produced and absorbed at any one time.

LACTULOSE Lactulose is an osmotic laxative. It reduces the number of colonic bacteria-producing neurotoxins. It also traps ammonia in its ionic form within the colon by acidifying the lumen. The dose of lactulose is 1–5 ml/kg every 8 h, adjusted to prevent diarrhoea.

ORAL ANTIBIOTICS Ampicillin (10 mg/kg orally every 8 h) is prescribed to modify the colonic flora and reduce neurotoxin production. Other antimicrobials that can be used include metronidazole, gentamicin, and amoxycillin.

Surgical management

The aim of surgery is to gradually attenuate the shunt to direct portal blood into the liver. Gradual attenuation devices such as the ameroid constrictor are used to close the anomalous vessel. Not all cases are amenable to surgery. Intra-operative haemorrhage, post-operative portal hypertension, and post-attenuation neurological syndrome are life-threatening perioperative complications. The mortality rate associated with surgery ranges from 5% (extrahepatic shunts) to 20% (intrahepatic shunts) and not all cases are suitable for surgery. Cases should be referred to specialist centres for surgical evaluation.

Outcomes

Both medical and surgical therapies can lead to marked improvement or complete resolution of signs, but surgery produces the best long-term results. Despite good outcomes in many patients, some show incomplete or no response to therapy and the prognosis must remain guarded.

Hepatic Tumours

Primary and secondary liver tumours are common in dogs and cats. Focal liver tumours may be amenable to resection by partial hepatectomy and, dependent on the type of tumour, the prognosis following resection may be good. Surgery can be challenging and there are risks of intra-operative bleeding and damage to the biliary tree or portal vein. Patients should be referred to specialist centres for evaluation for surgery.

Diseases of the Common Bile Duct and Gall Bladder

Surgery on the gall bladder and common bile duct is difficult and has a high complication rate. Patients should be referred to specialist centres.

Biliary tree rupture

Rupture of a hepatic duct, the common bile duct, or the gall bladder will lead to bile peritonitis. Rupture may be caused by trauma or may occur secondary to necrotizing cholecystitis or biliary mucocoele (see below). The onset of signs is insidious and several days may pass before the diagnosis is reached. The investigation of bile peritonitis is reviewed in Chapter 13.

Biliary obstruction

Obstructive jaundice occurs when flow of bile through the common bile duct is blocked. This may be caused by extraluminal lesions (e.g. proximal duodenal or pancreatic tumours), mural lesions (e.g. cholangiohepatitis; biliary tree neoplasia) or intraluminal lesions (e.g. choleliths). Obstructive jaundice can be relieved by performing cholecystoduodenostomy. This surgery creates a stoma between the gall bladder and the duodenum to provide an alternative route for drainage of bile. This is a high-risk surgery due to the potential for leakage of bile, stenosis of the surgery site, and progression of the inciting disease process.

Biliary mucocoele

Biliary mucocoele occurs in dogs. Bile becomes viscous and stops draining through the biliary tree. The hepatic ducts and gall bladder become congested leading to abdominal pain, obstructive jaundice, or cholangiohepatitis. Over time, the gall bladder wall becomes oedematous and thickened, and may rupture leading to bile peritonitis. Cases can be managed conservatively or surgically. Currently, there is no way of predicting which cases will not respond to medical management or will develop bile peritonitis, so early surgical intervention may be the safest option. Cholecystectomy or cholecystoduodenostomy is performed (Fig. 18.5).

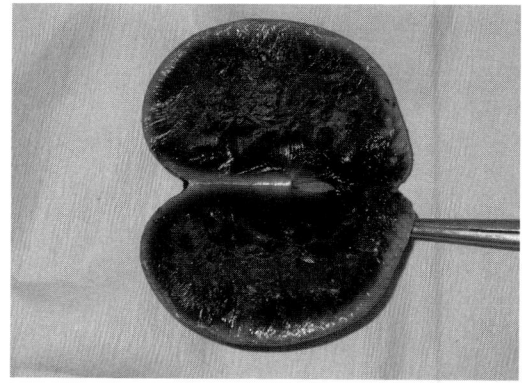

Fig. 18.5. Biliary mucocoele: this gall bladder has been removed and sectioned to show the consolidation of the lumen with inspissated bile.

Bibliography

Bacon, N.J and White, R.A. (2003) Extrahepatic biliary tract surgery in the cat: a case series and review. *Journal of Small Animal Practice* 44, 231–235.

Balkman, C. (2009) Hepatobiliary neoplasia in dogs and cats. *Veterinary Clinics of North America Small Animal Practice* 39, 617–625.

Berent, A.C. and Tobias, K.M. (2009) Portovascular anomalies. *Veterinary Clinics of North America Small Animal Practice* 39, 513–541.

Crews, L.J., Feeney, D.A., Jessen, C.R., Rose, N.D. and Matise, I. (2009) Clinical, ultrasonographic, and laboratory findings associated with gallbladder disease and rupture in dogs: 45 cases (1997–2007). *Journal of the American Veterinary Medical Association* 234, 359–366.

Evans, H.E. (1993) The liver. In: Evans, H.E. (ed.) *Miller's Anatomy of the Dog*, 3rd edn. W.B. Saunders, Philadelphia, Pennsylvania, pp. 451–462.

Greenhalgh, S.N., Dunning, M.D., McKinley, T.J., Goodfellow, M.R., Kelman, K.R., Freitag, T., O'Neill, E.J., *et al.* (2010) Comparison of survival after surgical or medical treatment in dogs with a congenital portosystemic shunt. *Journal of the American Veterinary Medical Association* 236, 1215–1220.

Kummeling, A., Vrakking, D.J., Rothuizen, J., Gerritsen, K.M. and Van Sluijs, F.J. (2010) Hepatic volume measurements in dogs with extrahepatic congenital portosystemic shunts before and after surgical attenuation. *Journal of Veterinary Internal Medicine* 24, 114–119.

Ludwig, L.L., McLoughlin, M.A., Graves, T.K. and Crisp, M.S. (1997) Surgical treatment of bile peritonitis in 24 dogs and 2 cats: a retrospective study (1987–1994). *Veterinary Surgery* 26, 90–98.

Pike, F.S., Berg, J., King, N.W., Penninck, D.G. and Webster, C.R. (2004) Gallbladder mucocele in dogs: 30 cases (2000–2002). *Journal of the American Veterinary Medical Association* 224, 1615–1622.

Rothuizen, J. (2009) Important clinical syndromes associated with liver disease. *Veterinary Clinics of North America Small Animal Practice* 39, 419–437.

Vasanjee, S.C., Bubenik, L.J., Hosgood, G. and Bauer, R. (2006) Evaluation of hemorrhage, sample size, and collateral damage for five hepatic biopsy methods in dogs. *Veterinary Surgery* 35, 86–93.

Weil, A.B. (2010) Anesthesia for patients with renal/hepatic disease. *Topics in Companion Animal Medicine* 25, 87–91.

Windsor, R.C. and Olby, N.J. (2007) Congenital portosystemic shunts in five mature dogs with neurological signs. *Journal of the American Animal Hospital Association* 43, 322–331.

Worley, D.R., Hottinger, H.A. and Lawrence, H.J. (2004) Surgical management of gallbladder mucoceles in dogs: 22 cases (1999–2003). *Journal of the American Veterinary Medical Association* 225, 1418–1422.

19 Ear Surgery

aural haematoma: haematoma within the cartilage of the pinna
ear cropping: cosmetic trimming of the pinna
lateral ear canal resection (Zepp's procedure, lateral wall resection): opening of the lateral wall of the ear canal
para-aural abscess: abscess around the base of the ear canal
pinnectomy: amputation of part of the pinna
total ear canal ablation with lateral bulla osteotomy (TECA-LBO): removal of the ear canal and curettage of the bulla
ventral bulla osteotomy (VBO): opening and curettage of the tympanic bulla

The reader should be able to:

- identify a suitable candidate for needle drainage of an aural haematoma and perform this procedure
- identify a suitable candidate for Penrose drain drainage of an aural haematoma and perform this procedure
- explain the technique of incisional drainage of an aural haematoma
- state the indications for lateral ear canal resection (LECR) in the dog
- state the indications for total ear canal ablation/lateral bulla osteotomy (TECA/LBO) in the dog
- recognize the radiographic features necessary to diagnose severe unilateral otitis externa/media in a dog from standard radiographic views
- instruct owners as to the relative advantages and disadvantages of TECA/LBO prior to their informed decision making

Diseases of the Pinna

Surgery to manage haematomas, lacerations, and tumours of the pinna is regularly performed in general practice. In some countries, cosmetic ear cropping is also performed but in others, such as the UK, it is considered to be an unnecessary form of mutilation and is banned.

Anatomy

The pinna is formed by the auricular cartilage and associated skin. The skin on the inner (concave) surface is firmly attached to the cartilage, and the two fascial planes cannot be separated. The skin on the outer (convex) surface of the pinna is separated from the cartilage by loose connective tissue and the two structures can be separated. Blood vessels run up the outer, convex surface of auricular cartilage from the base of the pinna and send perforating vessels through the auricular cartilage to supply the inner surface of the pinna.

Aural haematoma

Aural haematoma forms within the cartilage of the pinna, which splits to form a central cavity. Trauma is often implicated in the formation of the haematoma (e.g. scratching due to otitis externa). Animals present with painful, turgid swellings of the pinna.

Treatment

Treatment involves draining the haematoma to relieve pain and prevent scarring. If the haematoma is not drained, the blood clot that forms organizes into scar tissue that contracts and causes crumpling and distortion of the ear ('cauliflower ear'). This predisposes to local skin infection and irritation and can cause long-term discomfort to the patient. The haematoma can be drained within a few hours of forming, but drainage is often delayed for 3 or 4 days to give time for blood clots to mature, as this is thought to reduce the risk of recurrence. Following treatment, the ear is incorporated into a head bandage to help maintain apposition of the cartilages and to prevent further trauma. It is important to treat any underlying cause of self-inflicted trauma (e.g. otitis externa) to prevent further injury and recurrence. Corticosteroids are often prescribed systemically or instilled directly into the haematoma cavity, but their value is unknown. There are several techniques that can be used to manage aural haematomas.

DRAINAGE BY NEEDLE CENTESIS This is a very simple technique that can be performed under sedation. The concave surface of the pinna over the haematoma is aseptically prepared. The haematoma is drained using a needle and syringe. A second drainage may be required after 7–10 days, and several drainages are sometimes required until the problem resolves.

PENROSE DRAIN PLACEMENT This is a simple and quick technique that avoids the need to perform more invasive surgery. Anaesthetize the patient. Clip and prepare the pinna. Make small incisions at the top and at the bottom of the haematoma on the inner, concave surface of the pinna (Fig. 19.1). Evacuate the haematoma by squeezing blood and clots out of the drainage incisions. Pass a Penrose drain through the haematoma so that it exits through both holes, and secure it with two sutures, one at each drain exit site. Bandage the ear to prevent ascending infection and maintain the drain for 7–14 days.

INCISIONAL DRAINAGE Incisional drainage is the most effective treatment method but is often reserved for cases that have not responded to Penrose drain placement or needle drainage. The haematoma is drained through a sigmoid incision. The incision is sigmoid, rather than straight, as contracture of the incision will cause less crumpling of the ear as the incision shortens. The incision is left open to allow further drainage but a series of sutures is placed to obliterate the dead space to prevent recurrence.

Incise the skin and cartilage over the haematoma on the inner (concave) surface of the pinna in a sigmoid pattern. Evacuate the contents of the

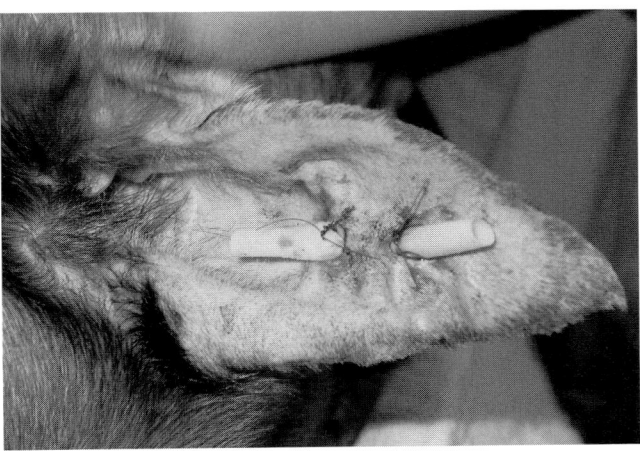

Fig. 19.1. Penrose drain placement.

haematoma. Place sutures running from the skin and cartilage of the inner surface of the pinna, across the haematoma cavity, and anchor them firmly in the cartilage on the opposite side of the haematoma cavity. Alternatively, pass the sutures through the full thickness of the ear. The sutures should be ~1 cm long and placed in staggered rows ~1 cm apart to prevent compromise to the blood supply of the pinna. Bandage the ear to keep the incision clean. Remove the sutures after 10–14 days (Fig. 19.2). Stents (e.g. buttons) have traditionally been used to distribute pressure from each suture over a wider area but these can be associated with pinna infection and necrosis, and are no longer recommended.

Complications

The main complication of treatment is recurrence of the haematoma. Pinna necrosis, deformity, and infection may also occur but are uncommon.

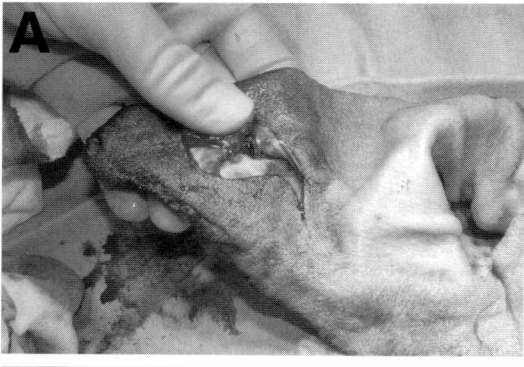

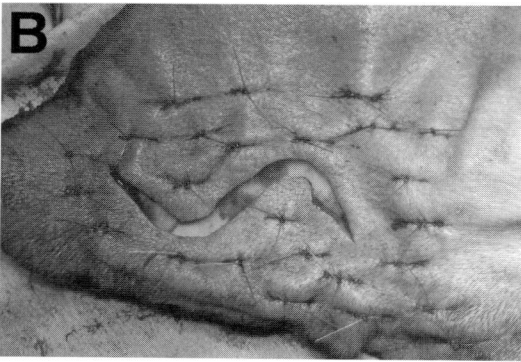

Fig. 19.2. Incisional drainage of aural haematoma: (A) sigmoid incision into cavity; (B) suture in place.

Lacerations of the pinna

Bite wounds, puncture wounds, and lacerations of the pinna are common. Small punctures and lacerations can be managed by clipping, cleaning, and leaving to heal by second intention. The lesions will contract as they heal and this may lead to some distortion of the pinna. Larger lesions can be debrided and sutured. Peripheral lesions can be managed by partial pinnectomy (see below).

Squamous cell carcinoma of the pinna

The pinna is a predisposed site for the development of squamous cell carcinoma (SCC). The condition is seen predominantly in white-haired cats that have unpigmented skin. It is thought to develop because of increased exposure of the pinna to ultraviolet radiation due to the sparse hair-coat, lack of pigment, and exposed position of the ear tip. These cats are also predisposed to eyelid and rhinarial SCC. Pinnal SCC is the end-stage of a series of transformations induced by solar radiation. Initially, actinic keratosis or carcinoma *in situ* develop as crusty, erythematous plaques that are confined to the epithelium. Over time, these lesions transform into SCC that invades into the surrounding tissue. At this stage, the tips of the ears become indurated and eroded (Fig. 19.3). Metastatic lesions are uncommon.

Treatment

SCC of the pinna can be treated surgically by partial or total pinnectomy. The lesions are excised with a 1 cm margin of grossly normal tissue. The procedure is simple and well tolerated but alters the appearance of the cat (Fig. 19.3). The prognosis is good providing that the entire tumour has been excised. Cryosurgery (freezing of diseased tissue), radiotherapy, and drug therapy have also all been used to control the condition. Recently, topical application of imiquimod, an immune modifier, has been described to control the lesions although local erythema and irritation may occur, and lesions may be resistant to therapy.

Pinnectomy

Clip the pinna and surrounding skin. Clean the ear canal with topical cleanser and rinse thoroughly with sterile saline. Do not use topical antiseptics to clean the ear canal, as agents such as chlorhexidine are ototoxic and may cause vestibular disease. Prepare the skin of both surfaces of the pinna using standard prepping guidelines.

First incise through the skin and cartilage of the inner (concave) surface of the pinna. As these are intimately apposed, this is performed in a single incision. Scallop the incision to ensure that no sharp edges of cartilage are left protruding at either end of the incision. Make a corresponding incision through the skin of the outer (convex) surface and ligate or cauterize vessels as they are encountered. Excise a margin of at least 1 cm of healthy tissue around neoplastic lesions. Suture the loose subcutaneous tissue of the outer surface of the pinna to the perichondrium of the cartilage. Suture the skin edges together using an interrupted pattern and use an Elizabethan collar to prevent scratching (Fig. 19.4). There is often crusting along the incision line postoperatively and portions are likely to dehisce. However, this can be managed by second intention healing, and major complications are uncommon.

Chronic Otitis Externa/Media

Chronic otitis externa is extremely common in dogs, and surgery is often performed to help improve medical therapy or alleviate signs. In contrast, chronic otitis externa is much less common in cats and surgery is generally only performed in cats that have otitis secondary to inflammatory polyps, neoplasia, or severe trauma. This section describes the assessment of patients with otitis externa and otitis media for surgery, and concentrates on the indications for lateral ear canal resection (LECR) and total ear canal ablation with bulla osteotomy in the dog. Both procedures are regularly performed in general practice but only LECR is suitable for an inexperienced surgeon to attempt.

Anatomy

The external ear canal is composed of two cartilages: (i) the auricular cartilage that forms the

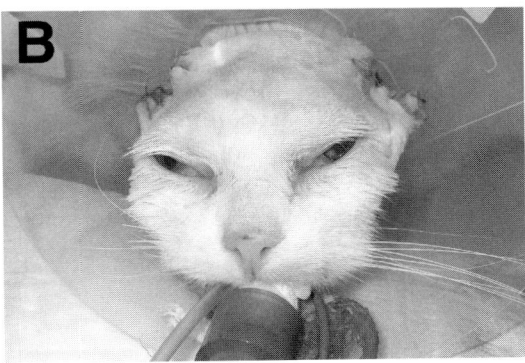

Fig. 19.3. Pinnectomy for management of SCC of the pinna. (A) before; (B) after.

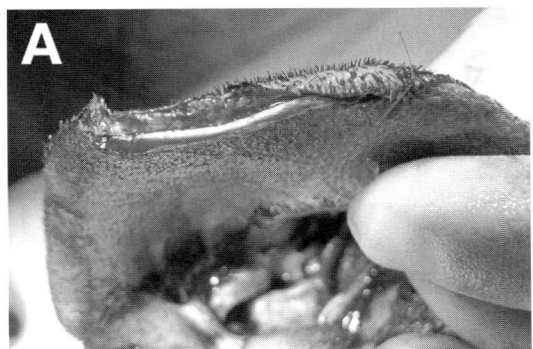
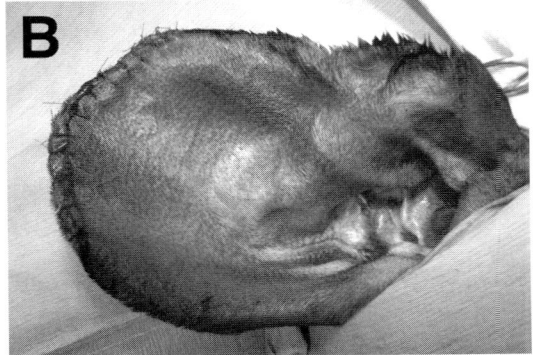

Fig. 19.4. Partial pinnectomy: (A) defect following amputation of tip of pinna; (B) sutures in place.

pinna and the vertical ear canal; and (ii) the annular cartilage that forms the horizontal ear canal. The vertical ear canal is formed by rolling of the auricular cartilage into a tube that starts at the base of the pinna. The external ear canal is covered with modified skin that extends onto the tympanic membrane. At the base of the external ear canal, the canal attaches to the external acoustic meatus, a bony rim on the lateral wall of the tympanic bulla that encircles the opening into the tympanic bulla. The facial nerve courses round the ventral aspect of the base of the horizontal ear canal. It emerges from the stylomastoid foramen immediately behind the external acoustic meatus, runs close to the ventral surface of the annular cartilage, and then branches to supply the base of the ear and other structures of the face. Immediately rostral to the external acoustic meatus is a large vein (retroglenoid vein). It emerges from the bone of the skull and is easily traumatized during bulla surgery.

The tympanic membrane divides the bulla and the external ear canal. It is covered with modified skin on its external surface and with modified respiratory epithelium on its inner surface. The first ossicle of the middle ear attaches to tympanic membrane and can be seen through the membrane. Most of the bulla is composed of a large, air-filled cavity that acts as a resonant chamber. The Eustachian tube connects the medial aspect of the bulla to the nasopharynx. Sympathetic nerve fibres supplying the orbit run through the bulla and can be damaged during surgery. Cats have a large septum that divides the bulla into two compartments that can be identified radiographically.

Aetiopathogenesis

Chronic otitis externa usually develops secondary to underlying skin disease (e.g. atopic dermatitis). Other predisposing causes include conformational abnormalities of the ear canal, infectious agents (ear mites; yeasts; bacteria), foreign bodies, and ear canal tumours. As otitis externa becomes established, the ear canal becomes occluded with exudate. The lumen is also constricted by hyperplasia of the epithelium and distortion of the cartilages. Dystrophic calcification leads to mineralization of the inflamed ear canal cartilage. Ultimately, otitis externa extends to affect the middle ear leading to secondary otitis media.

Investigating otitis externa/media

The medical management of otitis externa can be successful in the early stages of the disease but, as it becomes established, medical therapy becomes ineffective. Ear surgery can be performed early in the course of disease to prevent further progression, or later to salvage severe ear disease by removing affected tissues. Before performing surgery, it is important to carefully evaluate the ear to decide which, if any, surgery is appropriate. The major aims of evaluation are to:

1. identify factors that have contributed to otitis externa;
2. evaluate the horizontal ear canal for irreversible changes;
3. evaluate the middle ear for otitis media.

Physical examination (gross and otoscopic evaluation)

Animals with ear disease often resent examination. Sedate or anaesthetize the patient if necessary. Palpate and evaluate the ear canal for thickening, swelling, masses, distortion, or pain. Inspect the ear canal orifice, checking that it is patent and assessing the health of the skin of the pinna. Perform otoscopy to assess the ear canal. In normal dogs, the tympanic membrane should be visible at the base of the ear canal as a translucent, concave membrane divided into two components by the manubrium of the malleus that attaches to its inner surface (Fig. 19.5). In diseased ears, the tympanic membrane may be obscured by exudate or by stenosis of the canal. Otitis media can be identified by bulging and opacification of tympanic membrane. Rupture of the membrane also indicates extension of disease into the middle ear.

Cytology, culture, and biopsy

Exudate from the ear canal can be examined microscopically for infectious agents and submitted for bacterial culture. Perform biopsy of ear canal masses using grabbing forceps or punch biopsy knives.

Imaging

Radiography is useful for assessing the degree of damage to the external ear canal and the presence

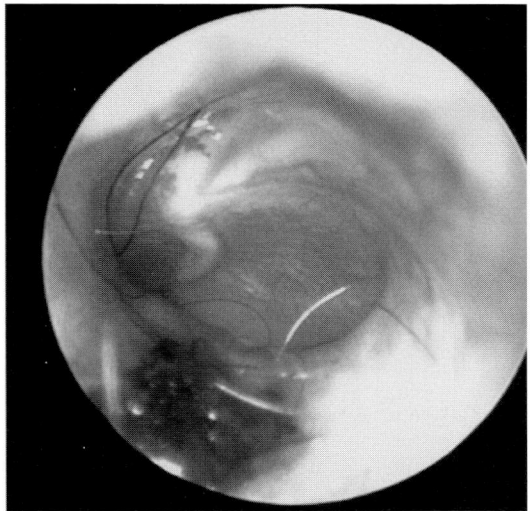

Fig. 19.5 Otoscopy of normal ear: the base of the ear canal and the tympanic membrane can be seen. The tympanic membrane is translucent and concave. The manubrium, which attaches to the medial surface, divides the membrane into a small cranial (to left) component and a larger caudal component. Some hair and exudate are seen in the ventral canal immediately above the membrane in this case. (Image courtesy of M. Kovalik.)

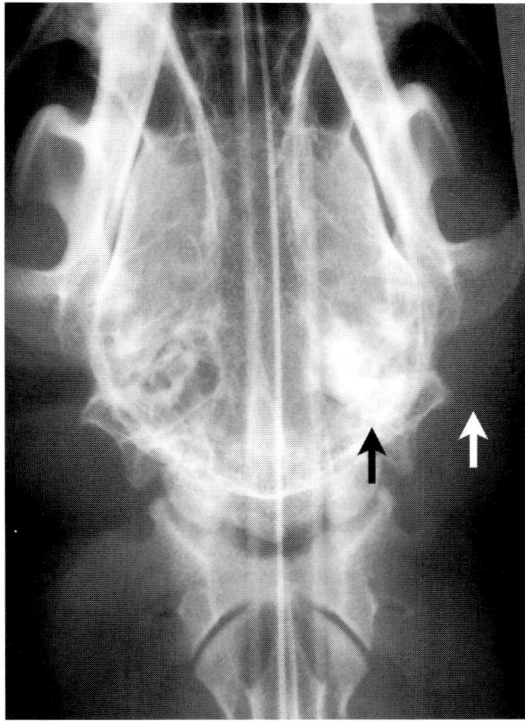

Fig. 19.6. Dorsoventral skull: unilateral ear disease. Compare left and right sides, noting sclerotic bulla (black arrow) and loss of ear canal air-shadow (white arrow) indicating otitis media and otitis externa.

of soft tissue or fluid within the middle ear, which indicates middle ear disease. The most useful projections are the *dorsoventral* and the *rostrocaudal open-mouth oblique* views.

The dorsoventral projection of the skull allows both external ear canals to be assessed for patency and for chronic inflammatory change. Normal ear canals have patent lumens identified by wide gas shadows running from the pinna to the base of the skull (Fig. 19.6). Obstruction of the ear canals is recognized by loss of the gas shadow within the ear canal lumen (Fig. 19.6). Mineralization of the ear canal cartilages indicates advanced ear disease (Fig. 19.7).

The rostrocaudal open-mouth oblique projection is difficult to obtain but produces a projection that skylines the bullae at the base of the skull (Fig. 19.8). It is the best radiographic projection for assessing the bullae. The wall of the tympanic bulla should be thin, smooth, and intact, and the cavity should be filled with air (Fig. 19.9). In cats, the septum dividing the bulla can be seen on this projection. When otitis media is present, the bulla wall becomes thickened and irregular and the lumen becomes opacified

with fluid or tissue (Fig. 19.10). If the wall of the bulla appears eroded, this indicates an aggressive bulla lesion (e.g. advanced otitis media; neoplasia). This projection increases the sensitivity of radiography in identifying middle ear disease, but is insensitive in comparison to CT or MRI. When available, either CT or MRI is used in preference, as both procedures provide far more detailed information about the external and middle ears.

Management of otitis externa/media

During the early stages of otitis externa, medical therapy can control and reverse the changes within the ear canal. However, once a patient has had persistent ear disease for more than a couple of months, an irreversible pattern of ear disease becomes established. Early during the course of otitis externa, *lateral ear canal resection* can be performed to improve airflow into, and drainage from, the horizontal ear canal. This surgery does

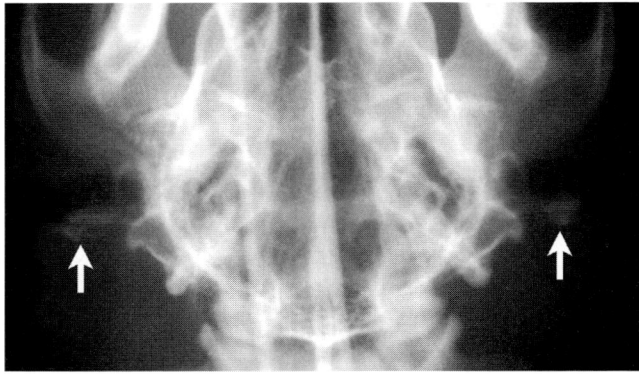

Fig. 19.7. Dorsoventral skull – mineralization of the ear canal cartilages (arrows).

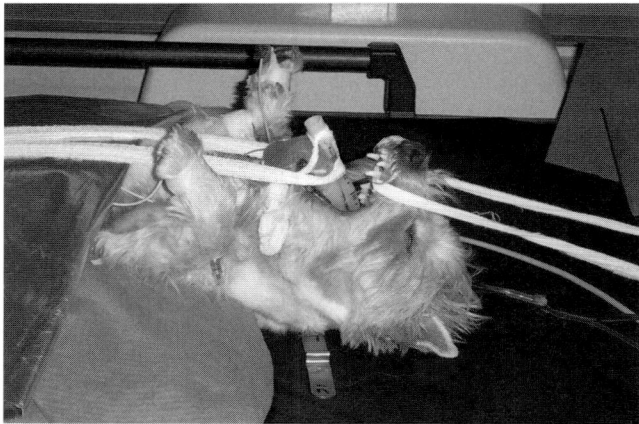

Fig. 19.8. Positioning for the rostrocaudal, open-mouth, oblique projection. Position the patient in dorsal recumbency with an X-ray plate centred on the atlanto-occipital joint. Elevate the jaw until the hard palate is perpendicular with the tabletop and secure it in this position. Hold the lower jaw open with a tie. Project the X-ray beam through the open mouth towards the X-ray plate angling the beam forwards by 10° (cats) to 20 or 30° (dogs). It may be necessary to extubate the patient before exposing the film as the endotracheal tube can become superimposed with the bullae.

not cure ear disease but it does facilitate treatment. Later in the course of ear disease, *total ear canal ablation with bulla osteotomy* can be performed to remove the diseased ear canal and infected material within the middle ear. This surgery permanently resolves signs associated with ear disease but necessitates sacrificing the ear canal and bulla.

Lateral ear canal resection

Lateral ear canal resection (LECR) is also known as lateral wall resection, or modified Zepp's procedure. Vertical ear canal resection is a similar technique.

Aims

The procedure opens up the lateral wall of the vertical ear canal to improve drainage and access to the horizontal ear canal, facilitating medical management.

Indications

LECR is indicated in the treatment of otitis externa when the horizontal ear canal is patent and there is no evidence of otitis media. To be of use in the treatment of otitis externa, it must be performed early in the course of the disease.

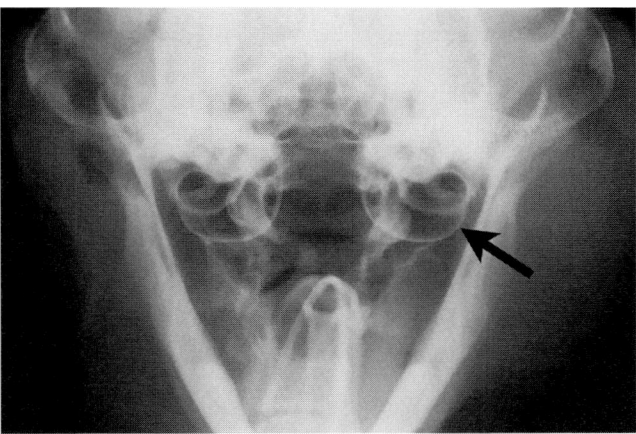

Fig. 19.9. Rostrocaudal, open-mouth, oblique projection of the feline bulla (arrow). Note the septum that divides the bulla into two compartments in the cat.

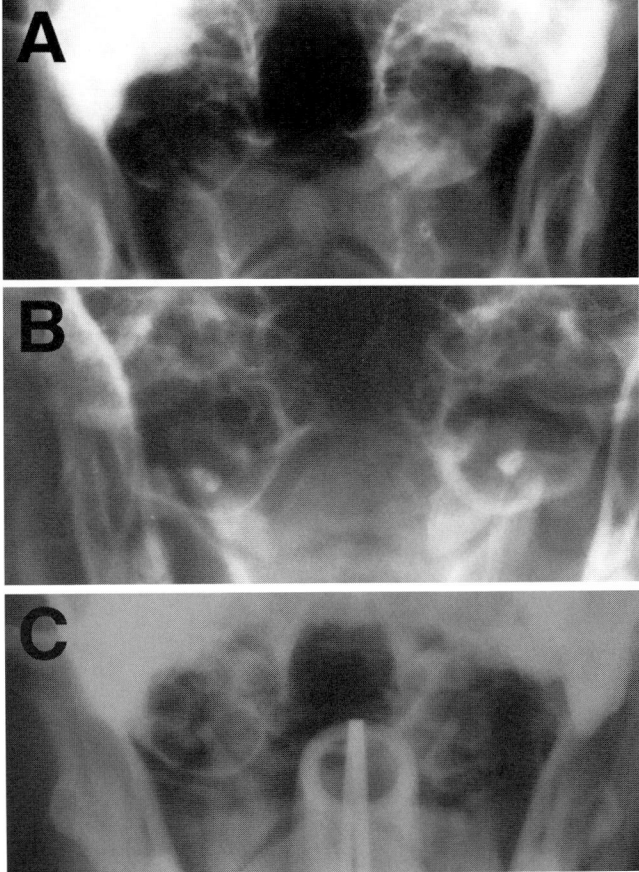

Fig. 19.10. Rostrocaudal, open-mouth, oblique projection – bulla pathology (healthy bulla on left): (A) opacification (fluid or neoplasia); (B) thickening of wall (otitis media); (C) erosion of bulla (e.g. neoplasia).

Contraindications

LECR is contraindicated when the horizontal ear canal is irreversibly obstructed as, even if LECR is performed, it will not improve the health of the horizontal ear canal. If otitis media is present, ear disease is likely to be too advanced for LECR to be effective.

Imaging findings to support surgery

Suitable patients will have patent horizontal ear canals that demonstrate no mineralization on radiography. There will be no indicators of otitis media (i.e. the tympanic membrane will be translucent and concave; there will be no changes in the tympanic bullae). Animals with inflamed, occluded horizontal ear canals may still be candidates for LECR if the patency of the ear canal improves with topical therapy.

Preparing the patient

Clip the entire pinna and skin surrounding the head from the dorsal midline to several centimetres below the base of the vertical ear canal, and from 3 cm rostral to 3 cm caudal to the pinna. Clean the ear with proprietary ear cleaner and flush it extensively with saline. Scrub the pinna and surrounding skin with chlorhexidine gluconate or povidone-iodine but ensure that chlorhexidine does not enter the ear canal as it is ototoxic.

Technique

The technique involves rotating the lateral wall of the vertical ear canal ventrally. This creates a direct entry into the horizontal ear canal. The repositioned lateral wall forms a drainage board (or baffle plate) onto which cerumen can collect before drying and flaking off. The drainage board is critical to the success of surgery. If one is not created, cerumen builds up around the new ear canal opening causing occlusion of the horizontal ear canal.

SKIN INCISION   Make a rectangular skin incision extending from 1 to 2 cm below the horizontal ear canal, up over the lateral aspect of the vertical ear canal. Start by identifying the pretragic incisure and the intertragic notch on the lateral rim of the opening to the external ear canal.

These mark the starting points of the rostral and caudal skin incisions (Fig. 19.11). Incise from these points through the skin to the vertical ear canal cartilage. Continue the incisions ventrally and parallel to each other, extending the incisions over the junction between the vertical and horizontal ear canals. Insert a haemostat into the vertical ear canal to help to locate the bottom of the vertical ear canal. Continue the incisions for a further 1–2 cm below this point to create a bed for the baffle plate to sit in. Complete the incision by joining the ventral points of the two incisions to generate a rectangular flap of skin. Elevate the skin from the base, bluntly dissecting it from the cartilage of the vertical ear canal as this is reached (this is a natural dissection plane which is easily established), but do not strip the perichondrium off the auricular cartilage (Fig. 19.12A).

CARTILAGE INCISION   Once the cartilage of the lateral aspect of the vertical ear canal is exposed, two parallel incisions are made from the pretragic and intertragic notches. These extend to the base of the vertical ear canal, to mobilize a parallel strip of auricular cartilage approximately one-third of the circumference of the vertical ear canal. Use the tip of a no. 10 scalpel blade to score the cartilage along the proposed incision sites. These score lines act as guides to complete the cartilage incision and ensure that a wide-based drainage board is produced. Complete the cartilage incision following the score line using either the scalpel or a pair of straight scissors (e.g. Mayo; iris). Continue the incisions down to the junction of the vertical and horizontal ear canals to mobilize the cartilage completely and reflect it ventrally (Fig. 19.12B). The blood supply to the drainage board runs through the base of the flap. Ensure that this remains wide while making the cartilage incisions. Amputate the distal half of the cartilage flap to generate a 1–2 cm rectangular plate of cartilage that will become the drainage board (Fig. 19.12B).

SUTURING THE DRAINAGE BOARD IN PLACE   Use 3-0 or 4-0 nylon or polypropylene suture material placed in a simple interrupted pattern (subcutaneous closure is not necessary). Place the first two sutures between the skin and ventral points of the rostral and caudal edges of exposed horizontal ear canal. Then secure the tips of the baffle plate to the ventral edges of the skin incision. Place additional

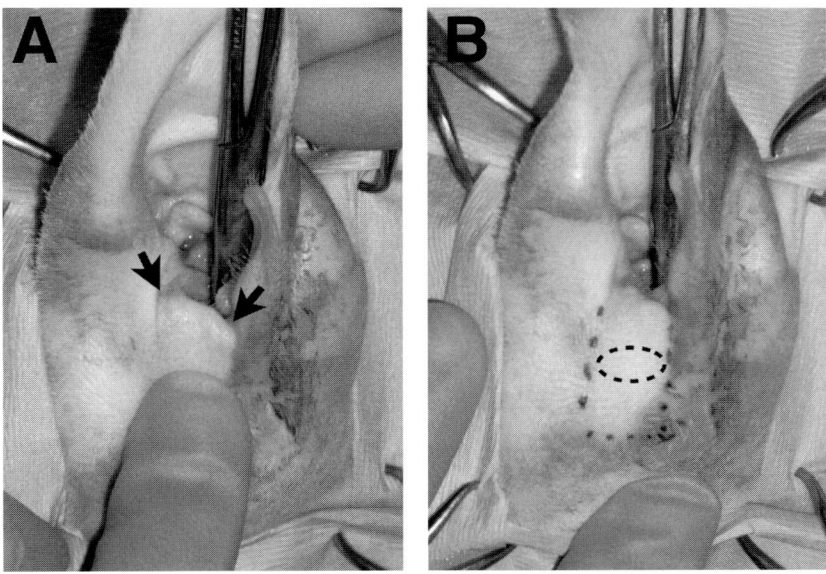

Fig. 19.11. LECR: (A) Identify the pretragic incisure (left arrow) and the intertragic notch (right arrow); (B) map two parallel skin incisions from these points running ventrally to below the base of the vertical ear canal (dotted circle). A haemostat has been placed in the ear canal as a guide to the junction between the horizontal and vertical canals.

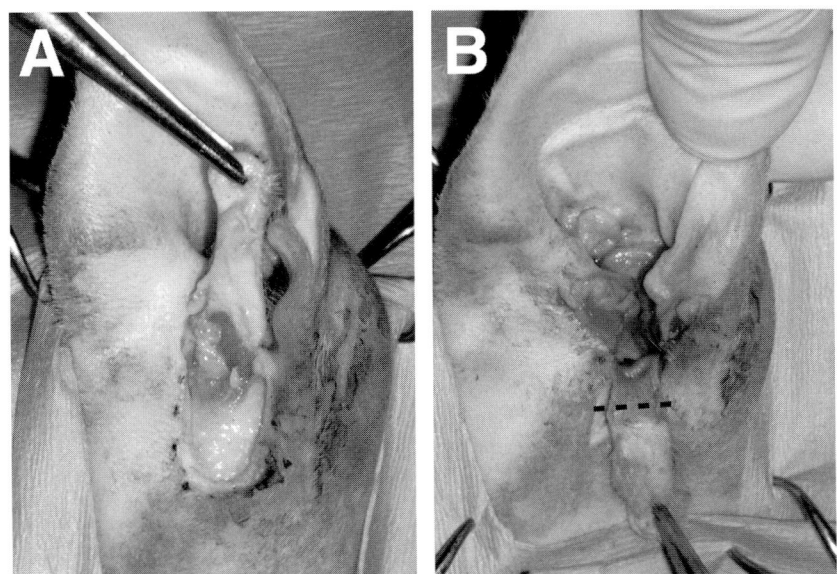

Fig. 19.12. LECR: (A) elevate the skin flap from the perichondrium to expose the lateral wall of the vertical ear canal; (B) Incise the cartilage and reflect the flap ventrally. Dashed line indicates site of cartilage resection.

sutures to secure the baffle plate to the skin ventrally and between the incised vertical ear canal and adjacent skin dorsally (Fig. 19.13).

Post-operative care

Prevent self-inflicted trauma by using an Elizabethan collar. Medical management of ear disease must be continued if the surgery is to be successful.

Complications

Dehiscence and infection of the suture line occurs in up to 27% of cases. Progression of ear disease is a major long-term complication. This may occur because of poor patient selection, because of failure to continue medical therapy post-operatively, or because of technical failures of the surgery. If the base of the drainage board is too narrow, the board may become necrotic. If the cartilage of the drainage board is not mobilized adequately, it may lift up post-operatively. Both these complications lead to failure of the surgery. Unfortunately, when major complications occur, total ear canal ablation with bulla osteotomy is generally required. Failure

rates of 40–50% are reported and may be as high as 85% in cocker spaniels.

Total ear canal ablation with lateral bulla osteotomy

Total ear canal ablation with lateral bulla osteotomy (TECA-LBO) is a protracted and technically demanding procedure. Many practitioners perform this surgery successfully but it should not be undertaken by inexperienced surgeons or with inadequate instrumentation or lighting. The rate of complications is likely to relate to the competency of the surgeon. In large-breed dogs and patients with extensive mineralization of the external ear canal or bulla thickening, the surgery can be very demanding, even for experienced surgeons. The core elements of the surgery are described here for illustration only.

Aims

To permanently alleviate signs of ear disease by removing the external ear canal and curetting infected tissue out of the middle ear.

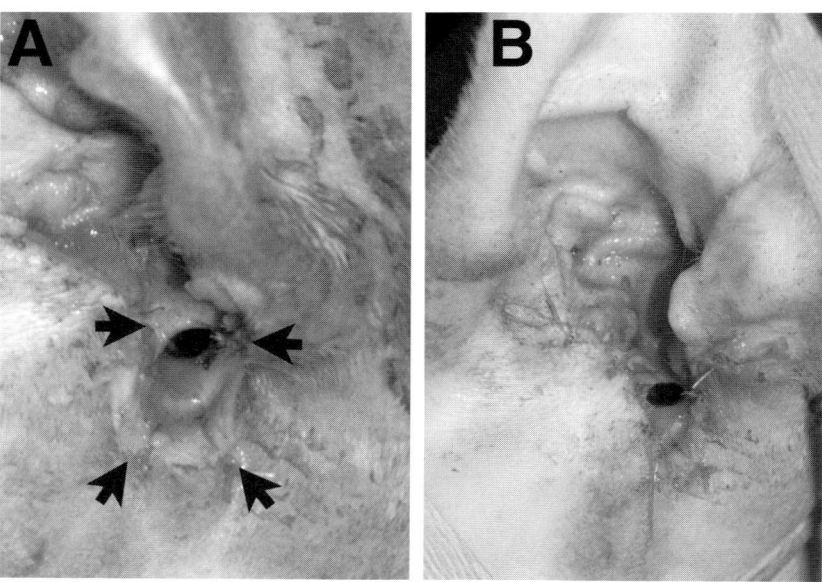

Fig. 19.13. LECR: (A) anchor the baffle plate to the skin with sutures where it joins the horizontal ear canal. Then anchor the tips of the baffle plate to the ventral edges of the skin incision. The arrows indicate the site of these first four sutures; (B) complete the procedures by suturing the rest of the cartilage and skin. A direct opening into the horizontal ear canal is created.

Indications

TECA-LBO is indicated in the treatment of otitis externa when the horizontal ear canal has irreversible changes or when chronic otitis media is also present. Other indications for TECA-LBO include revision of failed LECR, management of ear canal neoplasia, and management of ear canal separation.

Contraindications

There are no specific contraindications but, as this is a salvage procedure, it is worth pursuing other treatments first. Intra-operative bleeding can be extensive and this surgery should be performed with extreme caution in patients that have bleeding disorders. Animals with large swellings or draining sinuses at the base of their ear canals are likely to have para-aural abscesses. These are challenging to manage and these patients should be referred for advanced imaging and specialist surgery.

Imaging findings to support surgery

Imaging findings that demonstrate that TECA-LBO is indicated include occlusion of the horizontal ear canal, mineralization of the ear canal cartilages, and evidence of otitis media.

Core elements of surgery

The pinna is preserved but the rest of the ear canal is dissected free from the surrounding tissue and amputated. The lateral wall of the tympanic bulla is removed with rongeurs to provide access for curettage. The contents of the middle ear are removed by curetting, and the wound is reconstructed. During surgery, the facial nerve that passes around the base of the horizontal canal must be avoided. The retroglenoid vein may rupture leading to profuse bleeding. During bulla curettage, the inner ear structures must be avoided (Figs 19.14 and 19.15).

Outcome

Despite the radical nature of surgery, it is generally well tolerated and owner satisfaction with the procedure is high. It is reasonable to expect the patient to be much more comfortable post-operatively and to return to a normal lifestyle when sutures are removed. Hearing, which is likely to have been

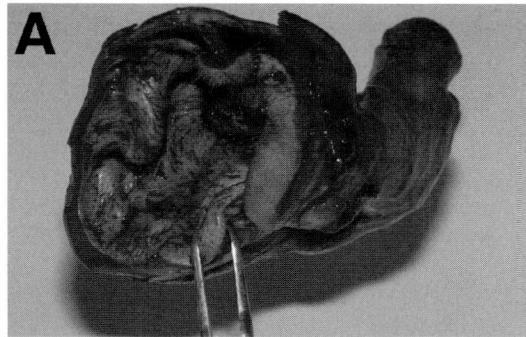

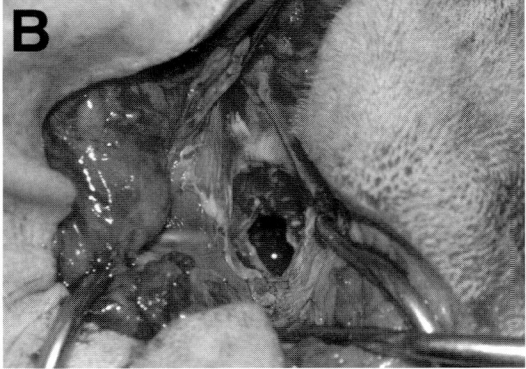

Fig. 19.14. TECA-LBO: (A) amputate the ear canal; (B) perform an osteotomy to open the bulla entrance for curettage. (Images courtesy of E. Welsh.)

poor due to the severity of ear disease preoperatively, will be further hampered by the loss of the external and middle ears, but as the inner ear is intact, it may not be completely lost. Warn owners that their pet is likely to have very poor hearing. If this surgery is performed (particularly bilaterally) on a cat, recommend that the cat is kept inside as its ability to avoid predators and vehicles will be impeded.

Complications

Dehiscence and wound infection are common following this surgery but generally are easily managed. Facial nerve paresis or paralysis affects 10–15% of patients but is well tolerated. Vestibular disease from inner ear injury during bulla curettage affects 5% of cases and generally improves over time. However, para-aural abscessation due to failure to remove all contaminated material from the middle ear is a major complication that may

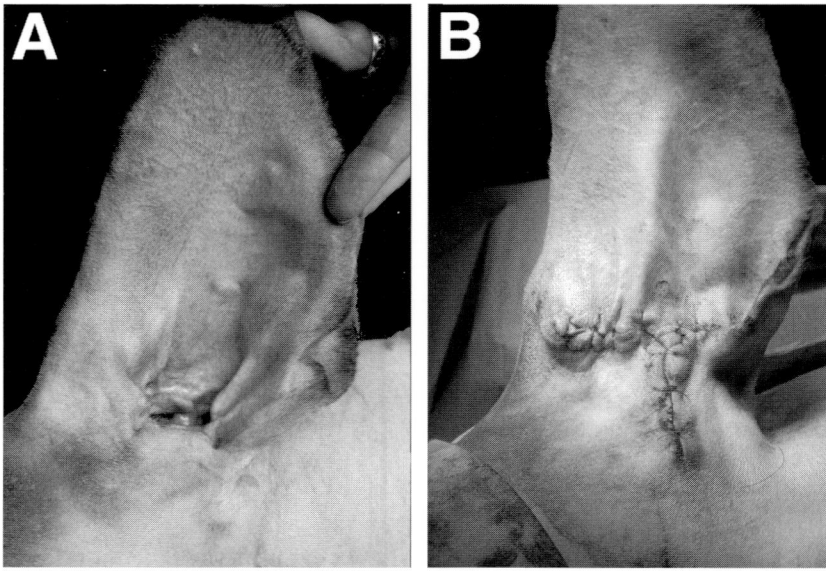

Fig. 19.15. TECA-LBO: (A) preoperative appearance; (B) post-operative appearance. (Images courtesy of E. Welsh.)

develop several months following surgery. It leads to severe clinical signs including pain and discharging sinuses at the surgery site and is extremely difficult to manage. This affects up to 10% of patients although, in the author's experience, the incidence is likely to reflect the competence and experience of the surgeon. The incidence of neurological complications (especially Horner's syndrome) may be higher in cats.

Ear Canal and Middle Ear Tumours

Ear canal tumours are common. The major differential diagnosis to consider for ear canal and middle ear tumours is middle ear inflammatory polyp, which is discussed separately below.

Aetiopathogenesis

Most aural tumours develop from the skin of the ear canal. Ceruminous gland adenocarcinomas are the commonest form in cats. These are malignant and can metastasize to the retropharyngeal lymph nodes or lungs. Ceruminous gland adenomas are the commonest ear canal tumours of dogs and are benign. Other forms of tumours include squamous cell carcinoma, poorly differentiated carcinoma, and soft tissue sarcoma.

Presentation

Ear canal tumours predominantly affect older dogs and cats. Common clinical signs include signs of otitis externa and the presence of a visible mass in the external ear canal. Tumours that involve the middle ear may cause Horner's syndrome or vestibular disease. Occasionally, ear canal tumours will lead to the formation of para-aural abscesses or sinuses due to destruction of the ear canal cartilage. Sometimes, enlarged retropharyngeal lymph nodes will be palpable dorsal to the larynx.

Investigation

Ear canal tumours are usually identified during the evaluation of otitis externa, as described above. Additional investigative steps include thoracic radiography to screen for metastatic lesions and advanced imaging to establish the extent of the primary tumour and involvement of the retropharyngeal lymph nodes.

Treatment

TECA-LBO is usually the surgery of choice for management of ear canal tumours and may provide a favourable outcome depending on the type and stage of the cancer. Radiotherapy has also been described as an adjunctive therapy following surgery.

Prognosis

TECA-LBO often achieves complete excision of the primary tumour as the ear canal cartilages act as good barriers to tumour invasion. The prognosis following complete excision of benign ear canal tumours is excellent. Malignant tumours may recur locally or metastasize, but many cases still progress well following surgery. In fact, dogs can have extended survival following removal of malignant ear canal tumours (median survival times of over 58 months have been reported). The prognosis for cats with malignant ear canal tumours is worse (median survival times of less than 12 months are typically reported). In both species, involvement of the bulla is a negative prognostic indicator.

Middle Ear Inflammatory Polyp

An inflammatory polyp is a benign, pedunculated mass that originates from the mucosa of the tympanic bulla or Eustachian tube. The polyp may remain in the middle ear, grow down the Eustachian tube into the pharynx, or extend through the tympanic membrane into the ear canal. The aetiology of polyps is unknown but both congenital lesions and chronic inflammation of the epithelium of the tympanic bulla have been suggested.

Presentation and clinical findings

Inflammatory polyps are common in young cats and they can be unilateral or bilateral. The median age at presentation is 2 years but animals as old as 13 years may develop them. In contrast, inflammatory polyps are rare in dogs.

Polyps isolated to the middle ear may cause signs of otitis media including aural pain, peripheral vestibular disease (by indirect involvement of the inner ear), and Horner's syndrome (through injury to the sympathetic nerve fibres running through the tympanic bulla). However, most are associated with signs of secondary otitis externa. Often the polyp can be seen extending along the horizontal ear canal.

Polyps that extend into the nasopharynx cause signs of upper respiratory tract obstruction including stertor (snoring), nasal discharge, and dyspnoea. If they cause ventral displacement of the soft palate, they may also cause dysphagia. Generally, they can only be visualized by retracting the soft palate or using a dental mirror or endoscope to examine the nasopharynx. However, large polyps may protrude beyond the caudal edge of the soft palate or cause ventral deviation of the palate.

Investigation

A high index of suspicion of inflammatory polyp is reached when young cats present with chronic otitis externa or media that is unresponsive to treatment, or with masses in the external ear canal. In older cats and dogs, other conditions are more likely to account for these signs but inflammatory polyp should still be considered as a possible diagnosis. Imaging studies demonstrate opacification of the tympanic bulla with or without involvement of the external ear canal or nasopharynx. The diagnosis can only be confirmed from histopathological assessment of the polyp to exclude other diagnoses such as nasopharyngeal and aural tumours.

Treatment

Treatment involves removing the polyp and treating any underlying inflammatory disease. The polyp can often be avulsed from the middle ear by applying traction. Alternatively, surgical debridement of the middle ear is required. In cats, this is achieved by performing ventral bulla osteotomy. There is little to be lost by attempting traction as it may be curative and provides tissue for histopathology to confirm the diagnosis. However, combining traction with ventral bulla osteotomy reduces the recurrence rate significantly.

Traction

To remove aural polyps, grasp the polyp with a forceps (e.g. crocodile forceps passed down an otoscope) and apply steady traction until the polyp avulses from its attachments to the middle ear. To remove nasopharyngeal polyps, pull the edge of the soft palate forwards using a spay hook, grasp the polyp with an Allis tissue forceps and apply steady traction until the polyp avulses. Following traction, prescribe prednisolone (1–2 mg/kg orally for 2 weeks then gradually reduce the dose).

Ventral bulla osteotomy

Ventral bulla osteotomy provides good access to both cavities of the feline tympanic bulla and enables bilateral bulla surgery to be performed without repositioning the patient. A hole is trephined into the ventral surface of the bulla, the septum dividing the two compartments is disrupted, and the bulla cavity is curetted. If the polyp is protruding into the ear canal or nasopharynx, it must also be removed from these sites by traction after the osteotomy has been performed.

Complications and prognosis

The main complications of treatment are recurrence of the polyp, vestibular disease, and Horner's syndrome. The prognosis for cats following ventral bulla osteotomy combined with traction is excellent, with recurrence rates of only 2% reported. Polyps recur in one-third to two-thirds of cats following traction alone, but prescribing prednisolone post-operatively reduces the recurrence rate. The prognosis following surgery to manage canine inflammatory polyp also appears to be good, although TECA-LBO is usually required.

Horner's syndrome affects approximately half of patients regardless of the method of treatment. However, it is of little clinical significance and usually resolves within 6 weeks. Vestibular dysfunction is more likely to lead to permanent neurological deficits but most patients adapt well to these.

Ear Canal Separation

Ear canal separation is an uncommon, traumatic lesion of dogs and cats.

It occurs when the auricular and annular cartilages become separated following trauma (e.g. being hit by a car). Left untreated, the damaged canal undergoes stenosis and para-aural abscessation develops from within the occluded horizontal ear canal.

Presentation

Immediately following injury, the pinna drops ventrally on the injured side, blood may be seen coming from the ear canal, and facial nerve paralysis has been reported. Chronic cases present with signs consistent with para-aural abscessation or sinus tract formation. Signs of otitis media may also be present (e.g. vestibular disease, Horner's syndrome).

Evaluation

Otoscopy at the time of injury reveals separation of the ear canal cartilages and tearing of the epithelial lining at the junction between the cartilages. Evaluation of chronic cases identifies occlusion of the base of the vertical ear canal and other signs consistent with para-aural abscessation and otitis media.

Treatment

Some cases can be successfully managed by primary repair but many require TECA-LBO. Surgery should not be undertaken by inexperienced surgeons and cases should be referred to an experienced colleague or specialist centre. The prognosis is good, with most cases responding well to surgery.

Bibliography

Anderson, D.M., Robinson, R.K. and White, R.A. (2000) Management of inflammatory polyps in 37 cats. *Veterinary Record* 147, 684–687.

Angus, J.C. (2004) Otic cytology in health and disease. *Veterinary Clinics of North America Small Animal Practice* 34, 411–424.

Bacon, N.J., Gilbert, R.L., Bostock, D.E. and White, R.A. (2003) Total ear canal ablation in the cat: indications, morbidity and long-term survival. *Journal of Small Animal Practice* 44, 430–434.

Boothe, H.W., Hobson, H.P. and McDonald, D.E. (1996) Treatment of traumatic separation of the auricular and annular cartilages without ablation: results in five dogs. *Veterinary Surgery* 25, 376–379.

Bradbury, C.A., Westropp, J.L. and Pollard, R.E. (2009) Relationship between prostatomegaly, prostatic mineralization, and cytologic diagnosis. *Veterinary Radiology and Ultrasound* 50, 167–171.

Bruyette, D.S. and Lorenz, M.D. (1993) Otitis externa and otitis media: diagnostic and medical aspects. *Seminars in Veterinary Medicine and Surgery* 8, 3–9.

Clarke, S.P. (2004) Surgical management of acute ear canal separation in a cat. *Journal of Feline Medicine and Surgery* 6, 283–286.

Cole, L.K. (2004) Otoscopic evaluation of the ear canal. *Veterinary Clinics of North America Small Animal Practice* 34, 397–410.

Connery, N.A., McAllister, H. and Hay, C.W. (2001) Para-aural abscessation following traumatic ear canal separation in a dog. *Journal of Small Animal Practice* 42, 253–256.

Donnelly, K.E. and Tillson, D.M. (2004) Feline inflammatory polyps and ventral bulla osteotomy. *Compendium of Continuing Education for the Practicing Veterinarian* 26, 446–454.

Garosi, L.S., Dennis, R. and Schwarz, T. (2003) Review of diagnostic imaging of ear diseases in the dog and cat. *Veterinary Radiology and Ultrasound* 44, 137–146.

Gross, T.L., Ihrke, P.J. and Walder, E.J. (2005) Epidermal tumours. In: Gross, T.L., Ihrke, P.J. and Walder, E.J. (eds) *Skin Diseases of the Dog and Cat: Clinical and Histopathological Diagnosis*, 2nd edn. Wiley-Blackwell, Oxford UK, pp. 561–603.

Hobson, H.P. (1988) Surgical management of advanced ear disease. *Veterinary Clinics of North America Small Animal Practice* 18, 821–844.

Joyce, J.A. (1994) Treatment of canine aural haematoma using an indwelling drain and corticosteroids. *Journal of Small Animal Practice* 35, 341–344.

Kirpensteijn, J. (1993) Aural neoplasms. *Seminars in Veterinary Medicine and Surgery* 8, 17–23.

Kudnig, S.T. (2002) Nasopharyngeal polyps in cats. *Clinical Techniques in Small Animal Practice* 17, 174–177.

Lanz, O.I. and Wood, B.C. (2004) Surgery of the ear and pinna. *Veterinary Clinics of North America Small Animal Practice* 34, 567–599, viii.

Layton, C.E. (1993) The role of lateral ear resection in managing chronic otitis externa. *Seminars in Veterinary Medicine and Surgery* 8, 24–29.

Little, C.J., Pearson, G.R. and Lane, J.G. (1989) Neoplasia involving the middle ear cavity of dogs. *Veterinary Record* 124, 54–57.

Little, C.J.L. and Lane, J.G. (1986) The surgical anatomy of the feline bulla tympanica. *Journal of Small Animal Practice* 27, 371–378.

London, C.A., Dubilzeig, R.R., Vail, D.M., Ogilvie, G.K., Hahn, K.A., Brewer, W.G., Hammer, A.S., *et al.* (1996) Evaluation of dogs and cats with tumors of the ear canal: 145 cases (1978–1992). *Journal of the American Veterinary Medical Association* 208, 1413–1418.

Moisan, P.G. and Watson, G.L. (1996) Ceruminous gland tumors in dogs and cats: a review of 124 cases. *Journal of the American Animal Hospital Association* 32, 448–452.

Owen, M.C., Lamb, C.R., Lu, D. and Targett, M.P. (2004) Material in the middle ear of dogs having magnetic resonance imaging for investigation of neurologic signs. *Veterinary Radiology and Ultrasound* 45, 149–155.

Peters-Kennedy, J., Scott, D.W. and Miller, W.H. Jr (2008) Apparent clinical resolution of pinnal actinic keratoses and squamous cell carcinoma in a cat using topical imiquimod 5% cream. *Journal of Feline Medicine and Surgery* 10, 593–599.

Pickrell, J.A., Oehme, F.W. and Cash, W.C. (1993) Ototoxicity in dogs and cats. *Seminars in Veterinary Medicine and Surgery* 8, 42–49.

Pratschke, K.M. (2003) Inflammatory polyps of the middle ear in 5 dogs. *Veterinary Surgery* 32, 292–296.

Rohleder, J.J., Jones, J.C., Duncan, R.B., Larson, M.M., Waldron, D.L. and Tromblee, T. (2006) Comparative performance of radiography and computed tomography in the diagnosis of middle ear disease in 31 dogs. *Veterinary Radiology and Ultrasound* 47, 45–52.

Smeak, D.D. (1997) Traumatic separation of the annular cartilage from the external auditory meatus in a cat. *Journal of the American Veterinary Medical Association* 211, 448–450.

Smeak, D.D. and Kerpsack, S.J. (1993) Total ear canal ablation and lateral bulla osteotomy for management of end-stage otitis. *Seminars in Veterinary Medicine and Surgery* 8, 30–41.

Theon, A.P., Barthez, P.Y., Madewell, B.R. and Griffey, S.M. (1994) Radiation therapy of ceruminous gland carcinomas in dogs and cats. *Journal of the American Veterinary Medical Association* 205, 566–569.

Tivers, M.S. and Brockman, D.J. (2009) Separation of the auricular and annular ear cartilages: surgical repair technique and clinical use in dogs and cats. *Veterinary Surgery* 38, 349–354.

Trevor, P.B. and Martin, R.A. (1993) Tympanic bulla osteotomy for treatment of middle-ear disease in cats: 19 cases (1984–1991). *Journal of the American Veterinary Medical Association* 202, 123–128.

Vail, D.M. and Withrow, S.J. (2007) Tumors of the skin and subcutaneous tissues. In: Withrow, S.J. and Vail, D.M. (eds) *Withrow and MacEwen's Small Animal Clinical Oncology*, 4th edn. Saunders Elsevier, London, pp. 375–401.

White, R.A.S. and Pomeroy, C.J. (1990) Total ear canal ablation and lateral bulla osteotomy in the dog. *Journal of Small Animal Practice* 31, 547–553.

Williams, J.M. and White, R.A.S. (1992) Total ear canal ablation combined with lateral bulla osteotomy in the cat. *Journal of Small Animal Practice* 33, 225–227.

20 Upper Respiratory Tract, Laryngeal, and Tracheal Surgery

brachycephalic: facial conformation with foreshortened nose

permanent tracheostomy: creation of a permanent stoma into the trachea to enable respiration to bypass the upper respiratory tract

staphylectomy: shortening of the palate

stertor: sonorous upper airway noise

stridor: harsh upper airway noise

temporary tracheotomy: insertion of a tube through an incision in the trachea to enable respiration to bypass the upper respiratory tract

tonsillectomy: removal of the tonsil

The reader should be able to:

- list the conditions that may cause stridor or stertor
- explain the difference between stridor and stertor and interpret what each indicates about the nature of the respiratory tract disease
- formulate an emergency treatment plan for the management of acute exacerbation of dyspnoea in a brachycephalic dog following overheating
- identify stenotic nares and brachycephalic conformation during physical examination of affected dogs
- list the anatomic landmarks necessary to diagnose overlong soft palate
- describe how to perform tonsillectomy
- classify the different forms of laryngeal paralysis
- list the key historical and clinical findings consistent with the diagnosis of laryngeal paralysis
- select candidates for arytenoid lateralization and instruct owners in order that they might make an informed decision regarding pursuing further investigation and treatment

---

Upper respiratory tract disease is common and usually causes *stridor* or *stertor*. Stridor is harsh respiratory noise associated with laryngeal disease. Stertor is sonorous respiratory noise similar to snoring that is characteristic of obstruction of the pharynx, nasopharynx, or nasal cavity. Generally, stridor is caused by laryngeal paralysis, which is seen predominantly in large, aged retriever breeds. In contrast, stertor is usually the result of brachycephalic airway conformation and is seen in small-breed dogs from an early age. These distinct syndromes will be discussed

in detail in this chapter but a host of other diseases may also lead to stridor or stertor and these are summarized in Table 20.1. Of particular note is nasopharyngeal polyp that produces signs of stertor in cats and is discussed in further detail in Chapter 19.

Management of Upper Respiratory Tract Obstruction

Animals with upper respiratory tract diseases are prone to episodes of severe dyspnoea caused by

Table 20.1. Causes of stertor and stridor in dogs and cats.

Anatomic area	Possible cause
Nares and nasal cavity	Chronic rhinitis
	Neoplasia
	Foreign body
	Stenotic nares*
Nasopharynx	Nasopharyngeal polyp
	Neoplasia
	Foreign body
	Nasopharyngeal stenosis
Pharynx	Neoplasia
	Foreign body
	Retropharyngeal lymphadenopathy
	Abscess
	Sialocoele
	Tonsillar neoplasia
	Tonsillar prolapse*
	Overlong soft palate elongation/ soft palate hypertrophy*
Larynx	Laryngeal paralysis
	Neoplasia
	Everted laryngeal saccules*
	Laryngeal collapse*
Trachea	Tracheal collapse
	Tracheal stenosis
	Foreign body

*Conditions grouped collectively as brachycephalic airway syndrome.

respiratory tract obstruction. They may require emergency treatment to relieve dyspnoea and they need careful management while hospitalized, particularly when being anaesthetized, to avoid precipitating a crisis. Regardless of the cause of dyspnoea, a range of general measures can be taken to manage these patients.

Respiratory crisis

Several factors, including overheating, excitement, stress, and increased exertion during exercise, can precipitate a respiratory crisis. Dyspnoea is often exacerbated by the development of pharyngeal and laryngeal oedema. Patients will often present in the middle of a respiratory crisis or develop one as they enter the veterinary hospital due to the stress and excitement of the visit. Several simple steps can be taken to help alleviate dyspnoea:

- provide supplemental oxygen (see p. 206);
- provide a cool environment;
- give the patient cage rest; and

- give an anti-inflammatory dose of rapid-onset, short-acting corticosteroid (e.g. dexamethasone sodium succinate).

Severely affected patients may require emergency anaesthesia and endotracheal intubation or temporary tracheotomy to bypass the area of obstruction.

General anaesthesia

Animals with upper respiratory tract disease are at increased risk of life-threatening respiratory obstruction when they are sedated or anaesthetized. The main risk periods are from premedication to intubation and from extubation to full recovery. At-risk patients require careful monitoring during these periods. Specific steps that can be taken to limit the risk include:

- modifying the anaesthetic protocol to limit the time from premedication to induction of general anaesthesia;
- pre-oxygenating the patient before inducing anaesthesia;
- using intravenous induction agents to induce anaesthesia rapidly and enable immediate endotracheal intubation;
- being prepared to perform emergency tracheotomy;
- being prepared to intubate the patient with small-diameter endotracheal tubes to accommodate luminal narrowing;
- considering performing elective tracheotomy;
- maintaining the endotracheal tube for as long as possible during the recovery period;
- positioning the patient carefully to help keep the airway open during recovery (e.g. neck stretched out); and
- monitoring the patient intensively after premedication and during recovery.

Temporary tracheotomy

A tracheotomy tube is a tube placed directly into the trachea to bypass the upper respiratory tract. Temporary tracheotomy may be performed as an elective procedure prior to airway surgery, or as an emergency to provide temporary relief of upper respiratory tract obstruction. Although tracheotomy tubes provide immediate and effective relief of respiratory obstruction, complications of tube use (particularly blockage and displacement) are dangerous and can also lead to respiratory obstruction.

Tubes require regular maintenance and patients require close, preferably continuous, monitoring while the tube is in place. Tracheotomy tubes should be removed as soon as they are no longer required, to limit the risk of these complications.

Tube selection

Single lumen tubes come in sizes that fit a range of patients from small cats to larger dogs. Double lumen tubes have an inner lining that can be removed easily for cleaning. These are easier to maintain but are also bulkier. They come in a range of sizes suitable for medium to large dogs (Fig. 20.1).

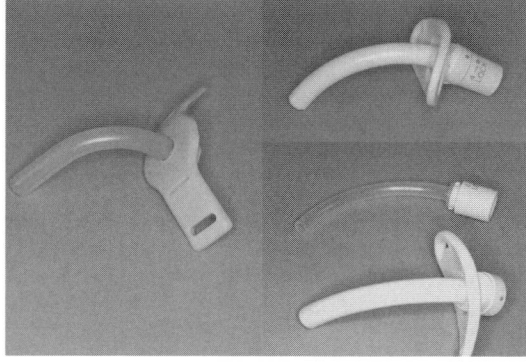

Fig. 20.1. Examples of single lumen and double lumen tracheotomy tubes.

The outer diameter of the tube should be two-thirds of the width of the trachea, to allow air to pass around the outside of the tube and to prevent pressure necrosis of the trachea. Use uncuffed tubes, unless the tube is being used to maintain general anaesthesia, as the inflated cuff can lead to pressure necrosis of the trachea over time. Uncuffed tubes of sizes 3, 4.5, 6, and 9 mm meet most requirements for dogs and cats.

Patient preparation

Temporary tracheotomy is performed under general anaesthesia. Clip and prepare the ventral neck from behind the angle of the jaw to the manubrium, and laterally beyond the jugular furrows. Position the patient in dorsal recumbency with the neck stretched out and legs tied back, ensuring that the neck is as straight as possible. Place a pad under the neck to facilitate exposure of the trachea (Fig. 20.2). In an emergency, patient preparation may have to be compromised in the interests of speed.

Technique

Make a midline skin incision from just distal to the larynx and extend it caudally for several centimetres. Identify the paired sternohyoideus muscles in midline and separate bluntly between them, ligating branches of the vessel that runs between

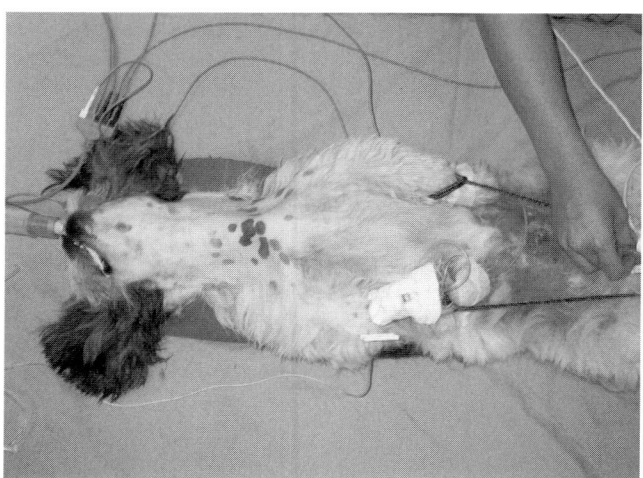

Fig. 20.2. Positioning for tracheotomy.

the muscle bellies as required. Place self-retaining retractors (e.g. Gelpi) to retract the sternohyoideus muscle bellies laterally. This exposes the ventral aspect of the trachea (Fig. 20.3).

Identify the second tracheal cartilage by counting back from the larynx. Palpate the ligament between the second and third tracheal cartilages. Make a transverse incision in the ligament running parallel to the tracheal cartilages using the tip of a scalpel blade (Fig. 20.4). Incise the ligament along a third of its ventral circumference. This ensures that the vessels and nerves of the neck are not damaged, as they lie more laterally.

Place two long loops of suture around the tracheal cartilages immediately above and below the tracheotomy site using 2-0 or 3-0 monofilament, non-absorbable material, and knot them to produce two long stay sutures for future manipulation of the tracheotomy site (Fig. 20.5). Pull the ventral suture upwards and insert the tip of the tracheotomy

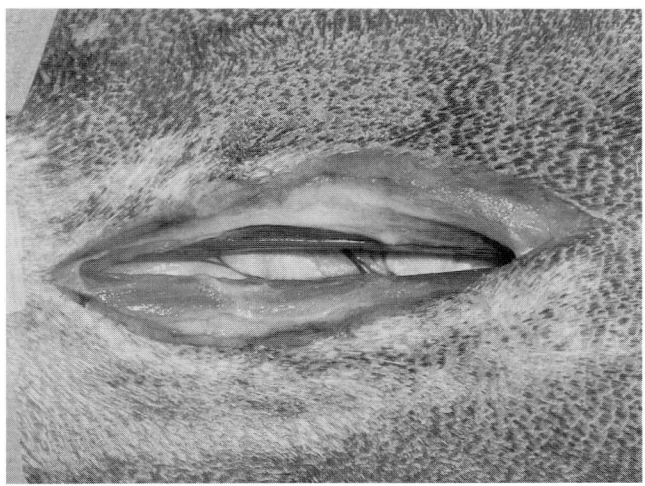

Fig. 20.3. Tracheotomy skin incision and the separated bellies of the sternohyoideus muscle.

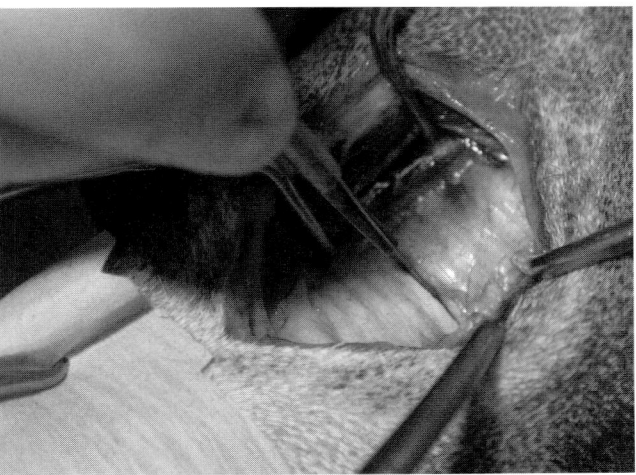

Fig. 20.4. Incise between tracheal rings.

tube into the tracheal lumen. If the patient is intubated, withdraw the endotracheal tube as the tracheotomy tube is placed (Fig. 20.6).

Switch the anaesthetic system to the tracheotomy tube. Partly close the muscle and skin incision above and below the tracheotomy site. Leave an open skin incision at least three times the width of the tube to facilitate tube removal and replacement. Ensure that the ends of the two stay sutures protrude through the incision so that they are accessible. Lastly, secure the tube by tying it snugly in position using tapes around the back of the patient's neck, and dress the surgical site.

Tube maintenance

The tracheotomy tube requires regular maintenance and, ideally, the patient should be constantly supervised. Tracheotomy tube displacement and blockage are common and both can lead to death. Single lumen tubes should be replaced with a clean tube several times each day. This gives time to clean and dry the dirty tube. To remove the tube, untie the tapes securing the tube and slip the tube out of the trachea. To replace the tube, have the patient held in a sitting position with its chin supported and head in a neutral position. Pull the two stay

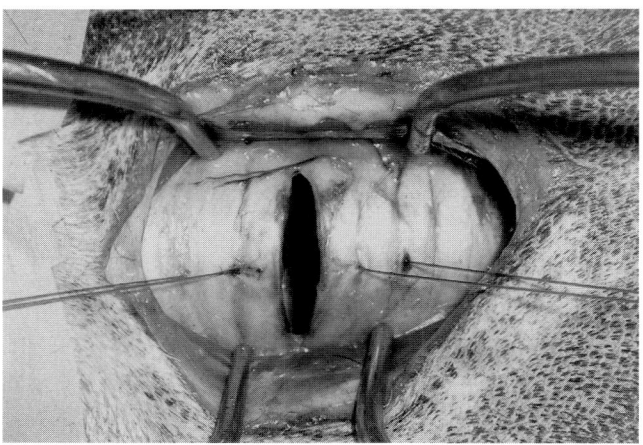

Fig. 20.5. Place stay sutures above and below tracheotomy to facilitate tube placement.

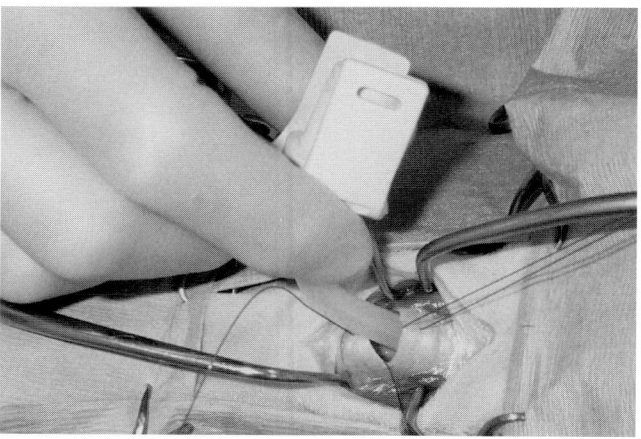

Fig. 20.6. Pull on the ventral stay suture and insert tube.

sutures forward and apart to lift the tracheotomy site towards the skin incision and separate the cartilages. Replace the tube by sliding it into the incision and check that it is positioned properly by assessing airflow through it. Most dogs and cats tolerate this well without sedation. Double lumen tubes are easier to maintain as the inner tube can be removed for regular cleaning (most kits come with a spare inner sleeve), but the entire tube should still be removed once daily for thorough cleaning.

Secretions collect and desiccate in the tube and airway and this can lead to obstruction. To reduce this, humidify the airway using a humidifier or by instilling sterile saline (1–2 ml) down the tracheotomy tube several times daily. Secretions should be suctioned from the trachea several times a day by passing a low-pressure, soft suction catheter down the trachea through the tube and withdrawing it slowly as suction is applied intermittently (continuous suction may injure the tracheal mucosa). A syringe and flexible catheter can be used if a suction device is not available.

Tube removal

Prior to removing the tube, evaluate how the patient copes with the tube occluded. Patients that cope with the tube occluded by breathing around the tube and through the larynx will generally cope well once the tube is removed. Remove the tube but leave the stay sutures in place for 1–2 days to enable rapid replacement of the tube if necessary. During this period, the patient should remain hospitalized. Allow the site to heal by second intention as this causes less wound problems than suturing the site. There may be some airflow through the site for the first 48 h following placement.

Complications

Tube occlusion leading to death is the most serious complication. Other complications include tracheal stenosis at the incision site, laryngeal paralysis due to iatrogenic recurrent laryngeal nerve injury during placement, and wound infection.

Permanent Tracheostomy

Permanent tracheostomy is creation of a permanent opening into the trachea to bypass the upper respiratory tract. It is a salvage procedure reserved for the management of severe respiratory tract disease causing obstruction of the upper respiratory tract or proximal trachea. The commonest indication for permanent tracheostomy is severe laryngeal obstruction (e.g. laryngeal collapse; laryngeal neoplasia). Stenosis of the site and occlusion of the airway with dried secretion both can lead to obstruction. Patients may sustain a good quality of life for a protracted period but the complication and mortality rates are high and owners require careful counselling before this is performed. Patients should be referred to a specialist centre for assessment and surgery if this procedure is required.

Anatomy and Function of Upper Respiratory Tract and Larynx

The upper respiratory tract includes the nares (nostrils), nasal cavity, nasopharynx, and common pharynx. The larynx marks the start of the lower respiratory tract. The nasal cavity is filled with nasal turbinates that warm and moisten inspired air and filter particulate matter from it. The nasopharynx is bordered by the pharyngeal muscles laterally, the base of the skull dorsally, and the hard and soft palates ventrally. The soft palate divides the caudal part of the nasopharynx from the oropharynx. It occludes the nasopharynx during swallowing to prevent food and fluid from running into the nasopharynx. The common pharynx contains the epiglottis, glottis (opening to the laryngeal lumen), and oesophageal ostium.

The larynx is composed of paired and unpaired cartilages. The 'V' shaped thyroid cartilage and the caudal cricoid cartilage provide structure to the laryngeal walls. The cricoid cartilage attaches to the first tracheal cartilage. The epiglottis sits at the opening to the larynx and acts as a baffle to prevent food entering the larynx during swallowing. Together, the arytenoid cartilages and vocal cords produce a diamond-shaped opening into the larynx called the glottis. The paired arytenoid cartilages (with their paired cuneiform and corniculate processes) form the dorsolateral walls of the laryngeal glottis. The vocal cords run from the cuneiform process of the arytenoids to the floor of the laryngeal lumen. They form the ventrolateral borders of the glottis. The dorsal cricoarytenoid muscle pulls the arytenoid cartilages laterally, opening the glottis during inspiration to allow air to enter. This muscle is innervated by the recurrent laryngeal nerve, which arises from the vagus nerve at the heart base and travels up the neck beside the trachea to innervate the laryngeal cartilages. The glottis also actively closes during swallowing to prevent aspiration of food.

Brachycephalic Airway Syndrome

Brachycephalic airway syndrome affects all brachycephalic animals to a lesser or greater extent. This conformation is common in a range of small-breed dogs but is also seen in some larger breeds of dog and in some cats (Table 20.2).

Table 20.2. Brachycephalic breeds of dog and cat.

Dog	Cat
Boston Terrier	Exotic shorthair
Boxer	Himalayan
Bulldogs (all breeds)	Persian
Cavalier King Charles spaniel	
Chow chow	
Dogue de Bordeaux	
Lhasa Apso	
Pekinese	
Pug	
Shar pei	
Shih tzu	

Aetiopathogenesis

Brachycephalic breeds have a foreshortened skull with a squat nasal cavity and nasopharynx. The soft tissues of the nostrils, nasal cavity, nasopharynx, and common pharynx are squashed out of position and are too large. Soft tissues compress the nasal and pharyngeal cavities compounding airway narrowing and increasing the resistance to airflow through the upper respiratory tract. As the upper respiratory tract accounts for 50% of the resistance to airflow during inspiration, obstruction markedly increases the resistance to airflow and the effort required to ventilate the lungs adequately. During inspiration, the negative pressure generated within the airway is excessive. Mobile parts of the upper respiratory tract, such as the nares, nasopharyngeal wall, and laryngeal glottis, collapse inwards and, over time, may sustain lasting damage.

All of these problems contribute to respiratory compromise and stertor that vary in degree depending on the anatomic abnormalities, conformation, and body weight of the individual. The main conditions are described individually.

Stenotic nares

The dorsolateral wings of the nares of brachycephalic dogs are often collapsed inwards. This leaves only a narrow slit opening into the nasal cavity and reduces air intake through the nose (Fig. 20.7).

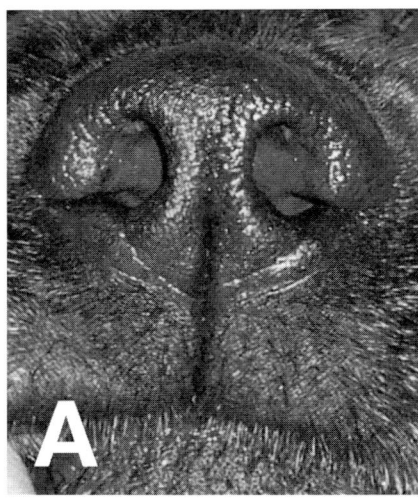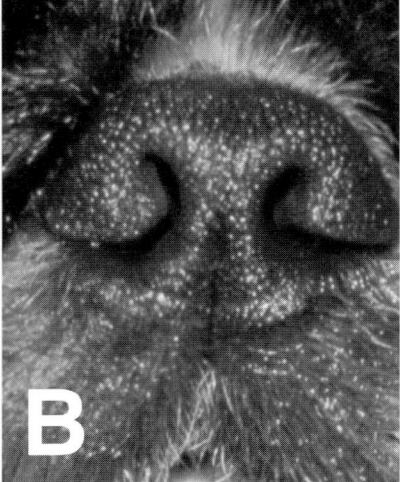

Fig. 20.7. Stenotic nares: (A) normally shaped nares; (B) stenotic nares.

Overlong soft palate

Overlong soft palate ('elongated soft palate') is a common primary problem of brachycephalic breeds. The palate is too long and extends beyond the caudal pole of the tonsil (the normal anatomic landmark for the caudal edge of the palate). Instead of reaching just to the tip of the epiglottis, the palate extends caudally over the epiglottis and obstructs the laryngeal lumen (Fig. 20.8). In the most severely affected cases, the soft palate is inhaled into the glottis during inspiration. The overlong soft palate also becomes hypertrophied and oedematous due to trauma during inspiration that compounds the problem.

Everted laryngeal saccules

The laryngeal ventricles are recesses located behind the vocal folds lined with mucosa (the laryngeal saccules). Increased inspiratory pressure can cause prolapse of the laryngeal saccules. These are identified as white globes of tissue protruding behind the vocal cords and obstructing the ventral half of the glottis. This condition is often classified as stage I laryngeal collapse (Fig. 20.9).

Laryngeal collapse

Laryngeal collapse stages II and III are the end stages of brachycephalic airway syndrome and

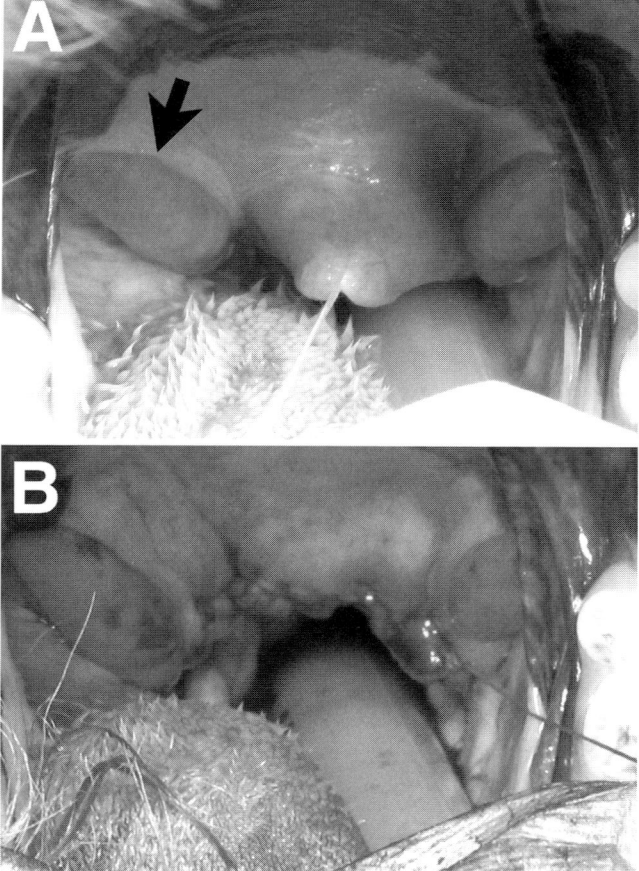

Fig. 20.8. Overlong soft palate and tonsillar prolapse: (A) the soft palate extends beyond the caudal poles of the tonsils (a stay suture is being used to pull the tip of the soft palate forward in preparation for shortening, demonstrating the redundant tissue). This dog also has tonsillar hypertrophy and prolapse (arrow); (B) the caudal edge of the palate now lies in a normal position following shortening.

produce severe dyspnoea. With increasing inspiratory effort, the dorsal glottis begins to collapse inwards as the arytenoid cartilages are placed under increasing strain. First the cuneiform processes that support the dorsolateral glottis collapse inwards and meet in midline (stage II collapse), then the corniculate processes that support the glottis dorsally collapse and the laryngeal lumen is completely obstructed (stage III collapse) (Fig. 20.9). Laryngeal collapse causes severe and progressive dyspnoea.

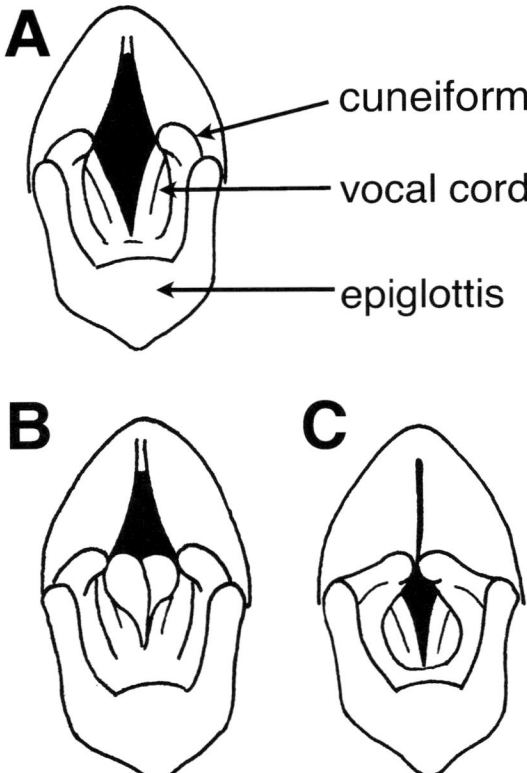

Fig. 20.9. Laryngeal collapse: (A) normal anatomy of the glottis in a neutral position (based on Fig. 20.12A) – note the diamond shaped glottis, clear vocal cords, and distance between the cuneiform cartilages; (B) everted laryngeal saccules (stage I laryngeal collapse) – the saccules protrude from behind the vocal cords, obstructing the ventral half of the glottis; (C) laryngeal collapse (stage II) – the cuneiform cartilages collapse inwards, closing the dorsal half of the glottis. In stage III collapse, the cuneiform cartilages fold in further and the glottis begins to crumple and shorten dorsoventrally, causing further obstruction of the ventral glottis.

Tonsillar prolapse

Tonsillar prolapse frequently occurs as a secondary problem in brachycephalic airway syndrome. The tonsils prolapse out of their crypts and become hypertrophied and oedematous (Fig. 20.8). The prolapsed tonsils contribute to obstruction of the common pharynx.

History

Most brachycephalic breeds exhibit some signs of respiratory compromise but this is often mistakenly considered to be normal in the affected breed. Stertor is the most consistent finding and is caused by turbulent airflow in the upper respiratory tract. It has often been present throughout the animal's life. Stertor is exacerbated when the patient is sleeping or relaxed or when respiratory effort increases during exercise or excitement. Exercise intolerance and respiratory distress get progressively worse as secondary changes develop. Initially, patients may only show reluctance to exercise but, as the condition progresses, cyanosis, syncope, and inspiratory dyspnoea are seen during exercise. In the worst-affected patients, cyanosis, dyspnoea, and collapse are seen at rest, and the patient's quality of life is severely impaired.

Physical findings

It is important to take care when handling brachycephalic patients, as stress during evaluation can precipitate a respiratory crisis. Brachycephalic conformation and stenotic nares are obvious physical features. Stertor and increased respiratory effort are usually present and many animals mouth-breathe during evaluation or at other times of stress. On auscultation, increased sonorous noise is heard over the pharynx, and nasal airflow may be reduced. Pharyngeal examination must be performed in the anaesthetized patient to catalogue the full extent of the problem (see below).

Investigation and management

Further investigation under anaesthesia and surgical correction of the airway are often scheduled together to limit the number of anaesthetics (and the risks involved) for the individual patient. Following induction of anaesthesia, position the patient in sternal recumbency. Ask an assistant to hold the upper jaw and use a laryngoscope blade to depress the base of the tongue and inspect the pharynx and larynx. Use the descriptions above to identify the various diseases.

Treatment

Correction of stenotic nares, elongated soft palate, tonsillar prolapse, and laryngeal saccule eversion are generally well tolerated and may lead to dramatic improvement in dyspnoea. Although the surgical techniques themselves are simple, accurate assessment of the condition and judgement of how much tissue to resect, particularly when shortening the soft palate, requires some experience.

Non-surgical management

Weight loss and restricting exercise, limiting stress, and preventing overheating can reduce signs of dyspnoea. Avoid using a collar and lead to restrain the patient. Use a body harness instead.

Timing of intervention

It is easy to recommend early intervention, because the syndrome is progressive. Early surgery may halt progression of the disease before life-threatening problems such as laryngeal collapse develop.

Preoperative preparation

Place the patient in sternal recumbency. Use a gag to hold the mouth open and position the head symmetrically and securely. Pack the pharynx with a pharyngeal sponge to prevent aspiration of blood. Prepare the oropharynx and nostrils with dilute povidone-iodine. Administer short-acting corticosteroid (e.g. dexamethasone sodium succinate) to reduce post-operative swelling.

Suture selection

Use 3-0 or 4-0 short-acting, absorbable suture material. Multifilament materials such as polyglactin 910 produce knots with soft ends in comparison to monofilament materials, and cause less pharyngeal irritation post-operatively.

Stenotic nares

Stenotic nares can be widened by resecting tissue from the dorsolateral wing of the nostril using a 2–6 mm, circular biopsy punch. Select a biopsy punch that will remove a plug of epithelium from the centre of wing of the nostril but will leave a rim of intact epithelium to suture. Use the biopsy punch to incise a plug of cartilage and epithelium to the full depth of the blade. Grasp the tissue with thumb forceps and detach the deep attachments with a no. 11 scalpel blade. Close the defect by suturing the medial edge to the lateral edge with two or three sutures, creating a vertical scar. This pulls the medial edge of the fold laterally, opening the nostril (Fig. 20.10).

Tonsillectomy

Grasp the prolapsed tonsil with forceps and retract it fully from the crypt. Place a curved haemostat across the base of the tonsil to act as a guide for suture placement. Place a transfixing ligature through the pedicle between the forceps and the tonsillar crypt, remove the forceps, and tighten the ligature. Excise the tonsil using Metzenbaum scissors and check for haemorrhage, placing additional sutures if required. The tonsillar pedicle should retract into the crypt as soon as it is released (Fig. 20.11).

Staphylectomy

Inexperienced surgeons should not perform staphylectomy (shortening of elongated soft palate), as excessive resection of tissue leads to nasopharyngeal regurgitation of food, rhinitis, and aspiration pneumonia. A wide range of techniques has been described. The basic technique is to grasp the tip of the soft palate and pull it forwards, apply right-angled forceps to crush the palate along a line between the caudal poles of the tonsillar crypts, amputate the redundant tissue, and suture the nasopharyngeal and oropharyngeal mucosa together to seal the defect (Fig. 20.8B).

Everted laryngeal saccule excision (stage I laryngeal collapse)

Grasp the everted laryngeal saccules with forceps and resect them with Metzenbaum scissors. There should be little bleeding as the blood supply to the saccules is minor. This procedure is easiest to perform if the patient is extubated. Do not cut the vocal folds.

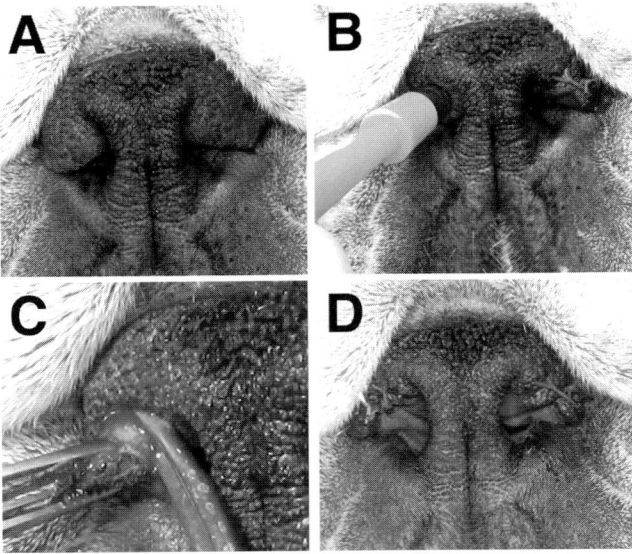

Fig. 20.10. Stenotic nares widening: (A) before surgery; (B) 4 mm circular skin punch is used to remove a core of tissue from the wing of the nostril; (C) the incised tissues is excised; (D) the defect is sutured, widening the nares.

Laryngeal collapse (stages II and III laryngeal collapse)

Advanced laryngeal collapse is a difficult condition to manage. A range of surgical techniques has been described but results are variable and may produce only short-lived improvement because of progressive collapse or scarring. Ultimately, permanent tracheostomy can be performed, but the prognosis is poor. A common approach to this problem is to correct the other abnormalities that are present in the hope that this will enable the patient to cope better with laryngeal collapse and reduce the rate of progression of the disease.

Aftercare

The main period of risk is in the first few hours following surgery as the patient is recovering from general anaesthesia. The patient should be continuously monitored until it is sitting and breathing without difficulty. Emergency tracheotomy may be necessary. Food and water should be withheld until the patient is fully recovered from anaesthesia and then given under supervision to ensure that the patient does not aspirate food.

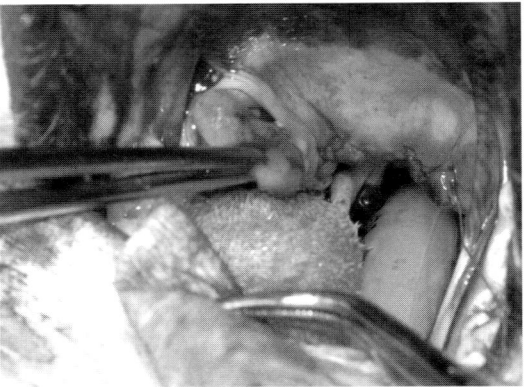

Fig. 20.11. Tonsillectomy: the tonsil has been pulled out of its crypt using forceps in preparation for clamping the base, ligating, and transecting it.

Prognosis and complications

The most serious complications are of respiratory obstruction during recovery from surgery and of over-shortening the soft palate, leading to nasopharyngeal aspiration of food and dyspnoea. However, the commonest problem encountered post-operatively is continuing stertor and respiratory compromise because of the numerous conformational problems that cannot be addressed surgically. It is reasonable to expect surgery to reduce stertor and dyspnoea in mildly affected patients and to improve quality of life and slow progression in severely affected patients.

Related conditions

Animals with brachycephalic conformation frequently also suffer from tracheal hypoplasia, a congenital condition in which the trachea has a very narrow diameter. This exacerbates dyspnoea and increases the risks of anaesthesia in these patients. It is untreatable and the condition is found frequently in bulldog breeds. When anaesthetizing brachycephalic animals, be prepared to intubate them with very small endotracheal tubes if required, as tracheal hypoplasia has often not been identified prior to general anaesthesia.

Laryngeal Paralysis

Laryngeal paralysis is a common acquired condition causing dyspnoea in older, large-breed dogs. It is occasionally diagnosed in small breed dogs, cats, and young animals.

Aetiopathogenesis

Laryngeal paralysis results from failure of the arytenoid cartilages to abduct on inspiration. This is caused by primary muscle disease or loss of innervation from the recurrent laryngeal nerve reducing function of the dorsal cricoarytenoid muscle. The failure to abduct cartilages during inspiration prevents the glottis from opening. This limits air intake and causes dyspnoea. In addition, control over the vocal cords is lost and these reverberate in the airstream during inspiration. This leads to stridor and dysphonia (loss of bark). The arytenoids also fail to adduct and close the glottis during swallowing, and this predisposes the patient to aspiration pneumonia. Laryngeal paralysis can be classified as idiopathic, secondary, or congenital.

Idiopathic laryngeal paralysis

Idiopathic laryngeal paralysis is the commonest form in dogs. It affects predominantly older, large-breed dogs and the retriever breeds are over-represented. The aetiology is unknown but recent work suggests that laryngeal paralysis may be an early manifestation of a more widespread, chronic neuropathy in geriatric dogs. Hypothyroidism has been implicated in the pathogenesis of disease but there is no strong link between the two conditions and they are probably unrelated in most patients.

Congenital laryngeal paralysis

Heritable congenital laryngeal paralysis has been identified in Bouvier des Flandres, huskies, and husky crosses and is caused by a defect in the brainstem nuclei controlling the recurrent laryngeal nerve. Laryngeal paralysis has also been identified in young Dalmatians, rottweilers and Pyrenean mountain dogs as part of more generalized polyneuropathy. An early-onset form of laryngeal paralysis affecting white German Shepherd dogs within the first 2 years of life has been described.

Acquired secondary laryngeal paralysis

Laryngeal paralysis can develop secondary to any condition affecting the function of the dorsal cricoarytenoid muscle or recurrent laryngeal nerve. Laryngeal paralysis may be an early manifestation of a generalized polyneuropathy, polymyopathy, or neuromuscular junction disorder (e.g. myasthenia gravis). In these cases, there may be concurrent megaoesophagus or ataxia indicating a more widespread problem. Laryngeal paralysis may also be caused by direct injury to the recurrent laryngeal nerve following neck trauma, surgery, or cranial thoracic pathology (where the nerve originates from the vagosympathetic trunk).

Feline laryngeal paralysis

Laryngeal paralysis is uncommon in cats but a similar range of presentations is reported. Most cases are classified as idiopathic, but iatrogenic injury to the recurrent laryngeal nerve has also been reported during thyroidectomy.

Signalment of idiopathic laryngeal paralysis

Idiopathic laryngeal paralysis occurs predominantly in middle or old aged, large- and giant-breed dogs. The Labrador retriever is over-represented and accounts for a third of cases. Males are diagnosed with the condition more frequently than females.

Historical findings

Patients usually present for evaluation of exercise intolerance or stridor but they may also be presented in crisis due to profound dyspnoea or aspiration pneumonia. Typical historical findings are of stridor, dyspnoea, dysphonia, coughing, and exercise intolerance. In animals that have widespread neuromuscular disease, other signs such as regurgitation, weakness, or ataxia may be reported.

Initially, stridor and dyspnoea are only noted during exercise but become increasingly apparent during mild activity or stress. Dyspnoea progressively worsens and can lead to profound exercise intolerance, collapse, and cyanosis. The signs generally disappear when the patient is sleeping or relaxed.

Physical examination

Inspiratory stridor and dyspnoea are the hallmarks of laryngeal paralysis and are often obvious during evaluation as they are exacerbated by stress. Noisy airflow is appreciable on auscultation of the larynx. There may be a harsh cough that can be induced by tracheal palpation. Always perform a full neurological examination to identify other signs of neuromuscular disease that may indicate an underlying aetiology of laryngeal paralysis.

Patients often present during a life-threatening respiratory crisis due to exacerbation of clinical signs by excitement, exercise, or periods of hot weather. These patients are cyanotic, have extreme inspiratory effort, and marked inspiratory stridor. If respiratory effort is large enough, expiratory stridor will also be heard. Animals with aspiration pneumonia are pyrexic, dull, and may show signs of septic shock (see Chapter 13). These patients have soft, productive coughs and adventitious lung sounds, particularly in the cranioventral lung fields.

Investigation

The diagnosis of laryngeal paralysis can only be confirmed by direct evaluation of the larynx to assess whether or not the glottis abducts on inspiration. Accurately confirming the diagnosis is difficult as the method of evaluation is prone to false-positive diagnosis and is easily over-interpreted by inexperienced operators.

To confirm the diagnosis, the patient is anaesthetized without premedication using a short-acting intravenous induction agent. It is positioned in sternal recumbency with mouth held open and direct laryngoscopy is performed as the patient recovers from anaesthesia. During assessment, normal laryngeal function is noted by active abduction of the glottis during inspiration. The diagnosis of laryngeal paralysis is reached by failing to demonstrate this as the patient regains consciousness. The biggest pitfall is the ease with which a false-positive diagnosis can be reached and the accuracy of evaluation is critically dependent on the induction and recovery from anaesthesia. The problem occurs because anaesthesia quickly ablates all normal laryngeal function and this only returns as the patient nears full consciousness. If laryngeal responses do not return before the patient regains sufficient consciousness to no longer tolerate being held, a false-positive diagnosis of laryngeal paralysis can be reached. A recent paper has evaluated various anaesthetic protocols and has concluded that thiopentone used for induction without premedication has least inhibitory effect on laryngeal function and is the preferred induction agent for performing this evaluation.

Perform thoracic radiography to identify secondary aspiration pneumonia and megaoesophagus.

Treatment

A range of non-surgical measures can help reduce signs in the early stages of the disease. Animals should be restrained with body harnesses or halter-style head collars, rather than collars around their necks. Exercise and stress are restricted to prevent exacerbating the condition. Obese animals are placed on weight-reduction diets. To reduce the risk of aspiration pneumonia, animals should not be fed sloppy or liquid diets. Tinned dog food has a good consistency as it tends to be swallowed in lumps and is not easily inhaled. However, as the condition is progressive and most patients will ultimately benefit from surgery, it is easy to recommend surgery early in the course of the disease.

Numerous surgeries have been described. All require a good knowledge of laryngeal anatomy and are technically demanding. Arytenoid lateralization (tie-back) is the most popular. It relieves signs of laryngeal paralysis by permanently suturing open one side of the glottis (Fig. 20.12). This is performed through a lateral or ventral approach to the larynx.

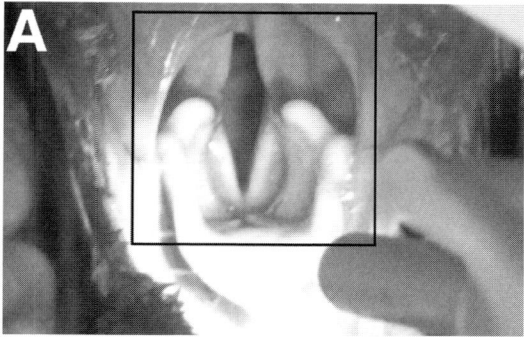

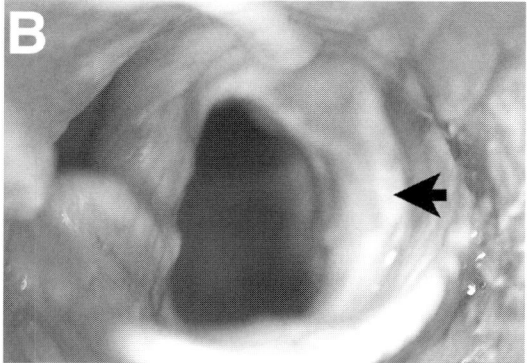

Fig. 20.12. Arytenoid lateralization: (A) normal glottis in neutral position (box defines equivalent area of view of next panel); (B) glottis following arytenoid lateralization – the left side (to right of image) has been abducted (arrow) widening the glottis.

Outcomes and complications

Arytenoid lateralization increases air intake during inspiration, relieving signs of dyspnoea. However, the glottis is still unable to close during swallowing and the increased width post-operatively increases the risk of aspiration. Vocal cord function is not improved, so stridor and dysphonia continue post-operatively.

The prognosis for animals with idiopathic laryngeal paralysis is good, as most recover from surgery and have improvement in their clinical signs. Over 90% of owners consider surgery to have been successful and their dog's quality of life to have been improved. It is reasonable to expect the patient to cope better with stress and exercise post-operatively, and to be at less risk of acute respiratory crisis. Most patients continue to have stridor and many have an intermittent, non-productive cough that appears to be of little significance. Animals recuperate quickly after surgery but require 4–6

weeks of exercise restriction while scar tissue forms, to improve stability of the arytenoids. The major risk of life-threatening complications post-operatively is aspiration pneumonia. Animals should not be fed sloppy or liquid diets post-operatively. Tinned dog food is a good diet as it tends to be swallowed in lumps and is not easily inhaled. A small proportion of patients have deterioration of signs due to failure of the sutures anchoring the arytenoid cartilage in place. Surgery can be repeated on the contralateral side.

Animals with laryngeal paralysis as part of a more generalized neuromuscular disorder have a guarded prognosis because of progression of the underlying disease. Young animals presenting with laryngeal paralysis should not be bred from as the condition may be inherited. Cats are rarely diagnosed with laryngeal paralysis but also respond well to arytenoid lateralization.

Tracheal Collapse

Tracheal collapse is a common syndrome affecting small-breed dogs that leads to progressive dyspnoea and a distinctive cough.

Aetiopathogenesis

Tracheal collapse is a progressive condition caused by inherent weakness of the tracheal cartilages that allows the trachea to flatten dorsoventrally over time (Fig. 20.13). Although the cartilages are abnormal from birth, tracheal collapse rarely becomes clinically apparent before middle age. Initially it affects the cervical trachea but over time the thoracic trachea and mainstem bronchi become involved. The condition is dynamic and collapse is induced by changes in airway pressures during inspiration (cervical trachea) and expiration (thoracic trachea). The condition causes severe dyspnoea that is exacerbated by increasing respiratory effort, and may become life-threatening.

Presentation and clinical signs

The condition affects small-breed dogs and the Yorkshire Terrier is predisposed. Dyspnoea is the commonest presenting signs and the median age at onset is 7 years. Dogs have a characteristic 'goose-honk', high-pitched cough. The cough can be induced by tracheal palpation. Animals can become profoundly dyspnoeic during evaluation or during bouts of coughing.

Investigation

Bronchoscopy can be used to confirm the diagnosis and to evaluate the full extent of collapse. Radiography may also be used but, as tracheal collapse is dynamic, the appearance varies with respiration and the severity of the problem may be underestimated (Fig. 20.14).

Treatment

Tracheal collapse can be treated medically or by stenting the trachea, but the prognosis is guarded. Medical management includes weight reduction, avoiding stress, use of a halter rather than a collar, antitussive medication, and brochodilators. Medical management is recommended as the first line of treatment because of the risks of stenting. Tracheal stenting involves placing stents to prevent the trachea from collapsing. These can be placed surgically (extraluminal stents) or endoscopically (intraluminal stents). Both methods require technical expertise and experience to be successful.

Prognosis

The prognosis for tracheal collapse is guarded. The condition is debilitating and medical management has limited effect in severely affected individuals. Following stenting, 91–95% of cases survive but all techniques have high complications rates and carry risk of life-threatening problems. Intraluminal stenting has only begun to be widely employed in

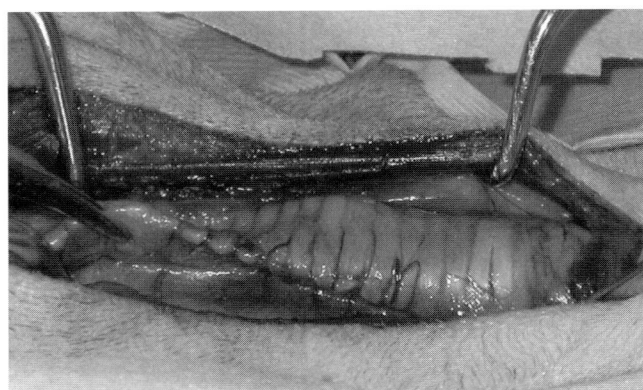

Fig. 20.13. Tracheal collapse of the cervical trachea of a small breed dog taken intra-operatively during tracheal stenting: forceps are holding a portion that has completely flattened dorsoventrally.

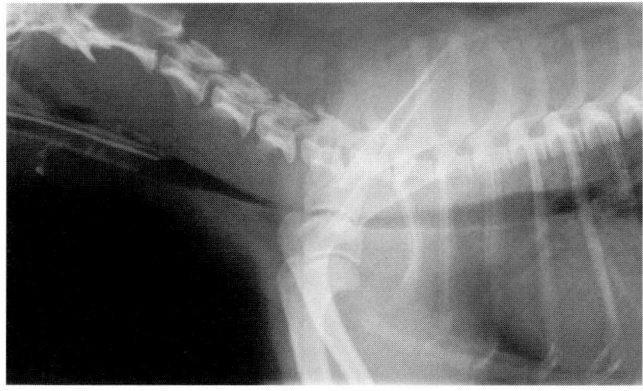

Fig. 20.14. Radiograph of tracheal collapse: the trachea can be seen collapsing at the thoracic inlet.

veterinary species in the last few years, and complications associated with this method may reduce as the technique is refined.

Devocalization

Devocalization is performed in some countries to prevent dogs and cats from making a noise, and involves resection of the vocal cords. However, the procedure provides no health advantages for the patient and many people considered it to be an unnecessary mutilation that prevents the patient from expressing normal behaviour. In addition, laryngeal scarring post-operatively may lead to laryngeal obstruction. It is illegal to perform devocalization in the UK.

Bibliography

Braund, K.G., Shores, A., Cochrane, S., Forrester, D., Kwiecien, J.M. and Steiss, J.E. (1994) Laryngeal paralysis-polyneuropathy complex in young Dalmatians. *American Journal of Veterinary Research* 55, 534–542.

Buback, J.L., Boothe, H.W. and Hobson, H.P. (1996) Surgical treatment of tracheal collapse in dogs: 90 cases (1983–1993). *Journal of the American Veterinary Medical Association* 208, 380–384.

Burbidge, H.M. (1995) A review of laryngeal paralysis in dogs. *British Veterinary Journal* 151, 71–82.

Davidson, E.B., Davis, M.S., Campbell, G.A., Williamson, K.K., Payton, M.E., Healey, T.S. and Bartels, K.E. (2001) Evaluation of carbon dioxide laser and conventional incisional techniques for resection of soft palates in brachycephalic dogs. *Journal of the American Veterinary Medical Association* 219, 776–781.

Demetriou, J.L. and Kirby, B.M. (2003) The effect of two modifications of unilateral arytenoid lateralization on rima glottidis area in dogs. *Veterinary Surgery* 32, 62–68.

Dewey, C.W., Bailey, C.S., Shelton, G.D., Kass, P.H. and Cardinet, G.H. 3rd (1997) Clinical forms of acquired myasthenia gravis in dogs: 25 cases (1988–1995). *Journal of Veterinary Internal Medicine* 11, 50–57.

Done, S.H. and Drew, R.A. (1976) Observations on the pathology of tracheal collapse in dogs. *Journal of Small Animal Practice* 17, 783–791.

Fasanella, F.J., Shivley, J.M., Wardlaw, J.L. and Givaruangsawat, S. (2010) Brachycephalic airway obstructive syndrome in dogs: 90 cases (1991–2008). *Journal of the American Veterinary Medical Association* 237, 1048–1051.

Gabriel, A., Poncelet, L., Van Ham, L., Clercx, C., Braund, K.G., Bhatti, S., Detilleux, J., *et al.* (2006) Laryngeal paralysis–polyneuropathy complex in young related Pyrenean mountain dogs. *Journal of Small Animal Practice* 47, 144–149.

Grubb, T. (2010) Anesthesia for patients with respiratory disease and/or airway compromise. *Topics in Companion Animal Medicine* 25, 120–132.

Hardie, R.J., Gunby, J. and Bjorling, D.E. (2009) Arytenoid lateralization for treatment of laryngeal paralysis in 10 cats. *Veterinary Surgery* 38, 445–451.

Harvey, C.E. (1982a) Everted laryngeal saccule surgery in brachycephalic dogs. *Journal of the American Animal Hospital Association* 18, 545–547.

Harvey, C.E. (1982b) Soft palate resection in brachycephalic dogs. *Journal of the American Animal Hospital Association* 18, 538–544.

Henrikson, D.M. (1969) Technique for devocalizing dogs. *Journal of the American Veterinary Medical Association* 155, 21–25.

Jackson, A.M., Tobias, K., Long, C., Bartges, J. and Harvey, R. (2004) Effects of various anesthetic agents on laryngeal motion during laryngoscopy in normal dogs. *Veterinary Surgery* 33, 102–106.

Jeffery, N.D., Talbot, C.E., Smith, P.M. and Bacon, N.J. (2006) Acquired idiopathic laryngeal paralysis as a prominent feature of generalised neuromuscular disease in 39 dogs. *Veterinary Record* 158, 17.

Johnson, L. (2000) Tracheal collapse. Diagnosis and medical and surgical treatment. *Veterinary Clinics of North America Small Animal Practice* 30, 1253–1266, vi.

Johnson, L.R. and McKiernan, B.C. (1995) Diagnosis and medical management of tracheal collapse. *Seminars in Veterinary Medicine and Surgery (Small Animal)* 10, 101–108.

MacPhail, C.M. and Monnet, E. (2001) Outcome of and postoperative complications in dogs undergoing surgical treatment of laryngeal paralysis: 140 cases (1985–1998). *Journal of the American Veterinary Medical Association* 218, 1949–1956.

Macready, D.M., Johnson, L.R. and Pollard, R.E. (2007) Fluoroscopic and radiographic evaluation of tracheal collapse in dogs: 62 cases (2001–2006). *Journal of the American Veterinary Medical Association* 230, 1870–1876.

Mahony, O.M., Knowles, K.E., Braund, K.G., Averill, D.R., Jr and Frimberger, A.E. (1998) Laryngeal paralysis-polyneuropathy complex in young Rottweilers. *Journal of Veterinary Internal Medicine* 12, 330–337.

Millard, R.P. and Tobias, K.M. (2009) Laryngeal paralysis in dogs. *Compendium of Continuing Education for the Practicing Veterinarian* 31, 212–219.

Nicholson, I. and Baines, S. (2010) Indications, placement and management of tracheostomy tubes. *In Practice* 32, 104–113.

Pink, J.J., Doyle, R.S., Hughes, J.M., Tobin, E. and Bellenger, C.R. (2006) Laryngeal collapse in seven brachycephalic puppies. *Journal of Small Animal Practice* 47, 131–135.

Polizopoulou, Z.S., Koutinas, A.F., Papadopoulos, G.C. and Saridomichelakis, M.N. (2003) Juvenile laryngeal paralysis in three Siberian husky x Alaskan malamute puppies. *Veterinary Record* 153, 624–627.

Ridyard, A.E., Corcoran, B.M., Tasker, S., Willis, R., Welsh, E.M., Demetriou, J.L. and Griffiths, L.G. (2000) Spontaneous laryngeal paralysis in four white-coated German shepherd dogs. *Journal of Small Animal Practice* 41, 558–561.

Riecks, T.W., Birchard, S.J. and Stephens, J.A. (2007) Surgical correction of brachycephalic syndrome in dogs: 62 cases (1991–2004). *Journal of the American Veterinary Medical Association* 230, 1324–1328.

Sis, R.F., Yoder, J.T. and Starch, C.J. (1967) Devocalization of cats by median laryngotomy and dissection of the vocal folds. *Veterinary Medicine (Small Animal Clinician)* 62, 975–980.

Snelling, S.R. and Edwards, G.A. (2003) A retrospective study of unilateral arytenoid lateralisation in the treatment of laryngeal paralysis in 100 dogs (1992–2000). *Australian Veterinary Journal* 81, 464–468.

Stanley, B.J., Hauptman, J.G., Fritz, M.C., Rosenstein, D.S. and Kinns, J. (2010) Esophageal dysfunction in dogs with idiopathic laryngeal paralysis: a controlled cohort study. *Veterinary Surgery* 39, 139–149.

Sun, F., Uson, J., Ezquerra, J., Crisostomo, V., Luis, L. and Maynar, M. (2008) Endotracheal stenting therapy in dogs with tracheal collapse. *Veterinary Journal* 175, 186–193.

Sura, P.A. and Krahwinkel, D.J. (2008) Self-expanding nitinol stents for the treatment of tracheal collapse in dogs: 12 cases (2001–2004). *Journal of the American Veterinary Medical Association* 232, 228–236.

Taylor, S.S., Harvey, A.M., Barr, F.J., Moore, A.H. and Day, M.J. (2009) Laryngeal disease in cats: a retrospective study of 35 cases. *Journal of Feline Medicine and Surgery* 11, 954–962.

Thieman, K.M., Krahwinkel, D.J., Sims, M.H. and Shelton, G.D. (2010) Histopathological confirmation of polyneuropathy in 11 dogs with laryngeal paralysis. *Journal of the American Animal Hospital Association* 46, 161–167.

Torrez, C.V. and Hunt, G.B. (2006) Results of surgical correction of abnormalities associated with brachycephalic airway obstruction syndrome in dogs in Australia. *Journal of Small Animal Practice* 47, 150–154.

Trostel, C.T. and Frankel, D.J. (2010) Punch resection alaplasty technique in dogs and cats with stenotic nares: 14 cases. *Journal of the American Animal Hospital Association* 46, 5–11.

Venker-Van Haagen, A.J., Hartman, W. and Goedegebuure, S.A. (1978) Spontaneous laryngeal paralysis in young Bouviers. *Journal of the American Animal Hospital Association* 14, 714–720.

Weinstein, J. and Weisman, D. (2010) Intraoperative evaluation of the larynx following unilateral arytenoid lateralization for acquired idiopathic laryngeal paralysis in dogs. *Journal of the American Animal Hospital Association* 46, 241–248.

White, R.A.S. (1989) Unilateral arytenoid lateralisation: an assessment of technique and long term results in 62 dogs with laryngeal paralysis. *Journal of Small Animal Practice* 30, 543–549.

White, R.N. (1995) Unilateral arytenoid lateralisation and extraluminal polypropylene ring prostheses for correction of tracheal collapse in the dog. *Journal of Small Animal Practice* 36, 151–158.

21 Upper Digestive Tract Surgery

glossectomy: removal of a portion of tongue
mandibulectomy: removal of a segment of mandible
maxillectomy: removal of a segment of maxilla
mediastinitis: inflammation/infection of the mediastinum
oronasal fistula: hole between the oral and nasal cavities
pyothorax: infection of the pleural cavity
ranula: synonym for submucosal sialocoele
sialocoele/mucocoele: collection of saliva under the skin or oral mucosa
sialolith: stone that forms in the saliva

The reader should be able to:

- classify the different forms of oronasal fistula in the dog
- identify animals with oronasal fistula that are suitable for surgical repair in general practice and those that are not
- define the terms mandibulectomy and maxillectomy
- derive a differential diagnosis list for a dog with a history of fluctuant cervical swelling and formulate and implement an investigation plan to reach a diagnosis
- list the therapeutic options for submandibular sialocoele and instruct an owner so that they can make an informed choice
- formulate a management plan for a dog that has just impaled itself on a stick that it was carrying in its mouth

Oronasal Fistula

An oronasal fistula is a direct communication between the oral and nasal cavities through the hard palate or dental arcade. Food and fluid can pass through the fistula into the nasal cavity during eating, leading to rhinitis. From here, food may move back into the nasopharynx and be inhaled, leading to aspiration pneumonia. A small fistula may cause only mild signs but large fistulas, particularly if they are positioned caudally, are debilitating and lead to malnourishment, severe rhinitis, and life-threatening pneumonia.

Aetiology

Oronasal fistulas may be congenital or acquired. Acquired fistulas occur secondary to trauma, dental disease, or oral cancer.

Congenital oronasal fistula

Congenital oronasal fistulas usually affect the midline region of the hard and soft palates and are often referred to simply as cleft palate (Fig. 21.1). There appears to be a recessive mode of inheritance and affected individuals are often euthanized at birth.

Traumatic cleft palates

Facial trauma often causes splitting of the palatine bones along the midline symphysis. This generates a traumatic midline cleft palate affecting both the hard and soft palates (Fig. 21.2). Gross instability is appreciable between the left and right maxillas and the split extends through the centre of the upper incisor arcade.

Dental disease

Periodontal disease leading to erosion around the upper tooth roots can lead to direct communication between the tooth root socket and the nasal cavity. Trauma during tooth extraction, particularly of the upper canine tooth, can cause iatrogenic oronasal fistula (Fig. 21.3A).

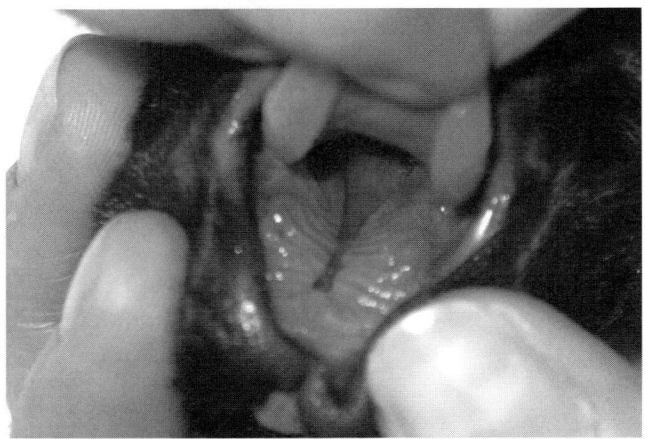

Fig. 21.1. Congenital oronasal fistula in a pug.

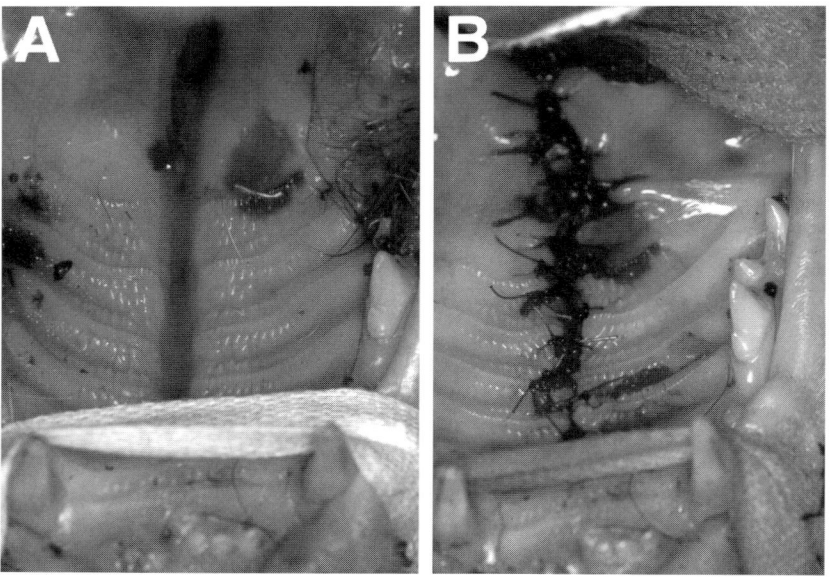

Fig. 21.2. Traumatic oronasal fistula: (A) midline defect in the hard and soft palates; (B) following closure of the soft tissue defects – the unstable maxilla was stabilized with cerclage wires anchored around the incisors and carnassial teeth.

Oral cancer

Oronasal fistulas can also develop secondary to erosive cancers affecting the hard palate and dental arcade. These fistulas are difficult to distinguish from fistulas associated with dental disease (Fig. 21.3B).

Clinical signs

All newborn puppies and kittens should be checked for congenital cleft palates at birth. If the fistula is not identified at birth, the animal may present because of failure to thrive and nasal regurgitation of food within the first few weeks of life.

Acquired oronasal fistulas produce varying signs depending on their location and size. Small fistulas at the front of the oral cavity may only cause signs of mild rhinitis (nasal discharge; sneezing). Large fistulas may lead to severe rhinitis or signs of aspiration pneumonia (soft, productive cough; pyrexia; dyspnoea). If large volumes of food move into the nasal cavity during eating, this can lead to food aversion and reduced food intake, causing malnutrition.

Large fistulas and midline fistulas are easily identified on gross inspection of the oral cavity. Small fistulas, particularly associated with tooth root cavities, can be difficult to identify without probing the area to identify a direct communication with the nasal cavity.

Management

Animals with acute, traumatic cleft palates are good candidates for surgery (see below) and are often treated successfully in general practice. The other forms of oronasal fistula are much more difficult to manage and should be referred to specialist centres or specialist veterinary dental surgeons. Surgery to repair chronic oronasal fistulas has high failure rates because the tissues are unhealthy and infected, and because there are usually bone defects under the fistulae that leave little support for the tissues to heal. The edge of the lesion should be biopsied before attempting repair, to identify if there is an underlying neoplastic process. Animals with congenital fistulas are usually euthanized at birth because the condition is debilitating and difficult to treat, often requiring multiple surgeries.

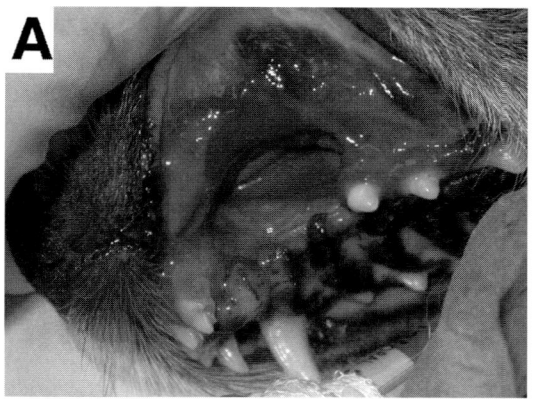

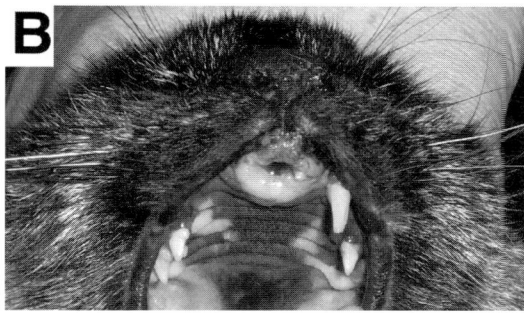

Fig. 21.3. (A) Acquired oronasal fistula at the site of canine tooth extraction; (B) acquired oronasal fistula at the site of oral squamous cell carcinoma in a cat.

Acute traumatic cleft palate repair

Traumatic cleft palates should be repaired before the nasomaxillary bones fuse, preferably within the first 2 or 3 days of trauma. If the palatine bones heal without being reduced, a bone defect is left under the cleft. This leaves a gap in the bony support under the suture line that increases the risk of dehiscence. There are two elements to acute traumatic cleft palate repair: (i) repair of the soft tissue; and (ii) reduction with stabilization of the fractured hard palate.

Sharply debride the edges of the soft tissue defects to remove devitalized tissue. Start at the caudal extent of the soft palate defect. Suture the soft palate defect closed in three layers. Incorporate the nasopharyngeal mucosa in the first layer, the palatine muscles in the second layer, and the oral mucosa in the third layer. In cats, it may only be possible to close the soft palate in two layers due to the thinness of the tissues. It is important that the palatine muscles are incorporated into one of these layers, as contraction of the muscles leads to dehiscence if they are not anchored to each other on midline. The mucoperiosteum of the hard palate is sutured in a single layer. Use a periosteal elevator to elevate it from the palatine bone along the edge of the defect if necessary, to reduce tension along the suture line. Use simple interrupted or continuous suture patterns of short-acting, absorbable suture material (3-0 or 4-0) for all layers. Multifilament materials such as polyglactin 910 produce soft suture ears that cause less intra-oral irritation than monofilament materials (Fig. 21.2).

After suturing the soft tissue defect closed, stabilize the two halves of the hard palate by placing cerclage wire around both upper canines and both upper carnassial teeth. Feed a soft diet for the first 3 weeks following surgery and do not allow the patient to play with hard toys. Remove the wires after 3 weeks, by which time the palatine bones should have healed.

Oral Cancer

Oral cancers are common in both dogs and cats. A range of different treatment protocols has been described but complete surgical excision remains one of the key elements to successful treatment. The surgical management of oral cancer is challenging and requires aggressive surgery that is generally performed at referral centres.

Presentation and clinical signs

Oral cancers cause dysphagia, drooling, oral bleeding, halitosis, oral pain, or disfigurement. Most tumours form proliferative lesions but some present as erosive plaques. Tumours affecting the dental arcades often lead to tooth loss and erosive tumours of the upper jaw may form oronasal fistulas (Fig. 21.3).

Investigation

Oral cancer should be staged before treatment is considered (see Chapter 9). Collect an incisional biopsy of the mass to assess the type and grade of tumour. Oral tumours are typically heterogeneous and the biopsy must include deep tissue and a border with normal mucosa to ensure that it is representative. Fine-needle aspiration of the submandibular lymph nodes and thoracic radiography should be performed to screen for metastatic spread.

Part of the initial investigation of the tumour includes evaluation of its local extent, as this is a key indicator of the type and value of surgery. Radiography provides information about the bone involvement but CT and MRI provide far more information about the soft tissue and bone changes, and are the preferred imaging modalities.

Treatment

Mandibulectomy (removal of a portion of the lower jaw) and maxillectomy (removal of a portion of the upper jaw) are performed to manage oral tumours affecting the bony parts of the jaw (Fig. 21.4). Occasionally, partial glossectomy is performed to manage lingual tumours.

Mandibulectomy is generally well tolerated. Large portions of the lower jaw can be removed while maintaining reasonable function, and patients

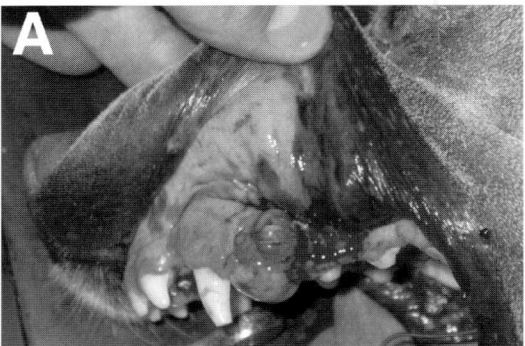

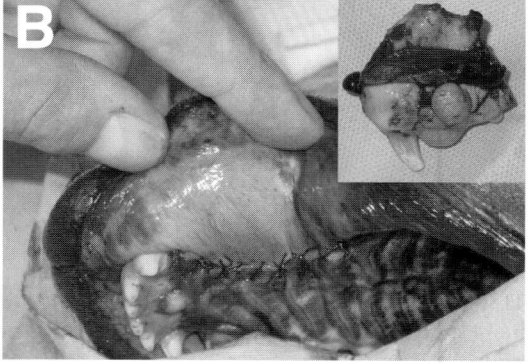

Fig. 21.4. Maxillectomy: (A) acanthomatous ameloblastoma forms a proliferative mass next to the canine; (B) the mass was removed with a margin of healthy tissue and the resultant oronasal fistula was repaired with a mucosal flap.

usually recover quickly. However, as the amount of tissue removed increases, jaw function is increasingly compromised. Common complications include drooling, tongue lolling, and messy eating although animals generally can still eat well and have a good quality of life. Wound dehiscence and infection may occur but are easily managed. Tumour recurrence is the most serious complication. Some experienced practitioners perform these surgeries but inexperienced surgeons should not attempt them.

Maxillectomy is also generally well tolerated but there is more risk of major complications developing. Intra-operative problems include profuse bleeding, difficulty reconstructing the oronasal defect created, and difficulty preserving the orbit and eye. Wound dehiscence is more difficult to manage as it may lead to the development of an oronasal fistula. However, the biggest complication following maxillectomy remains tumour regrowth. Tumour recurrence is more likely in comparison to mandibulectomy, probably because it is more difficult to achieve a wide margin of resection. Maxillectomy is a challenging surgery and cases are generally referred to specialist centres.

Owner satisfaction is high for both procedures.

Tumour types

The histopathological type of tumour has a strong influence on the prognosis and outcome.

Acanthomatous ameloblastomas

Acanthomatous ameloblastoma is a collective term used to describe odontogenic tumours (i.e. tumours of tooth origin). The classification of these tumours is complex and the terminology distinguishing between the various forms is confused. 'Epulis' (plural: epulides) has been used to describe these tumours but currently 'acanthomatous ameloblastoma' is the preferred terminology. These tumours share the same biological features in that they invade locally but do not metastasize. The acanthomatous ameloblastoma is the commonest form of oral cancer in dogs. Typically, these tumours form wide-based masses along the dental arcade causing displacement and loss of teeth and erosion of bone. Complete excision with a margin of normal tissue and bone is curative. Affected animals are good candidates for surgery.

Squamous cell carcinoma

Squamous cell carcinoma (SCC) is the second commonest form of malignant oral cancer in dogs and the commonest form of oral cancer in cats. The tumours may be proliferative or erosive, and erosive forms may develop oronasal fistulas (see above). SCCs on the mandible or maxilla have low metastatic rates but are locally invasive. In dogs, complete surgical excision of gingival tumours is curative in 90% of cases, and dogs are good candidates for surgery. Cats that undergo surgical removal of gingival SCCs have a guarded prognosis and one-year survival following mandibulectomy is reported to be 43%. This is because local recurrence is very common, probably due to the highly invasive nature of the primary tumour and limited capacity to achieve wide surgical margins in the feline oral cavity.

In both species, SCCs affecting non-gingival sites (tonsils and tongue) are more aggressive and have a poor prognosis. They are difficult to excise completely and often metastasize.

Malignant melanoma

Malignant melanomas are the commonest form of malignant oral cancer in dogs. These tumours are invasive and frequently metastasize. The prognosis is poor, even with surgical resection, as animals are likely to succumb to tumour regrowth or metastatic disease. With mandibulectomy alone, the median survival time is 10 months, and one-year survival is reported to be 21%.

Fibrosarcoma

Fibrosarcoma affects both dogs and cats. In the dog, the maxilla is a predisposed site. Fibrosarcomas have a low metastatic rate but often recur following excision because of their highly invasive nature. The prognosis is guarded due to the high rate of local recurrence within the first year following surgery.

Other tumours

A range of other tumours may affect the oral cavity. Oral mast cell tumours are quite common and tend to be high grade and malignant. Osteosarcoma is occasionally found affecting the mandible or maxilla and has a high metastatic rate. Other tumours occur sporadically.

Focal fibrous hyperplasia

Focal fibrous hyperplasia (also referred to as fibromatous or fibrous epulis) is a common condition in dogs (boxers may be predisposed). Focal fibrous hyperplasia results from chronic gingival hyperplasia and often forms pedunculated gingival masses along the gingival margin. It does not cause bone destruction and can be managed by addressing underlying dental disease (including tooth extraction) and trimming excessive gingival mucosa. As this lesion is often referred to as an epulis, there can be some confusion between this and the acanthomatous ameloblastomas.

Emerging therapies

A wide range of therapies has been evaluated for managing oral tumours including radical surgery, radiotherapy, cryosurgery, photodynamic surgery, and chemotherapy. New treatment protocols are emerging and combination therapies may improve outcomes in affected individuals. Consult a veterinary oncologist for current treatment recommendations.

Sialocoele

A sialocoele (mucocoele; ranula) is a subcutaneous or submucosal accumulation of saliva that forms following leakage of saliva from a salivary gland or duct.

Aetiopathogenesis

Dogs have four pairs of salivary glands that drain into the oral cavity through large ducts: the parotid, mandibular, sublingual, and zygomatic glands. Cats have a fifth pair of glands at the commissure of the lip, known as the molar glands. In addition, there is salivary tissue distributed widely throughout the oral mucosa and this empties directly into the oral cavity. Leakage of saliva can occur from any of the salivary glands or their ducts, but most sialocoeles form following leakage from the sublingual duct. Saliva accumulates initially at the point of leakage leading to sublingual mucosal swelling (submucosal sialocoele or 'ranula'), or subcutaneously leading to submandibular swelling. Over time, the pocket of saliva may migrate to a more dependent position. Most cases are classified as idiopathic, but trauma, foreign body, sialoliths, and salivary gland inflammation have all been identified as possible causes. The sialocoele itself is comparatively benign but may cause dysphagia or pharyngeal obstruction because of its size and location.

Presentation and clinical signs

Animals with sialocoeles may present because owners have noticed large swellings in the submandibular region or under the tongue, or because the patient is showing signs of dysphagia (Fig. 21.5). Rarely, submucosal sialocoeles form in the pharynx and cause pharyngeal and respiratory obstruction that can lead to signs of dyspnoea.

On physical exam, there may be a subcutaneous, fluctuant, non-painful swelling in the submandibular region. As the sialocoele sinks to a dependent position over time, the swelling migrates to the ventral neck. Alternatively, a fluid, fluctuant swelling may be seen pushing up from under the tongue. Animals with submucosal sialocoeles may have dysphagia, drooling, and blood tinged saliva

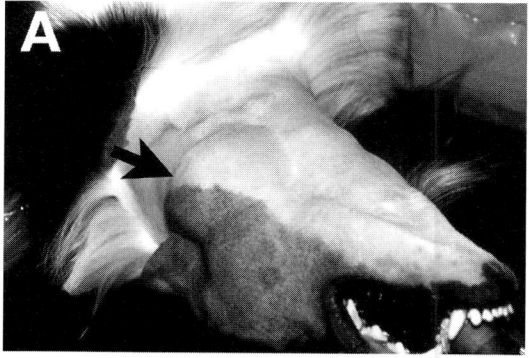

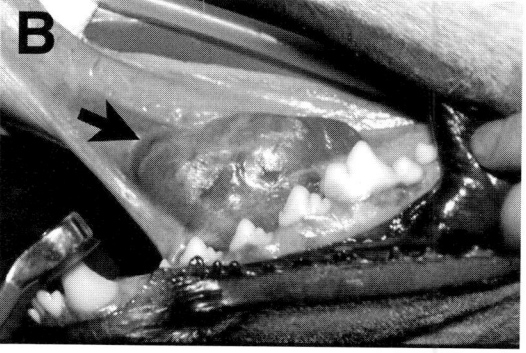

Fig. 21.5. Sialocoele: (A) submandibular; (B) submucosal ('ranula'). (Images courtesy of E. Welsh.)

because the sialocoele physically obstructs prehension and the mucosa over the sialocoele becomes traumatized. Some patients have both subcutaneous and submucosal sialocoeles.

Confirming the diagnosis

Differential diagnoses for cervical sialocoele include cervical abscess (see below), haematoma, and neoplasia. To confirm the diagnosis of sialocoele, an aspirate of fluid from the mass is collected. Sialocoeles contain saliva that has a distinctive honey-coloured appearance and is viscous.

Contrast radiographic studies (sialograms) produced by injecting contrast up the salivary gland ducts can demonstrate leakage directly from the affected tissue and are useful for planning surgery (Fig. 21.6). These studies are technically difficult to perform as salivary duct catheterization, particularly of the sublingual duct, is challenging.

Treatment

Sialocoeles are unlikely to resolve spontaneously. Management involves drainage of the sialocoele and removal of the salivary tissue (sialoadenectomy) that is contributing to saliva leakage. Excision of the mandibular and monostomatic sublingual salivary glands together is the commonest form of sialoadenectomy performed in dogs and cats. This is because most sialocoeles are caused by leakage from the sublingual duct and it is easier to resect both salivary glands together rather than to try to isolate the sublingual gland. This surgery is relatively straightforward and is often performed by experienced practitioners. Zygomatic and parotid sialoadenectomies are more challenging and less common. Cases are generally referred for treatment. Sialoadenectomy should not be performed by inexperienced clinicians without the assistance of an experienced colleague.

Complications and outcome

Recurrence occurs in less than 5% of cases and is probably the result of incomplete sialoadenectomy or removal of the wrong glands. Seroma may develop at the surgery site but other complications are rare. The prognosis for submandibular, cervical, and sublingual sialocoeles is good following sialoadenectomy.

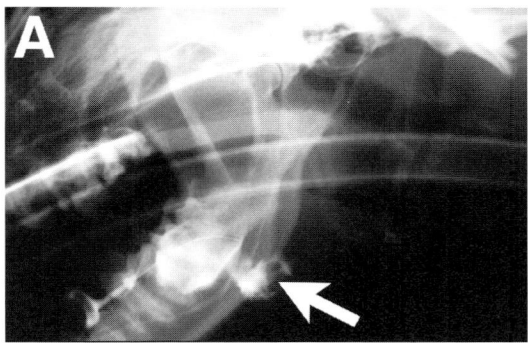

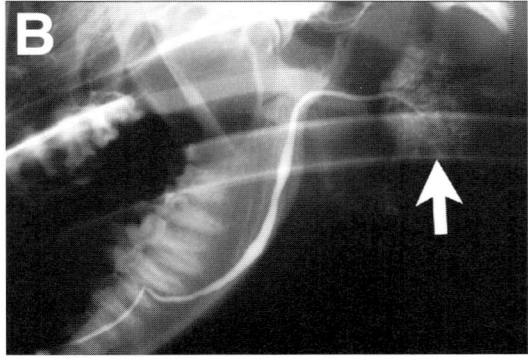

Fig. 21.6. Sialograms: (A) sublingual sialogram – contrast leaks from the duct into the ranula identifying this as the source of the sialocoele; (B) mandibular sialogram – contrast flows up to the gland and delineates the acinar structure (normal).

Oesophageal Foreign Body

Oesophageal foreign bodies are common. Most can be retrieved endoscopically but some require surgical removal.

Pathophysiology

The oesophagus is constricted by the structures surrounding it at the thoracic inlet, the heart base, and the diaphragm. Large objects that are swallowed (e.g. bones) may become lodged at these points leading to partial or complete oesophageal obstruction. The commonest point of obstruction is between the heart base and diaphragm but foreign bodies may get stuck anywhere along the length of the oesophagus. Smaller, sharp objects such as fishhooks may also lodge in the oesophageal wall. The oesophageal wall undergoes pressure necrosis over the foreign body leading to ulceration and, ultimately, perforation. Perforation causes life-threatening cellulitis, mediastinitis, pyothorax, pneumothorax, or pneumomediastinum. Aspiration pneumonia may develop due to regurgitation and inhalation of food.

Presentation and clinical signs

Dogs are more commonly affected than cats, reflecting their increased tendency to scavenge. Terrier breeds are over-represented. The main clinical signs are of passive regurgitation of undigested food, drooling of saliva, inappetence, and halitosis. Signs of dyspnoea, pneumonia, and sepsis may also develop.

Investigation

Cases of suspected oesophageal foreign body require emergency investigation and treatment before severe oesophageal injury develops.

The diagnosis can be confirmed radiographically if the foreign body is radiodense (Fig. 21.7). Contrast agents may help delineate radiolucent foreign bodies. The entire oesophagus (from pharynx to diaphragm) should be imaged. The clavicle, which is sometimes appreciated as a small sliver of bone overlying the thoracic inlet, may be mistaken for a foreign body. Similarly, cats have mucosal ridges in the terminal oesophagus that can retain contrast and be mistaken for a foreign body following contrast studies.

Oesophagoscopy is the imaging modality of choice as it is an extremely sensitive and fast method of identifying an oesophageal foreign body.

It also has the advantage that most foreign bodies can be retrieved at the same time.

Treatment

The majority of oesophageal foreign bodies can be removed endoscopically and this is the preferred treatment option. Occasionally, foreign bodies cannot be retrieved endoscopically because of their size and shape or because fishhooks have become lodged firmly in the wall of the oesophagus. If the foreign body cannot be removed endoscopically, oesophagotomy must be performed.

Cervical oesophagotomy

Confirm the position of the foreign body using radiography or endoscopy immediately before surgery to ensure that it has not moved. Position the patient in dorsal recumbency with the neck clipped, prepped, stretched out, and secured in position. Place a pad under the neck to elevate the surgical site. Make a skin incision from caudal to the larynx to just cranial to the manubrium. Identify and separate the midline raphe between the sternohyoideus muscles, ligating branches of the vessel running between the muscle bellies as they are encountered. Place a pair of self-retaining retractors to retract the muscle bellies. Develop a plane of dissection through the loose fascia on the left side of the trachea by blunt dissection to reveal the oesophagus that sits dorsolateral to the trachea. This approach to the ventral neck is illustrated in Chapter 22, Figs 22.2–22.4.

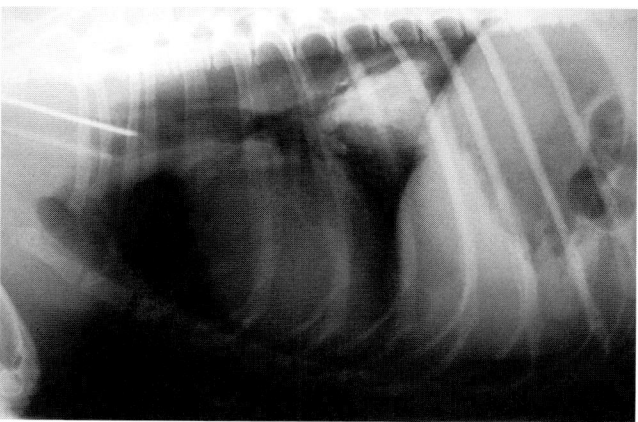

Fig. 21.7. Oesophageal foreign body (bone) in the distal oesophagus.

Once the foreign body is located through the oesophageal wall, the area around the oesophagus is packed with swabs. Stay sutures can be placed to pull the oesophageal wall away from the underlying tissues to reduce contamination. An area of wall distal or proximal to the foreign body is selected, ensuring that the recurrent laryngeal nerve and other neurovascular structures of the neck are not within the surgical field (Chapter 22, Fig. 22.1). Incise the oesophageal wall with a scalpel blade and extend the incision sharply, running longitudinally along the oesophagus. Grasp the foreign body with an Allis tissue forceps and remove it. Ensure the incision is long enough to allow foreign body retrieval without tearing the edges of the incision.

Close the oesophageal incision in two layers (mucosa and submucosa together; muscular layers together) using simple appositional suture patterns of 3-0 or 4-0 monofilament, absorbable suture material. Lavage the surgical field. Appose the sternohyoideus muscle bellies, subcutaneous fat, and skin separately.

Thoracic oesophagotomy

Thoracic oesophageal foreign bodies that cannot be retrieved endoscopically are removed by oesophagotomy following intercostal thoracotomy. The oesophagus weaves around the great vessels at the base of the heart and is intimately associated with the vagus nerves which branch over its surface. These cases are generally referred to specialist centres for management.

Fishhook oesophageal foreign body

The fishhook foreign body requires separate consideration. The hooks are often barbed and become firmly lodged in the oesophageal wall. They may also be attached to fishing line that occasionally acts as a linear foreign body and cause gastrointestinal obstruction (see Chapter 12). Despite these problems, most can still be removed endoscopically, ensuring that the hook is first manipulated to pull the barb out of the wall before it is pulled out of the oesophagus. If fishhooks are retrieved surgically, a standard approach to the oesophagus is made but, when the hook is identified, the barb is cut off using a pair of wire cutters and a small incision is made in the oesophagus to retrieve the remainder of the hook (Fig. 21.8).

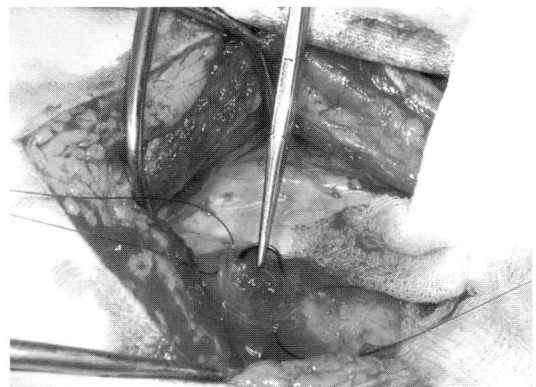

Fig. 21.8. Cervical oesophagostomy to retrieve a fishhook: the barb of the fishhook is located penetrating the oesophageal wall. A small incision in the oesophageal wall was all that was required to retrieve this foreign body. Stay sutures have been placed in the oesophageal wall to enable it to be tented up when it is incised, to limit spillage of its contents.

Post-operative management

Mucosal protectants (e.g. sucralfate) and antacids are prescribed to manage oesophagitis. If there is severe oesophageal ulceration, a gastrostomy tube may be placed for ten days, during which time no food or water is given orally.

Prognosis

The prognosis following prompt oesophageal foreign body removal is good with survival rates of over 90% reported. Outcomes following thoracic oesophagotomy for retrieval of foreign bodies are more variable but the majority of patients do well. Oesophageal stricture may develop following severe oesophageal ulceration, which can be debilitating and difficult to manage.

Oropharyngeal Penetrating Injuries

Penetrating oropharyngeal injuries (stick injuries) are common in dogs. Large, retriever breeds are over-represented but small dogs and cats can also be affected. Impalement on sticks is the commonest cause but injuries with fishhooks, grass awns, sewing needles, and bones have all been reported.

Pathophysiology

Penetrating oropharyngeal injuries result most commonly from impalement injuries through the mouth onto sticks that are being carried or retrieved. The stick may penetrate under the tongue, into the caudal recess of the angle of the jaw, or through the palate or tonsillar crypt. It may also penetrate more caudally into the dorsal pharyngeal wall near the larynx or even entering the oesophagus through the ostium and penetrating the oesophageal wall into the cervical soft tissues.

The immediate effects of the injury are to cause lacerations to the mucosa and bleeding. Bacteria and debris from the surface of the stick are inoculated into the oropharyngeal soft tissues, and fragments of stick detach and are left in the tissues. In the first few days after the injury, bacterial infection develops and air leaks into the soft tissues through the laceration in the wall of the oropharynx. Together these lead to cellulitis and emphysema that spreads into the cervical tissues and sometimes even onto the thoracic wall. In the most severely affected patients, cellulitis may track along tissue planes through the thoracic inlet into the mediastinum. Here, mediastinal infection quickly becomes established and leads to septic shock and dyspnoea. Finally, mediastinitis spreads into the pleural cavities causing pyothorax and pneumothorax that compound dyspnoea and sepsis.

Many patients that survive the original injury develop chronic abscesses or discharging sinus tracts around the pharynx, neck, and retrobulbar space. The abscesses are centred around foreign material left in the tissues, but the inflammatory capsule encroaches on neighbouring structures including the oesophagus, trachea, and neurovascular bundles.

Presentation and clinical signs

Less than 20% of patients present immediately following the injury. Often the trauma has been witnessed or the owner has had to physically remove the stick from the mouth of their dog because it has become lodged. However, in other cases, the impalement is not witnessed and patients are presented because their owners have noticed bloody saliva, pain on opening the mouth, subcutaneous emphysema around the neck, or report that the dog is reluctant to eat. A small number of patients (~6%) present with signs of septic shock, dyspnoea, and severe malaise associated with overwhelming infection or mediastinitis.

Over 80% of cases present weeks or months after the initial injury because of the development of cervical swellings or discharging sinus tracts. The original stick injury may never have been witnessed.

Occasionally, the stick penetrates dorsally behind the last molar and up into the retrobulbar space leading to signs of a retrobulbar mass including epiphora, ocular displacement, and pain on opening the jaw (due to temporomandibular impairment).

Investigation

The investigation of suspected oropharyngeal penetrating injury differs depending on whether the patient presents shortly after the injury or later when a cervical abscess develops. Animals with suspected acute oropharyngeal injury should be investigated immediately, as early intervention is associated with a better prognosis than delayed intervention.

Acute presentation

The goals of investigation are to confirm the diagnosis and assess the extent of the injury. Head, neck, and thoracic radiography are valuable diagnostic tools. Pieces of stick embedded in the oropharyngeal and cervical soft tissues are rarely identified radiographically, but radiographs give an indication of the extent and severity of cellulitis and emphysema. Radiographs may demonstrate displacement of the trachea or larynx, or distortion of the pharynx or cervical tissues due to swelling. Air tracking between tissue planes has a characteristic appearance and is easily distinguished from air in the oesophageal and tracheal lumens. When air is seen within the cervical soft tissues, this indicates that the pharyngeal or oesophageal wall is likely to be lacerated and should prompt further evaluation and surgery (having excluded other differential diagnoses such as tracheal rupture). Air may be seen tracking down beside the trachea and oesophagus into the mediastinum, which indicates that mediastinitis is likely to develop. Similarly, pneumothorax or pleural effusion may be present (Fig. 21.9).

All cases should be anaesthetized for evaluation of the pharynx and oral cavity for evidence of trauma. Oesophagoscopy is performed to assess for oesophageal perforation. Tracts that are found

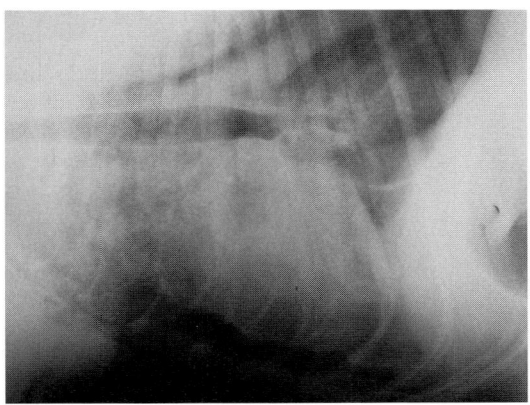

Fig. 21.9. Acute presentation with extension into the thorax: this radiograph demonstrates pneumomediastinum (with delineation of the aorta and other vessels in the dorsal thorax), pneumothorax, and mediastinitis (with loss of definition of the mediastinal structures including the heart). This patient had shock and died shortly after this radiograph was taken, within 6 h of the original injury (caused by carrying a stick).

should be probed and opened (see below) to evaluate their extent and to remove foreign material.

Chronic presentation

By the time that a cervical abscess develops, signs of the original oropharyngeal injury are likely to have disappeared and endoscopy may be of little value. The focuses of investigation are on confirming the diagnosis by distinguishing cervical abscess from sialocoele, evaluating the extent of the abscess and how it interacts with surrounding structures, and searching for foreign material.

Cytology of fluid collected by needle aspiration of the abscess is sufficient to distinguish cervical abscess from sialocoele and neoplasia. Fluid collected should be submitted for bacterial culture and sensitivity testing. The presence of a cervical abscess in a large-breed dog without a history of other injury to the neck or evidence of para-aural abscessation (see Chapter 19) is highly suggestive of the diagnosis.

Radiography provides limited information but cervical ultrasound enables the extent of the lesion to be assessed and may identify foreign material within the abscess cavity. CT or MRI provides most information about the extent and interaction of the abscess with other tissues and on the location of foreign material.

Treatment

Treatment of shallow penetrating injuries confined to the oral cavity is simple. More extensive acute injuries and cervical abscesses require extensive neck surgery to explore the tracts of tissue that have been compromised and to remove foreign material or abscesses that have formed. Although the majority of cases occur following stick injuries, foreign bodies are only identified in around 50% of cases. However, often the fragments of stick are only a few millimetres across, and the success of surgery is not affected by the failure to identify foreign material providing that all tracts have been explored or resected.

Surgery is classed as contaminated or dirty. Broad-spectrum antibiotics should be given perioperatively and continued as therapeutic courses.

Acute presentation

The basic principle of management of acute presentations of oropharyngeal penetrating injuries is to probe, open, and debride or lavage each tract to remove contaminants and foreign material. Penetrating injuries in the oral cavity can be managed from an intra-oral approach providing that there is no evidence of penetration extending into the cervical soft tissues. In preoperative imaging this is identified by cases that have no cervical emphysema or swelling. Each laceration is probed and incised to give access to the base of the tract. Debride and lavage the lining of the tract (e.g. using a spoon curette). The tracts are generally left open to heal by second intention healing (see Fig. 21.10).

Deeper penetrating injuries extending into the cervical soft tissues should be managed by a combination of probing from an intra-oral approach and exploration through a ventral midline neck approach. Although this surgery is similar to other approaches to the ventral neck such as thyroidectomy, local tissues are inflamed and may be disrupted by swelling and cellulitis, clear lines of dissection may be obscured, and dissection may necessitate deep dissection dorsal to the larynx avoiding the neurovascular structures in the area. These cases are best referred to an experienced colleague or specialist centre for management (Fig. 21.10).

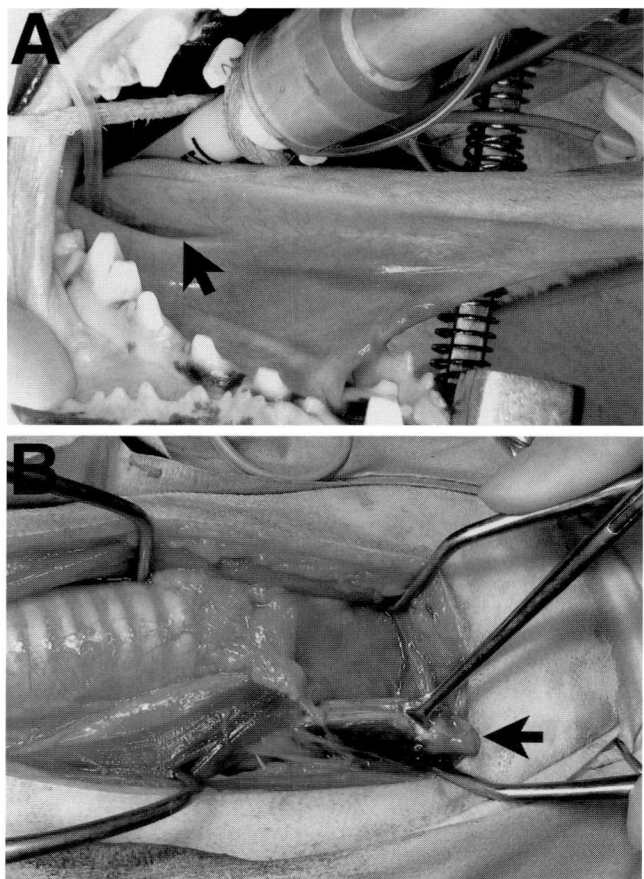

Fig. 21.10. Acute presentation: (A) laceration (arrow) and tract at base of tongue (a suction catheter has been placed in the tract); (B) ventral midline neck exploratory surgery in the same dog – a 6 cm stick (arrow) was removed from next to the oesophagus.

Chronic presentation

Animals presenting with cervical abscesses should be referred to an experienced colleague or specialist centre for management as dissection is difficult and iatrogenic injury to the carotid artery, recurrent laryngeal nerve, vagosympathetic trunk, oesophageal wall, or trachea can all lead to life-threatening complications intra-operatively or post-operatively. Recurrence of the abscess is common because of failure to remove all contaminated or infected tissues. The basic principles of surgery are to excise the abscess in its entirety while preserving the normal tissues in the area or, failing that, to excise most of the abscess and debride the lining of each fistulous tract (Fig. 21.11).

Aftercare

Feed patients soft food for 10 days after surgery and monitor them for signs of wound infection. Avoid using a collar and lead over this period.

Prognosis

Animals with acute presentations that have not developed mediastinitis and that undergo immediate surgery have a good prognosis. The prognosis for animals with cervical abscesses is guarded; recurrence rates of up to 40% have been reported following debridement or excision of the abscess. Animals with mediastinitis have a poor prognosis although some survive following aggressive therapy.

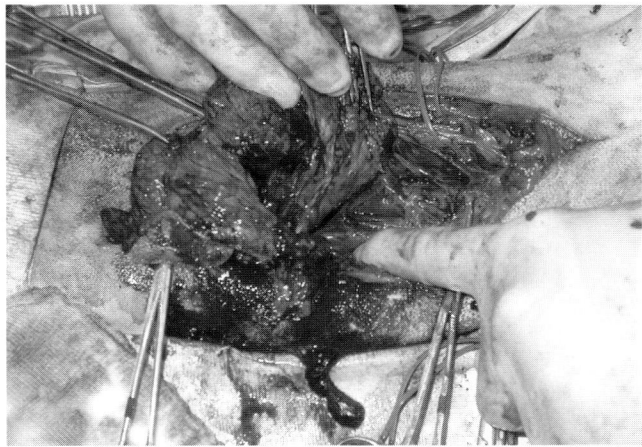

Fig. 21.11. Cervical abscess resection: this dog has a 4 cm piece of stick embedded in the abscess which is being excised. The normal tissue planes are disrupted by the extensive inflammation and scarring and the surgeon is pointing to the carotid artery, which is running through the abscess.

Bibliography

Bergman, P.J. (2007) Canine oral melanoma. *Clinical Techniques in Small Animal Practice* 22, 55–60.

Bright, S.R., Mellanby, R.J. and Williams, J.M. (2002) Oropharyngeal stick injury in a Bengal cat. *Journal of Feline Medicine and Surgery* 4, 153–155.

Dhaliwal, R.S., Kitchell, B.E. and Marretta, S.M. (1998) Oral tumors in dogs and cats. Part 1. Diagnosis and clinical signs. *Compendium of Continuing Education for the Practicing Veterinarian* 20, 1011–1022.

Doran, I.P., Wright, C.A. and Moore, A.H. (2008) Acute oropharyngeal and esophageal stick injury in forty-one dogs. *Veterinary Surgery* 37, 781–785.

Feinman, J.M. (1990) Pharyngeal mucocele and respiratory distress in a cat. *Journal of the American Veterinary Medical Association* 197, 1179–1180.

Fox, L.E., Geoghegan, S.L., Davis, L.H., Hartzel, J.S., Kubilis, P. and Gruber, L.A. (1997) Owner satisfaction with partial mandibulectomy or maxillectomy for treatment of oral tumors in 27 dogs. *Journal of the American Animal Hospital Association* 33, 25–31.

Gianella, P., Pfammatter, N.S. and Burgener, I.A. (2009) Oesophageal and gastric endoscopic foreign body removal: complications and follow-up of 102 dogs. *Journal of Small Animal Practice* 50, 649–654.

Glazer, A. and Walters, P. (2008) Esophagitis and esophageal strictures. *Compendium of Continuing Education for the Practicing Veterinarian* 30, 281–292.

Griffiths, L.G., Tiruneh, R., Sullivan, M. and Reid, S.W. (2000) Oropharyngeal penetrating injuries in 50 dogs: a retrospective study. *Veterinary Surgery* 29, 383–388.

Hamilton, M. (2006) Oral neoplasia part 1: diagnosis and staging. *UK Vet* 11, 37–46.

Harvey, C.E. (1987) Palate defects in dogs and cats. *Compendium of Continuing Education for the Practicing Veterinarian* 9, 404–418.

Harvey, H.J. (1981) Pharyngeal mucoceles in dogs. *Journal of the American Veterinary Medical Association* 178, 1282–1283.

Houlton, J.E.F., Herrtage, M.E., Taylor, P.M. and Watkins, S.B. (1985) Thoracic oesophageal foreign bodies in the dog: a review of ninety cases. *Journal of Small Animal Practice* 26, 521–536.

Jeffreys, D.A., Stasiw, A. and Dennis, R. (1996) Parotid sialolithiasis in a dog. *Journal of Small Animal Practice* 37, 296–297.

Kosovsky, J.K., Matthiesen, D.T., Marretta, S.M. and Patnaik, A.K. (1991) Results of partial mandibulectomy for the treatment of oral tumors in 142 dogs. *Veterinary Surgery* 20, 397–401.

Michels, G.M., Jones, B.D., Huss, B.T. and Wagner-Mann, C. (1995) Endoscopic and surgical retrieval of fishhooks from the stomach and esophagus in dogs and cats: 75 cases (1977–1993). *Journal of the American Veterinary Medical Association* 207, 1194–1197.

Moore, A.H. (2001) Removal of oesophageal foreign bodies in dogs: use of the fluoroscopic method and outcome. *Journal of Small Animal Practice* 42, 227–230.

Nicholson, I., Halfacree, Z., Whatmough, C., Mantis, P. and Baines, S. (2008) Computed tomography as an aid to management of chronic oropharyngeal stick injury in the dog. *Journal of Small Animal Practice* 49, 451–457.

Niemiec, B.A. (2008) Oral pathology. *Topics in Companion Animal Medicine* 23, 59–71.

Northrup, N.C., Selting, K.A., Rassnick, K.M., Kristal, O., O'Brien, M.G., Dank, G., Dhaliwal, R.S., *et al.* (2006) Outcomes of cats with oral tumors treated with mandibulectomy: 42 cases. *Journal of the American Animal Hospital Association* 42, 350–360.

Ritter, M.J., Von Pfeil, D.J., Stanley, B.J., Hauptman, J.G. and Walshaw, R. (2006) Mandibular and sublingual sialocoeles in the dog: a retrospective evaluation of 41 cases, using the ventral approach for treatment. *New Zealand Veterinary Journal* 54, 333–337.

Sale, C.S. and Williams, J.M. (2006) Results of transthoracic esophagotomy retrieval of esophageal foreign body obstructions in dogs: 14 cases (2000–2004). *Journal of the American Animal Hospital Association* 42, 450–456.

Schmidt, G.M. and Betts, C.W. (1978) Zygomatic salivary mucoceles in the dog. *Journal of the American Veterinary Medical Association* 172, 940–942.

Smith, M.M. (2000) Oronasal fistula repair. *Clinical Techniques in Small Animal Practice* 15, 243–250.

Verstraete, F.J., Ligthelm, A.J. and Weber, A. (1992) The histological nature of epulides in dogs. *Journal of Comparative Pathology* 106, 169–182.

Wallace, J., Matthiesen, D.T. and Patnaik, A.K. (1992) Hemimaxillectomy for the treatment of oral tumors in 69 dogs. *Veterinary Surgery* 21, 337–341.

Webb, J.L., Burns, R.E., Brown, H.M., Leroy, B.E. and Kosarek, C.E. (2009) Squamous cell carcinoma. *Compendium of Continuing Education for the Practicing Veterinarian* 31, 133–142.

White, R.A. and Gorman, N.T. (1989) Wide local excision of acanthomatous epulides in the dog. *Veterinary Surgery* 18, 12–14.

White, R.A.S. and Lane, J.G. (1988) Pharyngeal stick penetration injuries in the dog. *Journal of Small Animal Practice* 29, 13–35.

22 Endocrine Surgery

> **adrenalectomy:** removal of an adrenal gland
> **goitre:** enlargement of the thyroid gland
> **hypophysectomy:** removal of the pituitary gland
> **parathyroidectomy:** removal of a parathyroid gland
> **partial pancreatectomy:** removal of a portion of the pancreas
> **thyroidectomy:** removal of the thyroid gland (unilateral = one lobe; bilateral = both lobes)

The reader should be able to:

- define the terms adrenalectomy, parathyroidectomy, hypophysectomy, and partial pancreatectomy, and provide examples of specific and precise endocrine disorders where these procedures might be indicated
- define the term 'modified extracapsular thyroidectomy'
- describe the surgical approach to the thyroid glands and how to locate them in the cat
- list the key organs, nerves, and vessels that need be considered during thyroidectomy, and identify them intra-operatively
- describe the key elements of performing a modified extracapsular thyroidectomy
- formulate a plan for identifying and treating common complications of thyroidectomy in the cat
- compare the different treatment options for feline hyperthyroidism and instruct a pet owner in making an informed decision as to which to select

Thyroid Gland

Thyroidectomy is performed regularly in general practice to manage feline hyperthyroidism. Thyroidectomy is also occasionally performed to manage canine thyroid carcinoma but, in contrast to feline hyperthyroidism, these tumours are locally invasive and difficult to remove so affected animals should be referred to specialist practices.

Feline hyperthyroidism

Feline hyperthyroidism is the commonest endocrine disease of cats and is a major cause of disease and debility in older animals.

Aetiopathogenesis

Feline hyperthyroidism is caused by excess production of thyroid hormone, either from diseased thyroid glands or from ectopic thyroid tissue. Most cases are caused by benign adenomatous hyperplasia of one or both thyroid glands (the disease is bilateral in over 70% of cases). Malignant thyroid carcinoma is far less common, accounting for less than 2% of cases. Excess thyroid hormone leads to an increased metabolic rate associated with increased appetite, weight loss, and general debility. Secondary changes include hypertrophic cardiomyopathy and hypertension. Liver enzymes are often elevated although the exact mechanism for this is unknown.

Presenting signs

Feline hyperthyroidism is a disease that predominantly affects ageing cats. The average age at diagnosis is 13 years and any sex or breed may be affected. Most cats have signs of hypermetabolism including polyphagia, polyuria, polydipsia, tachycardia, hyperactivity, loss of body condition, weight loss, poor coat quality, behavioural changes (including aggression), and vomiting. However, occasionally hyperthyroid cats will have atypical presentations with signs including lethargy and anorexia.

Palpable thyroid enlargement (goitre) is found in most cats and is considered to be characteristic of the disease. When goitre cannot be palpated, it may be because the thyroid gland has sunk ventrally towards the thoracic inlet or because ectopic thyroid tissue within the thoracic cavity is diseased.

Most cats have elevated liver enzymes although this is usually associated with only mild liver pathology. Signs of hypertrophic cardiomyopathy are common and include tachycardia, murmurs and gallop rhythms. Occasionally, heart failure develops with pleural effusion and dyspnoea. Systemic hypertension is quite uncommon affecting less than 25% of cases but may lead to retinal haemorrhage and kidney damage.

Investigation and diagnosis

The presence of a palpable goitre in an aged cat with signs of hypermetabolism is highly suggestive of feline hyperthyroidism. Demonstration of elevated serum thyroxine levels is required to confirm the diagnosis and provides a useful benchmark to monitor response to treatment. Occasionally, cats with early hyperthyroidism will not have elevated thyroxine levels and repeated testing in 2–3 months may be required. Additional investigations include biochemical screening for concurrent renal and liver disease, blood pressure assessment, and cardiac evaluation.

Management

The mainstay of treatment of feline hyperthyroidism is reduction in thyroxine levels. Reducing thyroid hormone levels ultimately will stabilize and reverse many of the secondary effects of feline hyperthyroidism. However, severely affected cats may require specific therapy to control hypertension and hypertrophic cardiomyopathy before specific treatment of hyperthyroidism can be initiated (see below).

There are three approaches to reducing thyroid hormone levels; medical therapy, radioactive iodine therapy, and thyroidectomy. It is difficult to compare the costs of treatment directly but ultimately there may be little difference in the total cost of treatment between the three therapies for the 'average' patient.

1. Long-term medical management: carbimazole and methimazole block thyroid hormone production. These drugs avoid the risks of general anaesthesia and surgery but necessitate regular, life-long oral medication that may not be tolerated by the patient and involves ongoing costs. Side effects include gastrointestinal upset, facial excoriation, myelosuppression, and hepatoxicity. Although long-term drug therapy is not suitable for all patients, most cats receive at least a short course of medical management to control signs and stabilize cardiac and renal function prior to implementing other therapies.

2. Thyroidectomy: thyroidectomy is usually highly effective at curing feline hyperthyroidism. Bilateral thyroidectomy is recommended over unilateral surgery as between 70% and 94% of cats have bilateral disease. The main risk of surgery is the development of post-operative hypoparathyroidism. This can lead to life-threatening hypocalcaemia, although it is usually transient.

3. Radioactive iodine therapy: the radioisotope ^{131}I preferentially accumulates in thyroid tissue, where it destroys hyperfunctioning tissue. The therapy is highly effective and has the advantages that it is effective against all diseased thyroid tissue, including ectopic thyroid tissue, and that parathyroid function is preserved. The main disadvantages are the limited availability of facilities that are licensed to perform this treatment, and the reluctance of some owners to have radioisotopes injected into their pets.

Managing hypertrophic cardiomyopathy or hypertension

Some patients require therapy to stabilize cardiac function before anaesthesia and surgery can be performed. If the patient tolerates oral methimazole therapy, a 2–4-week course preoperatively may be sufficient. Alternatively, propanolol (0.5 mg/kg q8–12h orally for 3–5 days before surgery) may reduce the risks in animals with tachycardia and arrhythmias. Propanolol should be used with caution in animals with concurrent congestive heart failure. Amlodipine with or without angiotensin converting enzyme (ACE) inhibitor drugs (e.g. benazapril) may be prescribed in patients with systemic hypertension.

Anatomy

The paired thyroid glands lie on either side of the trachea embedded within the fascia between the trachea and the adjacent muscles (sternothyroideus and sternohyoideus muscles). The glands are usually located between the second and fifth tracheal cartilages but they can be mobile and the position may change with neck position or under the influence of gravity. The thyroid glands are flat, red/brown and elongated. They are enclosed within a distinct, well-vascularized capsule.

Each gland is intimately associated with the cranial (external) and caudal (internal) parathyroid glands. The cranial parathyroid gland is superficially positioned and can be seen on the surface of the thyroid capsule, typically at the cranial pole of the thyroid gland. However, the position of the cranial parathyroid gland is extremely variable and it may be located more centrally on the dorsal surface of the gland. The cranial parathyroid gland is a pale, flat disc usually less than 4 mm in diameter. It has a distinct blood supply arising from the cranial thyroid artery (see below) but it can be difficult to distinguish the gland from fat. The caudal (internal) parathyroid gland is embedded within the thyroid tissue. It cannot be seen externally and is typically located in the caudal half of the thyroid gland.

The thyroid gland receives a robust blood supply from the cranial thyroid artery, itself a branch of the common carotid artery, which runs onto the capsule from dorsolaterally at the cranial pole of the gland. Immediately before penetrating the thyroid capsule, the thyroid artery branches and supplies distinct smaller branches to the cranial parathyroid gland (this is a key anatomic landmark during thyroidectomy) (Fig. 22.1).

On the right, the carotid sheath (containing the vagosympathetic trunk, common carotid artery, and internal jugular vein) runs immediately laterally to the thyroid gland. The recurrent laryngeal nerve runs dorsolaterally to, and closely associated with, the gland. Medially, the gland is bordered by the trachea. On the left, the gland is bordered medially by the trachea and separated from the carotid sheath by the oesophagus. The left recurrent laryngeal nerve runs in the region of the ventral surface oesophagus between the carotid sheath and trachea. It passes close to the dorsal surface of the thyroid gland.

Ectopic thyroid tissue may be located anywhere along the trachea from the larynx to the heart base and accounts for disease in 12% of cats with hyperthyroidism.

Modified extracapsular thyroidectomy

This technique involves removing all of the thyroid tissue while preserving the cranial parathyroid gland. It has the advantages over other techniques of reducing the risk of local regrowth of diseased thyroid tissue and of making preservation of the cranial parathyroid gland easier. This technique is

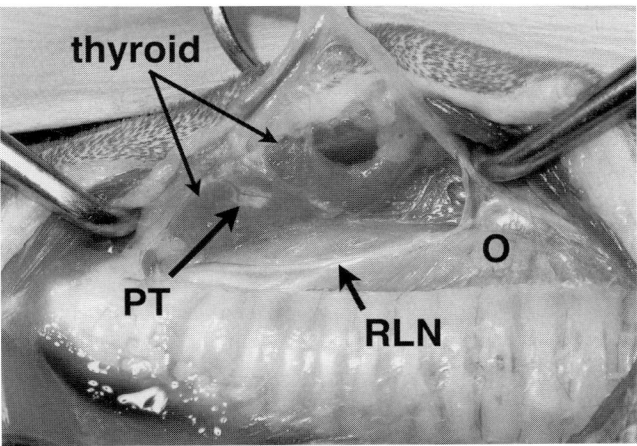

Fig. 22.1. Relationship of thyroid gland to other structures (head to left): PT – parathyroid gland with distinct blood supply; RLN – recurrent laryngeal nerve running over oesophagus; O – oesophagus.

greatly facilitated by the use of bipolar diathermy, self-retaining retractors (e.g. Gelpi retractors), and fine, sharp dissecting scissors (e.g. iris scissors).

Positioning

It is important to position the patient as straight as possible when performing ventral neck surgery, to preserve the anatomic landmarks. Position the patient in dorsal recumbency with the forelimbs tied back and the neck stretched. Place a pad under the neck to stabilize and lift it a little. Position pads on either side of the neck to help maintain position. Tape the muzzle to the table to increase stability (Fig. 22.2).

Approach

Incise the skin and subcutaneous fat from the larynx towards the manubrium to expose the sternohyoideus muscles and, caudally, the sterno-cephalicus muscles. The sternocephalicus muscles are the most superficial muscles and converge from laterally towards midline in the caudal extent of the incision. In the cat, the left and right muscle fibres merge and the division between the two muscle bellies may be indistinct. Separate these muscles on midline and place self-retaining retractors to help maintain exposure. The sternohyoideus muscles run on ventral midline from the manubrium to the hyoid. They are the most superficial layer of muscle in the proximal two-thirds of the neck but are covered by the more superficial sternocephalicus muscles caudally. Identify the septum between these two muscle bellies and bluntly separate them. To identify the septum, gently push the muscles apart to reveal the thin fascia of the septum and the distinctive unpaired blood vessel (the caudal thyroid vein) running parallel between the two muscle bellies. Separate the two muscle bellies, ligating branches of the vessel as required, and reposition the self-retaining retractors. This exposes the trachea (Fig 22.3). Bluntly dissect using gentle digital pressure along either side of the trachea. The thyroid glands can be identified associated with the muscle immediately lateral to the trachea as long red/brown glands between the caudal end of the larynx and the eighth tracheal ring (Fig 22.4).

Isolate the parathyroid

Identify the external (cranial) parathyroid gland. This is a pale, flat disc up to 4 mm in diameter that sits somewhere between the cranial pole of the thyroid gland and the mid body. It has a distinct blood supply branching from the cranial thyroid artery that helps to identify it. Using bipolar diathermy, cauterize the thyroid capsule 2 mm from the edge of the parathyroid gland and encircling it (Fig. 22.5). Use fine, sharp dissecting scissors (e.g. iris scissors) to incise the cauterized capsule and elevate the parathyroid gland from the thyroid tissue, ensuring that the blood supply to the parathyroid gland is preserved.

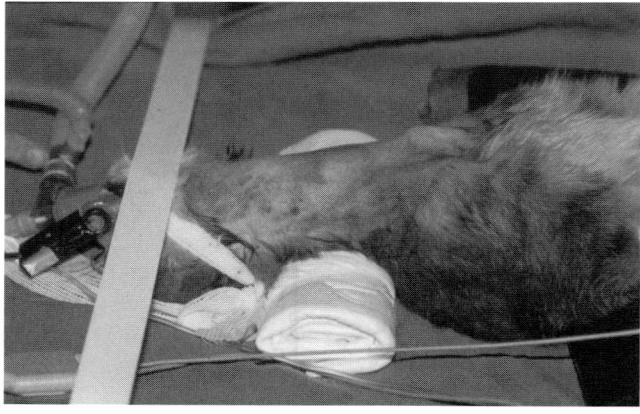

Fig. 22.2. Positioning for thyroidectomy.

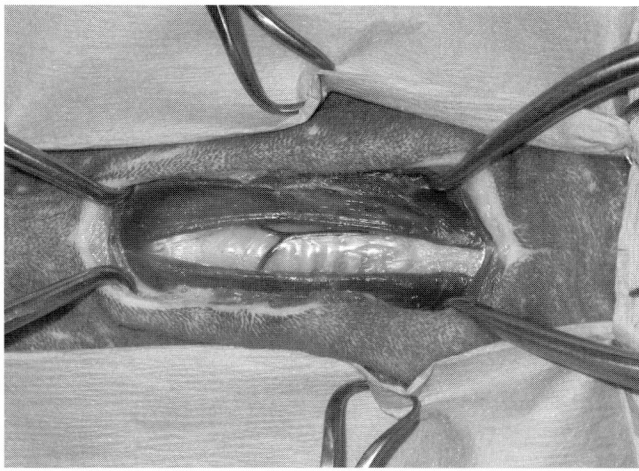

Chapter 22

Fig. 22.3. Separate the bellies of the sternohyoideus muscle.

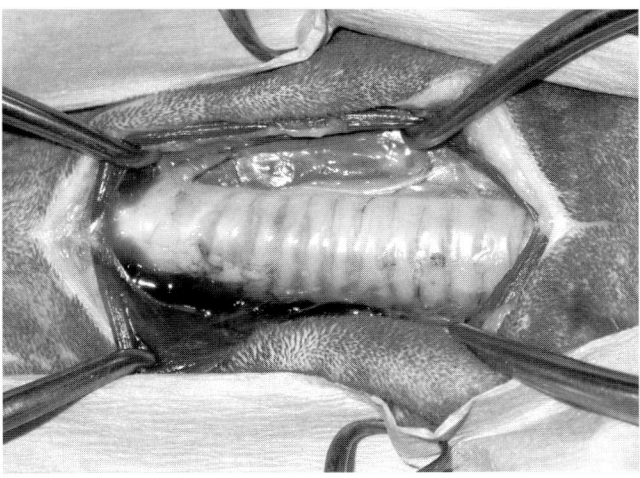

Fig. 22.4. Identify the thyroid glands lying beside the trachea distal to the larynx.

Remove the thyroid gland

Once the parathyroid gland is isolated, remove the thyroid gland by dissecting it from the surrounding fascia and ligating the vessels that enter it. Before starting the dissection, identify the recurrent laryngeal nerve that runs between the trachea and the gland, and ensure that it is preserved. This may require gentle dissection of the nerve away from the thyroid capsule using Halsted mosquito forceps. Ensure that the cranial thyroid vessels are ligated after they have branched to supply the parathyroid gland.

Closure

Appose the sternohyoideus muscle bellies and the sternothyroideus muscle bellies using 3-0 monofilament, absorbable suture material. Close subcutaneous fat and skin routinely.

Salvaging the parathyroid gland

If the blood supply to the parathyroid gland is inadvertently severed or the gland is accidentally removed, the parathyroid gland may be salvaged

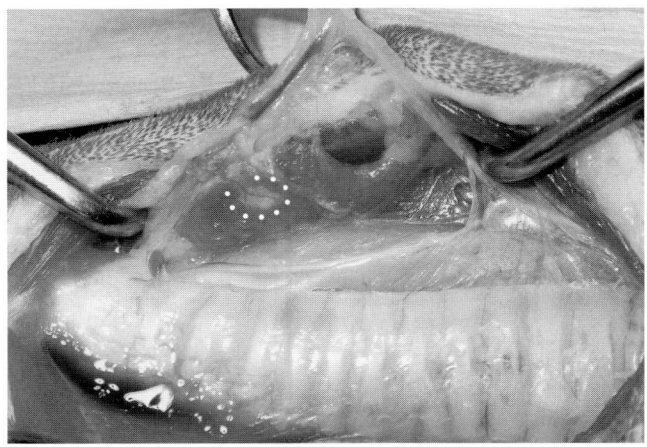

Fig. 22.5. Landmarks for isolating the parathyroid gland (dotted line indicates incision in thyroid capsule to elevate the parathyroid gland while preserving its blood supply).

by making a small incision in the belly of one of the sternohyoideus muscles (to create a small pocket) and inserting the parathyroid gland into this pocket. The gland may revascularize.

Post-operative monitoring

Hypoparathyroidism and hypococalcaemia develop 24–72 h after thyroidectomy in up to 23% of cats although the percentage showing signs is lower. Clinical signs range from mild irritability and inappetence to severe signs that may include facial twitching, muscle tremors, seizure, and collapse. Monitor patients for the first 72 h after surgery and assess serum calcium levels daily. If possible, measure ionized calcium in preference to total serum calcium as it provides a more accurate measure of hypocalcaemia.

Animals with severe signs of hypocalcaemia require intravenous calcium supplementation. Initially, 1 ml of 10% calcium gluconate solution is administered by slow intravenous injection over a minimum of 10 min (discontinue if bradycardia develops). This is followed by an infusion of calcium gluconate (10 ml of 10% calcium gluconate in 250 ml of 0.9% NaCl at 2.5 ml/kg/h for 8–12 h). Oral supplementation is started once the patient has stabilized.

Animals with mild signs can be treated with oral supplementation of calcium and a vitamin D analogue (200 mg/kg calcium gluconate three times daily plus dihydrotachysterol solution administered

at 0.03 mg/kg/day for 3 days and then reduced to 0.01–0.02 mg/kg/day). Oral medications are tapered as serum calcium concentrations increase, and, if possible, the patient is gradually weaned off medication over a 3–6 week period.

Complications

Hypocalcaemia is the most common and serious complication following feline thyroidectomy (see above). Hyperthyroidism recurs in ~5% of patients following bilateral thyroidectomy because of incomplete resection of the diseased gland or because ectopic thyroid tissue is diseased. Iatrogenic injury to the recurrent laryngeal nerve can also cause laryngeal paralysis and associated stridor and dyspnoea, although this is uncommon (see Chapter 20).

Parathyroid Gland

Parathyroidectomy (removal of the parathyroid gland) is indicated to manage primary hyperparathyroidism. This disease is caused by parathyroid hyperplasia, parathyroid adenoma or, rarely, parathyroid carcinoma. Uncontrolled production of parathyroid hormone (PTH) causes hypercalcaemia and a range of associated but vague clinical signs (calcium oxalate urolithiasis, polyuria/polydipsia, vomiting, constipation, seizure, muscle tremor, listlessness, and renal failure). The commonest clinical signs are associated with urolithiasis or with polyuria/polydipsia but many cases are diagnosed following the incidental finding of hypercalcaemia during the evaluation of unrelated conditions.

The major differential diagnoses for hypercalcaemia associated with primary hyperparathyroidism are secondary renal hyperparathyroidism, nutritional hyperparathyroidism, and pseudohyperparathyroidism. Pseudohyperparathyroidism is a paraneoplastic syndrome caused by the production of PTH-related proteins (PTHrp) from tumours. It is the commonest cause of hypercalcaemia in dogs and cats. Tumours associated with this syndrome include lymphoma, apocrine adenocarcinoma of the anal sac, and SCC of the head and neck.

Measuring levels of PTH, PTHrp, phosphate, and ionized calcium helps to distinguish pseudohyperparathyroidism from other forms. Primary hyperparathyroidism is diagnosed when high serum calcium levels are associated with an inappropriate PTH level (i.e. within or above the reference range) because other causes of hypercalcaemia are likely to lead to suppression of PTH production and low serum PTH concentration. In addition, primary hyperparathyroidism is usually associated with low or normal phosphate and low PTHrp levels. In contrast, pseudohyperparathyroidism leads to hypercalcaemia associated with low PTH and high PTHrp levels.

The prognosis following parathyroidectomy for primary hyperparathyroidism is good, with less than 10% of cases having ongoing hypercalcaemia.

Adrenal Gland

Adrenalectomy (adrenal gland removal) is performed to remove adrenal tumours. It is a high-risk surgery that should not be undertaken by inexperienced surgeons. Adrenal biopsy is not routinely performed.

Adrenalectomy is usually considered for the management of adrenal-dependent hyperadrenocorticism (Cushing's disease), although less than 20% of dogs with hyperadrenocorticism have a functional adrenal tumour and are candidates for adrenalectomy. Benign adrenal adenoma and malignant adrenal carcinoma occur with equal frequency. The mortality rate associated with adrenalectomy is ~20% and the median survival time is 690 days. The tumour may invade into the vena cava increasing the risk of haemorrhage intra-operatively. Perioperatively, thromboembolism and hypoadrenocorticism may also occur. There is also a risk of recurrence of signs due to incomplete

excision of the tumour or the development of metastatic disease. Long-term adrenal suppression with drugs such as trilostane can be considered as an alternative to adrenalectomy. However, surgery is often recommended if there is no evidence of metastatic disease, as it has the potential to cure affected dogs.

Other indications for adrenalectomy include the management of phaeochromocytoma (catecholamine-producing adrenal tumour) and mineralocorticoid-producing adrenal tumour. Adrenal tumours occur occasionally in cats but hyperadrenocorticism is uncommon.

Pituitary Gland

Hypophysectomy (removal of the pituitary gland) is occasionally performed for the management of pituitary-dependent hyperadrenocorticism and is an effective method of treatment in experienced hands. However, the procedure leads to a range of secondary endocrine disorders and is not widely recommended because of the good response to medical management of the condition.

Pancreas

Partial pancreatectomy (removal of a portion of the pancreas) is indicated to collect biopsy samples of pancreas and to manage insulin-secreting pancreatic tumours (insulinomas). Partial pancreatectomy is performed using a suture guillotine technique similar to that described for liver biopsy (see Chapter 18). Although iatrogenic pancreatitis following biopsy is cited as a potential complication, most biopsy techniques appear relatively safe.

Insulinoma is an uncommon tumour of dogs and has rarely been reported in cats. It causes episodic collapse or seizures associated with hypoglycaemia and the diagnosis is confirmed by demonstrating high serum insulin concentrations in association with hypoglycaemia. Canine insulinomas metastasize rapidly throughout the pancreas and to the liver and lungs. The tumours may also be microscopic, making identification impossible intra-operatively. However, removal of large insulin-secreting tumours is generally recommended, as surgery facilitates medical management of hypoglycaemia and improves the quality of life of the patient, even if metastatic disease is present. The investigation and management of patients with insulinoma is complex. Surgery can be challenging because of the difficulty in locating small insulinomas and the importance of preserving the common bile duct and duodenal blood supply that run through the pancreas. Cases should be referred to specialist centres for assessment.

Bibliography

Allen, S.W., Cornelius, L.M. and Mahaffey, E.A. (1989) A comparison of two methods of partial pancreatectomy in the dog. *Veterinary Surgery* 18, 274–278.

Birchard, S.J. (2006) Thyroidectomy in the cat. *Clinical Techniques in Small Animal Practice* 21, 29–33.

Broome, M.R. (2006) Thyroid scintigraphy in hyperthyroidism. *Clinical Techniques in Small Animal Practice* 21, 10–16.

Brown, C.G. and Graves, T.K. (2007) Hyperadrenocorticism: treating dogs. *Compendium of Continuing Education for the Practicing Veterinarian* 29, 132–134, 136, 138 passim; quiz 144–135.

Chiaramonte, D. and Greco, D.S. (2007) Feline adrenal disorders. *Clinical Techniques in Small Animal Practice* 22, 26–31.

Feldman, E.C., Hoar, B., Pollard, R. and Nelson, R.W. (2005) Pretreatment clinical and laboratory findings in dogs with primary hyperparathyroidism: 210 cases (1987–2004). *Journal of the American Veterinary Medical Association* 227, 756–761.

Flanders, J.A. (1999) Surgical options for the treatment of hyperthyroidism in the cat. *Journal of Feline Medicine and Surgery* 1, 127–134.

Foster, D.J. and Thoday, K.L. (2000) Tissue sources of serum alkaline phosphatase in 34 hyperthyroid cats: a qualitative and quantitative study. *Research in Veterinary Science* 68, 89–94.

Hanson, J.M., van't Hoofd, H.M., Voorhout, G., Teske, E., Kooistra, H.S. and Meij, B.P. (2005) Efficacy of transsphenoidal hypophysectomy in treatment of dogs with pituitary-dependent hyperadrenocorticism. *Journal of Veterinary Internal Medicine* 19, 687–694.

Harvey, A.M., Hibbert, A., Barrett, E.L., Day, M.J., Quiggin, A.V., Brannan, R.M. and Caney, S.M. (2009) Scintigraphic findings in 120 hyperthyroid cats. *Journal of Feline Medicine and Surgery* 11, 96–106.

Hermanson, J.W. and Evans, H.E. (1993) The muscular system. In: Evans, H.E. (ed.) *Miller's Anatomy of the Dog*, 3rd edn. W.B. Saunders, Philadelphia, Pennsylvania, pp. 258–384.

Hoenig, M. (2002) Feline hyperadrenocorticism – where are we now? *Journal of Feline Medicine and Surgery* 4, 171–174.

Hullinger, R.L. (1993) The endocrine system. In: Evans, H.E. (ed.) *Miller's Anatomy of the Dog*, 3rd edn. W.B. Saunders, Philadelphia, Pennsylvania, pp. 559–585.

Jepson, R.E. (2011) Feline systemic hypertension: classification and pathogenesis. *Journal of Feline Medicine and Surgery* 13, 25–34.

Liu, S.K., Peterson, M.E. and Fox, P.R. (1984) Hypertropic cardiomyopathy and hyperthyroidism in the cat. *Journal of the American Veterinary Medical Association* 185, 52–57.

Messinger, J.S., Windham, W.R. and Ward, C.R. (2009) Ionized hypercalcemia in dogs: a retrospective study of 109 cases (1998–2003). *Journal of Veterinary Internal Medicine* 23, 514–519.

Mooney, C.T. (2002) Pathogenesis of feline hyperthyroidism. *Journal of Feline Medicine and Surgery* 4, 167–169.

Naan, E.C., Kirpensteijn, J., Kooistra, H.S. and Peeters, M.E. (2006) Results of thyroidectomy in 101 cats with hyperthyroidism. *Veterinary Surgery* 35, 287–293.

Padgett, S. (2002) Feline thyroid surgery. *Veterinary Clinics of North America Small Animal Practice* 32, 851–859, vi.

Padgett, S.L., Tobias, K.M., Leathers, C.W. and Wardrop, K.J. (1998) Efficacy of parathyroid gland autotransplantation in maintaining serum calcium concentrations after bilateral thyroparathyroidectomy in cats. *Journal of the American Animal Hospital Association* 34, 219–224.

Peterson, M.E. (2006a) Diagnostic tests for hyperthyroidism in cats. *Clinical Techniques in Small Animal Practice* 21, 2–9.

Peterson, M.E. (2006b) Radioiodine treatment of hyperthyroidism. *Clinical Techniques in Small Animal Practice* 21, 34–39.

Radlinsky, M.G. (2007) Thyroid surgery in dogs and cats. *Veterinary Clinics of North America: Small Animal Practice* 37, 789–798, viii.

Reine, N.J. (2007) Medical management of pituitary-dependent hyperadrenocorticism: mitotane versus trilostane. *Clinical Techniques in Small Animal Practice* 22, 18–25.

Savary, K.C., Price, G.S. and Vaden, S.L. (2000) Hypercalcemia in cats: a retrospective study of 71 cases (1991–1997). *Journal of Veterinary Internal Medicine* 14, 184–189.

Schaefer, C. and Goldstein, R.E. (2009) Canine primary hyperparathyroidism. *Compendium of Continuing Education for the Practicing Veterinarian* 31, 382–390.

Schwartz, P., Kovak, J.R., Koprowski, A., Ludwig, L.L., Monette, S. and Bergman, P.J. (2008) Evaluation of prognostic factors in the surgical treatment of adrenal gland tumors in dogs: 41 cases (1999–2005). *Journal of the American Veterinary Medical Association* 232, 77–84.

Shiel, R.E. and Mooney, C.T. (2007) Testing for hyperthyroidism in cats. *Veterinary Clinics of North America Small Animal Practice* 37, 671–691, vi.

Stepien, R.L. (2011) Feline systemic hypertension: diagnosis and management. *Journal of Feline Medicine and Surgery* 13, 35–43.

Thoday, K.L. and Mooney, C.T. (1992) Historical, clinical and laboratory features of 126 hyperthyroid cats. *Veterinary Record* 131, 257–264.

Trepanier, L.A. (2006) Medical management of hyperthyroidism. *Clinical Techniques in Small Animal Practice* 21, 22–28

Welches, C.D., Scavelli, T.D., Matthiesen, D.T. and Peterson, M.E. (1989) Occurrence of problems after three techniques of bilateral thyroidectomy in cats. *Veterinary Surgery* 18, 392–396.

23 Management of Pleural Disease

chylothorax: chylous pleural effusion
pneumothorax: accumulation of air in the pleural cavity
pyothorax: purulent pleural effusion
thoracocentesis: needle drainage of the pleural cavity
thoracostomy tube: drain in the pleural cavity

The reader should be able to:

- list the different forms of pleural effusion and indicate how they might be differentiated from each other
- compare the possible aetiopathogenesis of pyothorax in the cat and dog and formulate a treatment plan for the medical management of pyothorax in the cat
- classify the different forms of pneumothorax and illustrate how these different classifications may influence the formulation of a treatment plan
- instruct assistants and perform needle thoracocentesis to remove air from the pleural cavity of a dog with pneumothorax
- identify clinical features that might prompt early referral for surgical assessment of pyothorax in the dog and pneumothorax in the dog or cat
- list treatment options for management of idiopathic chylothorax in the dog

Management of Pneumothorax

Pneumothorax is the accumulation of air in the pleural cavity. It can be classified based on its pathophysiology or on its aetiology. Both classifications are useful as they can be used to plan therapy and to predict the outcome to treatment.

Pathophysiological classification

Closed pneumothorax

Closed pneumothorax is the commonest form of pneumothorax. Air enters the pleural cavity from leakage of organs within the chest. Usually, this is from damaged lung tissue, but it may also develop from tracheal rupture or from oesophageal perforation. Air moves through the defect into the pleural cavity during inspiration and some air escapes through the same defect on expiration. Collapse of lung and reduced ventilatory capacity lead to dyspnoea, but dogs and cats can tolerate moderate volumes of air in their chests while maintaining tissue oxygenation.

Closed tension pneumothorax

Tension pneumothorax is a severe variant of closed pneumothorax that produces rapidly worsening respiratory compromise and life-threatening dyspnoea. Tension pneumothorax develops when the leaking area of lung is covered by a valve-like flap of tissue that prevents any air from escaping from the pleural cavity during exhalation. The lesion forms a one-way valve and the pleural cavity rapidly fills with air. Patients with tension pneumothorax are profoundly dyspnoeic and require rapid, often continuous, drainage to prevent death. Tension pneumothorax can be distinguished from other forms of pneumothorax radiographically (see below).

Open pneumothorax

Open pneumothorax is uncommon and often fatal. Air enters the thorax through a penetrating thoracic wall injury (Fig. 23.1). The pleural and atmospheric pressures equalize quickly making inspiratory effort ineffective at ventilating the lung. Patients are unlikely to survive open pneumothorax unless the injury in the thoracic wall leads to only intermittent leakage of air into the chest.

Aetiological classification

Traumatic pneumothorax

Trauma is the commonest cause of pneumothorax. Pneumothorax is usually caused by injury to the lung or the bronchial tree during blunt thoracic trauma. The sudden increase in intrathoracic pressure causes rupture of the inflated lung. Alternatively, a fractured rib may puncture a lung. Often there are concurrent thoracic injuries (e.g. fractured ribs;

pulmonary contusions; diaphragmatic rupture) that also contribute to dyspnoea.

Spontaneous pneumothorax

Spontaneous pneumothorax usually occurs following spontaneous rupture of diseased lung tissue. Most cases result from rupture of air-filled cavities known as bullae and blebs within the lung (Fig. 23.2). The bulla or bleb communicates directly with the alveoli or bronchioles and is covered by a thin lining of epithelium. When this ruptures, air is able to leak from the airway through the bulla or bleb, and into the pleural cavity. Bullae and blebs are generally considered to be primary lung lesions but their exact aetiologies are uncertain. Spontaneous pneumothorax may also develop secondary to destructive lung lesions (e.g. severe pneumonia; neoplasia) or, occasionally, oesophageal perforation.

Clinical signs

Animals with pneumothorax are dyspnoeic and typically have shallow, fast respiratory patterns. They may adopt an orthopnoeic stance (neck extended, elbows abducted) to maximize air intake. On auscultation, lung sounds are reduced or absent over the affected side of the thorax and the heart may sound muffled. On percussion, the chest is hyper-resonant.

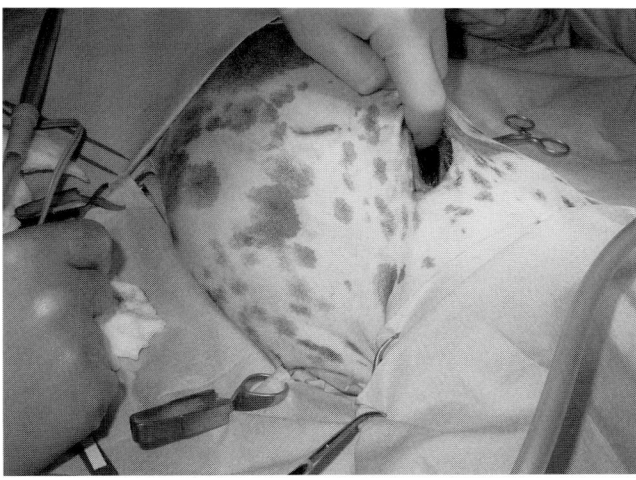

Fig. 23.1. Open pneumothorax: oblique tunnel from axilla to pleural cavity caused by impalement on a stick during exercise (patient in dorsal recumbency, head to right). The oblique nature of this injury caused the defect to close intermittently and enabled the dog to survive until it reached the veterinary clinic.

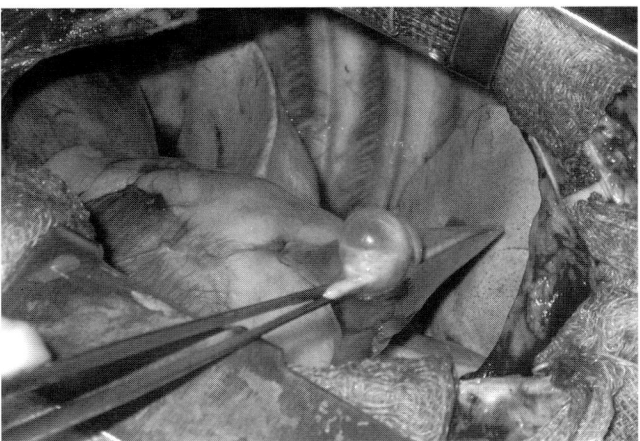

Fig. 23.2. Pulmonary bulla that ruptured and caused spontaneous pneumothorax in this dog (a median sternotomy has been performed to explore the chest).

Investigation

Pneumothorax can be confirmed radiographically although it is important not to exacerbate dyspnoea during sedation, handling, and positioning for radiography. It is often necessary to drain the pneumothorax by thoracocentesis (see below) to stabilize patients before the condition can be fully investigated. Animals tolerate being positioned in lateral or dorsoventral recumbency better than in ventrodorsal recumbency. Position the patient with the worst-affected lung lowermost, to maximize ventilation in the healthier lung.

Pneumothorax is diagnosed radiographically by demonstrating collapse of the lung and filling of the pleural cavity with air between the chest wall and the lung margin (Fig. 23.3). Other injuries such as fractured ribs, diaphragmatic rupture, and pulmonary contusion may also be identified. Tension pneumothorax is identified by the presence of these features in combination with marked flattening of the diaphragm and rounding of the thoracic cavity due to massive overinflation of the chest (Fig. 23.4).

In cases of spontaneous pneumothorax, radiography may identify cavitated lung lesions (Fig. 23.5), but it is insensitive for identifying bullae and blebs as they are often small or collapse once ruptured. In contrast, CT is sensitive for diagnosing bullae and blebs and is recommended for animals with spontaneous pneumothorax as it provides far more detail than standard thoracic radiography.

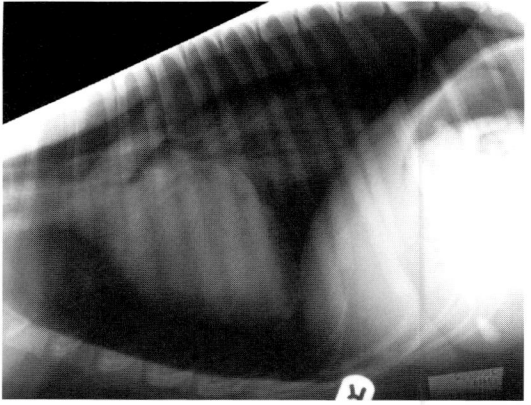

Fig. 23.3. Pneumothorax (tension) – lateral view: radiographic hallmarks of pneumothorax are a lack of vascular lung pattern extending to the edges of the thoracic cavity (being replaced with radiolucent air), collapse and dorsal displacement of the lungs, and lifting of the heart away from the sternum.

Management of pneumothorax

Most cases of traumatic pneumothorax resolve spontaneously as the lacerated lung lobe seals with fibrin within the first 72 h of injury. These cases may require repeated thoracic drainage to relieve dyspnoea over this period, but small quantities of air will resorb spontaneously over several days.

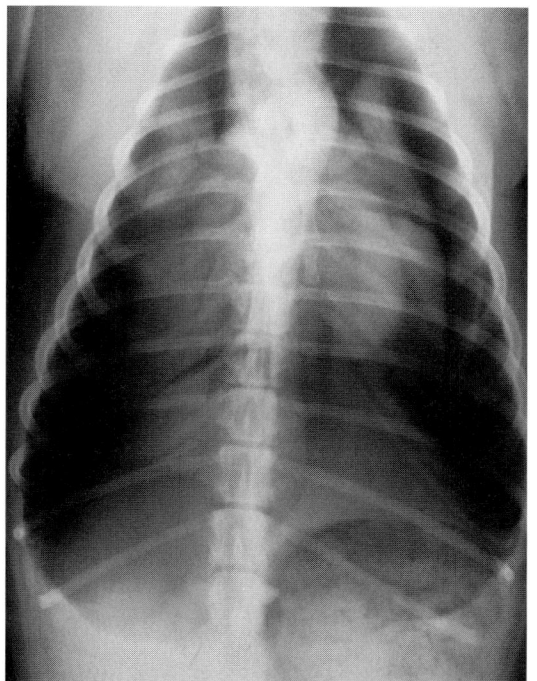

Fig. 23.4. Pneumothorax (tension) – ventrodorsal view: tension pneumothorax is identified by overinflation of the thorax, rounding of the costodiaphragmatic recess, and flattening of the diaphragm.

Supportive therapy

Animals with pneumothorax, like animals with other forms of respiratory compromise, benefit from cage rest and oxygen supplementation (see p. 206). Pain associated with thoracic trauma may limit chest movement and contribute to dyspnoea. Pain relief should be provided, but drugs must be titrated to limit secondary effects of respiratory compromise or sedation.

Thoracic drainage

Removing air from the thoracic cavity relieves dyspnoea rapidly in patients with pneumothorax. Most patients can be successfully managed by a single or repeated thoracocentesis (see below) and this is commonly performed in general practice. Rarely, animals have rapid re-accumulation of gas in the thorax, and intermittent thoracocentesis is ineffective at controlling dyspnoea. In these patients, chest drains can be placed to allow frequent or continuous drainage. Although chest tube placement is simple, it is rarely performed in general practice (see below).

Lung lobectomy

Surgery to remove damaged lung may be considered for animals with traumatic pneumothorax that do not resolve but, as intermittent thoracic drainage is successful at resolving the problem in

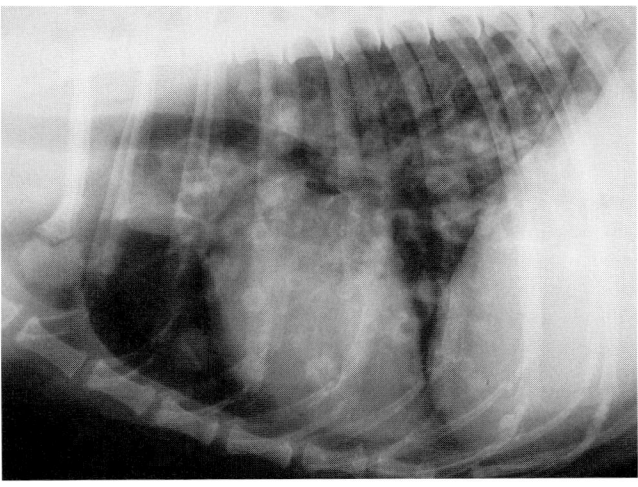

Fig. 23.5. Dog with spontaneous pneumothorax: radiographs identified diffuse, cavitated lung lesions that were subsequently confirmed to be neoplastic at post-mortem.

the majority of cases, this is rarely necessary. In contrast, surgery is usually required to resolve cases with spontaneous pneumothorax, and veterinarians should consider early referral of animals with spontaneous pneumothorax for assessment and surgery. Surgery involves exploratory median sternotomy and removal of diseased lung lobes (see Chapter 24).

Prognosis

The prognosis for traumatic pneumothorax is good. The prognosis for spontaneous pneumothorax caused by blebs or bullae is also good providing that the lesions are removed. However, the prognosis for animals with spontaneous pneumothorax caused by erosive lung lesions is generally poor, as disease tends to be widespread and unmanageable.

Pleural Effusions

Pleural effusions are commonly identified in dogs and cats, and develop for a variety of reasons. This section provides an overview of the different forms of pleural effusion and an outline of the approaches that may be used to manage the underlying condition. Cases that are considered potential candidates for surgery should be referred to a specialist centre early in the course of the investigation.

Classification

Pleural effusions may be classified on their physical characteristics.

Exudates

Inflammatory pleural effusions are common and are often associated with infectious agents. Infectious agents may enter the pleural cavity by a number of routes including through inhalation of oropharyngeal bacteria or foreign materials (e.g. grass awns), by extension from a diseased lung lobe, through haematogenous spread, or by direct thoracic wall injury. Collectively, pleural exudates are considered to be part of the syndrome of pyothorax.

Transudates and modified transudate

Modified transudate pleural effusions are common. They are produced by congested organs within the thorax (e.g. herniated liver lobe; lung lobe torsion),

thoracic neoplasia (e.g. mesothelioma), and congestive heart failure. In the cat, feline coronavirus infection leading to effusive feline infectious peritonitis (FIP) also commonly causes accumulation of modified transudates in the pleural cavity. In contrast, pure pleural transudates are uncommon but may be caused by congestive heart failure or hypoproteinaemia. When a pure transudate is identified, it is usually associated with a medical condition that will not benefit from surgery.

Chylothorax

Chylous effusions are opaque, white (or pink) effusions that develop as a result of leakage of lymph into the thorax. Chylothorax is often classified as being idiopathic but it is also associated with rupture of the thoracic duct, right-sided heart failure, thoracic neoplasia, pericardial effusion, and other thoracic pathology.

Haemothorax

Haemorrhagic pleural effusions may result from trauma or occur spontaneously in patients with bleeding disorders. Haemothorax has also been reported secondary to *Angiostrongylus vasorum* infection in a dog.

Clinical signs

Animals with pleural effusion are dyspnoeic and typically have shallow, fast respiratory patterns. They may adopt an orthopnoeic stance to maximize air intake. On auscultation, lung and heart sounds are muffled ventrally. The apex beat of the heart may be reduced. Percussion reveals a distinct line of reduced resonance separating the dorsal and ventral thorax on the affected side.

Additional findings may help establish the aetiology of pleural effusion. For example, animals with pyothorax are likely to be pyrexic and demonstrate malaise; animals with effusive FIP may have concurrent ascites; animals with congestive heart failure may have poor peripheral perfusion, weak pulses, tachycardia, peripheral oedema, distended jugular veins, and abnormalities on cardiac auscultation.

Investigation

The investigation of a patient with pleural effusion centres on accurately classifying the nature of the effusion and investigating thoracic and systemic diseases that may have contributed to its formation. Pleural fluid is collected by thoracocentesis (see below) and is analysed for its chemical composition, cytological features, and presence of infectious agents, using similar principles to those described for the investigation of ascites (see Chapter 13). Imaging of the thorax and heart is performed to identify intrathoracic pathology that may have caused the effusion. Other investigations are aimed at evaluating systemic disorders that may manifest as pleural effusion.

Treatment

Animals with pleural effusion are likely to require stabilization including thoracocentesis to relieve dyspnoea; cage rest; and oxygen. Additional therapy may include treatment of hypovolaemic or septic shock and stabilization of congestive heart failure.

Canine pyothorax

Pyothorax is common in dogs and is usually caused by bacterial infection. Bacteria enter the thorax through a variety of routes including migration of inhaled foreign bodies (e.g. grass awns), extension from a pulmonary abscess, or from haematogenous spread of bacteria. Many cases are classified as idiopathic, as the underlying cause cannot be determined despite extensive investigation. Pleural fluid from animals with pyothorax has the characteristics of a septic exudate and infectious agents may be seen. Facultative and obligate anaerobic infections are common. Often, sulfur granules (yellow, refractile particulate material floating in the fluid) are seen and are characteristic of *Actinomyces* infection. This is a particularly pathogenic organism causing severe pyothorax. Other common organisms include *Staphylococcus* spp., *E. coli*, *Nocardia* spp., and *Pasteurella* spp. Imaging studies may identify underlying lung pathology or, with advanced imaging, the presence of a foreign body within the thoracic cavity.

Canine pyothorax can be managed medically or surgically. Good candidates for medical management are animals that have no evidence of foreign body or other predisposing thoracic pathology. These animals can be treated by a combination of thoracic drainage, thoracic lavage (through chest drains), and systemic antibiotic therapy. Antibiotic selection should be based on culture or, if these results are not available, combination therapy using metronidazole and amoxicillin/clavulanic acid for a minimum of 6 weeks is commonly recommended.

Dogs that have evidence of pre-existing intrathoracic pathology or that do not respond to conservative therapy are candidates for surgery. Evidence of *Actinomyces* infection (e.g. sulfur granules in fluid) is also used as a criterion to select patients for surgery early in the course of the disease, as they may not respond well to medical therapy. Surgery involves exploration of the thorax through a median sternotomy, resection of infected pleura, extensive lavage, and management of underlying thoracic pathology or retrieval of a foreign body.

The prognosis for canine idiopathic pyothorax is reasonable, with more recent reports documenting high success rates for medically managed cases. However, death due to recurrence of signs or complications of treatment is still possible.

Feline pyothorax

Feline pyothorax shares many of the features of canine pyothorax but over 80% of cases are thought to develop through inhalation of oropharyngeal bacteria and migration of bacteria from the lower airways into the pleura. Medical management consists of pleural drainage, lavage, and systemic antibiotic therapy. As most organisms identified are facultative or obligate anaerobes, antibiotics with a broad spectrum of activity including efficacy against anaerobic organisms should be prescribed. The success rate with medical management of feline pyothorax is high. Similar criteria to those described for canine pyothorax can be used to select patients for surgery.

Effusive feline infectious peritonitis

Cats with feline coronavirus infection and effusive FIP often develop pleural effusions. The effusion has a distinctive gross appearance and is typically yellow, translucent, and very viscous. Fluid analysis demonstrates that it has a very high protein level but low nucleated cell counts (predominantly macrophages and neutrophils), classifying the fluid as a modified transudate. Animals with effusive FIP have a poor prognosis and most die or are euthanized shortly after diagnosis. Surgery has no part to play in the management of effusive FIP.

Chylothorax

Chylothorax has a characteristic appearance as it is opaque and white (or pink-tinged). It is generally classified as a modified transudate or exudate but has a high percentage of lymphocytes in comparison to other effusions. The key feature that distinguishes chylous effusion from other effusions is that its triglyceride level exceeds that in serum.

All patients with chylothorax require careful cardiac evaluation to distinguish cardiac causes from non-cardiac causes. If cardiac disease is present, treatment must be aimed at managing this. In animals without cardiac disease, idiopathic chylothorax must be differentiated from chylothorax secondary to other thoracic pathology such as neoplasia.

Idiopathic chylothorax is difficult to treat successfully. Medical and surgical therapies can be attempted. Medical management is based on feeding low-fat diets to reduce the production of chyle. The benzopyrone nutraceutical plant extract, rutin, can be prescribed as this is thought to reduce production and increase absorption of chyle. A range of techniques has been described for surgical management, and most procedures entail thoracic duct ligation through a caudal intercostal thoracotomy. Other procedures, including pericardiectomy and thoracic omentalization, have been tried concurrently with varying success. The prognosis for patients with chylothorax is guarded because many patients have recurrence of signs with both medical and surgical therapy, and because some animals succumb to the underlying disease that has caused the chylous effusion.

Thoracocentesis

Thoracocentesis is a simple technique performed routinely in general practice to collect pleural fluid for analysis and to remove air or fluid to relieve dyspnoea.

Equipment

- 20–24 gauge needle, butterfly needle or intravenous catheter.
- Extension set.
- Three-way tap.
- 10, 20, and 50 ml syringes.
- Container to collect fluid.

Preparation

Thoracocentesis requires a minimum of two people but is easiest to perform with three people (one to hold the patient, one to hold the needle, and one to operate the syringes and three-way tap). The thoracic wall is clipped widely, centred over the eighth intercostal space, and prepared aseptically. Thoracocentesis is performed using clean or aseptic technique (Fig. 23.6).

Technique

1. Assemble the needle, extension set, three-way tap, and syringe (in this order).
2. Hand the syringe to the assistant but retain the needle.
3. Identify the seventh or eighth intercostal space by counting backwards from the last rib.

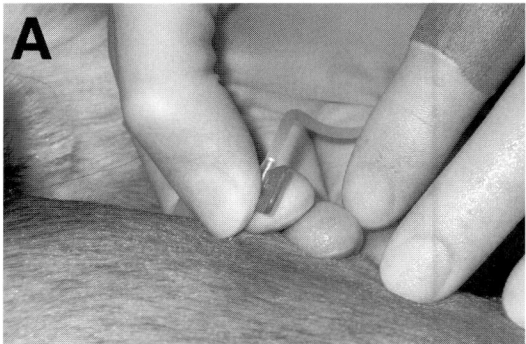

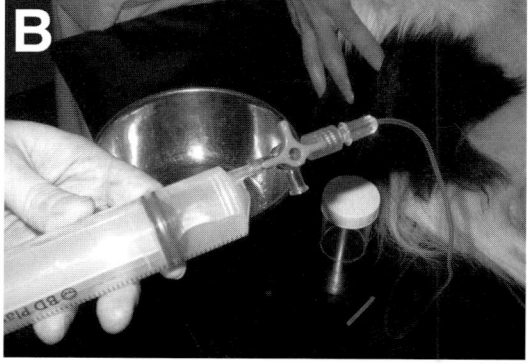

Fig. 23.6. Thoracocentesis: butterfly needle introduced through eighth intercostal space (A) and attached via an extension set to a syringe and three-way tap for drainage (B).

4. Insert the needle through the seventh or eighth intercostal space at an angle so that the bevel of the needle faces lung (to limit lung trauma); for pneumothorax introduce the needle two-thirds of the way up the intercostal space; for pleural fluid insert the needle one-third of the way up the thoracic wall.

5. Get the assistant to withdraw pleural fluid or air using the syringe and three-way tap. Ensure that the three-way tap is operated so that the egress port is never in direct communication with the extension set. If no gas or air is retrieved, reposition the needle and try again.

6. Repeat on the opposite side of the chest if the problem is bilateral.

Thoracic Drain Placement

Thoracic drains are placed to allow frequent thoracic drainage or thoracic lavage. Although thoracic drains are easy to place, they are rarely used in general practice and most patients requiring their use are referred to specialist centres. A range of techniques can be used to place thoracic drains, but recently guidewire-based chest drain kits have been developed for easy application in veterinary practice. The author recommends these drains for practitioners to use if they do not place thoracic drains regularly. These chest drains have the advantages of being easy to place, easy to secure to the patient, and comfortable. However, they are small-bore tubes and kinking and blockage may both lead to early failure. If performing this technique, purchase a veterinary guidewire chest tube kit designed specifically for the procedure, and review the manufacturer's instructions prior to use. Guidewire-based procedures are often marketed using the terminology 'Seldinger's technique'. Fig. 23.7 overviews the placement of one of these chest drains.

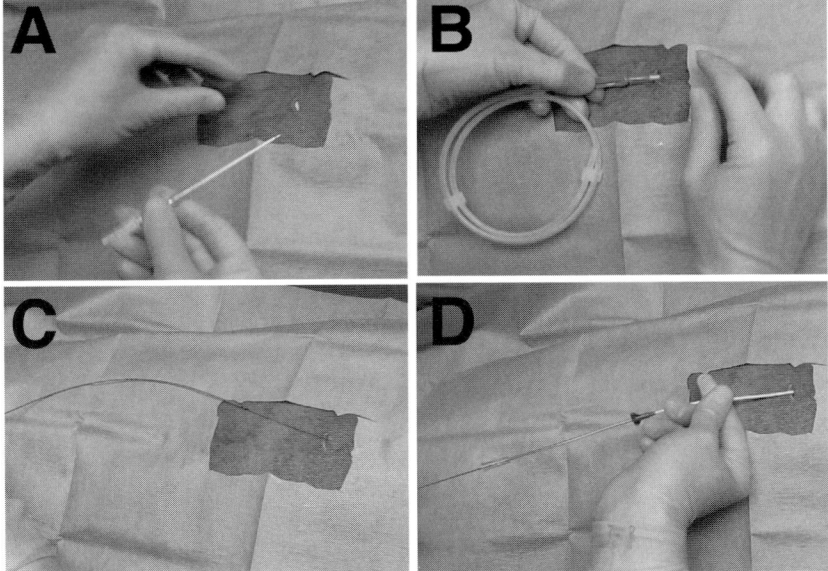

Fig. 23.7. Thoracic drain placement – Seldinger's technique (patient's head is towards the right): (A) a small stab incision is made over the appropriate intercostal space; a catheter is tunnelled under the skin for a short distance before being pushed into the thoracic cavity through an intercostal space; (B) the needle stylet of the catheter is removed and a guidewire is fed into the chest through the catheter (coiled device is the guidewire sheath); (C) the catheter is withdrawn over the guidewire leaving only the guidewire entering the thoracic cavity; (D) a small-bore thoracostomy tube is fed into the chest over the guidewire. Finally, the guidewire is removed and the drain is capped and sutured in place.

Management of Pleural Disease

Bibliography

Addie, D., Belák, S., Boucraut-Baralon, C., Egberink, H., Frymus, T., Gruffydd-Jones, T., Hartmann, K., *et al.* (2009) Feline infectious peritonitis: ABCD guidelines on prevention and management. *Journal of Feline Medicine and Surgery* 11, 594–604.

Au, J.J., Weisman, D.L., Stefanacci, J.D. and Palmisano, M.P. (2006) Use of computed tomography for evaluation of lung lesions associated with spontaneous pneumothorax in dogs: 12 cases (1999–2002). *Journal of the American Veterinary Medical Association* 228, 733–737.

Barrs, V.R. and Beatty, J.A. (2009a) Feline pyothorax – new insights into an old problem: part 1. Aetiopathogenesis and diagnostic investigation. *Veterinary Journal* 179, 163–170.

Barrs, V.R. and Beatty, J.A. (2009b) Feline pyothorax – new insights into an old problem: part 2. Treatment recommendations and prophylaxis. *Veterinary Journal* 179, 171–178.

Beatty, J. and Barrs, V. (2010) Pleural effusion in the cat: a practical approach to determining aetiology. *Journal of Feline Medicine and Surgery* 12, 693–707.

Carobbi, B., White, R.A. and Romanelli, G. (2008) Treatment of idiopathic chylothorax in 14 dogs by ligation of the thoracic duct and partial pericardiectomy. *Veterinary Record* 163, 743–745.

Demetriou, J.L., Foale, R.D., Ladlow, J., McGrotty, Y., Faulkner, J. and Kirby, B.M. (2002) Canine and feline pyothorax: a retrospective study of 50 cases in the UK and Ireland. *Journal of Small Animal Practice* 43, 388–394.

Forrester, S.D., Troy, G. and Fossum, T.W. (1988) Pleural effusions: pathophysiology and diagnostic considerations. *Compendium of Continuing Education for the Practicing Veterinarian* 10, 121–135.

Fossum, T.W. (2001) Chylothorax in cats: is there a role for surgery? *Journal of Feline Medicine and Surgery* 3, 73–79.

Fossum, T.W., Birchard, S.J. and Jacobs, R.M. (1986) Chylothorax in 34 dogs. *Journal of the American Veterinary Medical Association* 188, 1315–1318.

Fossum, T.W., Forrester, S.D., Swenson, C.L., Miller, M.W., Cohen, N.D., Boothe, H.W. and Birchard, S.J. (1991) Chylothorax in cats: 37 cases (1969–1989). *Journal of the American Veterinary Medical Association* 198, 672–678.

Fossum, T.W., Miller, M.W., Rogers, K.S., Bonagura, J.D. and Meurs, K.M. (1994) Chylothorax associated with right-sided heart failure in five cats. *Journal of the American Veterinary Medical Association* 204, 84–89.

Fossum, T.W., Mertens, M.M., Miller, M.W., Peacock, J.T., Saunders, A., Gordon, S., Pahl, G., *et al.* (2004) Thoracic duct ligation and pericardectomy for treatment of idiopathic chylothorax. *Journal of Veterinary Internal Medicine* 18, 307–310.

Gianella, P., Pfammatter, N.S. and Burgener, I.A. (2009) Oesophageal and gastric endoscopic foreign body removal: complications and follow-up of 102 dogs. *Journal of Small Animal Practice* 50, 649–654.

Johnson, M.S. and Martin, M.W. (2007) Successful medical treatment of 15 dogs with pyothorax. *Journal of Small Animal Practice* 48, 12–16.

Lipscomb, V.J., Hardie, R.J. and Dubielzig, R.R. (2003) Spontaneous pneumothorax caused by pulmonary blebs and bullae in 12 dogs. *Journal of the American Animal Hospital Association* 39, 435–445.

Mellanby, R.J., Villiers, E. and Herrtage, M.E. (2002) Canine pleural and mediastinal effusions: a retrospective study of 81 cases. *Journal of Small Animal Practice* 43, 447–451.

Milne, M.E., McCowan, C. and Landon, B.P. (2010) Spontaneous feline pneumothorax caused by ruptured pulmonary bullae associated with possible bronchopulmonary dysplasia. *Journal of the American Animal Hospital Association* 46, 138–142.

Pawloski, D.R. and Broaddus, K.D. (2010) Pneumothorax: a review. *Journal of the American Animal Hospital Association* 46, 385–397.

Piek, C.J. and Robben, J.H. (2000) Pyothorax in nine dogs. *Veterinary Quarterly* 22, 107–111.

Puerto, D.A., Brockman, D.J., Lindquist, C. and Drobatz, K. (2002) Surgical and nonsurgical management of and selected risk factors for spontaneous pneumothorax in dogs: 64 cases (1986–1999). *Journal of the American Veterinary Medical Association* 220, 1670–1674.

Sasanelli, M., Paradies, P., Otranto, D., Lia, R.P. and De Caprariis, D. (2008) Haemothorax associated with *Angiostrongylus vasorum* infection in a dog. *Journal of Small Animal Practice* 49, 417–420.

Schultz, R.M. and Zwingenberger, A. (2008) Radiographic, computed tomographic, and ultrasonographic findings with migrating intrathoracic grass awns in dogs and cats. *Veterinary Radiology and Ultrasound* 49, 249–255.

Stewart, K. and Padgett, S. (2010) Chylothorax treated via thoracic duct ligation and omentalization. *Journal of the American Animal Hospital Association* 46, 312–317.

Thompson, M.S., Cohn, L.A. and Jordan, R.C. (1999) Use of rutin for medical management of idiopathic chylothorax in four cats. *Journal of the American Veterinary Medical Association* 215, 339, 345–348.

Valtolina, C. and Adamantos, S. (2009) Evaluation of small-bore wire-guided chest drains for management of pleural space disease. *Journal of Small Animal Practice* 50, 290–297.

White, H.L., Rozanski, E.A., Tidwell, A.S., Chan, D.L. and Rush, J.E. (2003) Spontaneous pneumothorax in two cats with small airway disease. *Journal of the American Veterinary Medical Association* 222, 1547, 1573–1575.

24 Principles of Thoracic Surgery

> **intercostal thoracotomy:** incision between the ribs to enter the thorax
> **lung lobectomy:** removal of a lung lobe
> **median sternotomy:** incision through the sternum to enter the thorax
> **pericardiectomy (pericardectomy):** removal of a portion of the pericardium
> **pericardiocentesis:** needle drainage of the pericardial sac

The reader should be able to:

- define the terms intercostal thoracotomy, median sternotomy, lung lobectomy, and pericardiectomy
- identify clinical features consistent with patent ductus arteriosus in a puppy presenting for routine vaccination at 9 weeks of age
- instruct an owner on the benefit of occlusion of a patent ductus arteriosus (PDA) and recognize that both surgical and non-surgical approaches are possible

Thoracic surgery is more challenging and more complex than most surgeries. The anaesthetic management is complicated by the need to ventilate the animal throughout the procedure. Some specialist equipment is required to perform surgery, and the patients require intensive monitoring and care in the immediate post-operative period. For these reasons, with the exception of diaphragmatic rupture, thoracic surgery is rarely performed in general practice. The aim of this chapter is to provide sufficient background information for practitioners to advise owners before arranging referral. A brief description of the main surgical approaches to the thoracic cavity is given, followed by overviews of lung lobectomy, pericardiectomy, and patent ductus arteriosus (PDA) ligation.

Approaches to the Thoracic Cavity

Two approaches are used for most thoracic surgeries: (i) intercostal thoracotomy; and (ii) median sternotomy. Thoracoscopic surgery (placing a rigid endoscope into the pleural cavity) is occasionally performed for some thoracic procedures including thoracic duct ligation and pericardiectomy.

Intercostal thoracotomy

Intercostal thoracotomy is performed with the patient lying in lateral recumbency. An incision is made through the skin, latissimus dorsi muscle, and other external thoracic muscles to expose the selected intercostal space. The intercostal muscles and pleura are incised to give access to the thorax. To close the incision, circumcostal sutures encircle the ribs on either side of the incision, and the muscle, subcutaneous fat, and skin are closed in layers (Fig. 24.1).

Intercostal thoracotomy is well tolerated and gives good access to the heart base, hilus of the lung, and oesophagus on the side of surgery. However, it gives no access to the contralateral side of the thorax. It is indicated for cases in which exploration of the entire thorax is unnecessary because the lesion can be localized to an area accessible by this limited approach. It is the preferred approach for PDA ligation, lung lobectomy, thoracic duct ligation, and oesophageal foreign body removal.

Patients recover quickly from intercostal thoracotomy and often can be discharged within a few days of surgery. However, there may be transient lameness post-operatively, as the latissimus dorsi muscle has been cut and seromas often form ventral to the incision. Life-threatening complications, including pneumothorax, can occur but usually only in the immediate post-operative period. All patients require 4 weeks of recuperation with limited activity to ensure healing of the incision, but most animals appear comfortable within the first few days of surgery.

Median sternotomy

Median sternotomy is technically more demanding than intercostal thoracotomy. However, it enables most of the thoracic cavity to be explored. The patient is positioned in dorsal recumbency and the skin, subcutaneous tissues, and muscles are incised over the sternebrae (Fig. 24.2). Once the sternebrae

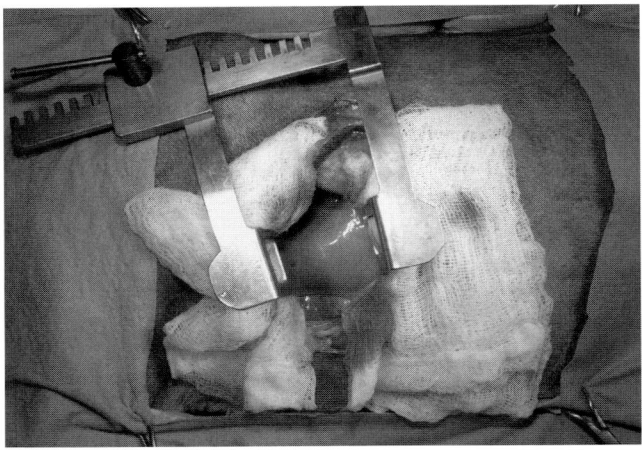

Fig. 24.1. Intercostal thoracotomy (head towards left): fourth left intercostal thoracotomy giving access to the heart base and cranial lung lobes.

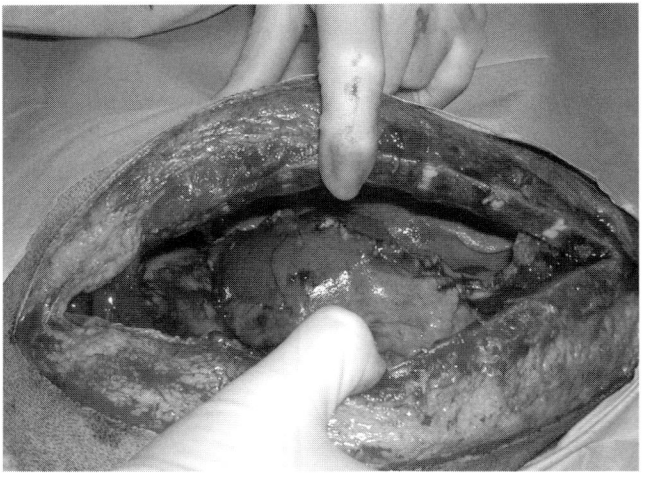

Fig. 24.2. Median sternotomy: the apex of the heart and one lung lobe can be seen. This dog had pyothorax and this image was collected once retractors had been removed. Note the split surfaces of the sternebrae.

are exposed, they are cut in longitudinal section to split the sternum, and self-retaining retractors are placed to spread the incision. This exposes both sides of the thorax and enables the whole chest to be explored. To close the incision, the sternebrae are wired together before the soft tissues are closed in layers.

Median sternotomy gives good access to the ventral thorax but it provides limited access to the dorsal thorax and is not suitable for PDA ligation, thoracic duct ligation, or oesophagotomy. The main indications for median sternotomy are for management of thoracic disease that cannot be localized preoperatively (e.g. pneumothorax) or for generalized pleural disease (e.g. pyothorax).

Recovery following median sternotomy is slower than following intercostal thoracotomy but, providing the sternum is reconstructed rigidly, patients still recover quickly and can often be discharged within a few days. Wound-healing complications are more common than following intercostal thoracotomy and include osteomyelitis of the sternebrae. Life-threatening complications such as pneumothorax can develop, but generally only in the immediate post-operative period. Patients require 4 weeks of exercise restriction while the sternebrae heal, but most appear to be comfortable within the first week or two of surgery.

Lung Lobectomy

The main indications for lung lobectomy are removal of infected lung lobes, management of bronchial foreign bodies, resolution of pneumothorax, and management of primary lung tumours. Often one or two lung lobes are removed and this is well tolerated in non-working animals. Occasionally, removal of the entire left or right lung field (pneumonectomy) is performed, but this is associated with a higher complication rate.

The outcome following lung lobectomy is dependent on the underlying disease process. The prognosis following removal of a primary lung tumour is variable and is dependent on the type of tumour and the stage at diagnosis. For example, dogs with metastatic lung tumours have a reported median survival time of 72 days following lobectomy in comparison to dogs with papillary adenocarcinoma without metastatic disease, which have a reported median survival time of 555 days.

Similar results are reported in cats. Unfortunately, it is difficult to establish what the histopathological type and stage of the tumour are prior to surgery, so surgery is often performed without prior knowledge of the long-term prognosis for the patient.

Pericardial effusions

Pericardial effusion is quite common and causes cardiac tamponade by compressing the right ventricle. This leads to signs of right heart failure including venous congestion, ascites, hepatomegaly, lethargy, and exercise intolerance. Most pericardial effusions are classified as being haemorrhagic but modified transudates and exudates also contribute to the condition.

In cats, pericardial effusions are usually caused by primary heart disease (89%) and tend to be of low volume. Treatment of the underlying heart condition is required, but the effusion rarely requires drainage. Pericardial effusions are also frequently associated with feline infectious peritonitis (FIP).

In dogs, pericardial effusions are usually classed as idiopathic or are associated with heart-base tumours and it is more likely that pericardiocentesis will be indicated. Idiopathic pericardial effusion predominantly affects large-breed dogs such as the golden retriever. The effusions are generally haemorrhagic but the aetiopathogenesis of the syndrome is unknown. The patient can be stabilized initially by draining the effusion through the right fifth intercostal space by pericardiocentesis, which rapidly resolves the signs of cardiac tamponade. Unfortunately, the effusion is prone to recur and this necessitates repeat drainage in many patients. If recurrent pericardial effusion causes persistent signs, long-term management can be achieved by removing a portion of the pericardium, a procedure called subtotal pericardiectomy. This allows fluid that would accumulate in the pericardium to drain into the pleural cavity where it is absorbed over the larger surface area. Pericardiectomy is well tolerated and controls signs in 72% of affected dogs.

Pericardial effusion secondary to heart-base tumours is usually haemorrhagic, and haemangiosarcoma of the right auricle is commonly identified. The long-term prognosis is generally poor although pericardiectomy, tumour removal, and chemotherapy can be performed and may extend the lifespan of the patient.

Patent Ductus Arteriosus

Patent ductus arteriosus (PDA) is the commonest congenital heart defect in dogs but is rarely diagnosed in cats. Without treatment, most animals develop heart failure but the prognosis following treatment is generally good.

Aetiopathogenesis and presenting signs

During fetal development, the ductus arteriosus allows blood to bypass the unexpanded lungs by flowing directly from the pulmonary artery into the descending aorta. At birth, the ductus arteriosus closes to allow blood from the pulmonary artery to flow into the lungs. Patients with PDA suffer from failure of the ductus arteriosus to close after birth, enabling blood to flow down the pressure gradient from the aorta into the pulmonary artery. This is termed left-to-right shunting, as oxygenated blood from the left side of the heart flows from the aorta into the pulmonary artery and mixes with deoxygenated blood from the right side of the heart. Initially, this causes no signs of heart failure as oxygenated blood still flows to the body. The only sign of disease is the characteristic continuous machinery murmur caused by turbulent blood flow through the PDA. Eventually, however, secondary heart failure will develop.

In some animals, pulmonary hypertension causes the pressure in the pulmonary artery to rise and this can lead to reversal of blood flow through the PDA. Right-to-left shunting results in poor tissue oxygenation, as aortic blood is diluted by deoxygenated blood from the pulmonary artery. Chronic hypoxia leads to a characteristic pattern of cyanosis and compensatory polycythaemia.

Early signs

Before signs of respiratory or heart dysfunction become apparent, the main clinical finding is the characteristic 'machinery murmur' that is present in most patients. The murmur is audible during systole and diastole and is often likened to the oscillating sound that an engine or pump makes. The point of maximum intensity is over the left heart base and there may be a precordial thrill. However, some patients have more focal murmurs that are only detected following careful evaluation, and many have concurrent systolic murmurs caused by mitral regurgitation.

Signs of heart failure

Left untreated, many patients develop signs of left heart failure that include adventitious lung sounds, coughing, exercise intolerance, lethargy, and dyspnoea.

Signs of right-to-left shunting

Once flow in the PDA reverses, the patient begins to show signs of hypoxia and becomes polycythaemic. Signs include cyanosis, exercise intolerance, lethargy, hind limb collapse, and seizures. The PDA enters the aorta distal to the left subclavian artery and brachiocephalic trunk. These vessels continue to receive well-oxygenated blood from the left atrium and carry the blood to the forelimbs and head. In some animals, this leads to the development of differential cyanosis: the gums and conjunctiva are pink, but the rectal mucosa and vulva/prepuce become cyanotic.

Management

Most patients with PDA will develop significant signs of cardiac dysfunction before reaching maturity unless the anomalous vessel is occluded. Occlusion of the PDA is recommended before right-to-left shunting occurs as it is associated with a good long-term prognosis and improvement in cardiac function. However, once right-to-left shunting has occurred, occlusion of the PDA is contraindicated, as the increased pressure in the pulmonary artery will cause life-threatening pulmonary hypertension as soon as the PDA is closed.

Left-to-right shunting PDA can be ligated surgically by intercostal thoracotomy and dissection of the vessel. This is associated with ~5% mortality rate, predominantly due to rupture of the vessel or intra-operative bradydysrhythmias. Alternatively, intravascular devices (e.g. thrombogenic coils) can be placed into the PDA by catheterization of the femoral or carotid artery. These lead to thrombus formation and occlusion of the PDA. These intravascular devices enable the PDA to be occluded without major surgery, but the overall mortality rates are similar to those associated with surgery. Ultimately, both surgery and intravascular strategies to occlude the PDA are very effective and are worth considering for affected animals.

Bibliography

Allman, D.A., Radlinsky, M.G., Ralph, A.G. and Rawlings, C.A. (2010) Thoracoscopic thoracic duct ligation and thoracoscopic pericardectomy for treatment of chylothorax in dogs. *Veterinary Surgery* 39, 21–27.

Aronsohn, M.G. and Carpenter, J.L. (1999) Surgical treatment of idiopathic pericardial effusion in the dog: 25 cases (1978–1993). *Journal of the American Animal Hospital Association* 35, 521–525.

Buchanan, J.W. (2001) Patent ductus arteriosus: morphology, pathogenesis, types and treatment. *Journal of Veterinary Cardiology* 3, 7–16.

Burton, C.A. and White, R.N. (1996) Review of the technique and complications of median sternotomy in the dog and cat. *Journal of Small Animal Practice* 37, 516–522.

Cote, E. and Ettinger, S.J. (2001) Long-term clinical management of right-to-left ("reversed") patent ductus arteriosus in 3 dogs. *Journal of Veterinary Internal Medicine* 15, 39–42.

Crumbaker, D.M., Rooney, M.B. and Case, J.B. (2010) Thoracoscopic subtotal pericardiectomy and right atrial mass resection in a dog. *Journal of the American Veterinary Medical Association* 237, 551–554.

Ehrhart, N., Ehrhart, E.J., Willis, J., Sisson, D., Constable, P., Greenfield, C., Manfra-Maretta, S., *et al.* (2002) Analysis of factors affecting survival in dogs with aortic body tumors. *Veterinary Surgery* 31, 44–48.

Gidlewski, J. and Petrie, J.P. (2005) Therapeutic pericardiocentesis in the dog and cat. *Clinical Techniques in Small Animal Practice* 20, 151–155.

Goodrich, K.R., Kyles, A.E., Kass, P.H. and Campbell, F. (2007) Retrospective comparison of surgical ligation and transarterial catheter occlusion for treatment of patent ductus arteriosus in two hundred and four dogs (1993–2003). *Veterinary Surgery* 36, 43–49.

Gordon, S.G. and Miller, M.W. (2005) Transarterial coil embolization for canine patent ductus arteriosus occlusion. *Clinical Techniques in Small Animal Practice* 20, 196–202.

Gordon, S.G., Saunders, A.B., Achen, S.E., Roland, R.M., Drourr, L.T., Hariu, C. and Miller, M.W. (2010) Transarterial ductal occlusion using the Amplatz Canine Duct Occluder in 40 dogs. *Journal of Veterinary Cardiology* 12, 85–92

Hahn, K.A. and McEntee, M.F. (1997) Primary lung tumors in cats: 86 cases (1979–1994). *Journal of the American Veterinary Medical Association* 211, 1257–1260.

Hahn, K.A. and McEntee, M.F. (1998) Prognosis factors for survival in cats after removal of a primary lung tumor: 21 cases (1979–1994). *Veterinary Surgery* 27, 307–311.

Hall, D.J., Shofer, F., Meier, C.K. and Sleeper, M.M. (2007) Pericardial effusion in cats: a retrospective study of clinical findings and outcome in 146 cats. *Journal of Veterinary Internal Medicine* 21, 1002–1007.

Jones, C.L. and Buchanan, J.W. (1981) Patent ductus arteriosus: anatomy and surgery in a cat. *Journal of the American Veterinary Medical Association* 179, 364–369.

Liptak, J.M., Monnet, E., Dernell, W.S., Rizzo, S.A. and Withrow, S.J. (2004) Pneumonectomy: four case studies and a comparative review. *Journal of Small Animal Practice* 45, 441–447.

Macdonald, K.A., Cagney, O. and Magne, M.L. (2009) Echocardiographic and clinicopathologic characterization of pericardial effusion in dogs: 107 cases (1985–2006). *Journal of the American Veterinary Medical Association* 235, 1456–1461.

McNiel, E.A., Ogilvie, G.K., Powers, B.E., Hutchison, J.M., Salman, M.D. and Withrow, S.J. (1997) Evaluation of prognostic factors for dogs with primary lung tumors: 67 cases (1985–1992). *Journal of the American Veterinary Medical Association* 211, 1422–1427.

Mellanby, R.J. and Herrtage, M.E. (2005) Long-term survival of 23 dogs with pericardial effusions. *Veterinary Record* 156, 568–571.

Moores, A.L., Halfacree, Z.J., Baines, S.J. and Lipscomb, V.J. (2007) Indications, outcomes and complications following lateral thoracotomy in dogs and cats. *Journal of Small Animal Practice* 48, 695–698.

Polton, G.A., Brearley, M.J., Powell, S.M. and Burton, C.A. (2008) Impact of primary tumour stage on survival in dogs with solitary lung tumours. *Journal of Small Animal Practice* 49, 66–71.

Pyle, R.L., Park, R.D., Alexander, A.F. and Hill, B.L. (1981) Patent ductus arteriosus with pulmonary hypertension in the dog. *Journal of the American Veterinary Medical Association* 178, 565–571.

Rush, J.E., Keene, B.W. and Fox, P.R. (1990) Pericardial disease in the cat: a retrospective evaluation of 66 cases. *Journal of the American Animal Hospital Association* 26, 39–46.

Shaw, S.P. and Rush, J.E. (2007) Canine pericardial effusion: pathophysiology and cause. *Compendium of Continuing Education for the Practicing Veterinarian* 29, 400–403; quiz 404.

Stafford Johnson, M., Martin, M., Binns, S. and Day, M.J. (2004) A retrospective study of clinical findings, treatment and outcome in 143 dogs with pericardial effusion. *Journal of Small Animal Practice* 45, 546–552.

Tattersall, J.A. and Welsh, E. (2006) Factors influencing the short-term outcome following thoracic surgery in 98 dogs. *Journal of Small Animal Practice* 47, 715–720.

Van Israel, N., French, A.T., Dukes-McEwan, J. and Corcoran, B.M. (2002) Review of left-to-right shunting patent ductus arteriosus and short-term outcome in 98 dogs. *Journal of Small Animal Practice* 43, 395–400.

Vicari, E.D., Brown, D.C., Holt, D.E. and Brockman, D.J. (2001) Survival times of and prognostic indicators for dogs with heart base masses: 25 cases (1986–1999). *Journal of the American Veterinary Medical Association* 219, 485–487.

Weisse, C., Soares, N., Beal, M.W., Steffey, M.A., Drobatz, K.J. and Henry, C.J. (2005) Survival times in dogs with right atrial hemangiosarcoma treated by means of surgical resection with or without adjuvant chemotherapy: 23 cases (1986–2000). *Journal of the American Veterinary Medical Association* 226, 575–579.

Appendix 1
Medical Terminology

> **elective procedure:** a planned (non-emergency) procedure (e.g. elective neutering)
> **diagnostic procedure:** a procedure to investigate a condition (e.g. incisional biopsy)
> **palliative procedure:** a surgery that aims to alleviate signs rather than to cure (e.g. splenectomy for bleeding splenic tumour that has metastasized)
> **prophylactic procedure:** a procedure to prevent disease (e.g. elective neutering)
> **salvage procedure:** a procedure that aims to salvage some function from an untreatable condition (e.g. hind limb amputation following failed fracture repair; total ear canal ablation with bulla osteotomy for chronic otitis externa)
> **therapeutic procedure:** a procedure to treat disease (e.g. ovariohysterectomy to treat pyometra)

Medical terminology is used extensively to describe conditions, procedures, and signs and provides a common frame of reference for clinicians to discuss aspects of veterinary surgery. Medical terms are generated by adding suffixes and prefixes to root words. The root word generally defines the organ or body system. The prefix is often descriptive of the appearance, physical features, or physical or temporal relationship to other objects or events. The suffix usually defines the action, pathology, or state.

Prefixes

brachy-	short	micro-	small
brady-	slow	neo-	new
dys-	defective; difficulty	oligo-	few; little
extra-	outside	para-	beside; near to
hyper-	more than; over	peri-	around
hypo-	less than; under	post-	after
infra-	below	pre-	before
inter-	between	pseudo-	false; fake
intra-	during; within	strang-	constricting painfully; straining
iso-	equal to	tachy-	fast
macro-	large; long		

Root words

aden(o)-	gland/glandular	mammo-	breast
adip(o)-	fat	mandibulo-	mandible/lower jaw
adren(o)-	adrenal	mast(o)-	breast
aer(o)-	air	maxillo-	maxilla/upper jaw
balan(o)-	glans of penis	metro-	uterus
brachi(o)-	arm	myel(o)-	bone marrow
bronch(o)-	bronchi	nephr(o)-	kidney
carcin(o)-	cancer	oesophag(o)-	oesophagus
cardi(o)-	heart	onycho-	nail
chol(e)-	bile	ophthalm(o)-	eye
cholecyst(o)-	gall bladder	orchi(o)-	testicle

choledoch(o)-	bile duct	oro-	mouth
coel-	cavity; hollow organ	ovario-	ovary
colo-	colon	ovariohyster-	ovary and uterus
colp(o)-	uterus	palato-	palate
cutaneo-	skin	pancreatico-	pancreas
cysto-	bladder	pancreato-	pancreas
dacryo-	tear	pericardio-	pericardium
derm(a)-	skin	pharyng(o)-	pharynx
dermat(o)-	skin	phrenic(o)-	diaphragm
duodeno-	duodenum	pneumon(o)-	lung
enter(o)-	intestinal	prostato-	prostate
episio-	vulva (pubic region)	py(o)-	pus
gastr(o)-	stomach	pyelo-	renal pelvis
gloss(o)-	tongue	pyloro-	pylorus
gonado-	testicle or ovary	reno-	kidney
haemangio-	blood vessel	rhin(o)-	nose
haemat(o)-	blood	sanguino-	blood
hepato-	liver	sanguineo-	blood
hydro-	water	spleno-	spleen
hypophyso-	pituitary	staphylo-	uvula in man – adopted to refer to palate in veterinary species
hystero-	uterus		
ile(o)-	ileum		
jejuno-	jejunum	tracheo-	trachea
lapar(o)-	flank	uretero-	ureter
laryng(o)-	laryngeal	urethro-	urethra
lip(o)-	fat	vagino-	vagina
lob-	lobe	vesico-	bladder
		vulvo-	vulva

Suffixes

-aemia	blood	-(o)stomy	create hole into; create permanent connection between; create a stoma
-centesis	aspiration or puncture		
-chezia	defecation		
-desis	binding together	-(o)tomy	incise into
-ectomy	excise	-paresis	weakness
-gram	record; picture	-pathy	disease
-graphy	act of recording	-pexy	fix to
-ism	disease	-phagia	eating; prehension
-itis	inflammation	-plasty	remodel; reconstruction
-lysis	destruction	-plegia	paralysis
-megaly	enlargement	-plication	folding
-oma	condition	-rrhoea	flowing; discharge
		-stasis	stop
		-uria	urine

There is substantial crossover of terminology between words of Latin and Greek origin, for example 'utero-' (Greek), and 'metro-' (Latin). In general, Greek root words are conjoined to Greek prefixes and suffixes, and Latin root words are conjoined to Latin prefixes or suffixes. There are also many inconsistencies: for example, 'tracheostomy' and 'tracheotomy' are used variably and interchangeably to refer to both temporary incision into and to permanent stoma in the trachea; 'pericardiectomy' is often truncated to 'pericardectomy'. Some terminology has been adopted from human medicine but species differences has led to some inaccuracy in its use. 'Staphylectomy', for example, has been adopted to mean excision of a portion of the palate, but 'staphyl-' actually relates to the uvula, an anatomic feature not present in any domestic species.

Other resources

Black's Veterinary Dictionary (2005): excellent general veterinary dictionary (21st revised edn. A & C Black Publishers Ltd, London, ISBN 978-0713663624).

Dorland's Medical Dictionary (2011): excellent general medical dictionary (32nd edn. W.B. Saunders, Philadelphia, Pennsylvania, ISBN 978-1416062578).

Nomina Anatomica Veterinaria: agreed international standard reference source of veterinary anatomy terminology (5th edn. www.wava-amav.org/nav_nev.htm, accessed 21 May 2011).

Oxford English Dictionary (2011): accepted standard for definitions and etymology (OED Online, Oxford University Press. www.oed.com, accessed 25 July 2011).

Recognised International Nonproprietary Names (rINN): international standard for drug names; guidelines for use (www.who.int/medicines/services/inn/innquidance/en/index.html, accessed 21 May 2011).

Other medical terminology and dictionary websites and on-line educational tools (accessed 21 May 2011).

- http://medical-dictionary.thefreedictionary.com;
- www.medilexicon.com/medicaldictionary.php;
- www.free-ed.net/sweethaven/MedTech/MedTerm/default.asp; and
- www4.caes.hku.hk/mt

Appendix 2
Self-Assessment

Chapter 1: Applying Halsted's Principles

1.1. Which of the following statements about diathermy is most accurate?

    A. Bipolar diathermy enables pinpoint haemostasis to be achieved.
    B. Diathermy is effective when applied to arteries of up to 4 mm diameter.
    C. Monopolar diathermy is less likely to cause burns than bipolar diathermy because it has a separate earth plate.
    D. Monopolar diathermy uses a heated probe to cauterize tissues.

1.2. Which of the following statements about chlorhexidine gluconate surgical scrub solution is most accurate?

    A. It is bacteriostatic.
    B. It has no cumulative effect.
    C. It has no residual effect.
    D. It has similar initial activity to povidone-iodine.

1.3. Which of the following statements about the sterile field is most accurate?

    A. It does not extend below the table top.
    B. It does not extend onto the surgeon's body.
    C. It extends to include the axillae.
    D. It never extends onto the instrument trolley.

1.4. Which of the following statements most accurately describes a Penrose drain?

    A. It is a fenestrated drain.
    B. It is a rigid drain.
    C. It is an active drain.
    D. It is an open drain.

1.5. Which of the following statements about surgical drains is most accurate?

    A. Closed active drains should not exit the wound through the primary incision.
    B. Closed active drains must be placed in dependent positions to be effective.
    C. Open passive drains act by displacing fluid with air.
    D. Open passive drains are associated with a low risk of ascending infection.

Chapter 2: Prophylactic, Perioperative Antimicrobials

2.1. Which of the following describes an optimum protocol for provision of perioperative, prophylactic antimicrobials for clean-contaminated surgery?

    A. Give a therapeutic dose intravenously 20 min before the start of surgery.
    B. Give a therapeutic dose intramuscularly 2 h before the start of surgery.
    C. Start oral dosing with a therapeutic dose 24 h before the start of surgery.
    D. Instill non-irritant antibiotics into the surgical wound at the end of surgery.

2.2. Which of the following statements describes best practice for uncomplicated, elective canine ovariohysterectomy?

    A. There is no indication for antibiotics.
    B. Give a single dose of antibiotics prior to the start of surgery.
    C. Give antibiotics for the first 24 h following the start of surgery.
    D. A therapeutic course of broad-spectrum antibiotics should be given.

2.3. Using the NRC wound classification system, how is elective cystotomy (incision into the bladder) classified?

    A. Clean.
    B. Clean-contaminated.
    C. Contaminated.
    D. Dirty.

2.4. Using the NRC wound classification system, how is elective ovariohysterectomy (neutering) classified?

    A. Clean.
    B. Clean-contaminated.
    C. Contaminated.
    D. Dirty.

2.5. Which of the following organisms is most frequently associated with surgical site infection in animals?

    A. *Escherichia coli.*
    B. *Proteus* sp.
    C. *Staphylococcus* spp.
    D. *Streptococcus* spp.

Chapter 3: Suture Materials, Staples, and Tissue Adhesive

3.1. Which of the following features is NOT desirable in the 'ideal suture material'?

    A. High memory.
    B. Low antigenicity.
    C. Low tissue drag.
    D. Synthetic material.

3.2. Which of the following materials is an example of a non-absorbable, synthetic suture material?

    A. Glycomer™ 631.
    B. Polyamide.
    C. Polydioxanone II.
    D. Polyglactin 910.

3.3. Which of the following suture materials is an example of a braided, synthetic suture material?

    A. Glycomer™ 631.
    B. Polyamide.
    C. Polydioxanone II.
    D. Polyglactin 910.

3.4. Which of the following statements about surgical gut is LEAST ACCURATE?

    A. It is composed of collagen.
    B. It has a consistent rate of absorption.
    C. It is a multifilament suture material.
    D. It is degraded by enzymatic digestion.

3.5. Which of the following statements about poliglecaprone is NOT ACCURATE?

    A. It is a monofilament, absorbable suture material.
    B. It degrades by enzymatic action.
    C. It loses most of its tensile strength within 14 days.
    D. It is suitable for intradermal and subcutaneous suturing.

Chapter 4: Suture Patterns and Knots

4.1. Which of the following suture patterns generally promotes the most rapid and healthy wound healing?

    A. Appositional.
    B. Crushing.
    C. Everting.
    D. Inverting.

4.2. Which of the following suture patterns is suitable for securing tubes to skin?

    A. Cushing pattern.
    B. Ford interlocking pattern.
    C. Purse-string suture.
    D. Roman sandal suture.

4.3. Which of the following knots is generally most secure?

    A. Granny knot.
    B. Slip knot.
    C. Square knot.
    D. Surgeon's knot.

4.4. What term is used to describe the basic unit of a surgical knot?

    A. Ear.
    B. Throw.
    C. Turn.
    D. Twist.

4.5. Which of the following rules for tying a square knot with instruments is INACCURATE?

    A. Apply even tension to both suture ends.
    B. Alternate which suture end is held by the instrument with each throw.
    C. Always place the instruments into the centre of the knot.
    D. Ensure that the suture ends change sides with each throw.

Chapter 5: Surgical Instruments

5.1. Which of the following instruments is a common type of thumb forceps?

    A. Brown-Adson.
    B. Gelpi.
    C. Gosset.
    D. Rochester-Pean.

5.2. Which of the following is suitable for fine, sharp dissection?

    A. Halsted mosquito forceps.
    B. Kelly forceps.
    C. Mayo scissors.
    D. Metzenbaum scissors.

5.3. Which of the following is suitable for holding stomach?

    A. Allis tissue forceps.
    B. Babcock forceps.
    C. Brown-Adson forceps.
    D. Rat-toothed forceps.

5.4. Which of the following is best suited to manipulating skin?

    A. Brown-Adson forceps.
    B. DeBakey forceps.
    C. Dressing forceps.
    D. Rat-toothed forceps.

5.5. Which of the following forceps is designed to occlude bowel during intestinal surgery?

    A. Crile.
    B. Doyen.
    C. Kocher.
    D. Pean.

Chapter 6: Nutritional Support

6.1. Where is the ideal point for an oesophagostomy tube to empty food into?

    A. Cervical oesophagus.
    B. Distal thoracic oesophagus.
    C. Gastric fundus.
    D. Gastris pylorus.

6.2. What is the earliest that a gastrostomy tube can be removed safely from a patient?

    A. Immediately after placement.
    B. Five days after placement.
    C. Ten days after placement.
    D. One month after placement.

6.3. What is the earliest an oesophagostomy tube can be removed safely from a patient?

    A. Immediately after placement.
    B. Five days after placement.
    C. Ten days after placement.
    D. One month after placement.

6.4. What part of the stomach is the ideal location for tube feeding via gastrostomy tube?

    A. Body.
    B. Cardia.
    C. Fundus.
    D. Pylorus.

6.5. The term parenteral nutrition means:

    A. Bypassing the small intestine and feeding into the colon.
    B. Introducing feed directly into the intestine.
    C. Introducing nutrients intravenously.
    D. Partly feeding by the enteric route.

Chapter 7: Wound Management

7.1. Which of the following is an example of an adherent wound dressing?

    A. Alginate.
    B. Foam.
    C. Hydrogel.
    D. Wet-to-dry.

7.2. Which of the following dressings fills irregular wounds well?

    A. Alginate.
    B. Foam.
    C. Hydrogel.
    D. Wet-to-dry.

7.3. You are presented with a case that your colleague has been managing. The dog has a partial degloving injury over the lateral aspect of digit 5 on its forelimb. You assess that the wound is healthy and free from infection or contamination although it has not formed granulation tissue. Which of the following contact layers would be most appropriate to promote progressive healing?

    A. Alginate.
    B. Foam with hydrogel.
    C. Gauze dressing impregnated with paraffin wax.
    D. Padded film dressing.

7.4. You are managing an infected wound. Which of the following dressings would be most likely to reduce the number of bacteria on the wound?

    A. Alginate dressing impregnated with Manuka honey.
    B. Foam dressing with hydrogel.
    C. Gauze dressing impregnated with paraffin wax.
    D. Nanocrystalline silver dressing presoaked with saline.

7.5. How frequently does a wet-to-dry dressing require changing?

    A. At least once a day.
    B. At least once every 3 days.
    C. At least once a week.
    D. When the outer surface becomes saturated.

Chapter 8: Reconstructive Surgery

8.1. How is secondary closure defined?

    A. Immediate closure of a surgical wound.
    B. Wound closure delayed but performed before granulation tissue has formed.
    C. Wound closure delayed until after granulation tissue has formed.
    D. Open wound management to achieve closure by contraction and epithelialization.

8.2. Which of the following is the least effective suture pattern at distributing tension?

    A. Cruciate mattress suture.
    B. Intradermal.
    C. Simple interrupted.
    D. Vertical mattress suture.

8.3. Which of the following is LEAST likely to lead to wound complications when used as the main method of relieving tension following resection of a mammary tumour in a dog?

    A. Meshed releasing incision.
    B. Stented horizontal mattress suture.
    C. Undermining and walking sutures.
    D. Vertical mattress sutures.

8.4. Which of the following methods of wound closure suffers from elastic recoil?

    A. Advancement flap.
    B. Axial pattern flaps.
    C. Free meshed skin graft.
    D. Transposition flap.

8.5. To avoid creating dog-ears when closing an elliptical wound, how long should the incision be in relation to the width of the wound?

    A. Width ×2.
    B. Width ×3.
    C. Width ×4.
    D. Width ×5.

Chapter 9: Oncological Surgery and Skin Tumours

9.1. Which regional lymph nodes are most likely to develop metastatic lesions from a perineal tumour?

    A. Axillary.
    B. Medial iliac.
    C. Parotid.
    D. Popliteal.

9.2. Which of the following statements provides the best definition for the term radical resection?

    A. Resection of the tumour and its pseudocapsule.
    B. Resection of the tumour with a 3 cm lateral margin of tissue and a margin of one deep fascial plane.
    C. Resection of the tumour with the tissue compartment within which it has developed.
    D. Resection of the tumour with requirement for advanced reconstructive surgery.

9.3. Which of the following biopsy methods is likely to cause fewest complications?

    A. Excisional biopsy.
    B. Fine-needle aspirate.
    C. Incisional biopsy.
    D. Needle-core biopsy.

9.4. What percentage of feline mammary tumours are malignant?

    A. 10%.
    B. 25%.
    C. 50%.
    D. 80%.

9.5. Which of the following statements is most accurate when treating a dog with a grade II mast cell tumour?

    A. Excision is likely to be curative in the absence of metastatic lesions.
    B. Excision with 1 cm lateral margins and extending to, but not through, the next fascial plane is recommended.
    C. The dog is likely to benefit from radiotherapy following surgery to slow progression of the disease.
    D. The dog is likely to die from metastatic disease.

Chapter 10: Principles of Abdominal Surgery

10.1. Which is the most accurate definition of laparotomy?

    A. Incision into the abdomen.
    B. Incision through the linea alba.
    C. Incision through the flank.
    D. Incision into a body cavity.

10.2. What structure provides most strength to the linea alba suture line?

    A. External rectus sheath.
    B. Internal rectus sheath.
    C. Rectus abdominis muscle.
    D. Transverse abdominis muscle.

10.3. What procedure can be performed to improve exposure of the right kidney?

    A. Colonic sling.
    B. Duodenal sling.
    C. Gastric sling.
    D. Omental sling.

10.4. Which structure can be excised to improve exposure of the cranial abdomen?

    A. Falciform fat.
    B. Inguinal fat.
    C. Round ligament.
    D. Suspensory ligament.

10.5. For removal of an enteric foreign body, what are the most appropriate landmarks for the abdominal incision?

    A. From the cranial to the caudal third of the linea alba.
    B. From the umbilicus to the pubis.
    C. From the xiphisternum to the pubis.
    D. From the xiphisternum to the umbilicus.

Chapter 11: Hernias and Ruptures

11.1. Which of the following hernias most commonly affects older, entire, male dogs?

    A. Femoral hernia.
    B. Umbilical hernia.
    C. Perineal hernia.
    D. Peritoneopericardial diaphragmatic hernia.

11.2. Which of the following is the least common form of hernia identified in dogs?

    A. Femoral hernia.
    B. Inguinal hernia.
    C. Umbilical hernia.
    D. Perineal hernia.

11.3. Which of the following nerves sometimes is damaged during perineal hernia repair?

    A. Femoral nerve.
    B. Genital nerve.
    C. Sciatic nerve.
    D. Trigeminal nerve.

11.4. Which of the following is classified as a false hernia?

    A. Inguinal.
    B. Femoral.
    C. Scrotal.
    D. Perineal.

11.5. What is the commonest organ to herniate through a diaphragmatic defect?

    A. Liver.
    B. Omentum.
    C. Spleen.
    D. Stomach.

Chapter 12: Gastrointestinal Surgery

12.1. Which layer of intestinal wall provides most support for sutures following enterotomy?

    A. Mucosa.
    B. Submucosa.
    C. Muscularis.
    D. Serosa.

12.2. Which of the following is a procedure that can be used to reduce the risk of post-operative leakage from an enterotomy incision?

    A. Colopexy.
    B. Enteroplication.
    C. Gastropexy.
    D. Omental wrap.

12.3. Which of the following suture materials is MOST appropriate for enterectomy closure in the dog?

    A. Collagen.
    B. Polydioxanone.
    C. Polyglactin 910.
    D. Polypropylene.

12.4. Which two structures must be joined together to provide protection against recurrence of GDV?

    A. Fundus and left body wall.
    B. Fundus and right body wall.
    C. Pylorus and left body wall.
    D. Pylorus and right body wall.

12.5. Following subtotal colectomy for the management of feline megacolon, which of the following statements is MOST accurate?

    A. Animals are likely to have persistent constipation post-operatively.
    B. Animals are likely to have persistent diarrhoea post-operatively.
    C. Persistent abdominal pain is a common long-term complication.
    D. Stricture of the surgery site is a common long-term complication.

12.6. The rate of dehiscence following gastrointestinal surgery in the dog is said to be in the region of:

    A. <1%.
    B. 1–5%.
    C. 5–10%.
    D. 10–20%.

Chapter 13: Peritonitis Management and the 'Acute Abdomen'

13.1. Which of the following is the common mechanism of all forms of shock?

    A. Cellular hypoxia.
    B. Poor cardiac output.
    C. Hypotension.
    D. Hypovolaemia.

13.2. What is the most effective method of providing supplemental oxygen to a shocked patient?

    A. Face mask.
    B. Flow-by supplementation.
    C. Nasal catheter.
    D. Oxygen cage.

13.3. What clinical feature consistently identified in dogs may not be seen in cats suffering from shock?

    A. Cold extremities.
    B. Pale mucous membranes.
    C. Prolonged capillary refill time.
    D. Tachycardia.

13.4. What feature of abdominal fluid analysis is most suggestive of septic peritonitis?

    A. High protein content.
    B. High white blood cell count.
    C. Predominance of neutrophils.
    D. Presence of intracellular bacteria.

13.5. What is the commonest cause of primary peritonitis in small animals?

    A. Ascending infection through the uterine tube.
    B. Feline coronavirus infection.
    C. Haematogenous spread of bacteria.
    D. Transmural spread of bacteria from the intestinal tract.

Chapter 14: Ovarian and Uterine Surgery

14.1. Which of the following conditions is canine ovariohysterectomy NOT protective against?

    A. Mammary tumour.
    B. Pyometra.
    C. Urinary incontinence.
    D. Vaginal leiomyoma.

14.2. What is the best time to perform elective ovariohysterectomy in the female dog?

    A. During anoestrus.
    B. During dioestrus.
    C. During oestrus.
    D. During pro-oestrus.

14.3. What are the landmarks for abdominal entry for canine ovariohysterectomy?

    A. From midway between the umbilicus and the pubis to the pubis.
    B. From midway between the xiphisternum and umbilicus to midway between the umbilicus and pubis.
    C. From the umbilicus to midway between the umbilicus and pubis.
    D. From the xiphisternum to umbilicus.

14.4. What is the function of the proximal clamp during triple-clamp technique for ovarian pedicle ligation?

A. To ensure all of the ovarian tissue is excised.
B. To generate a crush line for the circumferential ligature.
C. To prevent back-bleeding.
D. To secure the ovarian pedicle so that it can be checked for bleeding following transection.

14.5. Which ligament is disrupted to improve exposure to the ovarian ligament?

A. Broad ligament.
B. Round ligament.
C. Proper ligament.
D. Suspensory ligament.

14.6. What is the most important feature in the development of stump pyometra in the dog?

A. Failure to remove all ovarian tissue during ovariohysterectomy.
B. Failure to remove the entire uterine body during ovariohysterectomy.
C. Inappropriate suture selection during ovariohysterectomy.
D. Performing ovariectomy rather than ovariohysterectomy.

14.7. What is the earliest age that elective ovariohysterectomy can be performed in the dog?

A. 3 weeks.
B. 6 weeks.
C. 12 weeks.
D. 6 months.

Chapter 15: Testicular Surgery

15.1. What is the commonest form of castration in the dog?

A. Prescrotal.
B. Scrotal.
C. Perineal.
D. Castration by scrotal ablation.

15.2. What is the commonest form of castration in the cat?

A. Prescrotal.
B. Scrotal.
C. Perineal.
D. Castration by scrotal ablation.

15.3. What is the advantage of open castration over closed castration?

A. Improved haemostasis.
B. Improved pain management post-operatively.
C. Reduced risk of ascending infection.
D. Reduced risk of evisceration through scrotal herniation.

15.4. Which form of testicular tumour is most commonly associated with feminization in a percentage of dogs?

A. Hamartoma.
B. Interstitial cell tumour.
C. Seminoma.
D. Sertoli cell tumour.

Chapter 16: Urinary Tract Surgery

16.1. Which of the following suture materials is the best choice for closure of a cystotomy incision?

    A. Collagen.
    B. Glycomer™ 631.
    C. Polyglactin 910.
    D. Polypropylene.

16.2. Which of the following is the commonest cause of FLUTD?

    A. Feline idiopathic cystitis.
    B. Urethral plugs.
    C. Urethral stricture.
    D. Struvite urolithiasis.

16.3. What is the name of the technique used to return urethral stones to the bladder?

    A. Urethrostomy.
    B. Urethrotomy.
    C. Retrograde hydropulsion.
    D. Voiding hydropulsion.

16.4. What is the preferred site for urethrostomy in the dog?

    A. Perineal.
    B. Prescrotal.
    C. Prepubic.
    D. Scrotal.

16.5. Which technique is performed to gain access to the vestibule and vagina?

    A. Colposuspension.
    B. Episioplasty.
    C. Episiotomy.
    D. Urethropexy.

Chapter 17: Splenic Surgery

17.1. What structure DOES NOT receive part of its blood supply directly from the splenic artery?

    A. Gastric pylorus.
    B. Gastric fundus.
    C. Left limb of pancreas.
    D. Omentum.

17.2. What is the commonest type of splenic tumour in dogs?

    A. Haemangiosarcoma.
    B. Histiocytic sarcoma.
    C. Lipoma.
    D. Mast cell tumour.

17.3. Which of the following conditions has been linked to splenic torsion?

    A. Gastric dilatation and volvulus.
    B. Gastric necrosis.
    C. Mesenteric volvulus.
    D. Pancreatitis.

17.4. What breed of dog is thought to be predisposed to splenic torsion?

    A. Doberman pinscher.
    B. Husky.
    C. Great Dane.
    D. Rottweiler.

Chapter 18: Hepatic Surgery

18.1. Which two liver lobes does the gall bladder sit between?

    A. Right lateral and right medial.
    B. Right medial and quadrate.
    C. Quadrate and left medial.
    D. Left medial and left lateral.

18.2. Which procedure is most likely to be of benefit for management of extrahepatic biliary obstruction caused by occlusion of the common bile duct?

    A. Cholecystectomy.
    B. Cholecystoduodenostomy.
    C. Cholecystotomy.
    D. Pyloroplasty.

18.3. Which organs DO NOT have venous drainage into the portal circulation?

    A. Intestine.
    B. Kidney.
    C. Pancreas.
    D. Spleen.

18.4. Which of the following is NOT a common clinical finding in animals with portosystemic shunt?

    A. Dysuria.
    B. Jaundice.
    C. Stunting.
    D. Polydipsia.

Chapter 19: Ear Surgery

19.1. Which of the following surgeries would be most appropriate for a dog with chronic signs of otitis externa, patent horizontal ear canals, and mineralization of the ear canal cartilages?

    A. Lateral ear canal resection.
    B. Total ear canal ablation.
    C. Total ear canal ablation with lateral bulla osteotomy.
    D. Ventral bulla osteotomy.

19.2. Which of the following methods of managing aural haematoma produces the most reliable long-term results?

    A. Conservative management.
    B. Needle drainage.
    C. Penrose drain placement.
    D. Incisional drainage.

19.3. During incisional drainage of aural haematoma, why is a sigmoid incision made in preference to a linear incision?

A. It causes less crumpling as the scar contracts.
B. It causes less vascular injury as the incision can skirt around vessels.
C. It follows the natural contour of the inner surface of the pinna.
D. It provides a bigger area for drainage of the haematoma.

19.4. During total ear canal ablation with lateral bulla osteotomy, which of the following nerves is commonly injured?

A. Facial.
B. Hypoglossal.
C. Olfactory.
D. Trigeminal.

19.5. What is the treatment of choice for a ceruminous adenoma located on the medial wall of the vertical ear canal in a dog?

A. Local excision with 1 cm margin of grossly normal tissue.
B. Lateral ear canal resection.
C. Total ear canal resection.
D. Total ear canal resection with bulla osteotomy.

Chapter 20: Upper Respiratory Tract, Laryngeal, and Tracheal Surgery

20.1. Which of the following is the best description of stertor?

A. Harsh upper airway noise.
B. Noise associated with vocal cord reverberation.
C. Referred noise from the lower respiratory tract.
D. Sonorous upper airway noise.

20.2. Which of the following is NOT typically associated with brachycephalic airway syndrome?

A. Laryngeal paralysis.
B. Overlong soft palate.
C. Stenotic nares.
D. Tonsillar prolapse and hypertrophy.

20.3. Which of the following procedures is commonly performed for the management of laryngeal paralysis?

A. Arytenoid lateralization.
B. Tracheostomy.
C. Staphylectomy.
D. Vocal cord resection.

20.4. Which of the following describes the criteria for diagnosing laryngeal paralysis in the dog?

A. Failure to identify active abduction of the glottis as general anaesthesia is induced.
B. Failure to identify active abduction of the glottis as the animal recovers from anaesthesia.
C. Failure to identify active adduction of the glottis as general anaesthesia is induced.
D. Failure to identify active adduction of the glottis as the animal recovers from anaesthesia.

20.5. Which of the following procedures will NOT relieve upper respiratory tract obstruction?

A. Endotracheal intubation.
B. Nasal oxygen catheter placement.
C. Permanent tracheostomy.
D. Temporary tracheotomy.

Chapter 21: Upper Digestive Tract Surgery

21.1. Which of the following terms describes a submucosal collection of saliva?

    A. Abscess.
    B. Epulis.
    C. Ranula.
    D. Stoma.

21.2. Which of the following is the commonest form of oral cancer in the cat?

    A. Ameloblastoma.
    B. Fibrosarcoma.
    C. Mast cell tumour.
    D. Squamous cell carcinoma.

21.3. Where is the commonest location for an oesophageal foreign body to lodge?

    A. Cervical oesophagus.
    B. Diaphragm.
    C. Heart base.
    D. Thoracic inlet.

21.4. Which term describes making a linear incision into the oesophagus?

    A. Oesophagopexy.
    B. Oesophagectomy.
    C. Oesophagostomy.
    D. Oesophogotomy.

21.5. Which of the following statements about pharyngeal penetrating (stick) injuries is most accurate?

    A. Failure to identify stick at the time of surgery is common but does not influence response to surgery.
    B. Mediastinitis is common and can be managed medically.
    C. Resection of chronic foreign body reactions is simple and suitable for entry level veterinary surgeons to perform.
    D. Surgery for acute presentations is difficult to justify as the majority resolve spontaneously.

Chapter 22: Endocrine Surgery

22.1. Which of the following procedures would be most likely to be considered for the management of pituitary dependent hyperadrenocorticism?

    A. Adrenal biopsy.
    B. Adrenalectomy.
    C. Hyposphysectomy.
    D. Parathyroidectomy.

22.2. Which of the following complications is commonly reported following feline thyroidectomy?

    A. Hypercalcaemia.
    B. Hypoparathyroidism.
    C. Hypothyroidism.
    D. Hyperthyroidism.

22.3. Why is modified extracapsular thyroidectomy a recommended method of managing feline hyperthyroidism?

    A. It enables the caudal parathyroid gland to be preserved.
    B. It enables the cranial parathyroid gland to be preserved.

C. It enables the recurrent laryngeal nerve to be preserved.

D. It enables the vagosympathetic trunk to be preserved.

22.4. Where is the thyroid gland typically located in the cat?

A. Dorsal to the larynx.

B. Lateral to the trachea at the thoracic inlet.

C. Lateral to the trachea between rings 2 and 8.

D. Ventral to the trachea between rings 4 and 10.

22.5. What is the expected recurrence rate following unilateral thyroidectomy in a cat with hyperthyroidism?

A. Less than 5%.

B. 12%.

C. 40%.

D. 70%.

Chapter 23: Management of Pleural Disease

23.1. Which organism is commonly associated with the formation of sulfur granules in pleural effusion?

A. *Actinomyces pyogenes*.

B. Coronavirus infection.

C. *Escherichia coli*.

D. *Pasturella multocida*.

23.2. What term is used to describe placing a drain into the thorax?

A. Thoracocentesis.

B. Thoracoscopy.

C. Thoracostomy.

D. Thoracotomy.

23.3. Which of the following forms of pneumothorax is most likely to require placement of a thoracostomy tube?

A. Open pneumothorax.

B. Spontaneous pneumothorax.

C. Tension pneumothorax.

D. Traumatic pneumothorax.

23.4. Which intercostal space is thoracocentesis usually performed through?

A. Third.

B. Fifth.

C. Seventh.

D. Ninth.

23.5. What is the minimum number of people recommended to perform thoracocentesis with ease in a compliant dog?

A. One.

B. Two.

C. Three.

D. Four.

Chapter 24: Principles of Thoracic Surgery

24.1. What is the commonest classification of pericardial effusion in the dog?

A. Chylous.

B. Idiopathic.

    C. Neoplastic.

    D. Septic.

24.2. Which intercostal space is pericardiocentesis performed through?

    A. Left third.

    B. Left fifth.

    C. Right third.

    D. Right fifth.

Answers

1.1	A	5.1	A	9.1	B	12.6	C	16.4	D	21.1	C
1.2	D	5.2	D	9.2	C	13.1	A	16.5	C	21.2	D
1.3	A	5.3	B	9.3	B	13.2	D	17.1	A	21.3	B
1.4	D	5.4	A	9.4	D	13.3	D	17.2	A	21.4	D
1.5	A	5.5	B	9.5	A	13.4	D	17.3	A	21.5	A
2.1	A	6.1	B	10.1	C	13.5	B	17.4	C	22.1	C
2.2	A	6.2	C	10.2	A	14.1	C	18.1	B	22.2	B
2.3	B	6.3	A	10.3	B	14.2	A	18.2	B	22.3	B
2.4	A	6.4	C	10.4	A	14.3	C	18.3	B	22.4	C
2.5	C	6.5	C	10.5	C	14.4	B	18.4	B	22.5	D
3.1	A	7.1	D	11.1	C	14.5	D	19.1	C	23.1	A
3.2	B	7.2	C	11.2	A	14.6	A	19.2	D	23.2	C
3.3	C	7.3	B	11.3	C	14.7	B	19.3	A	23.3	C
3.4	B	7.4	A	11.4	D	15.1	A	19.4	A	23.4	C
3.5	B	7.5	A	11.5	A	15.2	B	19.5	D	23.5	C
4.1	A	8.1	C	12.1	B	15.3	A	20.1	D	24.1	B
4.2	D	8.2	C	12.2	D	15.4	D	20.2	A	24.2	D
4.3	C	8.3	C	12.3	B	16.1	B	20.3	A		
4.4	E	8.4	A	12.4	D	16.2	A	20.4	B		
4.5	E	8.5	B	12.5	B	16.3	C	20.5	B		

Index